Emergency Echocardiography

Echocardiography is the most powerful and cost-effective imaging technique for assessing patients suffering from unstable cardiovascular diseases. This didactically structured third edition of *Emergency Echocardiography* contains fully rewritten chapters by well-known, internationally recognized contributors. It includes new chapters on echo-guided patient management in the ICU, lung ultrasound, and complications of percutaneous interventions. Special attention is given to Focus Cardiac Ultrasound (FoCUS) in emergency settings. This book uses over 600 video loops of illustrative cases to interest a wide readership of all medical professionals involved in diagnostics and treatment of emergency cardiovascular patients.

Key Features

- Covers the role of cardiac ultrasound in most cardiovascular emergencies and emergency settings
- Offers clinically useful information to a wide range of medical professionals dealing with cardiovascular emergencies, including cardiologists, emergency physicians, anesthesiologists, intensivists, and related fellows
- Features over 600 carefully chosen videos of illustrative cases with detailed explanations and highlights key decision management points

T0383930

Emergency Echocardiography

THIRD EDITION

EDITED BY

Aleksandar N. Neskovic, MD, PhD, FESC, FACC

Professor of Medicine and Cardiology
Chief of Department of Cardiology
Clinical Hospital Center Zemun
Faculty of Medicine
University of Belgrade
Belgrade, Serbia

Frank A. Flachskampf, MD, PhD, FESC, FACC

Professor of Cardiology
Department of Medical Sciences
Uppsala University
and
Department of Cardiology and Clinical Physiology
Uppsala University Hospital
Uppsala, Sweden

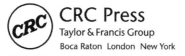

CRC Press
Taylor & Francis Group
Boca Raton London New York

CRC Press is an imprint of the
Taylor & Francis Group, an **informa** business

Cover picture: upper left panel: from Video 3.32A; upper right panel: from Video 22.7; lower left panel: from Video 12.11; lower right panel: from Video 13.42

Third edition published 2024
by CRC Press
6000 Broken Sound Parkway NW, Suite 300, Boca Raton, FL 33487–2742

and by CRC Press
4 Park Square, Milton Park, Abingdon, Oxon, OX14 4RN

CRC Press is an imprint of Taylor & Francis Group, LLC

© 2024 selection and editorial matter, Aleksandar N. Neskovic and Frank A. Flachskampf; individual chapters, the contributors

First edition published by Informa Healthcare 2005
Second Edition published by Taylor & Francis 2016

ISBN: 9781032157016 (hbk)
ISBN: 9781032157009 (pbk)
ISBN: 9781003245407 (ebk)

DOI: 10.1201/9781003245407

Typeset in Times
by Apex CoVantage, LLC

Contents

Preface to the Third Edition

The editors are proud and pleased to present the third edition of this textbook of echocardiography in cardiovascular emergency situations. The continuing demand for the book makes us confident that its concept is adequate and readers find here what they expect. As in the previous edition, we have further expanded topics, now including new chapters on lung ultrasound, percutaneous interventions, and intensive care. Figures and, crucially, videos have also been increased, the latter by 30%, and importantly, everything is also accessible electronically. The image material is truly a treasure trove of instructive cases, to which the editors can attest by themselves frequently using examples from the book for talks and presentations.

Needless to say, echocardiography, focus cardiac ultrasound, and recently, lung ultrasound have become diagnostic workhorses in cardiovascular emergencies, re-emphasizing the critical need for education and training in these techniques. We hope readers and, most importantly, prospective patients will benefit from the in-depth knowledge and insight that our outstanding expert authors have brought to this new edition.

We are proud to offer the contributions of so many excellent authors, far surpassing the expertise of any one expert, and sincerely thank them for their generously provided time and effort.

Aleksandar N. Neskovic
Frank A. Flachskampf

Preface to the Second Edition

The use of echocardiography in cardiovascular emergency situations continues to expand. Since the first edition of this book, cardiac ultrasound has become more widely available by introducing truly mobile, often pocket-sized devices that offer surprisingly good image quality. It has become more sophisticated by improving image quality and adding tissue Doppler, strain imaging, and real-time 3D imaging, as well as many electronic post-processing capabilities. Finally, its versatility and easy logistics are now harnessed by more medical specialists than ever, such as anesthesiologists, intensive care physicians, and emergency physicians.

Most of these aspects are represented in this book. The authors have added an enormous wealth of often stunning video examples that brings the book much nearer to imaging reality than still-frame illustrations can. New chapters, like that on mechanical circulatory assist devices and the FoCUS routine, have been also added, and all chapters have been rewritten and updated.

The editors are proud of this much-enhanced second edition and thank the authors and numerous colleagues who contributed their experience and material. The authors continue to be a truly international and intercontinental band of friends that make this book much better than any single author could.

We hope it will again be found useful by the readers.

Aleksandar N. Neskovic
Frank A. Flachskampf
Michael H. Picard

Preface to the First Edition

A unique feature of current echocardiography machines is their mobility, which allows examinations to be carried out wherever necessary—from echocardiographic laboratories to emergency departments, wards, catheterization labs, electrophysiology labs, and operating theatres. Information about the structure and function of the heart and its hemodynamics can be obtained relatively rapidly and such information is of incomparable value for decision-making in cardiovascular emergencies and the critically ill.

This book is intended to outline specific echocardiographic features and procedures pertinent to emergency situations, in particular cardiologic severe acute illnesses. Thus, it is not an introduction into echocardiography in general and assumes a basic knowledge of the technique. It should serve as a guide to rapid, up-to-date echocardiographic evaluation of life-threatening clinical situations.

Emergency Echocardiography consists of state-of-the-art reviews on the role of cardiac ultrasound in emergency clinical settings. International experts discuss the use of echocardiography in acute coronary syndromes, acute native and prosthetic valve disease, cardiac tamponade, acute diseases of the great vessels, cardiac-related embolism, cardiac arrest, chest trauma and cardiogenic shock. Specific problems related to intraoperative echocardiography, echocardiography in the emergency room, and the use of portable echo machines in the emergency setting are also addressed. Since echocardiography is already incorporated into patient management algorithms for the majority of cardiac emergencies, special efforts were made by the contributors to underline its diagnostic power. Importantly, the limitations of echocardiography in specific clinical situations are also discussed. Additionally, the role and potential advantages of special echocardiographic techniques, such as transesophageal echocardiography, are discussed whenever appropriate.

The book is illustrated by carefully selected echocardiographic images and schematics. At times some of the images may appear to be of relatively poor technical quality; however, we included them in the book because they represent images that are obtained under challenging conditions. Some of these are real rarities and contain exciting information.

While we aimed to focus this book toward all members of the healthcare team, it should be noted that echocardiographic examination in unstable patients in the emergency setting is a highly demanding procedure that requires both excellent technical skills to obtain adequate images in a stressful environment and the ability to interpret findings quickly and accurately. Therefore, despite efforts made to give complete overview of the field to the readers, the importance of appropriate echocardiographic training and personal experience in the evaluation of emergency patients should not be neglected.

Finally, we express our gratitude to all contributors, who generously and enthusiastically linked their talent and experience with this project.

The authors sincerely hope that this book will be found useful in everyday clinical practice and encourage feedback, criticism, and suggestions.

Aleksandar N. Neskovic
Frank A. Flachskampf
Michael H. Picard

Editors

Aleksandar N. Neskovic went to the Faculty of Medicine, University of Belgrade, Serbia, where he also completed his training in internal medicine and cardiology. He continued his education in echocardiography at the Massachusetts General Hospital and Cleveland Clinic in the United States and in interventional cardiology at Careggi Hospital in Florence, Italy. During his career he served as a chair of Cardiology Clinic and Dr A.D. Popovic Cardiovascular Research Center at the Dedinje Cardiovascular Institute and a chief of the Coronary Care Unit, Interventional Cardiology, and Department of Cardiology at the University Clinical Hospital Center Zemun, in Belgrade. He is a professor of medicine and cardiology at the Faculty of Medicine, University of Belgrade.

His major clinical and research interests include acute coronary syndrome, left ventricular function and remodeling, heart failure, and emergency cardiac ultrasound.

He has been a long-time board member of the European Association of Echocardiography/Cardiovascular Imaging.

He is married and has two daughters and Buddy.

Frank A. Flachskampf went to medical school in Bonn, Germany, followed by training in internal medicine/cardiology at the University of Aachen, Germany.

He completed fellowships in the United States at the Massachusetts General Hospital and at the Cleveland Clinic. He continued at the University of Erlangen, Germany, as a staff cardiologist with both invasive and non-invasive work and research.

Since 2010, he has been a professor of cardiology/cardiac imaging at the University of Uppsala, Sweden. Currently, he is pursuing research in the field of valvular heart disease and left ventricular function.

He has been a long-time board member of the European Association of Echocardiography/Cardiovascular Imaging, as well as a fellow of the American College of Cardiology and the European Society of Cardiology. He is an associate editor at the *Journal of the American College of Cardiology: Cardiovascular Imaging* and *European Heart Journal Open*.

He is married and has three children and one cat.

Contributors

Maria João Andrade, MD, FESC
Cardiology Department
Hospital de Santa Cruz
Carnaxide, Portugal

George Athanassopoulos, MD, PhD, FESC
Noninvasive Diagnostics Department
Cardiology Section
Onassis Cardiac Surgery Center
Athens, Greece

Tomasz Baron, MD, PhD
Department of Medical Sciences
Uppsala Clinical Research Center
Uppsala University
and
Department of Cardiology and Clinical Physiology
Uppsala University Hospital
Uppsala, Sweden

Leonardo Bolognese, MD, FESC, FACC
Director
Cardiovascular and Neurological Department
San Donato Hospital
Azienda Ospedaliera Arezzo
Arezzo, Italy

Nuno Cardim, MD, PhD, FESC, FACC
Professor of Cardiology
Faculdade de Ciências Médicas
    da Universidade Nova de Lisboa
Hospital CUF Descobertas Lisbon
Lisbon, Portugal

Quirino Ciampi, MD, PhD, FESC
Head of Echocardiography Laboratory
Division of Cardiology
Ospedale Fatebenefratelli
Benevento, Italy

Patrick Collier, MD, PhD, FASE
Assistant Professor of Medicine
Cleveland Clinic Lerner College of Medicine
Case Western Reserve University
Robert and Suzanne Tomisch Department of Cardiovascular
    Medicine
Sydell and Arnold Miller Family Heart and Vascular Institute
The Cleveland Clinic Foundation
Cleveland, Ohio, USA

Costanza Natalia Julia Colombo, MD
Anaesthesia, Intensive Care and Pain Therapy
Fondazione IRCCS Policlinico San Matteo
Pavia, Italy

Valentino Dammassa, MD
Adult Intensive Care Unit
Royal Brompton Hospital
London, United Kingdom

Elena Romero Dorta, MD
Head of the Echocardiography Laboratory
Department of Cardiology, Angiology and Intensive
    Care Medicine
Deutsches Herzzentrum Charité (DHZC), Campus Mitte
Berlin, Germany

Frank A. Flachskampf, MD, PhD, FESC, FACC
Professor of Cardiology
Department of Medical Sciences
Uppsala University
and
Department of Cardiology and Clinical Physiology
Uppsala University Hospital
Uppsala, Sweden

Luna Gargani, MD
Department of Surgical, Medical and Molecular Pathology and
    Critical Care Medicine
University of Pisa
Pisa, Italy

Brian P. Griffin, MD, FACC
The John and Rosemary Brown Endowed Chair
Director of Cardiovascular Imaging
Robert and Suzanne Tomisch Department of Cardiovascular
    Medicine
Sydell and Arnold Miller Family Heart and Vascular
    Institute
The Cleveland Clinic Foundation
Cleveland, Ohio, USA

Andreas Hagendorff, MD, FESC
Professor of Cardiology
Department für Innere Medizin
Neurologie und Dermatologie Abteilung für Kardiologie
    und Angiologie
Universitätsklinikum Leipzig AöR
Leipzig, Germany

Fabian Knebel, MD
Professor of Cardiology
Head of the Cardiology Department
Sana Klinikum Lichtenberg
Berlin, Germany

Katarzyna Kurnicka, MD, PhD
Head of Echocardiography Laboratory
Department of Internal Medicine and Cardiology
Medical University of Warsaw
Warsaw, Poland

Agatha Y. Kwon, BSc (Hons), PGDip (Cardiac Ultrasound)
Heart Care Partners
Wesley Hospital
Brisbane, Queensland, Australia

Nicolas Merke, MD
Head of the Echocardiography Laboratory
Clinic for Cardiac, Thoracic and Vascular Surgery
Deutsches Herzzentrum Charité (DHZC)
Berlin, Germany

Predrag M. Milicevic, MD
Head of Division of Heart Failure
Department of Cardiology
Clinical Hospital Center Zemun
Belgrade, Serbia

Manuela Muratori, MD
Centro Cardiologico Monzino IRCCS
Milan, Italy

Sean P. Murphy, MD
Corrigan Minehan Heart Center
Cardiology Division
Massachusetts General Hospital
Harvard Medical School
Boston, Massachusetts, USA

Aleksandar N. Neskovic, MD, PhD, FESC, FACC
Professor of Medicine and Cardiology
Chief of Department of Cardiology
Clinical Hospital Center Zemun
Faculty of Medicine
University of Belgrade
Belgrade, Serbia

Mauro Pepi, MD, FESC
Clinical Director
Centro Cardiologico Monzino IRCCS
Milan, Italy

Eugenio Picano, MD, PhD, FESC
Research Director
Institute of Clinical Physiology, CNR
Pisa, Italy

Michael H. Picard, MD, FACC, FAHA, FASE
Professor of Medicine
Corrigan Minehan Heart Center
Cardiology Division
Massachusetts General Hospital
Harvard Medical School
Boston, Massachusetts, USA

David G. Platts, MBBS, MD, FRACP, FCSANZ, FESC, FASE
Associate Professor of Medicine
School of Medicine
University of Queensland
Department of Echocardiography
Queensland Advanced Heart Failure and Cardiac
    Transplant Unit
The Prince Charles Hospital
Brisbane, Queensland, Australia

Zoran B. Popovic, MD, PhD
Associate Professor of Medicine
Cleveland Clinic Lerner College of Medicine
Case Western Reserve University
and
Robert and Suzanne Tomisch Department of Cardiovascular
    Medicine
Sydell and Arnold Miller Family Heart and
    Vascular Institute
The Cleveland Clinic Foundation
Cleveland, Ohio, USA

Susanna Price, MD, PhD, MBBS, BSc, FRCP, EDICM, FFICM, FESC
Professor of Practice in Cardiology and Intensive Care
Adult Intensive Care Unit
Royal Brompton Hospital
and
National Heart and Lung Institute
Imperial College London
London, United Kingdom

Piotr Pruszczyk, MD, FESC
Professor of Medicine
Department of Internal Medicine and Cardiology
Medical University of Warsaw
Warsaw, Poland

Gregory M. Scalia, MBBS (Hons), MMedSc, FRACP, FACC, FCSANZ, FASE, JP
Professor of Medicine
University of Queensland
and
Director of Echocardiography
The Prince Charles Hospital
Heart Care Partners
Wesley Hospital
Brisbane, Queensland, Australia

Christopher Shirley, MD
Betsi Cadwaladr University Health Board
Wales, United Kingdom

Henry Skinner, MD
Consultant Cardiac Anaesthetist
Nottingham University Hospitals NHS Trust
Nottingham, United Kingdom

Hatem Soliman-Aboumarie, MD, MBBS, MRCP, MSc, EDICM, FHEA, FASE, FEACVI
Consultant in Cardiothoracic Intensive Care
Department of Cardiothoracic Intensive Care
School of Cardiovascular Sciences and Medicine
Royal Brompton and Harefield Hospitals
London, United Kingdom

Sebastian Spethmann, MD
Senior Consultant
Department of Cardiology, Angiology and Intensive
    Care Medicine
Deutsches Herzzentrum Charité (DHZC), Campus Mitte
University of Berlin
Berlin, Germany

Ivan Stankovic, MD, PhD
Director of Echocardiography
Department of Cardiology
Clinical Hospital Center Zemun
and
Faculty of Medicine
University of Belgrade
Belgrade, Serbia

Justiaan Swanevelder, MBChB, FCA (SA), MMED (Anes), FRCA
Professor
Head of Department of Anaesthesia and Perioperative Medicine
Groote Schuur and Red Cross War Memorial
Children's Hospitals
and
Faculty of Health Sciences
University of Cape Town
Cape Town, South Africa

Gloria Tamborini, MD
Director of Echocardiography
Centro Cardiologico Monzino IRCCS
Milan, Italy

Guido Tavazzi, MD, PhD
Assistant Professor in Intensive Care
Anaesthesia and Intensive Care
Fondazione IRCCS Policlinico San Matteo
and
Department of Clinical-Surgical, Diagnostic and
    Pediatric Sciences
Unit of Anesthesia and Intensive Care
University of Pavia
Pavia, Italy

Adam Torbicki, MD, FESC
Professor of Medicine
Department of Pulmonary Circulation and Thromboembolic
    Diseases
Medical Center for Postgraduate Education
ECZ-Otwock, Poland

Gabriele Via, MD, EDIC
Senior Consultant
Cardiac Anesthesia and Intensive Care
Istituto Cardiocentro Ticino
Lugano, Switzerland

Emily K. Zern, MD
Corrigan Minehan Heart Center
Cardiology Division
Massachusetts General Hospital
Harvard Medical School
Boston, Massachusetts, USA

Image and Video Contributors[*]

Maria João Andrade, MD, FESC (MJA)
Cardiology Department
Hospital de Santa Cruz
Carnaxide, Portugal

Svetlana Apostolovic, MD, PhD, FESC (SA)
Department of Cardiology
University Clinical Center Nis
Nis, Serbia

George Athanassopoulos, MD, PhD, FESC (GA)
Noninvasive Diagnostics Department
Cardiology Section
Onassis Cardiac Surgery Center
Athens, Greece

Luigi P. Badano, MD, PhD, FESC, FACC (LB)
School of Medicine and Surgery
University of Milano Bicocca
Milan, Italy

Maja Cikes, MD, PhD (MC)
Department of Cardiovascular Diseases
University Hospital Center Zagreb
University of Zagreb School of Medicine
Zagreb, Croatia

Vojkan Cvorovic, MD (VC)
Acibadem/Belmedic General Hospital
Belgrade, Serbia

Branka Gakovic, MD (BG)
Department of Cardiology
Clinical Hospital Center Zemun
Belgrade, Serbia

Andreas Hagendorff, MD, FESC (AH)
Department für Innere Medizin
Neurologie und Dermatologie Abteilung für Kardiologie
    und Angiologie
Universitätsklinikum Leipzig AöR
Leipzig, Germany

Bojan Ilisic, MD (BI)
Acibadem/Belmedic General Hospital
Belgrade, Serbia

Srdjan Kafedzic, MD (SK)
Department of Cardiology
Clinical Hospital Center Zemun
Faculty of Medicine
University of Belgrade
Belgrade, Serbia

Dragana Kosevic, MD (DK)
Dedinje Cardiovascular Institute
Belgrade, Serbia

Mila Kovacevic, MD, PhD (MK)
Institute of Cardiovascular Diseases of Vojvodina
Faculty of Medicine
University of Novi Sad
Novi Sad, Serbia

Gordana Krljanac, MD, PhD (GK)
University Clinical Center of Serbia
Faculty of Medicine
University of Belgrade
Belgrade, Serbia

Aleksandar Lazarevic, MD, PhD, FESC, FACC (AL)
Faculty of Medicine
University of Banja Luka
Banja Luka, Bosnia and Herzegovina

Miloje Marjanovic, MD (MM)
Emergency Department
Clinical Hospital Center Zemun
Belgrade, Serbia

Stefan Mijatovic, MD (SM)
Department of Cardiology
Clinical Hospital Center Zemun
Belgrade, Serbia

Predrag M. Milicevic, MD (PMM)
Department of Cardiology
Clinical Hospital Center Zemun
Belgrade, Serbia

---

[*] In addition to the images and videos provided by the authors for their chapters, listed contributors also provided images and/or videos that are presented in different chapters of the book. These contributions are indicated by the initials of the contributor (e.g., GA, AH, LB) at the end of the caption for the corresponding image or video.

Aleksandar N. Neskovic, MD, PhD, FESC, FACC (ANN)
Department of Cardiology
Clinical Hospital Center Zemun
Faculty of Medicine
University of Belgrade
Belgrade, Serbia

Slobodan Obradovic, MD, PHD (SO)
Military Academy
Faculty of Medicine
University of Defense
Belgrade, Serbia

Milos Panic, MD (MMP)
Department of Cardiology
Clinical Hospital Center Zemun
Belgrade, Serbia

Teodora Pantic, MD (TP)
Institute of Cardiovascular Diseases of Vojvodina
Novi Sad, Serbia

Sinisa U. Pavlovic, MD, PhD (SUP)
Pacemaker Center
University Clinical Center of Serbia
Faculty of Medicine
University of Belgrade
Belgrade, Serbia

Mauro Pepi, MD, FESC (MP)
IRCCS Centro Cardiologico Monzino
University of Milan
Milan, Italy

Viktor Persic, MD, PhD (VP)
Clinic for Treatment, Rehabilitation and Prevention of
    Cardiovascular Disease
Opatija, School of Medicine Rijeka
University of Rijeka
Opatija, Croatia

Michael H. Picard, MD, FACC, FAHA, FASE (MHP)
Corrigan Minehan Heart Center
Cardiology Division
Massachusetts General Hospital
Harvard Medical School
Boston, Massachusetts, USA

**Bogdan A. Popescu, MD, PhD, FESC, FACC,
FASE (BAP)**
University of Medicine and Pharmacy
"Carol Davila," Euroecolab
Institute of Cardiovascular Diseases
"Prof. Dr. C. C. Iliescu"
Bucharest, Romania

Marija Popovic, MD (MPo)
Cardiology Clinic
University Clinical Center Kragujevac
Kragujevac, Serbia

Biljana Putnikovic, MD, PhD (BP)
Policlinic Euromedik
Belgrade, Serbia

Gopalan Nair Rajesh, MD, DNB, DM (GNR)
Government Medical College Calicut (Kozhikode)
Kerala, India

Srdjan Raspopovic, MD (SR)
Department of Cardiology
Clinical Hospital Center Zemun
Belgrade, Serbia

Elizabeta Srbinovska Kostovska, MD, PhD, FESC (ES)
Diagnostic Center
University Clinic of Cardiology
Medical Faculty University "St. Cyril and Methodius"
Skopje, Macedonia

Ilija Srdanovic, MD, PhD (ISr)
Institute of Cardiovascular Diseases of Vojvodina
Faculty of Medicine
University of Novi Sad
Novi Sad, Serbia

Ivan Stankovic, MD, PhD (IS)
Department of Cardiology
Clinical Hospital Center Zemun
Faculty of Medicine
University of Belgrade
Belgrade, Serbia

Maja Stefanovic, MD, PhD (MS)
Institute of Cardiovascular Diseases of Vojvodina
Faculty of Medicine
University of Novi Sad
Novi Sad, Serbia

Milica Stefanovic, MD (MSt)
Department of Cardiology
Clinical Hospital Center Zemun
Belgrade, Serbia

**Justiaan Swanevelder, MBChB, FCA (SA), MMED (Anes),
FRCA (JS)**
Department of Anaesthesia and Perioperative Medicine
Groote Schuur and Red Cross War Memorial
Children's Hospitals
Faculty of Health Sciences
University of Cape Town
Cape Town, South Africa

Gabriele Via, MD, EDIC (GV)
Cardiac Anesthesia and Intensive Care
Istituto Cardiocentro Ticino
Lugano, Switzerland

Radosav Vidakovic, MD, PhD (RV)
Department of Cardiology
Clinical Hospital Center Zemun
Faculty of Medicine
University of Belgrade
Belgrade, Serbia

Alja Vlahovic Stipac, MD, PhD (AVS)
Mediclinic Middle East
Dubai, UAE

Ivona Vranic, MD (IV)
Department of Cardiology
Clinical Hospital Center Zemun
Belgrade, Serbia

Lale Zastranovic, MD (LZ)
Cardiology Department
Medical Center Zajecar
Zajecar, Serbia

Aleksandra Zivanic, MD (AZ)
Department of Cardiology
Clinical Hospital Center Zemun
Belgrade, Serbia

Important Technical Note

Readers should be aware that every effort has been made to provide fully accessible video material through the QR codes and URLs. Please note that newer versions of mobile phone browsers and QR code readers should be used to play videos flawlessly.

https://routledgetextbooks.com/textbooks/9781032157009/videos.php

Abbreviations

2CH	two-chamber (view)	CT	computed tomography
4CH	four-chamber (view)	CTPA	computed tomography pulmonary angiography
5CH	five-chamber (view)		
2D	two-dimensional	CUS	cardiac ultrasound examination
3D	three-dimensional	CVP	central venous pressure
A	late transmitral velocity (i.e., A-wave)	DA	descending aorta
A4CH	apical four-chamber (view)	DAo	descending aorta
AAo	ascending aorta	dIVC	inferior vena cava diameter
ADHF	acute decompensated heart failure	DICOM	digital imaging and communications in medicine (standard)
ACLS	Advanced Cardiac Life Support		
ACS	acute coronary syndrome	DT	deceleration time of the E-wave
ACP	acute core pulmonale	DVT	deep venous thrombosis
AcT	acceleration time	E	early transmitral velocity (i.e., E-wave)
AF	atrial fibrillation		
AI	artificial intelligence	e′	mitral annular early diastolic velocity
AI	aortic insufficiency		
ALAX	apical long-axis (view)	E/A	E-to-A-wave ratio
ALI	acute lung injury	ECG	electrocardiogram
ALMV	anterior leaflet of mitral valve	ECMO	extracorporeal membrane oxygenation
AMI	acute myocardial infarction		
AMI-CS	acute myocardial infarction cardiogenic shock	ED	emergency department
		EDD	end-diastolic diameter
Ao	aorta	EDPVR	end-diastolic pressure volume relationship
AoV	aortic valve		
AR	aortic regurgitation	E/e′	ratio of the early transmitral flow velocity and early diastolic velocity of the mitral valve annulus
ARDS	acute respiratory distress syndrome		
ASA	atrial septal aneurysm		
Asc Ao	ascending aorta	E/e′sr	early mitral inflow velocity to global diastolic strain rate
AT	acceleration time		
AT/ET	acceleration time to ejection time ratio	EMD	electromechanical dissociation
		EP	electrophysiology
ATLS	Advanced Trauma Life Support	EROA	effective regurgitant orifice area
AVC	aortic valve closure	ESD	end-systolic diameter
AVPO	aortic valve prosthetic obstruction	ESPVR	end-systolic pressure-volume relationship
BCT	blunt chest trauma		
BNP	brain natriuretic peptide	ET	ejection time
BSA	body surface area	ETCO$_2$	end tidal CO$_2$
CABG	coronary artery bypass grafting	FAST	Focused Assessment with Sonography for Trauma
CCU	coronary care unit		
COPD	chronic obstructive pulmonary disease	FEEL	Focused Echocardiography Evaluation in Life support
CPB	cardiopulmonary bypass	FL	false lumen
CPR	cardiopulmonary resuscitation	FoCUS	focus cardiac ultrasound
CRT	cardiac resynchronization therapy	fTEE	focused transesophageal echocardiography
CS	cardiogenic shock		

GLS	global longitudinal strain	**NSTE**	non-ST-segment elevation
HALT	hypoattenuated leaflet thickening	**NSTEMI**	non-ST-segment elevation myocardial infarction
HF	heart failure		
HFpEF	heart failure with preserved ejection fraction	**OR**	operating room
		P	pericardial effusion
HFrEF	heart failure with reduced ejection fraction	**PA**	pulmonary artery
		PA	pulmonary artery systolic pressure
HOCM	hypertrophic obstructive cardiomyopathy	**PCI**	percutaneous coronary intervention
hs Tn	high-sensitive troponin	**PCT**	penetrating cardiac trauma
HUD	handheld ultrasound device	**PE**	pulmonary embolism or pericardial effusion
IA	innominate artery		
ICD	implantable cardioverter defibrillator	**PEA**	pulseless electrical activity
		PISA	proximal isovelocity surface area
ICU	intensive care unit	**PLAX**	parasternal long-axis (view)
INR	international normalized ratio	**PLMV**	posterior leaflet of mitral valve
IOE	intraoperative echocardiography	**PMVA**	percutaneous mitral valve annuloplasty
IVC	inferior vena cava		
IVCCI	inferior vena cava collapsibility index	**POCUS**	point-of-care ultrasound
		PSAX	parasternal short-axis (view)
LA	left atrium	**PSS**	postsystolic shortening
LAA	left atrial appendage	**PST**	postsystolic thickening
LAP	left atrial pressure	**PV**	prosthetic valve
LAX	long-axis (view)	**PVR**	pulmonary vascular resistance
LPA	left pulmonary artery	**PW**	pulsed-wave (Doppler)
LV	left ventricle	**RA**	right atrium
LVAD	left ventricular assist device	**RAP**	right atrial pressure
LVEDA	left ventricular end-diastolic area	**RHT**	right heart thrombi
LVEDP	left ventricular end-diastolic pressure	**ROA**	regurgitant orifice area
		ROSC	return of spontaneous circulation
LVEDV	left ventricular end-diastolic volume	**RPA**	right pulmonary artery
		RV	right ventricle
LVEF	left ventricular ejection fraction	**RVAD**	right ventricular assist device
LVESA	left ventricular end-systolic area	**RWMA**	regional wall motion abnormality
LVESV	left ventricular end-systolic volume	**SAM**	systolic anterior motion
LVOT	left ventricular outflow tract	**SAX**	short-axis (view)
MAPSE	mitral annular plane systolic excursion	**SAVR**	surgical aortic valve replacement
		SE	stress echocardiography
MCE	myocardial contrast echocardiography	**SEC**	spontaneous echo contrast
		SIVC	subcostal inferior vena cava (view)
MCS	mechanical circulatory support	**SLAX**	subcostal long-axis (view)
MDCT	multidetector computed tomography	**SPECT**	single-photon emission computed tomography
MI	myocardial infarction		
MPA	main pulmonary artery	**STEMI**	ST-segment elevation myocardial infarction
MPG	mean (transvalvular) pressure gradient		
		SV	stroke volume
MPI	myocardial perfusion imaging	**TA**	tricuspid annulus
MR	mitral regurgitation	**TAH**	total artificial heart
MSCT	multislice computed tomography	**TAPSE**	tricuspid annular plane systolic excursion
MV	mitral valve		
MVA	mitral valve area	**TAVI**	transcatheter aortic valve implantation
MVAL	mitral valve–anterior leaflet		
MVIV	transcatheter mitral valve-in-valve	**TAVR**	transcatheter aortic valve replacement
MVIR	transcatheter mitral valve-in-ring		
MVPL	mitral valve–posterior leaflet	**TDI**	tissue Doppler imaging

TEE	transesophageal echocardiography	**VAD**	ventricular assist device
TEER	transcatheter edge-to-edge repair	**VA ECMO**	venoarterial extracorporeal membrane oxygenation
t-ET	total ejection time		
t-FT	total filling time	**VHV**	valvular heart disease
THV	transcatheter heart valve	**VIV**	valve-in-valve
TIA	transitory ischemic attack	**VIR**	valve-in-ring
t-IVT	total isovolumic time	**VS**	ventricular septum
TL	true lumen	**VSR**	ventricular septal rupture
TMVIR	transcatheter mitral valve-in-ring	**VTE**	venous thromboembolism
TTE	transthoracic echocardiography	**VTI**	velocity-time integral
T-TEER	tricuspid transcatheter edge-to-edge repair	**VUS**	venous ultrasound
		VV ECMO	venovenous extracorporeal membrane oxygenation
TTVr	transcatheter tricuspid valve repair		
TR	tricuspid regurgitation	**UEA**	ultrasound-enhancing agents
TV	tricuspid valve	**WMA**	wall motion abnormality
V	video (e.g., V4.4B, V6.17)	**WMSi**	wall motion score index

Emergency echocardiography
General considerations

1

Ivan Stankovic, Andreas Hagendorff,
and Aleksandar N. Neskovic

Truth is one, paths are many.
—Mahatma Gandhi

The pure and simple truth is rarely pure and never simple.
—Oscar Wilde

Competence makes the difference.
—Motto of emergency medicine physicians

Key Points

- Emergency echocardiography is a comprehensive diagnostic ultrasound examination of the heart performed by cardiologists or adequately trained non-cardiologists who are able to independently perform and interpret the study.
- Echocardiography in the emergency setting is a highly demanding procedure, and because of the serious implications of the examination results, it should not be attempted by inexperienced healthcare providers without supervision.
- Standards are proposed for ultrasound equipment, execution, documentation, and interpretation, as well as for education and training of physicians performing echocardiography in the emergency setting.
- Acute chest pain, acute dyspnea, hemodynamic instability, new murmur, syncope, chest trauma, and cardiac arrest are the main clinical situations in which emergency echocardiography is required.

Rapid and accurate evaluation of unstable patients presenting with symptoms suggestive of cardiovascular pathology is a crucial task in a busy emergency department (ED). A focused history taking, physical examination, and 12-lead electrocardiogram (ECG) remain essential first steps of guideline-proposed algorithms, but additional laboratory tests and imaging studies are required in a sizeable number of patients. Among the currently available imaging techniques, echocardiography seems perfectly fitted for demanding emergency settings because of its availability, portability, and accuracy. It can be performed promptly virtually everywhere, and the results of examination are

DOI: 10.1201/9781003245407-1

immediately available, allowing initiation of appropriate treatment without unnecessary delay.

It should be noted that although requirements and recommendations proposed in this chapter are based on international guidelines,[1,2] models for use of emergency echocardiography in everyday clinical practice depend on local human and technological resources and *may differ* among institutions and countries.

In this chapter, we provide a brief overview of practical and medicolegal aspects pertinent to emergency echocardiography[1]; specific considerations related to handheld imaging devices (HUDs) and focused cardiac ultrasound (FoCUS) in the emergency setting, as well as echocardiographic features of particular cardiac emergencies, are detailed in corresponding chapters of this book (Chapters 18 and 19).

Importantly, both cardiologists and non-cardiologists can perform either echocardiographic examinations or FoCUS, depending on clinical circumstances, existing equipment, and expertise. Thus, although FoCUS is typically used by non-cardiologists who have undergone minimal training, it can also be performed by fully trained cardiologists in emergency settings.

Furthermore, FoCUS and emergency echocardiography can be both used in unstable patients at different phases of diagnostic process, as shown in (Figure 1.1). For instance, in a patient presenting with shock, the emergency physician may use an HUD to perform FoCUS in search for cardiac causes of patient's instability; if diagnostic uncertainty persists after FoCUS, comprehensive emergency echocardiography (transthoracic and transesophageal) can be subsequently performed to obtain a correct diagnosis.

TERMINOLOGY

The current trend of rapidly increasing use of echocardiography in emergency settings by non-cardiologists or cardiologists without specific expertise[1] occurs in parallel with an evolving trend of using the cardiac ultrasound examination as a bedside, point-of-care diagnostic test in emergency settings. This examination has been named *focus(ed) cardiac ultrasound* (FoCUS). It is important to distinguish emergency echocardiography, goal-oriented echocardiography, and FoCUS for practical, logistic, educational, and medicolegal reasons.[3]

Echocardiography is a comprehensive investigation requiring maximum technical skills along with expertise in cardiovascular pathophysiology and cardiovascular diseases. Thus, the term *echocardiography* refers to comprehensive standard echocardiography in emergency settings—that is, *emergency echocardiography*, which always represents a full echocardiographic investigation of cardiac morphology and function, using fully equipped echocardiographic machines, performed by a sufficiently trained operator who is able to independently perform the study and interpret its results.[1,3]

The term *FoCUS* defines the point-of-care cardiac ultrasound examination, performed according to a standardized but restricted scanning protocol to add information to the physical examination findings, by an operator who is not necessarily fully trained in echocardiography but rather appropriately trained in FoCUS and who is at the same time usually responsible for immediate decision-making and/or treatment.[3]

Furthermore, FoCUS should be distinguished from *goal-oriented (targeted)* echocardiographic examination, performed by a fully trained echocardiographer who is capable to use full range of echocardiographic techniques, attempting to obtain an answer to a specific, often critical and frequently complex clinical dilemmas (e.g., failure to wean from mechanical ventilation, thrombosis of mechanical valve prosthesis, exclusion of inter-ventricular dyssynchrony, echocardiography in mechanical circulatory support).[3]

ECHOCARDIOGRAPHY IN THE EMERGENCY SETTING

Even under the best possible conditions for the evaluation of patients, echocardiography is a highly operator-dependent technique, and human factors (e.g., ability, training, and experience) account for the vast majority of diagnostic errors. In the stressful emergency situation, critically ill patients are typically scanned in minimal time, and potentially catastrophic errors are even more likely to occur, especially if the examination is performed by an inexperienced operator. Echocardiography is already a widely available imaging modality, but with the advent of HUDs, even wider dissemination of the technique is expected, with increasing use by non-experts (emergency physicians, intensivists, anesthesiologists, cardiac surgeons). Medical professionals involved in emergency echocardiography must be able not only to obtain adequate images under challenging conditions but also to interpret them accurately. A failure to either obtain the appropriate image or understand what is imaged may result in misleading and dangerous conclusions. A failure of inexperienced echocardiographers to distinguish normal variants and artifacts from serious pathology may result in unnecessary hospital admissions and further costly investigations (Figure 1.2) (V1.1, V1.2A, and V1.2B), and serious pathology can be missed because of suboptimal scanning technique (Figure 1.3) (V1.3A and V1.3B).

Apart from difficulties in image acquisition and interpretation, non-cardiologists performing emergency echocardiography may also be challenged by lack of appropriate knowledge that is required to view echocardiographic findings in the clinical context. A pattern recognition approach is useful for diagnosing obvious pathology, such as pericardial effusion or severe left ventricular (LV) dysfunction, whereas the assessment of complicated emergency cases (e.g., severe hypotension caused by dynamic LV tract obstruction) requires the comprehensive understanding of cardiovascular pathology to establish the underlying cause of the patient's instability.

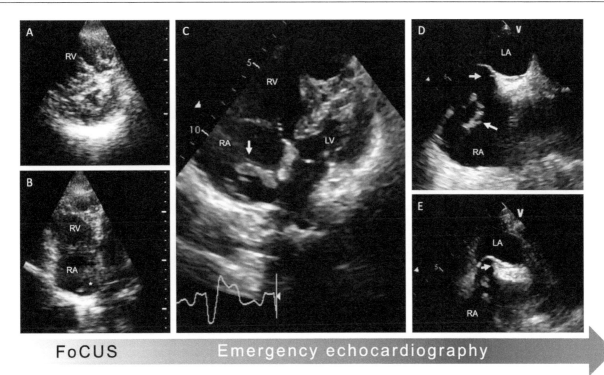

FIGURE 1.1   An example of sequential use of FoCUS and emergency echocardiography in a patient presenting with syncope and hypotension. FoCUS performed using an HUD showing right ventricular (RV) dilatation and dysfunction, septal flattening (A), and mobile structure (*) within the right atrium (RA), initially interpreted as prominent Chiari network in a patient with acute cor pulmonale (B). Transthoracic emergency echocardiography confirmed FoCUS findings but also clearly depicted a highly mobile right atrial thrombus (arrow) (C). Since it was unclear whether the thrombus was entrapped in a patent foramen ovale (PFO), emergency transesophageal echocardiography (TEE) was immediately performed (D). TEE revealed the thrombus (white arrow) entrapped within Chiari network (D), but there was a thrombotic fragment within the foramen ovale (yellow arrows) suggesting that the thrombotic mass had been initially trapped in PFO (D and E).

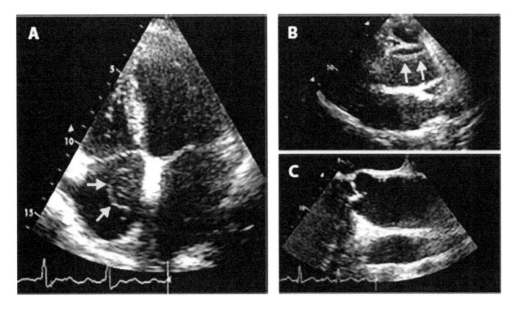

FIGURE 1.2   Challenging image interpretation in patients with suspected cardiac emergencies. (A) Unusually prominent Chiari's network (an embryologic remnant normally seen in approximately 2% of the population; arrows) was initially interpreted as right heart thrombus (V1.1). (B) Ultrasound artifact mimicking intimal flap in the ascending aorta on transthoracic examination (arrows, see V1.2A) required transesophageal study (C) to rule out aortic dissection (V1.2B).

(V1.2A and V1.2B provided by VC.)

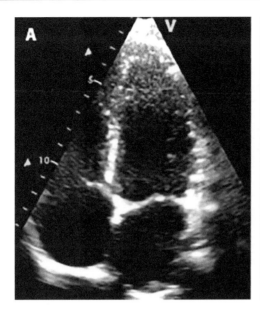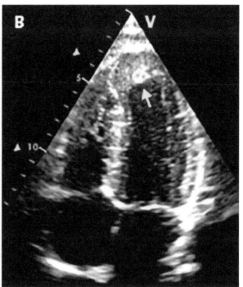

FIGURE 1.3 Challenging image acquisition in the emergency setting. Important findings may be overlooked because of poor scanning technique resulting in apical foreshortening (A) (see V1.3A). Apical dyskinesia and thrombus (arrow) became obvious only when a full-length image of the left ventricle was obtained (B) (see V1.3B).

TABLE 1.1   ABCD Approach in Performing Emergency Echocardiography

A	**A**wareness	• Fight against routine
		• Think beyond apparent explanations
B	**B**e suspicious	• Referral diagnosis may be misleading
		• Never trust; confirm
C	**C**omprehensiveness	• Do as complete an examination as suitable
		• Carefully interpret
D	**D**ouble R	• The study should be **R**ecorded and **R**eviewed
		• Teamwork is crucial

(With permission from Oxford University Press from Neskovic AN, et al.[1])

As an aid to adequate assessment of cardiac emergencies, an ABCD approach[1] consisting of four practical steps in performing emergency echocardiography has been proposed (Table 1.1).

TRAINING AND EDUCATION REQUIREMENTS

An accurate diagnosis of cardiac emergency is essential because it often triggers immediate aggressive treatment. Although "quick look" echocardiography performed by an experienced operator using an HUD may sometimes be life-saving in resource-limited situations, it carries a substantial risk of both over- and underdiagnosing serious cardiac pathology.

It should be noted that recent developments in ultrasound technology narrowed the gap between HUDs and high-end ultrasound machines. In line with this, new generations of handheld imaging platforms overcome limitations of first devices with regard to image quality and technical characteristics. The latest versions of tablet-based handheld devices are equipped with full Doppler capabilities (color, pulsed-wave, and continuous-wave Doppler), while some probes also offer ECG, digital auscultation, and advanced artificial intelligence (AI)-driven functions. Examples of AI-empowered capabilities include stroke volume, left ventricular ejection fraction and cardiac output calculations, as well as AI-guided image acquisition. For instance, AI-driven software may detect suboptimal image quality and show the guidance message to the operator to improve it; once the sufficient image quality is reached, the image is automatically captured and processed by the system.

Adequate training and competence of all medical professionals using ultrasound devices in critically ill cardiovascular patients is required to ensure proficient use of echocardiography in the emergency setting. Both the European Association of Cardiovascular Imaging (EACVI) and the American Society of Echocardiography (ASE) proposed standards for adequate

TABLE 1.2 Minimal Training Requirements for Physicians Performing Adult Emergency Echocardiography

LEVEL OF COMPETENCE IN ADULT TTE	MINIMAL NUMBER OF EXAMINATIONS PERFORMED (TTE)	LEVEL OF COMPETENCE IN EMERGENCY ECHOCARDIOGRAPHY	ADDITIONAL TRAINING REQUIREMENTS
ACC/AHA/ASE			
Level 1	75	Assist with emergent image acquisition	N/A
Level 2	150	Independent operator	No
Level 3	300	Independent operator	No
ESC/EACVI			
Cardiologist Basic echo, level 3	350	Independent operator	Highly recommended
Non-cardiologist Basic echo, level 3	350	Independent operator	Mandatory (theoretical and practical part)
Cardiologist Advanced echo, level 3	750	Expert operator	No

Abbreviations: ACC, American College of Cardiology; AHA, American Heart Association; ASE, American Society of Echocardiography; EACVI, European Association of Cardiovascular Imaging; ESC, European Society of Cardiology; N/A, not applicable; TTE, transthoracic echocardiography.

(Modified with permission from Oxford University Press from Neskovic AN, et al.[1])

training and education of physicians performing emergency echocardiography.[1–4] Minimal numbers of transthoracic echocardiography (TTE) studies required for reaching the certain level of competence as determined by expert consensus are shown in Table 1.2.

Competence requirements for emergency echocardiography are essentially the same for cardiologists and non-cardiologists, meaning that non-cardiologists should reach the same level of expertise through a training program similar to the training program for general cardiologists, with additional theoretical knowledge on certain cardiovascular diseases and conditions.[1]

A basic level of competence in classic adult echocardiography is required for all medical professionals performing emergency echocardiography, but it is not considered sufficient for unaided use of echocardiography in the emergency setting. For cardiologists with a basic level of competence, additional training consisting of 150 emergency cases is highly recommended; for non-cardiologists with a basic level of competence, both additional theoretical and practical training are mandatory before they are considered *independent operators*.[1] Only for cardiologists with an advanced level of expertise in echocardiography is no additional training in emergency echocardiography required. Healthcare providers (non-cardiologists, fellows, or sonographers) with a basic level of competence can assist in acquiring emergent images, which must be subsequently reviewed and interpreted by competent independent operators (Table 1.2). Depending on local logistics, supervision, and interpretation of acquired images can be personal, on-site, or, if there are network solutions to provide a connection between the operator and the expert, remote. To maintain competence in emergency echocardiography,

both cardiologists and qualified non-cardiologists should be exposed to at least 50 emergency cases per year with adequate diversity.[1]

EMERGENCY ECHOCARDIOGRAPHY SERVICE

Human resources and local availability of equipment, networks, and information systems will indisputably dictate organization of emergency echocardiography services in various institutions. However, teamwork, supervision, and quality control are essential for establishing an efficient emergency echocardiography service, which should ideally have the following characteristics[1]:

- Around-the-clock availability of a physician with an independent level of competence in emergency echocardiography
- An efficient on-call service providing second opinion for special echocardiographic techniques by a physician with an expert operator level in emergency echocardiography
- Continuous supervision by a physician with an expert operator level in emergency echocardiography (Supervision should be mandatory for all cases performed by sonographers and fellows and is strongly recommended for cardiologists and non-cardiologists.)
- Quality control for systematic detection, handling, and correction of errors

If available, network or web-based audiovisual connections from the examination room to the supervisor laboratory should be used to provide direct visualization of the echocardiographic images and enable immediate discussion with the most competent colleague in the hospital (preferably a cardiologist with an expert operator level in emergency echocardiography).[1] Ideally, the emergency echocardiographic laboratory should be accredited in TTE and TEE, and continuing education through courses and additional training in basic and advanced TTE and TEE should be organized.[1]

MEDICOLEGAL ISSUES AND EMERGENCY ECHOCARDIOGRAPHIC STUDY REPORT

Physicians performing emergency echocardiography should be aware of potential medicolegal consequences because the time-critical nature of the decision-making and the stressful environment may increase the chances for diagnostic errors.

For quality assurance purposes, all emergency echocardiograms should be performed by competent physicians using high-quality machines and must be recorded and stored in an appropriate format.[1,2] Well-documented and fully retrievable studies should not only provide evidence of reported findings but also be used for educational purposes.

The report should be reflective of observed findings and signed by the physician who is formally competent to perform and interpret emergency echocardiography.[1,5,6] In the case of critical findings requiring urgent treatment, the preliminary report comprising the most important results of the study should be issued and communicated directly to the treating physician; the final report should be issued shortly after the patient is transferred for further care.[1]

ECHOCARDIOGRAPHIC TECHNIQUES FOR ASSESSING CARDIAC EMERGENCIES

Transthoracic echocardiography

Conventional TTE, consisting of grayscale and blood flow Doppler imaging, plays the most important role in the emergency setting; other echocardiographic techniques, such as TEE and stress and contrast echocardiography, may be useful under special circumstances and in specific patient populations.[1,2,5–9] It should be noted that physicians performing emergency echocardiography must be able to obtain and interpret images from nonstandard imaging planes and acoustic windows (e.g., subcostal) that are sometimes the only planes

and windows available. For instance, TTE can be particularly challenging and sometimes impossible in unconscious, sedated, or intubated patients who are not able to cooperate and can be examined only in the supine position. The decision whether to perform TEE or computed tomography (CT) to rule out aortic dissection in such patients should be guided by local availability of both imaging modalities and expertise to perform these studies.

The usefulness and feasibility of novel echocardiographic techniques, such as three-dimensional echocardiography and strain imaging, have not yet been validated in the emergency setting, and their added value in the acute setting is currently only anecdotal.[10–12]

Transesophageal echocardiography

TEE is the preferred echocardiographic modality for the emergent patient in whom standard TTE is nondiagnostic because of poor image quality or expected inferiority of TTE in providing adequate visualization of certain cardiac structures of interest (thoracic aorta, pulmonary artery, native and prosthetic heart valves).[13] As in the case of TTE, emergency TEE should be performed only by physicians with appropriate training and experience in acquiring and interpreting TEE images.

Contrast echocardiography

Visual assessment of regional wall motion abnormalities (WMAs) in emergency situations is often a difficult task even for the most skillful cardiologists, but it can be facilitated by the use of a contrast agent. A slow bolus of an ultrasound contrast agent not only improves delineation of the endocardial border but also allows assessment of myocardial perfusion, resulting in higher accuracy of detection of regional LV dysfunction than with conventional echocardiography alone.[14] Furthermore, bubble appearance within pericardial effusion after injection of agitated saline (V1.4) through a needle is a simple and useful procedure to confirm the position of the needle during echocardiographically guided pericardiocentesis.[15] Several other applications of contrast echocardiography (e.g., ruling out LV pseudoaneurysm or thrombus formation) may also have a role in the emergency setting,[16] provided that adequate instrument settings and experienced physicians are available for correct acquisition and interpretation of images.

Stress echocardiography

Because it is performed only in clinically stable patients, stress echocardiography formally does not belong in the spectrum of emergency echocardiographic techniques. It is, however, a guideline-proposed, predischarge test in patients with chest pain, nondiagnostic ECG, and normal troponin values to resolve the remaining uncertainty regarding the presence of significant coronary artery disease.[17]

Owing to an excellent negative predictive value, use of early exercise and dobutamine stress echocardiography (see Chapter 17) provides valuable timely information for early risk stratification and allows safe discharge from the ED of troponin-negative patients.[18,19]

CLINICAL APPLICATIONS OF ECHOCARDIOGRAPHY IN THE EMERGENCY SETTING

When performed by a competent operator, emergency echocardiography may facilitate the evaluation of patients presenting to the ED with acute chest pain, dyspnea, hemodynamic instability, syncope, or a new heart murmur. In addition, it may provide crucial diagnostic information in patients who present with chest trauma or under cardiopulmonary resuscitation.

Table 1.3 summarizes recommendations for the use of echocardiography in cardiac and cardiac-like emergencies. Most of these are addressed in other chapters of this book.

Acute chest pain

Chest pain is one of the most common symptoms in patients presenting to the ED and may be caused by either benign (e.g.,

musculoskeletal chest pain) or life-threatening cardiac conditions. The essential role of emergency echocardiography is to help distinguish potentially lethal cardiac causes from other, noncardiac sources of chest pain syndrome. It is also imperative to make a clear distinction among a wide range of cardiac emergencies with similar presentation but with markedly different therapeutic approaches (e.g., acute myocardial infarction versus acute aortic dissection).

Patients with acute chest pain, nondiagnostic ECG, and negative cardiac biomarkers are those who can benefit most from emergency echocardiography. In the ischemic cascade, regional WMAs occur well before ECG changes and, if present on resting echocardiogram, are useful markers of myocardial ischemia (V2.3A and V2.3B). It should be noted that WMAs are not a specific marker of acute myocardial ischemia; they may also be found in patients with previous myocardial infarction, LV dyssynchrony, myocarditis, or stress cardiomyopathy. To improve detection of regional LV dysfunction in patients with poor LV endocardial border delineation, the application of ultrasound contrast agent can be considered, whereas in patients with no WMAs at rest, an early stress echocardiographic test could facilitate the decision regarding whether to admit or discharge the patient from the ED.

Acute aortic dissection may mimic other, more frequent conditions, and a high index of suspicion is critical for accurate diagnosis at initial presentation. Because mortality in acute dissection may be as high as 1% per hour during the

TABLE 1.3   Summary of Recommendations for the Use of Echocardiography in Cardiac and Cardiac-Like Emergencies

EMERGENCY CLINICAL PRESENTATIONS	CAUSES[a]	ECHOCARDIOGRAPHY RECOMMENDED[b, c]	ECHOCARDIOGRAPHY NOT RECOMMENDED[c]
Acute chest pain	Frequent: ACS, AoD, PE, MP, Ptx Less frequent: ADHF, T, AVR/PVD	1 Evaluation of acute chest pain in patients with suspected myocardial ischemia or infarction and nondiagnostic ECG and cardiac enzymes, and when resting echocardiogram can be performed during the pain 2 Evaluation of acute chest pain in patients with known underlying cardiac disease (valvular, pericardial, or primary myocardial disease) 3 Evaluation of patients with chest pain and hemodynamic instability unresponsive to simple therapeutic measures 4 Evaluation of chest pain in patients with suspected acute aortic syndromes, pulmonary embolism, myopericarditis, and Takotsubo cardiomyopathy 5 As an initial imaging modality for diagnosis of suspected aortic dissection in the emergency setting 6 Guiding the therapeutic approach in patients with known pulmonary embolism (e.g., thrombectomy and thrombolytics) 7 In patients with suspected pericardial disease, including effusion, constriction, or effusive-constrictive process 8 In patients with suspected bleeding in the pericardial space (e.g., trauma, perforation) 9 Guidance and monitoring of pericardiocentesis	1 Evaluation of chest pain when noncardiac cause is apparent 2 Evaluation of chest pain in patients with confirmed diagnosis of myocardial ischemia or infarction 3 In patients with suspected pulmonary embolism to rule out the diagnosis 4 As an elective diagnostic strategy in hemodynamically stable, normotensive patients with suspected pulmonary embolism

(Continued)

TABLE 1.3   Summary of Recommendations for the Use of Echocardiography in Cardiac and Cardiac-Like Emergencies (continued)

EMERGENCY CLINICAL PRESENTATIONS	CAUSES[a]	ECHOCARDIOGRAPHY RECOMMENDED[b, c]	ECHOCARDIOGRAPHY NOT RECOMMENDED[c]
Acute dyspnea	Frequent: ADHF, PE, T, AVR/PVD, ACS Less frequent: AoD, PTx, MP	1 Distinguishing cardiac versus noncardiac etiology of dyspnea in patients whose clinical and laboratory findings are ambiguous 2 Assessment of LV size, shape, and global and regional function in patients with suspected clinical diagnosis of heart failure 3 Detection of echocardiographic signs of tamponade 4 Detection of acute valvular regurgitation and/or prosthetic valve dysfunction 5 Detection of suspected complication of myocardial ischemia/infarction, including but not limited to acute mitral regurgitation, ventricular septal defect, free-wall rupture/tamponade, right ventricular involvement, and heart failure	
Hemodynamic instability or shock	Frequent: ADHF, T, AVR/PVD, PE, ACS Less frequent: AoD, PTx, MP	1 For differential diagnosis of the cause of hypotension or shock, by detecting cardiac or noncardiac causes 2 Rapid identification of pericardial effusion, LV or RV dysfunction, and acute valvular dysfunction 3 Rapid assessment of intravascular volume status	1 In patients in shock of apparently noncardiac cause (e.g., anaphylactic, neurogenic, hemorrhagic)
New murmur	Frequent: AVR/PVD, ACS, AoD Less frequent: MP, ADHF, PE	1 In patients with cardiac murmurs and symptoms or signs of or suggestive of heart failure, myocardial ischemia or infarction, syncope, thromboembolism, or infective endocarditis, or clinical evidence of structural heart disease 2 Detection of valvular vegetations indicating infective endocarditis	
Chest trauma	Frequent: T, AoD, PTx Less frequent: ACS, AVR/PVD	1 Detection of pericardial effusion, myocardial contusion or laceration, regional wall motion abnormalities, acute valvular regurgitation, and aortic dissection in patients with severe deceleration injury or chest trauma	1 Routine evaluation in the setting of mild chest trauma with no electrocardiographic changes or biomarker elevation
Cardiac arrest or CPR	Frequent: ACS, PE, T Less frequent: AoD, MP, AVR/PVD, PTx	1 Identification of the reversible or unexpected cause of cardiac arrest to guide CPR and therapy (e.g., tamponade, pulmonary embolism, hypovolemic heart, hypertrophic cardiomyopathy)	1 As a routine procedure during CPR, or if it interferes with CPR

[a] In case of chest trauma, consequences are listed, not causes.

[b] Transesophageal echocardiography (TEE) is indicated when transthoracic echocardiography (TTE) is nondiagnostic.

[c] Recommendations related to specific conditions are applicable for all emergency clinical presentations patients may have; after initial recommendation, recommendations are not repeated in subsequent emergency clinical presentation sections in the table.

Abbreviations: ACS, acute coronary syndrome; ADHF, acute decompensated heart failure; AoD, aortic dissection; AVR/PVD, acute valvular regurgitation/prosthetic valve dysfunction; CPR, cardiopulmonary resuscitation; ECG, electrocardiogram; LV, left ventricular; MP, myopericarditis; PE, acute pulmonary embolism; PTx, pneumothorax; RV, right ventricular; T, cardiac tamponade.

(Modified and reproduced with permission from Oxford University Press from Neskovic AN, et al.[1])

first 24 hours, early diagnosis and prompt treatment are essential.[20] Many echocardiographic features of aortic dissection (pericardial effusion, aortic regurgitation, and dilation) may be revealed by TTE, but it should be noted that a negative TTE study cannot rule out aortic dissection. In fact, TTE has poor sensitivity for detecting acute aortic dissection. The choice of imaging study (TEE, multislice CT, or magnetic resonance imaging) to establish or exclude the diagnosis of aortic dissection depends on local availability and expertise (see also Chapter 6).

Standard TTE or lung ultrasound may also be of value in diagnosing other conditions associated with chest pain as a chief complaint, such as acute myopericarditis, stress cardiomyopathy, pneumothorax, and pleurisy.

Acute dyspnea

Echocardiography may help to distinguish between cardiac (e.g., acute pulmonary embolism, heart failure, cardiac tamponade) and noncardiac conditions (e.g., worsening of chronic obstructive pulmonary disease [COPD], massive pleural effusion) associated with dyspnea.

Echocardiography should not be considered a diagnostic test for acute pulmonary embolism, but rather its use should be reserved for the assessment of the hemodynamic effects of the pulmonary embolism, such as right ventricular strain, that might dictate specific therapy. Nevertheless, for making the definitive diagnosis of acute pulmonary embolism, especially in hemodynamically stable patients, CT pulmonary angiography is the preferred imaging modality. Standard TTE, and particularly TEE, can be used for detection of right ventricular dysfunction and other signs of high-risk acute pulmonary embolism (right-sided heart thrombi and patent foramen ovale) (see Chapter 7).

Other reasons for cardiac dyspnea, such as severe LV dysfunction and cardiac tamponade, are also easily detectable by echocardiography, whereas lung ultrasound (Chapter 20) has proven to be useful for making the distinction between acute decompensated heart failure and worsening COPD (V1.5).

Chest trauma

Patients with chest trauma who are presenting to the ED with ECG abnormalities or symptoms suggestive of cardiac pathology may benefit from emergency echocardiography to rule out myocardial contusion, valvular or aortic rupture, coronary artery dissection, and cardiac tamponade. Suspected pathology (e.g., aortic or tricuspid valve rupture) and/or a patient's condition (polytrauma, mechanical ventilation) may require TEE for the definitive diagnosis to be reached (see Chapter 16).

Hemodynamic instability and cardiac arrest

Echocardiography plays a central role in the evaluation of patients presenting with hemodynamic instability and/or under cardiopulmonary resuscitation because all cardiac emergencies may eventually lead to shock and cardiac arrest (see Chapters 4 and 5). Depending on the suspected pathology, the patient's condition, and imaging windows, TEE may be the preferred echocardiographic technique for determining the underlying reason for the patient's instability.

MACHINE LEARNING AND ARTIFICIAL INTELLIGENCE

In recent years, AI is slowly but steadily being integrated in image acquisition and analysis in different fields of medicine, including emergency settings.[21] Maybe earlier than one would imagine, AI-augmented HUDs became commercially available, with capability of guiding inexperienced users to obtain and optimize echocardiographic images by analyzing the current image and then navigate the user to adjust the position of the probe on the chest, if required.[22] In addition, AI-guided systems can automatically calculate LVEF with excellent agreement with the reference values provided by human experts.[23]

On the other hand, AI-augmented ultrasound devices and applications will truly revolutionize the use of echocardiography in the emergency setting only if they become able to reliably perform qualitative assessments and identify diseases based on the integration of imaging and clinical data. Current advances are encouraging and suggest it is only a matter of time before these new capabilities become commercially available. For instance, a deep learning approach for assessment of regional WMA from echocardiographic images had an accuracy similar to that of cardiologist and superior to that of resident readers.[24] In addition, in a cohort study that included clinical and TTE data, a real-time system for fully automated interpretation of echocardiographic loops was more accurate than cardiologists in differentiating Takotsubo syndrome from myocardial infarction.[25]

However, in all aforementioned studies, machines were imperfect, just like humans. Although we are approaching the era of AI-augmented clinical decision-making, several ethical and legal issues must be resolved before AI-assisted emergency echocardiography becomes a routine clinical tool.

CONCLUSIONS AND FUTURE PERSPECTIVES

Emergency echocardiography is both a life-saving and cost-effective technique, and its application in acute settings will continue to grow. Further miniaturization and reduction of cost of the devices will contribute to even wider use of ultrasound in the emergency setting, and the examinations will be frequently performed by non-cardiologists. Precise and strict requirements consisting of a carefully prepared curriculum have to be defined to preserve the quality and the accuracy of the data provided by echocardiography, especially in the emergency setting.[1] The examinations performed by non-experts should remain simple and goal oriented, with the intention of answering clear, bimodal (yes or no) clinical questions. Comprehensive emergency echocardiography must stay in the hands of trained independent operators because this imaging technique can reach its full potential only if performed by fully competent users able to resolve the most complicated emergency cases by putting imaging data in a clinical context. Finally, we believe there is a real hope that AI will prove to be a valuable tool in clinical decision-making in emergency settings in the near future.

LIST OF VIDEOS

https://routledgetextbooks.com/textbooks/9781032157009/chapter-1.php

VIDEO 1.1   Unusually prominent Chiari's network: Chiari's network (an embryologic remnant normally seen in approximately 2% of the population) in the right atrium; this was initially interpreted as right heart thrombus.

VIDEO 1.2A   Ultrasound artifact mimicking intimal flap (1/2): This finding in the dilated ascending aorta on transthoracic examination required transesophageal study (see Video 1.2B) to rule out aortic dissection. *(Video provided by VC.)*

VIDEO 1.2B   Ultrasound artifact mimicking intimal flap (2/2): Transesophageal echocardiography (TEE) study of a patient with ultrasound artifact mimicking intimal flap in the dilated ascending aorta on transthoracic examination (see Video 1.2A) performed to rule out aortic dissection. No intimal flap is noted in the lumen of the ascending aorta. *(Video provided by VC.)*

VIDEO 1.3A   Poor scanning technique (1/2): Important findings may be overlooked because of poor scanning technique resulting in apical foreshortening. In this transthoracic echocardiography (TTE) four-chamber view, true apex is missed (see also Video 1.3B).

VIDEO 1.3B   Poor scanning technique (2/2): In contrast to foreshortened view of the left ventricle (see Video 1.3A), apical dyskinesia and thrombus became apparent when a full-length image of the left ventricle was obtained.

VIDEO 1.4   Echocardiographically guided pericardiocentesis: An injection of agitated saline (microbubbles) is performed to confirm the pericardial location of the tip of the needle before fluid removal.

VIDEO 1.5   Lung comets: In a patient with acute decompensated heart failure, the presence of extravascular lung water can be detected by lung ultrasound as multiple diffuse bilateral hyperechogenic vertical B-lines spreading from the pleural line to the edge of the screen, resembling comet tails ("lung comets").

NOTE

*   Record and Review.

REFERENCES

1. Neskovic AN, Hagendorff A, Lancellotti P, et al. Emergency echocardiography: the European Association of Cardiovascular Imaging recommendations. Eur Heart J Cardiovasc Imaging 2013; 14(1):1–11.
2. Stewart WJ, Douglas PS, Sagar K, et al. Echocardiography in emergency medicine: a policy statement by the American Society of Echocardiography and the American College of Cardiology. The Task Force on Echocardiography in Emergency Medicine of the American Society of Echocardiography and the Echocardiography TPEC Committees of the American College of Cardiology. J Am Soc Echocardiogr 1999; 12(1):82–4.
3. Neskovic AN, Skinner H, Price S, et al. Focus cardiac ultrasound core curriculum and core syllabus of the European Association of Cardiovascular Imaging European Heart Journal. Eur Heart J Cardiovasc Imaging 2018; 19:475–81.
4. Evangelista A, Flachskampf F, Lancellotti P, et al. European Association of Echocardiography recommendations for standardization of performance, digital storage and reporting of echocardiographic studies. Eur J Echocardiogr 2008; 9(4):438–48.
5. Quiñones MA, Douglas PS, Foster E, et al. ACC/AHA clinical competence statement on echocardiography: a report of the American College of Cardiology/American Heart Association/American College of Physicians—American Society of Internal Medicine Task Force on Clinical Competence. J Am Coll Cardiol 2003; 41(4):687–708.
6. Neskovic AN, Hagendorff A. Echocardiography in the emergency room. In: Galiuto L, Badano L, Fox K, Sicari R, Zamorano JL (eds). The EAE Textbook of Echocardiography. New York: Oxford University Press, 2011.
7. Piérard LA, Lancellotti P. Echocardiography in the emergency room: non-invasive imaging. Heart 2009; 95(2):164–70.
8. Oh JK, Meloy TD, Seward JB. Echocardiography in the emergency room: is it feasible, beneficial, and cost-effective? Echocardiography 1995; 12(2):163–70.
9. Van Dantzig JM. Echocardiography in the emergency department. Semin Cardiothorac Vasc Anesth 2006; 10(1):79–81.
10. Ciobanu AO, Griffin SC, Bennett S, et al. Catastrophic mitral prosthesis dehiscence diagnosed by three-dimensional transesophageal echocardiography. J Clin Ultrasound 2014; 42(4):249–51.
11. Sasaki S, Watanabe H, Shibayama K, et al. Three-dimensional transesophageal echocardiographic evaluation of coronary involvement in patients with acute type A aortic dissection. J Am Soc Echocardiogr 2013; 26(8):837–45.
12. Stankovic I, Cvorovic V, Putnikovic B, et al. Two-dimensional speckle tracking-derived strain to distinguish acute coronary syndrome from a marked early repolarization in a patient with chest pain: a fancy gadget or a useful tool? Echocardiography 2014; 31(2):E48–51.
13. Douglas PS, Khandheria B, Stainback RF, et al. ACCF/ASE/ACEP/ASNC/SCAI/SCCT/SCMR 2007 appropriateness criteria for transthoracic and transesophageal echocardiography: a report of the American College of Cardiology Foundation Quality Strategic Directions Committee Appropriateness Criteria Working Group, American Society of Echocardiography, American College of Emergency Physicians, American Society of Nuclear Cardiology, Society for Cardiovascular Angiography and Interventions, Society of Cardiovascular Computed Tomography, and the Society for Cardiovascular Magnetic Resonance endorsed

by the American College of Chest Physicians and the Society of Critical Care Medicine. J Am Coll Cardiol 2007; 50(2):187–204.

14. Senior R, Becher H, Monaghan M, et al. Contrast echocardiography: evidence-based recommendations by European Association of Echocardiography. Eur J Echocardiogr 2009; 10(2):194–212.

15. Tibbles CD, Porcaro W. Procedural applications of ultrasound. Emerg Med Clin North Am 2004; 22(3):797–815.

16. Yong Y, Wu D, Fernandes V, et al. Diagnostic accuracy and costeffectiveness of contrast echocardiography on evaluation of cardiac function in technically very difficult patients in the intensive care unit. Am J Cardiol 2002; 89(6):711–8.

17. Hamm CW, Bassand JP, Agewall S, et al. ESC Guidelines for the management of acute coronary syndromes in patients presenting without persistent ST-segment elevation: the Task Force for the management of acute coronary syndromes (ACS) in patients presenting without persistent ST-segment elevation of the European Society of Cardiology (ESC). Eur Heart J 2011; 32(23):2999–3054.

18. Jeetley P, Burden L, Senior R. Stress echocardiography is superior to exercise ECG in the risk stratification of patients presenting with acute chest pain with negative troponin. Eur J Echocardiogr 2006; 7(2):155–64.

19. Nucifora G, Badano LP, Sarraf-Zadegan N, et al. Comparison of early dobutamine stress echocardiography and exercise electrocardiographic testing for management of patients presenting to the emergency department with chest pain. Am J Cardiol 2007; 100(7):1068–73.

20. Hiratzka LF, Bakris GL, Beckman JA, et al. American College of Cardiology Foundation/American Heart Association Task Force on Practice Guidelines; American Association for Thoracic Surgery; American College of Radiology; American Stroke Association; Society of Cardiovascular Anesthesiologists; Society for Cardiovascular Angiography and Interventions; Society of Interventional Radiology; Society of Thoracic Surgeons; Society for Vascular Medicine. Guidelines for the management of patients with thoracic aortic disease. Circulation 2010; 121:e266–369.

21. Stewart J, Sprivulis P, Dwivedi G. Artificial intelligence and machine learning in emergency medicine. Emerg Med Australas 2018; 30(6):870–74.

22. Schneider M, Bartko P, Geller W, et al. A machine learning algorithm supports ultrasound-naïve novices in the acquisition of diagnostic echocardiography loops and provides accurate estimation of LVEF. Int J Cardiovasc Imaging 2021; 37(2):577–86.

23. Asch FM, Poilvert N, Abraham T, et al. Automated echocardiographic quantification of left ventricular ejection fraction without volume measurements using a machine learning algorithm mimicking a human expert. Circ Cardiovasc Imaging 2019; 12(9):e009303.

24. Kusunose K, Abe T, Haga A, et al. A deep learning approach for assessment of regional wall motion abnormality from echocardiographic images. JACC Cardiovasc Imaging 2020; 13(2 Pt 1):374–81.

25. Laumer F, Di Vece D, Cammann VL, et al. Assessment of artificial intelligence in echocardiography diagnostics in differentiating Takotsubo syndrome from myocardial infarction. JAMA Cardiol 2022; 7(5):494–503.

Echocardiography in acute myocardial infarction

2

Aleksandar N. Neskovic, Leonardo Bolognese, and Michael H. Picard

Key Points

- Echocardiography is valuable in all patients with acute myocardial infarction (MI) for diagnosis, functional assessment, detection of complications, and/or prognosis.
- Echocardiography may miss small, nontransmural infarctions.
- Regional wall motion abnormality associated with preserved wall thickness in diastole, which is an echocardiographic hallmark of acute MI, may be caused by conditions other than infarction (e.g., ischemia or acute myocarditis).
- The value of echocardiography as a diagnostic tool is highest in patients with acute coronary syndrome with atypical clinical presentation, nondiagnostic electrocardiogram, and/or normal or only slightly increased cardiac enzymes.
- Measuring ejection fraction in the acute phase of the infarction may not reflect true functional loss, although a low postinfarction ejection fraction is a strong predictor of poor outcome.
- Dyssynergic myocardial regions may be viable and may have the potential of functional recovery. Viability can be assessed early by echocardiography-based techniques.
- Initial left ventricular volumes, wall motion score index, infarct zone viability, and diastolic filling carry important prognostic information.
- Echocardiographic examination must not induce unnecessary delays in triage of patients to reperfusion therapy.

In patients with suspected or evolving acute myocardial infarction, echocardiography facilitates diagnosis and differential diagnosis, detects complications (Chapter 3), and provides valuable information regarding the infarct-related artery, functional infarct size, prognosis, and effects of therapy (Table 2.1). As a handy, widely available, and cost-effective imaging technique, echocardiography is commonly used in almost all patients with acute myocardial infarction for at least one of the aforementioned reasons. The collected information, whether assessed quantitatively or qualitatively, is of incomparable value for accurate estimation of risk and for guiding management, especially in hemodynamically unstable patients. Even in patients traditionally considered to be at low risk, echocardiography may reveal unexpected left ventricular (LV) dysfunction because of an extensive dyssynergic zone. However, it should be emphasized that echocardiographic examination in unstable patients with ongoing chest pain in the emergency setting is a highly demanding procedure that requires both excellent technical skills to obtain adequate images in a stressful environment and the ability to interpret findings quickly and accurately.

Technological developments (harmonic imaging, intravenous contrast agents) improve endocardial definition by two-dimensional (2D) echocardiography, which is crucial for accurate regional wall motion analysis. Experienced supervisors are able

DOI: 10.1201/9781003245407-2

TABLE 2.1   The Role of Echocardiography in Acute Myocardial Infarction

- Diagnosis
- Differential diagnosis
- Assessment of functional infarct size
- Identification of infarct-related artery
- Assessment of left ventricular function
- Assessment of right ventricular function
- Detection of myocardial viability
- Prognosis assessment
- Evaluation of the effects of therapy

to provide training that may result in improvement in regional wall motion abnormality (WMA) readings in a short period of time. In addition, intracoronary or intravenous myocardial contrast echocardiography (MCE) may provide important data regarding the area at risk after coronary occlusion, regional coronary flow reserve, myocardial viability, and functional outcome.

Although in almost all cases standard 2D and Doppler transthoracic examinations provide information that may be effectively used for decision-making, transesophageal echocardiography (TEE) may also be helpful, especially in critically ill patients. In experienced hands, TEE is safe and feasible. It may be of value particularly in differential diagnosis, to exclude other life-threatening conditions with similar clinical presentation, such as aortic dissection (Chapter 6) or massive pulmonary embolism (Chapter 7).

Because the clinical course of acute myocardial infarction is highly variable, *serial echocardiographic studies* may be needed to assess actual risk and to modify therapeutic strategy throughout the acute phase. In addition, *follow-up studies* provide unique insight into the natural history of LV systolic and diastolic function and the effects of reperfusion and revascularization therapies.

Finally, cardiologists are not the only health professionals involved in diagnosis and treatment of patients with acute coronary syndrome (ACS). In an attempt to obtain essential diagnostic information in a variety of clinical situations, many non-cardiologists (Chapter 19), including emergency physicians, anesthesiologists, intensive care specialists, trainees, and sonographers, are performing cardiac ultrasound scanning in patients with suspected ACS.[1,2] Often, they use portable or handheld imaging devices (Chapter 18). Of note, essential information, no matter who obtained it and how it was obtained, if accurate and used thoughtfully, may direct patient management and save lives. Important issues related to training and competence in the field are discussed in Chapter 1.

ECHOCARDIOGRAPHIC SIGNS OF MYOCARDIAL ISCHEMIA AND INFARCTION

Myocardial ischemia or infarction causes WMAs of the left ventricle[3] that can be easily documented by echocardiography.

The key echocardiographic sign of acute myocardial ischemia or necrosis is *regional WMA (dyssynergy) associated with preserved wall thickness in diastole*[3] (V2.1). Over time, necrotic myocardial segments typically become thin and highly reflective (V2.2). In contrast to infarction, short-lasting ischemia, by definition, causes transient WMA (V2.3A, V2.3B).

In patients with ongoing myocardial infarction, 2D echocardiography may reveal *different degrees of WMA:* hypokinesis, akinesis, or dyskinesis. The degree and the magnitude of WMA caused by actual infarction are related to the location of the culprit lesion in the infarct-related artery, the presence or absence of collateral circulation, and the extent of coronary artery disease (CAD). It has been shown that WMA detectable by echocardiography occurs if resting coronary flow is reduced by >50%,[4] if >20% of myocardial thickness is jeopardized by actual ischemia or necrosis,[5] or if at least 1–6% of the LV mass is involved.[6] Thus, echocardiography may miss myocardial infarction if it is very small and/or limited to the thin endocardial layer (small nontransmural infarctions).[3,6]

When standard visual assessment of regional wall motion fails to detect WMA, *myocardial strain analysis* (deformation imaging) may potentially reveal subtle abnormalities (including postsystolic shortening/thickening phenomenon) (Figure 2.1) (V2.4A, V2.4B, V2.4C, V2.4D, V2.26) that could be clinically relevant.[7–9] Recent developments in ultrasound technology and software make it possible to quantify both global and regional LV deformation (or function) with myocardial strain analysis. Although strain can be assessed by both tissue Doppler and 2D echocardiographic speckle tracking technique, the latter approach is preferred in the clinical setting because it is independent of angle of insonation, has lower interobserver variability, and allows semiautomatic quantification. Myocardial strain may be useful for detection of CAD both at rest and during stress echocardiography, for making a diagnosis of myocardial infarction and distinguishing between nontransmural and transmural infarction, and for assessing myocardial viability and the patient prognosis.[10] Furthermore, it has been reported that longitudinal strain, reflective of deformation of subendocardial fibers that are most susceptible to ischemia, is useful for exclusion of significant CAD in patients with suspected ACS, especially when electrocardiographic findings are confusing and cardiac biomarkers are normal.[11] In a small, single-center study, global peak systolic longitudinal strain (with a cutoff value of −20%) was superior to Global Registry of Acute Coronary Events (GRACE) risk score and conventional echo parameters in detecting significant CAD, with a negative predictive value of 92%.[11] However, it should be noted that longitudinal strain values may be decreased in conditions other than CAD (e.g., nonischemic cardiomyopathies, diabetes mellitus, significant valvular heart disease, hypertension) and also may be affected by age and sex differences (with lower values being observed in male and in elderly subjects).[12]

Despite a plethora of studies suggesting the ability of myocardial strain to describe even subtle changes in myocardial contraction, it is *not commonly used* in daily practice, and its clinical usefulness has not yet been addressed in clinical

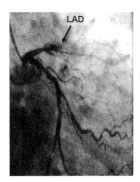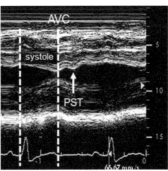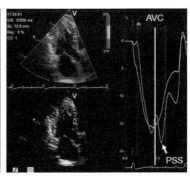

FIGURE 2.1   Altered deformation of the anteroseptal wall in a patient with suspected acute coronary syndrome without actual chest pain and normal standard two-dimensional echocardiogram (V2.4A, V2.4B, V2.4C). In transthoracic long-axis views (V2.4D), the "shivering" of the septum was noted. M-mode recording (middle panel) showing the "double peak" contraction pattern of the septum (arrow pointing at postsystolic thickening of the septum, not detectable in the posterior wall). Tissue Doppler-derived segmental longitudinal strain curves depict on the right panel normal posterior wall mechanics (yellow curve with a single peak occurring at aortic valve closure) and ischemic anteroseptal wall mechanics (double peak green curve with the latter postsystolic peak occurring after the aortic valve closure). Coronary angiography (left panel) revealed proximally occluded (arrow) left anterior descending coronary artery (LAD) with moderate collateral circulation. AVC: aortic valve closure; PSS: postsystolic shortening; PST: postsystolic thickening.

(Image and videos provided by IS.)

guidelines. Prior to routine clinical use of strain in ACS, there need to be harmonized standards for strain measurements to establish appropriate cut-off values across different vendors' equipment and also large-scale multicenter studies that demonstrate the feasibility, accuracy, and usefulness of these strain-derived parameters. In the meantime, when using strain in patients with suspected ACS, we believe it is more feasible (and less confusing) to look for specific patterns of contraction and deformation and relative differences between segments rather than to rely on numbers.[9]

ECHOCARDIOGRAPHY IN DIAGNOSIS OF ACUTE MYOCARDIAL INFARCTION

In patients with suspected acute myocardial infarction, accuracy of diagnostic information obtained by echocardiography is related to local expertise, image quality, clinical circumstances, and specific patient population evaluated. It is well known that sensitivity, specificity, and accuracy of any diagnostic technique are strongly influenced by the pretest likelihood of the disease (Bayesian theory). Therefore, different results can be expected in the coronary care unit patient population than in a much less selected group of individuals such as patients examined in the emergency department. Successful technique, however, should identify low-risk patients without compromising the detection of those at high risk for coronary events and complications.[13]

As pointed out earlier, in acute myocardial ischemia or necrosis, echocardiography reveals *regional WMA associated with preserved wall thickness in diastole and normal myocardial reflectivity*. Thin, dyssynergic, bright or highly reflective

myocardial wall strongly suggests scar from old infarction. However, in patients with acute chest pain, it is often impossible to differentiate on 2D transthoracic echocardiography the regional WMA caused by ischemia (V2.5A, V2.5B), necrosis (V2.6), or myocardial inflammation (V2.7).[14,15]

Echocardiography seems to be sensitive in the diagnosis of acute infarction or ischemia during anginal pain.[13,14,16] The incremental value of echocardiography as a diagnostic tool is highest in patients with suspected acute myocardial infarction with atypical clinical presentation, nondiagnostic electrocardiogram (ECG), and/or normal or only slightly increased cardiac enzymes.[17] Overall, sensitivity of the technique is high (over 90%), but specificity and positive predictive value are more variable and less convincing,[16–18] indicating interpretation difficulties in the emergency setting. As a consequence, confusion and frequent overdiagnosis (false positive diagnosis) may occur in attempts not to miss those with true infarction. On the other hand, the absence of segmental WMA in a patient with prolonged chest pain without history of prior infarction or known CAD has negative predictive value as high as 99% and practically excludes major myocardial ischemia.[19] Although it should be expected that a few small subendocardial injuries will be missed by echocardiography, importantly, prognosis in patients with ACS and normal echocardiogram is favorable.[16–19]

ECHOCARDIOGRAPHY IN DIFFERENTIAL DIAGNOSIS OF ACUTE MYOCARDIAL INFARCTION

Echocardiography provides critical information for differentiation of other conditions that may be associated with acute

TABLE 2.2 Common Causes of Acute Chest Pain in the Emergency Department

- Acute coronary syndrome
- Acute aortic syndrome
- Acute pulmonary embolism
- Takotsubo cardiomyopathy
- Myocarditis
- Acute pericarditis
- Pneumothorax
- Aortic stenosis
- Hypertrophic cardiomyopathy
- Mitral valve prolapse

Note: The list is not in order of frequency.

TABLE 2.3 Conditions That May Present with Resting Regional Wall Motion Abnormalities Mimicking Myocardial Ischemia or Infarction

- Acute myocarditis
- Takotsubo cardiomyopathy
- Left bundle branch block*
- Left ventricular pre-excitation*
- Paced heart rhythm*
- Cardiomyopathies*
- Right ventricular pressure or volume overload*

* May also be related to coronary artery disease to a certain extent.

chest pain (Table 2.2) and/or hemodynamic instability when recommended therapeutic strategies are strikingly different and when misdiagnosis and mistreatment may be life threatening (e.g., acute aortic syndrome versus acute ST-elevation myocardial infarction) (V2.27A, V2.27B). The situation may become even more puzzling when these conditions occur simultaneously, as in the case of acute coronary artery obstruction caused by dissection of the vessel wall or ostial coronary artery obstruction by intimal flap in patients with acute proximal aortic dissection (Chapter 6) (V2.8A, V2.8B).

Apart from acute myocardial infarction, resting regional WMA caused by CAD can be detected in patients with other forms of ACS, during transient anginal attack, in chronic ischemia (hibernated myocardium), in myocardial stunning, or in patients with old infarctions (myocardial scar). In addition, there are *conditions other than CAD* that may be associated with resting regional WMAs (Table 2.3), indistinguishable from those that occur as a result of obstructive coronary lesions.

Echocardiography may also be helpful in identifying the rare cause of non-atherosclerotic coronary artery obstruction (e.g., coronary artery embolization—see Chapter 13) (V2.28A, V2.28B), as well as the underlying cause of ischemia-like ST segment changes in patients presenting with atypical chest pain (e.g., hypertrophic cardiomyopathy) (V2.29).

Echocardiography may assist in *clarifying potentially confusing situations* in the emergency department related to imperfect sensitivity and specificity of electrocardiography in detecting CAD. The ECG is normal or nondiagnostic in a substantial proportion of patients with ACS and may show ST-segment elevation in conditions not inevitably linked with ACS (LV hypertrophy, acute pericarditis, left bundle branch block, cardiomyopathies, hyperkalemia, Brugada syndrome), or ST elevation may be typical but misleading, as in the aforementioned situation of acute aortic syndrome complicated by coronary artery obstruction.

Acute myocarditis and pericarditis

Of note and contrary to common opinion, many patients with clinically significant acute myocarditis reveal *segmental rather than diffuse WMA*, quite similar to typical echocardiographic presentation of an acute coronary event[20] (V2.9A, V2.9B, V2.9C). Clinical presentation of acute myocarditis may be indistinguishable from ACS,[20] and these patients should often undergo coronary angiography or cardiac computed tomography to exclude CAD. Various degrees of global LV dilation or dysfunction can be present. Regional heterogeneity in contractility (V2.10A, V2.10B, 2.10C) (Figure 2.2) and thickened myocardium in affected regions (interstitial myocardial edema)

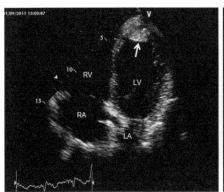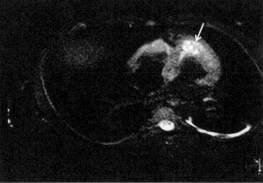

FIGURE 2.2 Acute myocarditis with apical akinesis and thrombus formation. Left ventricular thrombus in the apex (left panel, arrow) (V2.10B) in a patient with acute myocarditis and clinical course resembling acute myocardial infarction (V2.10A). Magnetic resonance imaging, performed 3 weeks after initial presentation, demonstrated good global left ventricular function (V2.10C) with late gadolinium enhancement confined to mid-myocardial layers (right panel, arrow), consistent with postmyocarditis scar. LA: left atrium; LV: left ventricle; RA: right atrium; RV: right ventricle.

may also be found.[21] In the majority of cases regional WMAs are transient, while subtle changes can be appreciated with deformation imaging (V2.30A, V2.30B). Interestingly, aneurysms are not seen in myocarditis (except in cases of Chagas myocarditis).

In patients with *acute pericarditis*, presence of chest pain, ECG changes, and slightly elevated troponin level may lead to confusion with ACS. On the other hand, acute myocardial infarction itself can be complicated by pericarditis. The most common echocardiographic finding in pericarditis is a normal echocardiogram. Echocardiography detects pericardial effusion when present. Regional WMAs are found in associated myocarditis or infarction. Pericardial effusion seen in acute aortic dissection is a warning sign, suggesting imminent aortic rupture and cardiac tamponade. Echo-free space around the heart as a result of pericardial effusion should be distinguished from a pericardial fat pad and pleural effusion (see Chapter 3, Figure 3.12).

Takotsubo cardiomyopathy

Takotsubo cardiomyopathy (also known as *stress-induced cardiomyopathy, apical ballooning syndrome*, or *broken heart syndrome*), a cardiac syndrome that can occur after various types of stress, is also seen in patients presenting to the emergency department with chest pain or dyspnea.[22–28] Accompanying ECG changes and elevation of serum cardiac troponin are often similar to those seen in ACS. The incidence of the syndrome is relatively high and, by some reports, reaches up to 2% in patients presenting with ACS.[22]

Echocardiography typically reveals transitory left ventricular WMAs encompassing more than one coronary vascular territory, and in the majority of cases, complete recovery occurs within 2 weeks. The most common echocardiographic presentation is *apical ballooning* (apical form, see the following paragraph).

In a majority of cases the absence of significant CAD should be confirmed by coronary angiography or cardiac computed tomography. In some cases, however, detection of preserved distal coronary flow in the LAD by transthoracic coronary artery Doppler may strongly suggest a noncoronary cause (V2.14B). Complications such as LV thrombus formation, profound cardiogenic shock, pericardial effusion with cardiac tamponade, LV rupture, and life-threatening arrhythmias have been reported during the acute phase of illness.

Based on echocardiographic appearance, several morphologic forms of Takotsubo cardiomyopathy have been described:

- *Apical* form—"apical ballooning," the most common; characterized by hypokinesis, akinesis, or dyskinesis of the apical one-half to two-thirds of the left ventricle with hyperkinesis of basal segments (Figure 2.3) (V2.11A, V2.11B, V5.14A, V5.14B).
- *Midventricular* form—less common; characterized by hypokinesis, akinesis, or dyskinesis of midventricular segments of the left ventricle and

sparing of apical and basal segments (V2.12A, V2.12B). "Apical nipple" sign—that is, mid-ventricular ballooning with preserved contractility of the apex—may help to discriminate between stress cardiomyopathy and anterior acute myocardial infarction.[29]
- *Basal (reversed)* form—rarest; only the basal third of the left ventricle is affected (V2.13A, V2.13B).

According to one series, up to 29% of patients with Takotsubo cardiomyopathy have evidence of *right ventricular* involvement[23] (V2.14A, V2.14B, V2.14C, V2.14D). Also, in approximately 16% of patients with Takotsubo cardiomyopathy, *transient LV outflow obstruction* may occur because of the compensatory hyperdynamic motion of the LV outflow tract myocardium, leading to significant narrowing of the outflow tract[24] (V2.15).

Pneumothorax

Pneumothorax may be suspected in patients with chest pain and a poor echocardiographic window because the air in the pleural space in front of the heart makes it impossible to image it by ultrasound. However, *lung ultrasound* is more accurate and typically reveals the absence of a normal lung sliding pattern (if sliding is present, negative predictive value is 100%). Also, the *lung point sign* (V2.16) can be noted, indicating the area of the chest wall where the regular reappearance of the lung sliding replaces the pneumothorax pattern (sensitivity 65%, specificity 100%).[30]

IDENTIFICATION OF THE INFARCT-RELATED ARTERY

Actual *distribution of dyssynergic segments* on two-dimensional echocardiogram reflects the location of the *culprit* coronary artery lesion (Figure 2.4). If the left anterior descending coronary artery (LAD) is involved, dyssynergy of the anterior wall, anterior septum, and LV apex is present. The *extent of dyssynergy* is determined by the level of the infarct-related artery obstruction (the more proximal the lesion, the more extensive the WMAs) and the presence of collateral circulation (if present, less extensive WMAs are expected). Lateral wall dyssynergy points to the left circumflex artery (LCx) as an infarct-related artery, whereas dyssynergy of the inferior wall and inferior septum suggests a right coronary artery (RCA) lesion.[31] Of note, there is *substantial overlap* in segmental distribution of the territories supplied by the RCA and LCx, depending on the coronary artery dominance in a particular patient. *Dyssynergy* (V2.17) detected in segments that do not fit a single coronary artery perfusion zone (remote dyssynergy) typically indicates multivessel coronary disease.[31]

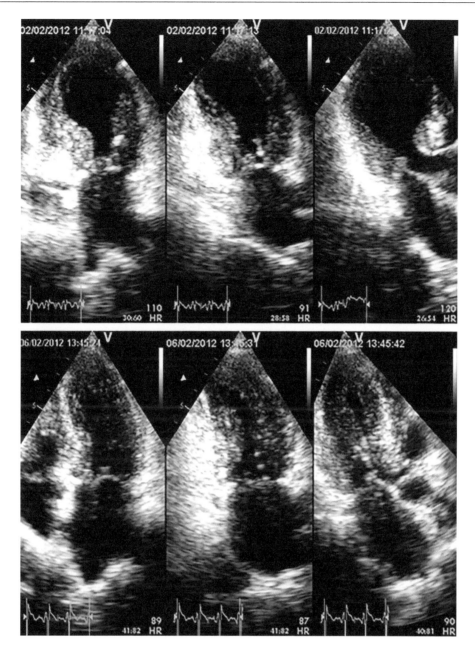

FIGURE 2.3   Apical form of Takotsubo cardiomyopathy. Typical apical ballooning with hypercontractility of the basal segments of the left ventricle at initial presentation (upper panels, systolic frames) (V2.11A). Note the normalization of the left ventricular function 4 days after admission (lower panels, systolic frames) (V2.11B). Upper and lower left panels: apical four-chamber view. Upper and lower middle panels: apical two-chamber view. Upper and lower right panels: apical long-axis view.

ASSESSMENT OF FUNCTIONAL INFARCT SIZE

The extent of dyssynergic myocardium in evolving myocardial infarction determines its *functional size* and has direct impact on the degree of hemodynamic compromise and prognosis (Figure 2.5) (V2.18A, V2.18B, V4.5, V4.7). The extent of dyssynergy correlates well with the anatomic size of the infarction or jeopardized myocardium.[32] However, information obtained by segmental wall motion analyses tends to overestimate true anatomic infarction size.[32,33] The nonfunctional zone consists of the actual necrosis zone, segments jeopardized by actual ischemia, stunned and hibernated segments, and scars from previous infarctions. Thus, functional infarct size is often *considerably larger* than the anatomic size of the actual necrosis.[33] Frequently, *hypercontractility* of the segments not affected by actual infarction can be noted (see later), and as a consequence, global ejection fraction (EF) can be maintained in the normal range or is only slightly reduced during the acute phase.

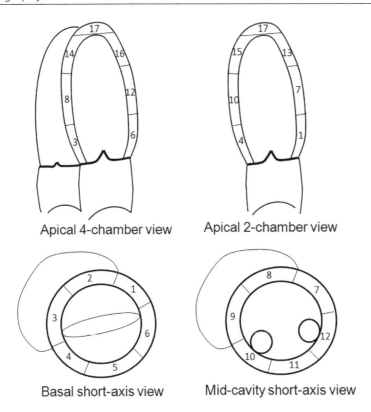

FIGURE 2.4 Coronary artery territories. *Left anterior descending coronary artery* supplies anteroseptal and apical septal segments (2, 8, and 14), anterior free wall (1 and 7), anterior apical segment (13), and true apex (17). *Right coronary artery* supplies inferior free wall (4 and 10), inferior septum (3 and 9), and inferior apical segment (15). *Left circumflex coronary artery* supplies inferolateral (5 and 11), anterolateral (6 and 12), and lateral apical segment (16). There is an overlap between the right coronary artery and left circumflex coronary artery territories, according to the coronary artery dominance.

In patients with a complicated clinical course, *repeated echocardiographic examinations* in the coronary care unit may serve as a substitute for hemodynamic monitoring because they provide useful information on changes in LV function, detect complications, assist in decisions regarding therapeutic interventions, and assess response to treatment.

Of note, many patients without clinical evidence of hemodynamic instability may have significant WMAs, indicating a risk for early LV remodeling and an associated worse prognosis. These patients identified by serial echocardiographic examinations will benefit from an aggressive management strategy.

Finally, it is important to remember that there is frequent *discordance* between severity of electrocardiographic changes and true extent of myocardial damage. The ECG may overestimate or underestimate (V2.19) the amount of dysfunctional myocardium in both acute and chronic phases.

ASSESSMENT OF LEFT VENTRICULAR FUNCTION

Functional impairment of the left ventricle in acute myocardial infarction may be assessed in different ways. Changes in

different parameters of LV systolic and diastolic function are important features of acute myocardial infarction. *Serial echocardiographic assessment* can be helpful for early detection of deterioration or to document improvement of these parameters over time and/or after therapeutic interventions. In addition, the absolute value of these parameters as well as the pattern of their changes carries prognostic information in postinfarction survivors (see later).

The *improvement of segmental function* over time is a well-known phenomenon after myocardial infarction, especially in the reperfusion/revascularization era. This improvement has been shown to be related mainly to timely administered reperfusion therapy, a percutaneous coronary intervention, infarct-related artery patency, effective tissue reperfusion, and viability of the infarcted segments. These factors are obviously interrelated. They most likely, in different ways, reflect the same basic principle—that is, preserved myocardial viability and halting of the necrosis process.

Systolic function

Global LV function, assessed by EF, may be preserved even in large infarctions during the acute phase as a consequence of compensatory hypercontractility of non-infarcted segments.

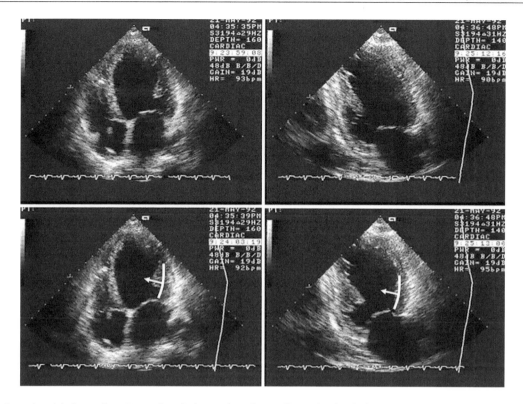

FIGURE 2.5 Functional infarct size. Example of the patient in cardiogenic shock from extensive anterior myocardial infarction (V2.18A, V2.18B). Note that only basal parts of the anterior and lateral wall are moving in systole (marked with arrow). Upper panels: diastolic frames, apical four-chamber (left) and two-chamber view (right). Lower panels: systolic frames, apical four-chamber (left) and two-chamber view (right).

This *hyperkinesia* of the remote (noninfarcted) areas has been reported in up to two-thirds of patients after acute myocardial infarction (V2.20, V2.21, V2.22), with the incidence related to the time when the examination was performed (it declines with time after infarction) and the extent of the CAD (lower incidence in multivessel disease).[34] Hyperkinesia may disappear during the first days after an infarction, especially after successful revascularization in patients with single-vessel disease. In some studies hyperkinesia was observed more often in patients with anterior infarction,[35] probably because of easier visual detection of hyperkinesia in the inferior wall. In addition, the presence of bundle branch block makes the detection of hyperkinesia more difficult. Also, it can be seen more often in patients treated with reperfusion therapy,[35] correlating with increased TIMI (thrombolysis in myocardial infarction) grade flow in the infarct-related artery.[36] Therefore, measuring EF in the acute phase may not reflect *true functional loss*, although low postinfarction EF is a strong predictor of poor outcome.[37] Of note, LV volumes and EF should be measured by either the biplane method of discs or three-dimensional echocardiography.

Infarction size is a major determinant of LVEF. Because anterior infarctions tend to be larger and are more frequently coupled with infarct expansion, they often cause greater reduction in global LVEF.[38] For infarctions of similar size, *apical involvement* is associated with lower LVEF.[39] These findings indicate that *infarction site*, independently of its size, may have an important impact on LV systolic function.

A high *wall motion score index* (WMSi), which reflects extensive and severe actual dyssynergy, is associated in general with lower global LV function and indicates a potentially complicated course and worse prognosis.[15,40]

Increased initial *LV end-diastolic and end-systolic volumes* indicate extensive myocardial damage. In these cases, serial echocardiographic evaluation can identify the early presence and estimate the degree of adverse LV remodeling.[41–43]

Failure to achieve *adequate microvascular reperfusion at tissue level* (the so-called no-reflow phenomenon) as detected with MCE during acute myocardial infarction[44] is consistently associated with impaired functional recovery of affected myocardial segments and a worse clinical outcome.[44] Of note, *contractile reserve* elicited by low-dose dobutamine is a more accurate predictor of regional functional recovery after reperfused acute myocardial infarction than microvascular integrity.[45] *Contractile recovery* occurs earliest in well-reperfused segments, involving 40% of these segments before the end of the second week.[46] However, significant recovery can still be observed at 6 weeks in segments with homogeneous contrast enhancement, indicating resolved myocardial stunning.[47] Importantly, up to 25% of segments with heterogeneous contrast enhancement also reveal wall motion recovery within the first 6 weeks, whereas the absence of tissue perfusion is highly predictive of the permanent contractile impairment of infarcted segments.[46]

It has been recently shown that *global longitudinal strain* (GLS) reflects impairment of global LV systolic function in patients with acute myocardial infarction and that values of GLS > −15% early in the course of the disease are associated with worse short- and long-term outcome.[48] Of note, compared with WMSi, the advantage of GLS that is a semiautomated quantitative measure (Figure 2.6) (V2.23A, V2.23B, V2.23C, V2.23D, V2.23E, V2.23F).

Finally, the assessment of *right ventricular function* should always go together with assessment of LV function, especially in patients with inferior myocardial infarction with suspected right ventricular involvement or in cases of cardiogenic shock without clear reason (see Chapters 3 and 4). The most common approaches to measure right ventricular systolic function on 2D transthoracic echocardiography are fractional area change, tricuspid annular plane systolic excursion (TAPSE), and tricuspid valve annular peak systolic velocity.[49]

Diastolic function

A few *important caveats* should be noted in the assessment of LV diastolic function in the setting of acute myocardial infarction. LV filling is affected by numerous factors that may have influence on the left atrial to LV pressure gradient in diastole. Therefore, it is very difficult to assess diastolic function in individual patients by looking at ventricular filling only because it may appear similar in different clinical settings that change the pressure gradient in the same way.

Almost all Doppler indices of LV diastolic function are affected by a number of *physiologic factors*,[50,51] such as heart rate, that can change ventricular filling regardless of diastolic function. In addition, these indices are dependent on LV *systolic function*, and finally, *therapy* may produce major changes in indices of diastolic function simply by varying loading conditions.[52] However, it appears that *early filling deceleration* time is less dependent on heart rate, contractility, and afterload and reliably reflects LV chamber stiffness.[53]

Biphasic changes of *LV chamber stiffness* after acute myocardial infarction have been demonstrated by Doppler echocardiography. Increased LV chamber stiffness (denoted by short early filling deceleration time) can be detected 24–48 hours after myocardial infarction, but it returns to normal within several days.[54] The increase in chamber stiffness is higher in large or anterior infarcts and appears to be independent of LV systolic function.[54] Importantly, it has been shown that a normal ratio of early passive to late active filling (E/A ratio) can be found in half of the patients after myocardial infarction.[52] Because very few patients (with the largest infarcts) have a marked increase of E/A ratio of >2, the appearance of the E/A ratio after myocardial infarction may be misleading in differentiating patients with normal and impaired LV diastolic function.[54] In clinical practice, it seems that deceleration time of <150 ms and E/e′ ratio >15 have reasonable accuracy in predicting both increased LV filling pressures and poor prognosis.[55,56]

ASSESSMENT OF MYOCARDIAL VIABILITY

As a consequence of myocardial infarction, alterations in myocardial tissue structure and composition occur, leading to changes in acoustic properties of affected myocardial segments.[57] With a standard resting two-dimensional echocardiographic examination, however, early differentiation of irreversibly damaged from reperfused, stunned, or hibernating myocardium with potential for functional recovery is not possible.

Principal therapeutic aims in acute myocardial infarction are directed toward preserving as much jeopardized myocardium as possible. To determine further management strategy after infarction, information about infarcted tissue properties—that is, whether infarcted segments are still viable or not—should be collected *early*. These data are as important as information on vessel patency because patent infarct-related artery on coronary angiogram does not guarantee viability of perfused segments. Echocardiographic modalities for detection of viability include low-dose dobutamine (V2.24A, V2.24B, V2.24C) and dipyridamole echocardiography, tissue characterization, myocardial deformation imaging, and detection of functional improvement of previously dyssynergic segments on follow-up studies. Viability can indicate therapeutic success of acute intervention, and it has a beneficial impact on survival in those suitable for revascularization.[58]

In patients with coronary artery disease, impaired LV function at rest is not necessarily an irreversible process because dyssynergic myocardial regions may be viable and may have the potential to recover function. This can occur in different states: during a short period of reversible ischemia, in nontransmural infarction, in myocardial stunning, and in hibernation.[59] Identification of these abnormal myocardial conditions may be challenging and usually requires more than one diagnostic modality.[60] The occurrence of pure transmural stunning or hibernation is infrequent, and commonly there is a mixing of subendocardial scar with a variable amount of viable subepicardium.

The identification of viable myocardium with *dobutamine echocardiography* is based on the principle that the presence of contractile reserve of dyssynergic segments may be evoked by low-dose inotropic stimulation.[61,62] It has been recently shown that viability early after acute myocardial infarction detected by low-dose dobutamine echocardiography is associated with improvement in LV function after revascularization: when viable myocardium is not revascularized, the left ventricle tends to remodel without improvement of EF, whereas the absence of viability results in LV dilation and deterioration of EF, irrespective of revascularization status.[63]

In patients with either successful pharmacologic or mechanical reperfusion, the response of postischemic myocardium to dobutamine is influenced by the extent of necrosis, the severity of residual stenosis, the size of the risk area, and the extent and magnitude of collateral blood flow.[64] Thus, in the absence of significant residual stenosis, as is the case

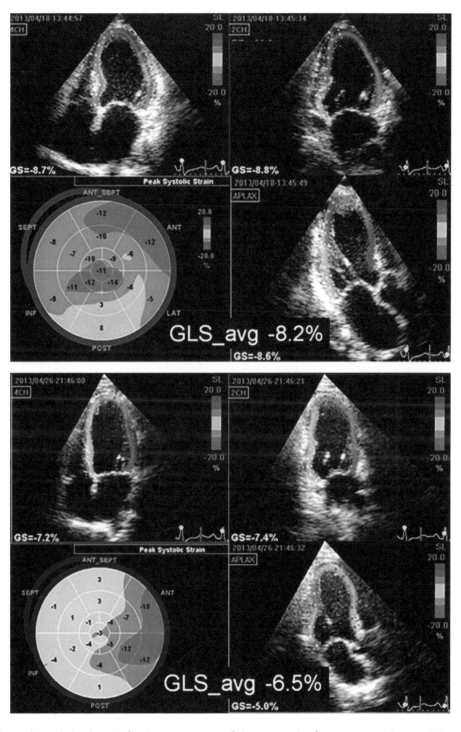

FIGURE 2.6   Speckle tracking-derived strain for the assessment of the prognosis after acute anterior non-ST-segment elevation rein-farction in a 72-year-old man with a history of previous inferior infarction. At admission, reduced segmental peak systolic longitudinal strain values (pale red segments) could be observed in almost all segments, resulting in a global longitudinal strain (GLS) of −8.2% (upper panels). There was a relative sparing of basal anterior and anteroseptal segments (bright red segments) but also positive strain values of basal and mid posterior segments (blue shading, indicative of dyskinesia) resulting from previous inferoposterior infarction (upper panels). The patient underwent percutaneous coronary intervention (PCI) and stenting of the tight proximal left anterior descending coronary artery (LAD) lesion complicated by perforation of the diagonal branch, requiring implantation of a covered stent. However, 3 hours after the PCI the stent thrombosis occurred, associated with cardiogenic shock. Repeat PCI was successful, and with intra-aortic balloon pump support, the patient was transferred back to the coronary care unit. Urgent echocardiographic assessment demonstrated no pericardial effusion but reduced contractility of the basal septum (see V2.23D, V2.23E, V2.23F). Hypercontractility of the lateral wall was also noted. Repeated strain analysis (lower panels) revealed the decline of segmental strain values in almost all (particularly septal) segments, along with the decrease of GLS to −6.5%, indicating large functional infarct size and poor long-term prognosis.

(Image and videos provided by IS.)

of a patient successfully treated by primary PCI, no response at any dose of dobutamine suggests nonviable myocardium.[64] In patients successfully treated with primary PCI and no flow-limiting residual stenosis in the infarct-related artery, low-dose dobutamine echocardiography (up to 10 µg/kg per min) performed early (3 days) after index infarction could identify the presence and the extent of viable myocardium. The extent of contractile reserve, expressed as infarct zone WMSi changes at peak dobutamine, correlated well with the spontaneous recovery at late follow-up.[65] This relationship may be compromised if the infarct-related artery is severely stenotic. In this case, jeopardized myocardium can be identified by a *biphasic* response (improvement of contractility at low dose and worsening at high dose) or by a *new dyssynergy* in adjacent segments within the infarct-related area. In the presence of a flow-limiting stenosis, ischemia may occur, and wall thickening diminishes despite the presence of viable myocardium. Therefore, the induction of ischemia in a dysfunctional segment suggests the presence of both viable myocardium and significant residual stenosis even in the absence of a biphasic response. For the same reasons, it must be recognized that persistence of akinesis in the affected region during dobutamine testing does not necessarily imply the absence of residual viability. Finally, ischemia at a distance from the affected area, detected by new dyssynergy in response to high-dose dobutamine, correlates with the presence of multivessel CAD.

The relation between myocardial viability and clinical outcome is complex. It is generally postulated that only recovery of resting regional function denotes clinically relevant viability. However, although recovery in resting function is the best clinical outcome, there may be other advantages of having nonischemic viable myocardium. The presence of viable myocardium in the outer layers of the ventricular wall may in fact contribute to maintenance of LV shape and size by preventing infarct expansion, LV remodeling, and subsequent heart failure and thus reducing late ventricular arrhythmias and mortality after myocardial infarction.[66,67]

Apart from dobutamine echocardiography, it has been recently shown that *myocardial deformation imaging* (global and regional longitudinal and circumferential strain) provides an accurate assessment of the presence of segments with transmural extent of necrosis[68,69] and predicts global functional recovery as well as LV remodeling after acute myocardial infarction, with accuracy comparable to that of late gadolinium enhancement cardiac magnetic resonance imaging.[70] Furthermore, layer-specific analysis of endocardial deformation may improve accuracy in prediction of segmental functional recovery.[70]

Finally, information regarding microvascular integrity, obtained with MCE, and response to low-dose dobutamine infusion, assessed with echocardiography, may be used for predicting irreversible damage and chances for functional recovery.[45] Patients with no myocardial contrast opacification revealed no response to dobutamine and no functional recovery, whereas various degrees of myocardial contrast opacification may be detected in those with or without contractile improvement elicited by dobutamine.[45]

ASSESSMENT OF PROGNOSIS

Numerous echocardiographic parameters have been used for risk stratification after acute myocardial infarction (Table 2.4).

It has been known for years that a two-dimensional echocardiogram obtained immediately after admission in the coronary care unit[71] and/or before hospital discharge yields important prognostic information.[72–75]

Reduced LVEF is associated with increased morbidity and mortality.[73] However, among patients with similar reduction of LVEF after infarction, long-term prognosis is worse in those with higher *LV end-systolic volume*.[76]

Large initial end-diastolic and end-systolic volumes are important predictors of LV remodeling.[41,42,65,74] Importantly, relatively small increases in LV volumes are associated with a fivefold to sixfold increase of the risk for cardiac death.[75,76] Quantitative measurements of LV volume may predict complications after acute myocardial infarction; an *end systolic volume index of >35 mL/m²* is associated with LV thrombus formation during the acute phase.[77]

Infarct expansion, which can be easily detected by serial echocardiographic studies during first days after acute myocardial infarction (see Chapter 3),[42,78–80] is associated with consequent LV remodeling, aneurysm formation, development of heart failure, and myocardial rupture.[79]

Change of LV shape toward *increased sphericity*, assessed by three-dimensional echocardiography, can identify early postinfarction LV remodeling.[81]

Extensive WMAs and/or *high WMSi* are predictors of increased mortality and indicate susceptibility for hypotension, pump failure, severe heart failure, serious dysrhythmias, reinfarction, and cardiogenic shock.[34,40,73,82–84] Although the positive predictive value is <50%, these patients should be followed up carefully for development of complications. On the other hand, the presence of a small dyssynergic zone is highly

TABLE 2.4 Echocardiographic Parameters That May Be Used for *Early* Prognostic Assessment after Acute Myocardial Infarction

- Left ventricular ejection fraction
- Left ventricular volumes
- Infarct perimeter (infarct expansion)
- Left ventricular shape (sphericity index)
- Wall motion score index
- Remote dyssynergy
- Hyperkinesia of noninfarcted segments
- Infarct zone viability
- Mitral regurgitation
- Microvascular reperfusion (by MCE)
- Early filling deceleration time
- Left atrial volume
- E/e′ ratio
- Global longitudinal strain (GLS)

Abbreviations: E/e′, ratio of the early transmitral flow velocity and early diastolic velocity of the mitral valve annulus; MCE, myocardial contrast echocardiography.

suggestive of an uncomplicated course.[34,40,73,82–84] A high WMSi at hospital discharge is associated with a poor prognosis.[84,85] *Remote WMAs* indicate multivessel disease and worse prognosis.[86]

Hyperkinesia of noninfarcted segments is associated with lower 30-day and 1- and 3-year mortality.[35] Although hyperkinesia is detected less frequently if echocardiography is performed later in the course of infarction, its prognostic importance appears to be unrelated to the time of echocardiographic evaluation.[35]

Even mild *mitral regurgitation* detected in the first 48 hours in patients with acute myocardial infarction is an independent marker of 1-year mortality.[87]

Lack of infarct zone viability by low-dose dobutamine echocardiography is associated with higher mortality.[65]

Effective microvascular reperfusion by MCE predicts functional recovery, prevents LV remodeling,[88] and has beneficial impact on clinical outcome,[89] whereas abnormal perfusion identified 2 days after admission strongly predicts late mortality.[90]

Among Doppler parameters, it has been demonstrated that *short transmitral E-wave deceleration time* on day 1 after infarction (Figure 2.7) predicts the development of congestive heart failure better than the EF.[91] Also, *restrictive filling* has been reported as the single best predictor of cardiac mortality after myocardial infarction, adding significantly to the predictive power of clinical and echocardiographic markers of systolic dysfunction.[92] A strong association of short deceleration time on day 3 after infarction and subsequent 6-month LV dilation was reported in a selected group of patients with reperfused acute anterior myocardial infarction.[93] The degree of LV dilation was related to the severity of impairment of LV filling, and, importantly, a restrictive filling pattern was the most powerful predictor of LV remodeling even after controlling for infarct size.[93] This observation was recently extended to unselected patients after infarction, in whom short transmitral early filling deceleration time detected as early as day 1 after infarction clearly identified patients who were likely to undergo LV remodeling in the following year.[55] Extensive LV remodeling observed in these patients was associated with higher 1- and 5-year mortality.[55] It has also been reported that short deceleration time detected in the early phase of anterior infarction in patients treated with primary PCI still retains its prognostic significance even after optimal recanalization of the infarct-related artery and late persistent vessel patency. During a follow-up period of more than 2½ years, cardiac death was observed only in patients with restrictive filling. They also had more frequent hospital readmissions for heart failure and higher cumulative 2-year mortality and hard cardiac events rates.[94] Simple Doppler parameters, such as early filling deceleration time, may have some advantages over LV volumes and EF in acute settings. Deceleration time not only was found to be a superior prognostic parameter to EF after acute myocardial infarction,[92] but is also less time-consuming to measure and more reproducible (subjected to an almost twofold-lower intraobserver and interobserver variability than end-systolic volume index).[55] Finally, although deceleration time measurement is subject to selection bias because it is more difficult to measure in the sickest patients with acute myocardial infarction (those with tachycardia, atrial fibrillation, or significant mitral regurgitation), short initial deceleration time on day 1 can still identify patients who are at increased risk for cardiac death and in whom short- and long-term LV remodeling is likely to occur.[55,92]

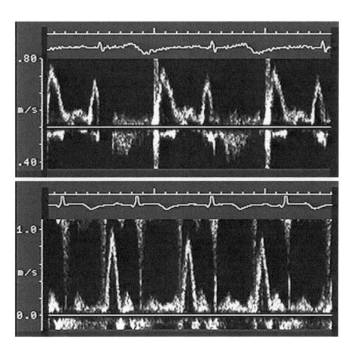

FIGURE 2.7   Examples of a normal (or pseudonormal) (upper panel) and restrictive pattern (lower panel) of transmitral flow assessed by pulsed-wave Doppler in patients with acute myocardial infarction immediately after admission to the coronary care unit.

Left atrium volume index of >32 mL/m² assessed during admission for acute myocardial infarction independently predicts long-term mortality.[95] Left atrium volume can be measured on apical views by either the area-length method or biplane method of discs.

Recently, it has been shown that the *ratio of the early transmitral flow velocity to early diastolic velocity of the mitral valve annulus (E/e')* correlates well with mean LV end-diastolic pressure; E/e' ratio of >15 was found to be a powerful predictor of survival after acute myocardial infarction, providing incremental prognostic information to other clinical or echocardiographic features.[56] Also, the ratio of *early mitral inflow velocity (E) to global diastolic strain rate (E/e'sr)* has been independently related to poor outcome in a large group of patients with acute myocardial infarction.[96]

Reduced GLS with values of >−14% can identify high-risk individuals among patients with myocardial infarctions with relatively preserved LVEF (>40%),[97] in particular those who are prone to in-hospital hemodynamic deterioration and heart failure in the acute phase of myocardial infarction.[98] Furthermore, in patients treated with primary PCI, reduced GLS has been repeatedly reported to be predictive of LV remodeling and cardiac events.[99,100] It is comparable to WMSi and superior to EF and end-systolic volume index for

early (in the first 24 hours) postinfarction risk assessment[48] (Figure 2.6).

ASSESSMENT OF EFFECTS OF THERAPY

Evaluation of natural history[41] of acute myocardial infarction and the effect of reperfusion therapy on systolic and diastolic LV function revealed that *serial echocardiographic studies* are useful in detecting changes in LV size, shape, and function in the earliest phase and during long-term follow-up. Progressive and complex LV dilation and changes in LV architecture, a process known as *LV remodeling*, is clearly associated with infarct expansion in the earliest phase of infarction and large initial LV end-systolic volume[42,43] (see Chapter 3).

In patients with *successful reperfusion*, either by thrombolysis or PCI, contractile improvement of initially dyssynergic segments could be detected, and the extent of adverse remodeling could be limited (Figures 2.8 and 2.9) (V2.25A, V2.25B, V2.25C, V2.25D).[42,101] Finally, the presence of *viability of the infarct zone* clearly indicates therapeutic success.

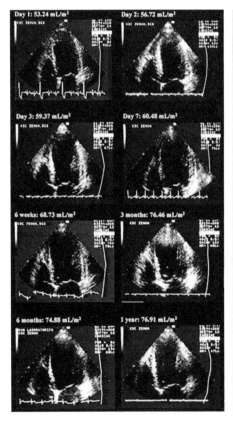 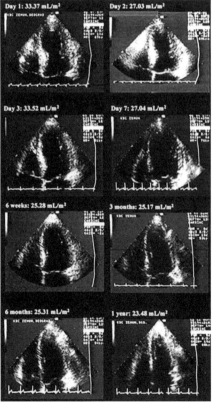

FIGURE 2.8   Serial two-dimensional echocardiograms in a patient with occluded infarct-related artery and adverse left ventricular remodeling (left panel). Note the increase in left ventricular end-diastolic volumes over time (from 53.24 mL/m² on day 1 to 76.91 mL/m² after 1 year). In a patient treated with thrombolysis and patent infarct-related artery (right panel), the left ventricle did not dilate over the one-year follow-up period (33.37 mL/m² on day 1 and 23.48 mL/m² after 1 year).

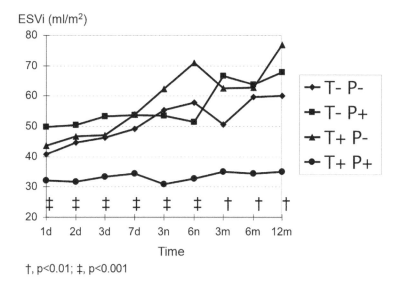

ESVi (ml/m²)

†, p<0.01; ‡, p<0.001

FIGURE 2.9 Combined impact of thrombolysis (T) and infarct-related artery patency (P) on changes in end-systolic volume index (ESVi) more than 1 year after acute myocardial infarction. Note that left ventricular dilation did not occur only in patients who received thrombolysis and who had patent infarct-related artery (T+ P+).[42]

LIST OF VIDEOS

https://routledgetextbooks.com/textbooks/9781032157009/chapter-2.php

VIDEO 2.1   Acute anterior myocardial infarction: Upper left panel: transthoracic parasternal long-axis view showing akinesis of the septum with preserved wall thickness in diastole. Upper right panel: apical four-chamber view showing akinesis of the left ventricular apex. Lower left panel: apical two-chamber view showing hypokinesis of the distal half of the anterior wall. Lower right panel: apical long-axis view showing akinesis of the anterior septum and left ventricular apex. Note preserved wall thickness in diastole in all akinetic segments, which is the hallmark of acute infarction.

VIDEO 2.2   Old inferoposterior and acute lateral myocardial infarction: A patient with a history of previous inferior infarction, presenting with acute chest pain and electrocardiographic signs of lateral ST-segment elevation myocardial infarction. Upper left panel: transthoracic parasternal long-axis view showing akinesis of the posterior wall, which is thinner than septum, with hyperechogenic zones in the basal and middle segments of the posterior wall, indicating fibrosis. Upper right panel: apical four-chamber view showing akinesis of the distal half of the lateral wall with preserved wall thickness in diastole, indicating actual infarction. Lower left panel: apical two-chamber view showing akinesis of the basal two-thirds of the inferior wall with

subendocardial fibrosis. Lower right panel: apical long-axis view showing akinesis of the posterior wall, which appears thin and fibrotic.

VIDEO 2.3A   Transitory left ventricular wall motion abnormality (1/2): Brief history: A 64-year-old woman came to the emergency department complaining of chest pain at rest that had occurred 4 hours before, radiating to the left shoulder, with a duration of approximately 15 minutes. The electrocardiogram was nondiagnostic. At the time of presentation, she was free of chest pain, and transthoracic apical four-chamber view revealed a discrete hypokinesis of the left ventricular apex that could be easily overlooked (shown here). This discrete apical hypokinesis could be easily missed by an inexperienced operator. However, during echo examination, the patient experienced a new episode of chest pain with marked deterioration of regional left ventricular function in the apical zone (see also Video 2.3B). Coronary angiography revealed tight thrombotic mid-LAD lesion. *(Video provided by AVS.)*

VIDEO 2.3B   Transitory left ventricular wall motion abnormality (2/2): Brief history: A 64-year-old woman came to the emergency department complaining of chest pain at rest that had occurred 4 hours before, radiating to the left shoulder, with a duration of approximately 15 minutes. The electrocardiogram was nondiagnostic. At the time of presentation, she was free of chest pain. This transthoracic apical four-chamber view during a new episode of chest pain that occurred during echocardiographic examination revealed a large apical akinesis that extended toward the mid and apical part of the septum. Note marked deterioration of regional left ventricular function compared with the loop obtained 1 minute before (see Video 2.3A). Coronary angiography revealed tight thrombotic mid-LAD lesion. *(Video provided by AVS.)*

VIDEO 2.4A   Postsystolic shortening in a patient with suspected acute coronary syndrome without actual chest pain (1/4): In a patient with suspected acute coronary syndrome without actual chest pain, with nondiagnostic electrocardiogram and normal initial troponin values, transthoracic echocardiography in apical four-chamber view (shown here), apical two-chamber view (see Video 2.4B), and parasternal short-axis view (see Video 2.4C) revealed no wall motion abnormalities. However, in parasternal and apical long-axis views (see Video 2.4D), "shivering" of the septum can be appreciated, and M-mode and longitudinal strain analyses revealed a postsystolic septal thickening and shortening (see Figure 2.1 in the book). Coronary angiography showed proximal occlusion of the left anterior descending coronary artery with moderate collateral circulation. *(Video provided by IS.)*

VIDEO 2.4B   Postsystolic shortening in a patient with suspected acute coronary syndrome without actual chest pain (2/4): In a patient with suspected acute coronary syndrome without actual chest pain, with nondiagnostic electrocardiogram and normal initial troponin values, transthoracic echocardiography in apical four-chamber view (see Video 2.4A), apical two-chamber view (shown here), and parasternal short-axis view (see Video 2.4C) revealed no wall motion abnormalities. However, in parasternal and apical long-axis views (see Video 2.4D), "shivering" of the septum can be appreciated, and M-mode and longitudinal strain analyses revealed a postsystolic septal thickening and shortening (see Figure 2.1 in the book). Coronary angiography showed proximal occlusion of the left anterior descending coronary artery with moderate collateral circulation. *(Video provided by IS.)*

VIDEO 2.4C   Postsystolic shortening in a patient with suspected acute coronary syndrome without actual chest pain (3/4): In a patient with suspected acute coronary syndrome without actual chest pain, with nondiagnostic electrocardiogram and normal initial troponin values, transthoracic echocardiography in apical four-chamber view (see Video 2.4A), apical two-chamber view (see Video 2.4B), and parasternal short-axis view (shown here) revealed no wall motion abnormalities. However, in parasternal and apical long-axis views (see Video 2.4D), "shivering" of the septum can be appreciated, and M-mode and longitudinal strain analyses revealed a postsystolic septal thickening and shortening (see Figure 2.1 in the book). Coronary angiography showed proximal occlusion of the left anterior descending coronary artery with moderate collateral circulation. *(Video provided by IS.)*

VIDEO 2.4D   Postsystolic shortening in a patient with suspected acute coronary syndrome without actual chest pain (4/4): In a patient with suspected acute coronary syndrome without actual chest pain, with nondiagnostic electrocardiogram and normal initial troponin values, transthoracic echocardiography in apical four-chamber view (see Video 2.4A), apical two-chamber view (see Video 2.4B), and parasternal short-axis view (see Video 2.4C) revealed no wall motion abnormalities. However, in parasternal and apical long-axis views (shown here), "shivering" of the septum can be appreciated, and M-mode and longitudinal strain analyses revealed a postsystolic septal thickening and shortening (see Figure 2.1 in the book). Coronary angiography showed proximal occlusion of the left anterior descending coronary artery with moderate collateral circulation. *(Video provided by IS.)*

VIDEO 2.5A   Akinesis caused by an anginal attack (acute myocardial ischemia) (1/2): Transthoracic apical four-chamber view performed during an episode of chest pain, showing large apical akinesis. After administration of nitroglycerin, the chest pain subsided and few minutes later the complete recovery of the apical wall motion abnormality was noted (see Video 2.5B). *(Video provided by VC.)*

VIDEO 2.5B   Akinesis caused by an anginal attack (acute myocardial ischemia) (2/2): Transthoracic apical four-chamber view performed a few minutes after relieving of an acute chest pain episode with nitroglycerin, showing normal segmental wall motion (see also Video 2.5A). *(Video provided by VC.)*

VIDEO 2.6   Akinesis caused by acute myocardial infarction: Transthoracic apical four-chamber view showing akinesis of the medial and apical segments of septum and left ventricular apex.

VIDEO 2.7   Akinesis caused by acute myocarditis: Transthoracic apical four-chamber view showing akinesis of the distal half of the lateral wall caused by acute myocarditis.

VIDEO 2.8A   Acute myocardial infraction caused by acute aortic dissection (1/2): Brief history: A 53-year-old man was brought to the emergency department by paramedics because of severe chest pain. The electrocardiogram showed ST-segment elevation in leads II, III, aVF, and V4–V6. The patient was immediately transferred to the catheterization laboratory. Coronary angiography revealed occlusion and dissection of both LAD and LCx with stasis of the contrast (shown here). Because of suspected aortic dissection, emergency transthoracic and transesophageal echocardiography was performed (see Video 2.8B).

VIDEO 2.8B   Acute myocardial infarction caused by acute aortic dissection (2/2): Brief history: A 53-year-old man was brought to the emergency department by paramedics because of severe chest pain. The electrocardiogram showed ST-segment elevation in leads II, III, aVF, and V4–V6. The patient was immediately transferred to the catheterization laboratory. Coronary angiography revealed occlusion and dissection of both LAD and LCx with stasis of the contrast (see Video 2.8A). Because of suspected aortic dissection emergency transthoracic and transesophageal echocardiography was performed. Upper left panel: transthoracic parasternal long-axis view showing substantial thickening of the posterior wall of the ascending aorta at sinotubular junction. Upper right panel: modified apical four-chamber view showing akinesis of the lateral wall. Lower left panel: apical long-axis view showing akinesis of the posterior wall. Lower right panel: transesophageal long-axis view showing intramural hematoma and dissection of the posterior wall of the ascending aorta. The patient underwent emergent aortic surgery and coronary artery bypass grafting.

VIDEO 2.9A   Acute myopericarditis (1/3): A 37-year-old man with acute respiratory tract infection and fever came to the emergency department with chest pain, which was getting worse on deep inspiration. The electrocardiogram showed diffuse ST-segment elevation up to 1 mm, and initial troponin was slightly elevated. Transthoracic echocardiography was performed on admission and showed mild global left ventricular dysfunction with some regional heterogeneity in contractility. Upper left panel: apical four-chamber view showing a hypokinesis of the distal lateral wall. Upper right panel: apical two-chamber view showing hypokinesis of the apical segment of anterior wall, the apex, and inferior wall, along with mild spontaneous echo contrast (smoke sign). Lower left panel: apical long-axis view showing hypokinesis of the posterior wall and apex. The septum appears "hyperkinetic." Lower right panel: parasternal short-axis view at the papillary muscle level showing global hypocontractility. The next day, the patient started to feel shortness of breath and progressive dyspnea, and transthoracic echocardiography was repeated (see Video 2.9B).

VIDEO 2.9B Acute myopericarditis (2/3): This is the repeated transthoracic echocardiogram on the second day of hospitalization of a patient with suspected acute myocarditis on the basis of medical history and global left ventricular dysfunction with regional heterogeneity in contractility detected on initial presentation (see Video 2.9A). The patient started to complain of progressive dyspnea and shortness of breath, and transthoracic echocardiography was repeated (shown here). The echocardiogram showed the deterioration of global left ventricular systolic function as a result of severe diffuse hypocontractility of myocardial segments and pronounced spontaneous echo contrast (see also Video 2.9A). The patient underwent multislice computed tomography, which revealed normal coronary arteries. Upper left panel: apical four-chamber view. Upper right panel: apical two-chamber view. Lower left panel: apical long-axis view. Lower right panel: parasternal short-axis view at the papillary muscle level.

VIDEO 2.9C Acute myopericarditis (3/3): This is a transthoracic echocardiogram performed on the fifth day of hospitalization in a patient with suspected acute myocarditis. Initially he had mild left ventricular dysfunction (see Video 2.9A) with significant deterioration on the second day of hospitalization (see Video 2.9B), associated with symptoms of acute heart failure. This echocardiogram shows full recovery of left ventricular function only 5 days after initial presentation.

VIDEO 2.10A Acute myocarditis with apical akinesis and thrombus formation (1/3): A 33-year-old man with no previous history of cardiovascular disease was admitted to the coronary care unit because of sudden onset of chest pain and dyspnea. Shortly after admission, he developed ventricular fibrillation, which was successfully terminated with DC shock. The electrocardiogram showed significant ST elevation in precordial leads. Initial troponin was high. Transthoracic echocardiography was performed and in this apical four-chamber view showed poor global left ventricular (LV) function with regional heterogeneity in contractility, which was worst in apex and apical lateral segments. At this point, coronary angiography was performed, and no obstructive coronary lesions were found. After 5 days, repeated transthoracic echocardiography showed further deterioration of global LV function with apical akinesis and thrombus formation (see also Video 2.10B). Magnetic resonance imaging performed 3 weeks later demonstrated good global LV function (see Video 2.10C), with late gadolinium enhancement confined to mid-myocardial layers (see Figure 2.2 in the book), consistent with post-myocarditis scar.

VIDEO 2.10B Acute myocarditis with apical akinesis and thrombus formation (2/3): A 33-year-old man with no previous history of cardiovascular disease was admitted to the coronary care unit because of sudden onset of chest pain and dyspnea. Shortly after admission, he developed ventricular fibrillation, which was successfully terminated with DC shock. The electrocardiogram showed

significant ST elevation in precordial leads. Initial troponin was high. Transthoracic echocardiography was performed and in this apical four-chamber view showed poor global left ventricular (LV) function with regional heterogeneity in contractility, which was worst in apex and apical lateral segments (see Video 2.10A). At this point, coronary angiography was performed, and no obstructive coronary lesions were found. After 5 days, repeated transthoracic echocardiography showed deterioration of global LV function with apical akinesis and thrombus formation (shown here). Magnetic resonance imaging performed 3 weeks later (see Video 2.10C) demonstrated good global LV function, with late gadolinium enhancement confined to mid-myocardial layers (see Figure 2.2 in the book), consistent with post-myocarditis scar.

VIDEO 2.10C Acute myocarditis with apical akinesis and thrombus formation (3/3): A 33-year-old man with no previous history of cardiovascular disease was admitted to the coronary care unit because of sudden onset of chest pain and dyspnea. Shortly after admission, he developed ventricular fibrillation, which was successfully terminated with DC shock. The electrocardiogram showed significant ST elevation in precordial leads. Initial troponin was high. Transthoracic echocardiography was performed and, in this apical four-chamber view, showed poor global left ventricular (LV) function with regional heterogeneity in contractility, which was worst in apex and apical lateral segments (see Video 2.10A). At this point, coronary angiography was performed, and no obstructive coronary lesions were found. After 5 days, repeated transthoracic echocardiography showed deterioration of global LV function with apical akinesis and thrombus formation (see Video 2.10B). Magnetic resonance imaging performed 3 weeks later (shown here) demonstrated good global LV function, with late gadolinium enhancement confined to mid-myo-cardial layers (see Figure 2.2 in the book), consistent with postmyo-carditis scar.

VIDEO 2.11A Apical form of Takotsubo cardiomyopathy (1/2): Transthoracic echocardiography showing typical echocardiographic appearance of the apical form of Takotsubo cardiomyopathy with akinesis of the apical two-thirds of the left ventricle and hypercontractility of the basal segments (see also Video 2.11B). Left panel: apical four-chamber view. Middle panel: apical two-chamber view. Right panel: apical long-axis view.

VIDEO 2.11B Apical form of Takotsubo cardiomyopathy (2/2): Video shows normalization of left ventricular function 4 days after admission in a patient with the typical apical form of Takotsubo cardiomyopathy (see also Video 2.11A). Left panel: apical four-chamber view. Middle panel: apical two-chamber view. Right panel: apical long-axis view.

VIDEO 2.12A Midventricular form of Takotsubo cardiomyopathy (1/2): Transthoracic apical four-chamber view showing akinesis of the mid segments of the septum and lateral wall, with hypercontractility of both basal and apical segments (see also Video 2.12B).

VIDEO 2.12B Midventricular form of Takotsubo cardiomyopathy (2/2): Transthoracic apical four-chamber view showing complete recovery of left ventricular function 30 days after admission in a patient with midventricular form of Takotsubo cardiomyopathy (see Video 2.12A).

VIDEO 2.13A   Reversed Takotsubo cardiomyopathy (1/2): Transthoracic echocardiography showing akinesis of the basal segments with preserved contractility of the distal two-thirds of the left ventricle. Upper left panel: parasternal long-axis view. Upper right panel: parasternal short-axis view at the level of papillary muscles. Lower left panel: parasternal short-axis view at the level of left ventricular apex. Lower right panel: apical four-chamber view (see also Video 2.13B). *(Video provided by VC and IS.)*

VIDEO 2.13B   Reversed Takotsubo cardiomyopathy (2/2): Transthoracic echocardiography showing normalization of left ventricular function. Upper left panel: parasternal long-axis view. Upper right panel: parasternal short-axis view at the level of papillary muscles. Lower left panel: parasternal short-axis view at the level of LV apex. Lower right panel: apical four-chamber view (see also Video 2.13A). *(Video provided by VC and IS.)*

VIDEO 2.14A   Biventricular Takotsubo cardiomyopathy (1/4): A 57-year-old man was admitted to the coronary care unit because of suspected acute anterior myocardial infarction, with chest pain and dyspnea with an electrocardiogram showing ST-segment elevation in the leads I, aVL, and precordial series. Initial brain natriuretic peptide (BNP) and troponin levels were high. The patient reported a history of asthma with extensive use of bronchodilators during the last several days before admission. Transthoracic apical four-chamber view revealed akinesis of the distal two-thirds of the left ventricle and hypercontractility of the basal segments. Note the presence of spontaneous echo contrast in the left ventricle and small pericardial effusion. Also, there is akinesis of the apical segment of the right ventricular free wall. Quick transthoracic assessment of flow through the left anterior descending coronary artery (see Video 2.14B) suggested that the artery is patent. The patient was transferred to the catheterization laboratory (see also Videos 2.14C and 2.14D).

VIDEO 2.14B   Biventricular Takotsubo cardiomyopathy (2/4): Quick transthoracic coronary flow assessment by color Doppler revealed normal diastolic flow (appears as a small circle, colored in red) in the distal part of the left anterior descending coronary artery, indicating its patency (see also Videos 2.14A, 2.14C, and 2.14D).

VIDEO 2.14C   Biventricular Takotsubo cardiomyopathy (3/4): Coronary angiography performed after initial assessment in the coronary care unit revealed no significant stenoses in the left coronary artery tree (shown here) and minor right coronary artery (see also Videos 2.14A, 2.14B, and 2.14D).

VIDEO 2.14D   Biventricular Takotsubo cardiomyopathy (4/4): On the 11th day of hospitalization, control transthoracic echocardiography showed recovery of left and right ventricular function (see Video 2.14A for comparison). Note also larger pericardial effusion over the right heart ventricle as compared with initial presentation.

VIDEO 2.15   Apical form of Takotsubo cardiomyopathy with left ventricular outflow tract obstruction: Transthoracic echocardiography showing apical form of Takotsubo cardiomyopathy with akinesis of distal two-thirds of the left ventricle and hypercontractility of the basal segments, causing systolic anterior motion of the mitral valve and left ventricular outflow tract obstruction. Upper left panel: apical four-chamber view showing akinesis of distal two-thirds of left ventricle. Upper right panel: color Doppler apical five-chamber view showing a turbulence in the left ventricular outflow tract. Lower left panel: apical long-axis view showing systolic anterior motion of the mitral leaflet causing the left ventricular outflow tract obstruction. Lower right panel: zoom view of the left ventricle outflow tract.

VIDEO 2.16   Lung point: This video clip illustrates the lung point, represented by the inspiration-synchronous appearance of lung sliding (the respirophasic shimmering of the pleural line, yellow arrow) on the left half of the pleural line, otherwise immobile for the remaining part of the respiratory cycle. The right half of the pleural line is immobile throughout the entire respiratory cycle. The lung point marks the exact place on the chest wall where a partially deflated lung rises beneath the probe with partial inflation at each inspiration. This sign has 100% specificity for pneumothorax. See also text in the book for further explanation. *(Video provided by GV.)*

VIDEO 2.17   Remote dyssynergy: A 69-year-old man with a history of an old inferior myocardial infarction was admitted to the coronary care unit because of reinfarction of the inferior wall, with ST-segment elevation in leads II, III, and aVF and depression in leads V4–V3. Transthoracic echocardiography revealed akinesis of the basal inferior septum, basal half of the inferior wall, and the whole posterior wall. Inferior wall appears thin (old infarction). However, there was also akinesis of the apex with hypokinetic apical segments of the anterior and lateral wall. These findings reflect actual acute reinfarction of the inferior wall, associated with remote dyssynergy (possibly ischemia) in the myocardial region supplied by the left anterior descending coronary artery. Upper left panel: parasternal long-axis view. Upper right panel: apical four-chamber view. Lower left panel: apical two-chamber view. Lower right panel: apical long-axis view. Outcome: Coronary angiography revealed right coronary artery occlusion and 95% stenosis of the medial segment of the left anterior descending coronary artery.

VIDEO 2.18A   Functional infarct size (1/2): Example of a patient in cardiogenic shock from extensive anterior myocardial infarction. Note that only the basal part of the lateral wall is moving in systole (transthoracic four-chamber view). A temporary pacemaker electrode can be noted in the right side of the heart (see also Video 2.18B).

VIDEO 2.18B   Functional infarct size (2/2): Example of a patient in cardiogenic shock from extensive anterior myocardial infarction. Note that only the basal part of the anterior wall is moving in systole (transthoracic two-chamber view) (see also Videos 2.18A).

VIDEO 2.19   Large left ventricular asynergy in a patient with minimal electrocardiographic changes: A 38-year-old man presented to the emergency department because of chest pain. His electrocardiogram (ECG) showed horizontal ST depression up to 0.1 mV in leads V3–V6. Transthoracic echocardiography revealed akinesis of the anterior septum, distal half of the anterior wall, and left ventricular apex with moderate to severe global left ventricular dysfunction. There is a frequent discordance between severity of electrocardiographic changes and true extent of myocardial damage. The ECG may overestimate or underestimate the amount of dysfunctional myocardium both in acute and in chronic phase. Upper left panel: parasternal long-axis view. Upper right panel: apical four-chamber view. Lower left panel: apical two-chamber view. Lower right panel: apical long-axis view.

VIDEO 2.20 Hypercontractility of a noninfarcted region in a patient with acute anterior myocardial infarction: Upper left panel: parasternal long-axis view showing akinesis of the septum and hypercontractility of the posterior wall. Upper right panel: apical four-chamber view showing akinesis of the mid and apical segments of the septum and the apical segment of the lateral wall, with marked hypercontractility of the basal lateral wall. Lower left panel: apical two-chamber view showing akinesis of the distal half of the anterior wall and apex with hypercontractility of the basal segments. Lower right panel: apical long-axis view showing akinesis of the septum and hypercontractility of the posterior wall.

VIDEO 2.21 Hypercontractility of a noninfarcted region in a patient with acute inferior myocardial infarction: Upper left panel: parasternal long-axis view showing akinesis of the posterior wall and hypercontractility of the septum. Upper right panel: apical four-chamber view showing akinesis of the basal septum and hypercontractility of all other segments. Lower left panel: apical two-chamber view showing akinesis of the basal and mid segment of the inferior wall and hypercontractility of the anterior wall. Lower right panel: apical long-axis view showing akinesis of the posterior wall and hypercontractility of the septum. Note that regardless of inferoposterior akinesis, global left ventricular function is preserved because of hypercontractility of noninfarcted segments.

VIDEO 2.22 Hypercontractility of a noninfarcted region with left ventricular outflow tract obstruction: In a patient with acute anterior ST-segment elevation myocardial infarction, transthoracic four-chamber view (upper left panel) and apical long-axis view (upper right panel) revealed akinesis of the apex, with marked hypercontractility of the basal two-thirds of the septum and lateral wall, associated with systolic anterior motion (SAM) of the mitral valve and resulting left ventricular outflow tract (LVOT) obstruction. Note the turbulent flow in the LVOT (lower left panel), with a maximal LVOT gradient of 36 mmHg (lower right panel).

VIDEO 2.23A Comprehensive echocardiographic assessment of the prognosis after acute myocardial infarction (1/6): A 72-year-old man was admitted to the coronary care unit (CCU) because of anterior non-ST-segment elevation myocardial infarction (NSTEMI). He had a history of an old inferior infarction. At admission, transthoracic apical four-chamber (shown here), two-chamber (see Video 2.23B), and long-axis views (see Video 2.23C) revealed akinesis of the apex and the distal two-thirds of the septum and lateral and anterior wall, with akinetic and aneurysmatic inferior wall (old infarction), and visually estimated global ejection fraction of 25%. Also, moderately severe mitral regurgitation resulting from papillary muscle dysfunction was observed. Measured wall motion score index (WMSi) was 2.3, global longitudinal strain (GLS) was −8.2, and E/e′ was 27. The patient underwent percutaneous coronary intervention (PCI) and stenting of the tight proximal left anterior descending artery lesion; during intervention, perforation of the diagonal branch with a guidewire occurred, requiring implantation of a covered stent. However, 3 hours after the PCI the stent thrombosis occurred, associated with cardiogenic shock. Repeat PCI was successful, and with intra-aortic balloon pump support, the patient was transferred back to the CCU. Urgent echocardiographic assessment demonstrated no pericardial effusion, but reduced contractility of the basal septum (see Videos 2.23D, 2.23E, and 2.23F). Hypercontractility of the lateral wall was also noted. Repeated measurements revealed left ventricular (LV) dilation with

deterioration of the regional LV systolic function (WMSi increased to 2.6), poor global LV systolic function (end-diastolic volume [EDV] = 170 mL; end-systolic volume [ESV] = 128 mL; ejection fraction [EF] = 25%, by Simpson biplane method; GLS decreased to −6.5) (see Figure 2.6 in the book), and diastolic function (E/e′ increased to 31) with severely affected hemodynamics (calculated Doppler-derived cardiac output was 2.6 L/min). These measurements indicate large functional infarct size, high filling pressures, high risk for LV remodeling, and poor short- and long-term prognosis. *(Video provided by IS.)*

VIDEO 2.23B Comprehensive echocardiographic assessment of the prognosis after acute myocardial infarction (2/6): Transthoracic apical two-chamber view in a patient with non-ST-segment elevation anterior reinfarction, recorded before percutaneous coronary intervention (PCI). Note the akinetic and aneurysmatic inferior wall (old infarct) and akinetic distal two-thirds of the anterior wall (actual infarction). For more details, see Video 2.23A (see also Videos 2.23C, 2.23D, 2.23E, and 2.23F). *(Video provided by IS.)*

VIDEO 2.23C Comprehensive echocardiographic assessment of the prognosis after acute myocardial infarction (3/6): Transthoracic apical long-axis view in a patient with non-ST-segment elevation anterior reinfarction, recorded before percutaneous coronary intervention (PCI). Note the akinesis of distal two-thirds of the septum and posterior wall. For more details, see Video 2.23A (see also Videos 2.23B, 2.23D, 2.23E, and 2.23F). *(Video provided by IS.)*

VIDEO 2.23D Comprehensive echocardiographic assessment of the prognosis after acute myocardial infarction (4/6): Transthoracic apical four-chamber view in a patient with non-ST-segment elevation anterior reinfarction, recorded after percutaneous coronary intervention (PCI). Note the lost contractions of the basal septum and hyperkinetic basal lateral wall; for direct comparison, see Video 2.23A (see also Videos 2.23B, 2.23C, 2.23E, and 2.23F). *(Video provided by IS.)*

VIDEO 2.23E Comprehensive echocardiographic assessment of the prognosis after acute myocardial infarction (5/6): Transthoracic apical two-chamber view in a patient with non-ST-segment elevation anterior reinfarction, recorded after percutaneous coronary intervention (PCI). Note the hyperkinetic basal anterior wall; for direct comparison, see Video 2.23B (see also Videos 2.23A, 2.23C, 2.23D, and 2.23F). *(Video provided by IS.)*

VIDEO 2.23F Comprehensive echocardiographic assessment of the prognosis after acute myocardial infarction (6/6): Transthoracic apical long-axis view in a patient with non-ST-segment elevation anterior reinfarction, recorded after percutaneous coronary intervention (PCI). Note the lost contraction of the proximal septum; for direct comparison, see Video 2.23C (see also Videos 2.23A, 2.23B, 2.23D, and 2.23E). *(Video provided by IS.)*

VIDEO 2.24A Stunned postinfarction myocardium detected by dobutamine echocardiography test (1/3): A 71-year-old man underwent successful primary percutaneous coronary intervention for anterior ST-segment elevation myocardial infarction. Low-dose dobutamine testing was performed on day 4 before discharge. Apical four-chamber view (quad screen) revealed the akinetic mid part of the septum at rest that improved gradually and significantly on low- and high-dose dobutamine. This response indicates the presence of stunned myocardium, perfused by the patent infarct-related artery. There was no new wall motion abnormality during the test (see also Videos 2.24B and 2.24C). Upper left panel: rest. Upper right panel: low-dose dobutamine. Lower left panel: high-dose dobutamine. Lower right panel: recovery.

VIDEO 2.24B   Stunned postinfarction myocardium detected by dobutamine echocardiography test (2/3): A 71-year-old man underwent successful primary percutaneous coronary intervention for anterior ST-segment elevation myocardial infarction. Low-dose dobutamine testing was performed on day 4 before discharge. Apical two-chamber view (quad screen) revealed the hypokinetic apical part of anterior wall at rest that improved gradually and significantly on low- and high-dose dobutamine. This response indicates the presence of stunned myocardium, perfused by the patent infarct-related artery. There was no new wall motion abnormality during the test (see also Videos 2.24A and 2.24C). Upper left panel: rest. Upper right panel: low-dose dobutamine. Lower left panel: high-dose dobutamine. Lower right panel: recovery.

VIDEO 2.24C   Stunned postinfarction myocardium detected by dobutamine echocardiography test (3/3): A 71-year-old man underwent successful primary percutaneous coronary intervention for anterior ST-segment elevation myocardial infarction. Low-dose dobutamine testing was performed on day 4 before discharge. Apical long-axis view (quad screen) revealed the akinetic mid part of the septum at rest that improved gradually and significantly on low- and high-dose dobutamine. This response indicates the presence of stunned myocardium, perfused by the patent infarct related artery. There was no new wall motion abnormality during the test (see also Videos 2.24A and 2.24B). Upper left panel: rest. Upper right panel: low-dose dobutamine. Lower left panel: high-dose dobutamine. Lower right panel: recovery.

VIDEO 2.25A   Favorable effect of timely percutaneous coronary intervention on left ventricular function (1/4): A 79-year-old man experienced anterior ST-segment elevation myocardial infarction with signs of acute heart failure (Killip 2) during hospitalization for noncardiac reason. While he was waiting for the transfer to the catheterization laboratory, quick transthoracic echocardiography revealed akinesis of the distal half of the septum and apex (shown here, four-chamber view) and distal half of the anterior wall (see Video 2.25B). A primary percutaneous coronary intervention was performed (20 minutes from the onset of pain), and thrombotic occlusion of the proximal left anterior descending coronary artery was successfully recanalized and stented. Five days after the intervention, complete recovery of the regional left ventricular function was observed (see Videos 2.25C and 2.25D).

VIDEO 2.25B   Favorable effect of timely percutaneous coronary intervention on left ventricular function (2/4): A 79-year-old man experienced anterior ST-segment elevation myocardial infarction with signs of acute heart failure (Killip 2) during hospitalization for noncardiac reason. While he was waiting for the transfer to the catheterization laboratory, quick transthoracic echocardiography revealed akinesis of the distal half of the septum and apex (see Video 2.25A) and distal half of the anterior wall (shown here, two-chamber view). A primary percutaneous coronary intervention

was performed (20 minutes from the onset of pain), and thrombotic occlusion of the proximal left anterior descending coronary artery was successfully recanalized and stented. Five days after the intervention, complete recovery of the regional left ventricular function was observed (see Videos 2.25C and 2.25D).

VIDEO 2.25C   Favorable effect of timely percutaneous coronary intervention on left ventricular function (3/4): A 79-year-old man experienced anterior ST-segment elevation myocardial infarction with signs of acute heart failure (Killip 2) during hospitalization for noncardiac reason. While he was waiting for the transfer to the catheterization laboratory, quick transthoracic echocardiography revealed akinesis of the distal half of the septum and apex (see Video 2.25A) and distal half of the anterior wall (see Video 2.25B). A primary percutaneous coronary intervention was performed (20 minutes from the onset of pain), and thrombotic occlusion of the proximal left anterior descending coronary artery was successfully recanalized and stented. Five days after the intervention, complete recovery of the regional left ventricular function was observed (shown here and in Video 2.25D).

VIDEO 2.25D   Favorable effect of timely percutaneous coronary intervention on left ventricular function (4/4): A 79-year-old man experienced anterior ST-segment elevation myocardial infarction with signs of acute heart failure (Killip 2) during hospitalization for noncardiac reason. While he was waiting for the transfer to the catheterization laboratory, quick transthoracic echocardiography revealed akinesis of the distal half of the septum and apex (see Video 2.25A) and distal half of the anterior wall (see Video 2.25B). A primary percutaneous coronary intervention was performed (20 minutes from the onset of pain), and thrombotic occlusion of the proximal left anterior descending coronary artery was successfully recanalized and stented. Five days after the intervention, the complete recovery of the regional left ventricular function was observed (shown here and in Video 2.25C).

VIDEO 2.26   Postsystolic shortening in a patient with significant LAD stenosis. In a patient with suspected acute coronary syndrome, "shivering" of the septum, consistent with post-systolic shortening, can be noted in transthoracic apical long-axis view. Coronary angiography revealed significant LAD stenosis. *(Video provided by BG.)*

VIDEO 2.27A   Aortic dissection DeBakey type I (Stanford A) (1/2). In a patient presented in the emergency department with sudden severe chest pain irradiating to the back and palpable difference in left and right radial pulse, cardiac ultrasound examination performed with a handheld imaging device revealed intimal membrane (flap) in the ascending aorta from parasternal long-axis view (see also Video 2.27B), indicating aortic dissection. *(Video provided by SR and MM.)*

VIDEO 2.27B   Aortic dissection DeBakey type I (Stanford A) (2/2). In a patient presented in the emergency department with sudden severe chest pain irradiating to the back and palpable difference in left and right radial pulse, and intimal membrane (flap) in the ascending aorta (see Video 2.27A), a "double lumen" separated by the intimal membrane can be appreciated in the descending aorta from subcostal view, with brisk (red) and slow (blue) flows in opposite directions, in the true and the false lumen, respectively. Aortic dissection DeBakey type I (Stanford A) was confirmed by computed tomography. *(Video provided by SR and MM.)*

VIDEO 2.28A   Obstruction of RCA ostium and RCA embolism caused by thrombus lodged in the right sinus Valsalva (1/2). In a patient with active Crohn's disease and ECG signs of acute inferior infarction, a mass in the right sinus Valsalva consistent with thrombus involving right coronary cusp was detected by TTE in a parasternal long-axis view (see also Video 2.28B). *(Video provided by TP and MS.)*

VIDEO 2.28B   Obstruction of RCA ostium and RCA embolism caused by thrombus lodged in the right sinus Valsalva (2/2). In a patient with active Crohn's disease and ECG signs of acute inferior infarction, a mass in the right sinus Valsalva consistent with thrombus involving right coronary cusp was detected by TTE in a parasternal short-axis view of the base of the heart (see also Video 2.28A). *(Video provided by TP and MS.)*

VIDEO 2.29   Apical hypertrophic cardiomyopathy mimicking acute coronary syndrome. Transthoracic echocardiogram performed in a lady with presented with atypical chest pain and deep negative T-waves in precordial ECG leads revealed apical myocardial hypertrophy (upper left panel: apical 4-chamber view; upper right panel: apical two-chamber view). Note complete obliteration of the left ventricular cavity in systole in a parasternal short-axis view at apical level (lower right panel), as compared to papillary muscle level (lower left panel). *(Video provided by IV.)*

VIDEO   2.30A   Acute myocarditis, acute phase (1/2). Transthoracic echocardiography performed on admission showed global left ventricular dysfunction with regional heterogeneity in contractility. Upper left panel: apical four-chamber view showing akinesis of distal two-thirds of the lateral wall. Upper right panel: apical two-chamber view showing akinesis of distal two-thirds of the anterior wall and apex and hypokinesis of the inferior wall. Lower left panel: apical long-axis view showing hypokinesis of the septum and inferoposterior wall. Lower right panel: Longitudinal strain "bull's-eye" showing regional differences in contractility, with worse deformation notable in the lateral (pale red) and apical segments (blue color). Five days later, visual normalization of contractility of all segments could be noted; however, subtle differences in longitudinal strain could still be detected (pale red in lateral segments) (see Video 2.30B). *(Video provided by PMM.)*

VIDEO 2.30B   Acute myocarditis, recovery phase (2/2). Although visual normalization of contractility of all segments could be noted 5 days after onset of the disease, subtle differences in longitudinal strain were still present (pale red in lateral segments). Transthoracic echocardiography performed on admission showed global left ventricular dysfunction with regional heterogeneity in contractility (see Video 2.30A). *(Video provided by PMM.)*

REFERENCES

1. Neskovic AN, Hagendorff A, Lancellotti P, et al. Emergency echocardiography: the European Association of Cardiovascular Imaging recommendations. Eur Heart J Cardiovasc Imaging 2013;14(1):1–11.

2. Neskovic AN, Edvardsen T, Galderisi M, et al. Focus cardiac ultrasound: the European Association of Cardiovascular Imaging viewpoint. Eur Heart J Cardiovasc Imaging 2014;15(9):956–60.

3. Horowitz RS, Morganroth J, Parroto C, et al. Immediate diagnosis of acute myocardial infarction by two-dimensional echocardiography. Circulation 1982;65:323–9.

4. Kerber RE, Marcus ML, Ehrhardt J, et al. Correlation between echocardiographically demonstrated segmental dyskinesis and regional myocardial perfusion. Circulation 1975;52:1097–114.

5. Lieberman AN, Weiss JL, Jugdutt BI, et al. Two-dimensional echocardiography and infarct size: relationship of regional wall motion and thickening to the extent of myocardial infarction in the dog. Circulation 1981;63:739–46.

6. Pandian NG, Skorton DJ, Collins SM. Myocardial infarct size threshold for two-dimensional echocardiographic detection: sensitivity of systolic wall thickening and endocardial motion abnormalities in small versus large infarcts. Am J Cardiol 1985;55:551–5.

7. Eek C, Grenne B, Brunvand H, et al. Strain echocardiography predicts acute coronary occlusion in patients with non-ST-segment elevation acute coronary syndrome. Eur J Echocardiogr 2010;11:501–8.

8. Grenne B, Eek C, Sjoli B, et al. Acute coronary occlusion in non-ST-elevation acute coronary syndrome: outcome and early identification by strain echocardiography. Heart 2010;96:1550–6.

9. Stankovic I, Putnikovic B, Cvjetan R, et al. Visual assessment vs. strain imaging for the detection of critical stenosis of the left anterior descending coronary artery in patients without a history of myocardial infarction. Eur Heart J Cardiovasc Imaging 2015;16(4):402–9.

10. Hoit BD. Strain and strain rate echocardiography and coronary artery disease. Circ Cardiovasc Imaging 2011;4(2):179–90.

11. Dahlslett T, Karlsen S, Grenne B, et al. Early assessment of strain echocardiography can accurately exclude significant coronary artery stenosis in suspected non-ST-segment elevation acute coronary syndrome. J Am Soc Echocardiogr 2014;27(5):512–9.

12. Cheng S, Larson MG, McCabe EL, et al. Age- and sex-based reference limits and clinical correlates of myocardial strain and synchrony: the Framingham Heart Study. Circ Cardiovasc Imaging 2013;6(5):692–9.

13. Lancellotti P, Price S, Edvardsen T, et al. The use of echocardiography in acute cardiovascular care: recommendations of the European Association of Cardiovascular Imaging and the Acute Cardiovascular Care Association. Eur Heart J Cardiovasc Imaging 2015;16(2):119–46.

14. Peels CH, Visser CA, Kupper AJ, et al. Usefulness of two-dimensional echocardiography for immediate detection of myocardial ischemia in the emergency room. Am J Cardiol 1990;65:687–91.

15. Jaarsma W, Visser CA, Eenige van MJ, et al. Predictive value of two-dimensional echocardiographic and hemodynamic measurements on admission with acute myocardial infarction. J Am Soc Echocardiogr 1988;1:187–93.

16. Zabalgoitia M, Ismaeil M. Diagnostic and prognostic use of stress echocardiography in acute coronary syndromes including emergency department imaging. Echocardiography 2000;17:479–93.

17. Ibanez B, James S, Agewall S, et al. 2017 ESC Guidelines for the management of acute myocardial infarction in patients presenting with ST-segment elevation: the Task Force for the management of acute myocardial infarction in patients

presenting with ST-segment elevation of the European Society of Cardiology (ESC). Eur Heart J 2018;39(2):119–77.

18. Ioannidis JP, Salem D, Chew PW, et al. Accuracy of imaging technologies in the diagnosis of acute cardiac ischemia in the emergency department: a meta-analysis. Ann Emerg Med 2001;37:471–7.

19. Gibler WB, Runyon JP, Levy RC, et al. A rapid diagnostic and treatment center for patients with chest pain in the emergency department. Ann Emerg Med 1995;25:1–8.

20. Narula J, Khaw BA, Dec W, et al. Brief report: recognition of acute myocarditis masquerading as acute myocardial infarction. N Engl J Med 1993;328:100–4.

21. Felker G, Boehmer J, Hruban R, et al. Echocardiographic findings in fulminant and acute myocarditis. J Am Coll Cardiol 2000;36:227–32.

22. Kurowski V, Kaiser A, von Hof K, et al. Apical and mid-ventricular transient left ventricular dysfunction syndrome (Takotsubo cardiomyopathy): frequency, mechanisms, and prognosis. Chest 2007;132(3):809.

23. Haghi D, Athanasiadis A, Papavassiliu T, et al. Right ventricular involvement in Takotsubo cardiomyopathy. Eur Heart J 2006;27(20):2433.

24. Gianni M, Dentali F, Grandi AM, et al. Apical ballooning syndrome or Takotsubo cardiomyopathy: a systematic review. Eur Heart J 2006;27(13):1523.

25. Lyon AR, Citro R, Schneider B, et al. Pathophysiology of Takotsubo syndrome: JACC state-of-the-art review. J Am Coll Cardiol 2021;77(7):902–21.

26. Hurst R, Prasad A, Askew J, et al. Takotsubo cardiomyopathy: a unique cardiomyopathy with variable ventricular morphology. JACC Cardiovasc Imaging 2010;3:641–9.

27. Akashi YJ, Tejima T, Sakurada H, et al. Left ventricular rupture associated with Takotsubo cardiomyopathy. Mayo Clin Proc 2004;79:821–24.

28. Sharkey SW, Windenburg DC, Lesser JR, et al. Natural history and expansive clinical profile of stress (Takotsubo) cardiomyopathy. J Am Coll Cardiol 2010;55(4):333–41.

29. Desmet W, Bennett J, Ferdinande B, et al. The apical nipple sign: a useful tool for discriminating between anterior infarction and transient left ventricular ballooning syndrome. Eur Heart J Acute Cardiovasc Care 2014;3(3):264–7.

30. Volpicelli G, Elbarbary M, Blaivas M, et al. International evidence-based recommendations for point-of-care lung ultrasound. Intensive Care Med 2012;38:577–91.

31. Stamm RB, Gibson RS, Bishop HL, et al. Echocardiographic detection of infarct-localized asynergy and remote asynergy during acute myocardial infarction: correlation with the extent of angiographic coronary disease. Circulation 1983;67:233–44.

32. Wyatt HL, Meerbaum S, Heng M, et al. Experimental evaluation of the extent of myocardial dyssynergy and infarct size by two-dimensional echocardiography. Circulation 1981;63:607–14.

33. Buda AJ, Zotz RJ, Pace DP, et al. Comparison of two-dimensional echocardiographic wall motion and wall thickening abnormalities in relation to the myocardium at risk. Am Heart J 1986;111:587–92.

34. Jaarsma W, Visser CA, Eenige van MJ, et al. Prognostic implications of regional hyperkinesia and remote asynergy of non-infarcted myocardium. Am J Cardiol 1986;58:394–98.

35. Kjøller E, Køber L, Jørgensen S, et al. Long-term prognostic importance of hyperkinesia following acute myocardial infarction. Am J Cardiol 1999;83:655–59.

36. Grines CL, Topol EJ, Califf RM, et al. Prognostic implications and predictors of enhanced regional wall motion of the noninfarct zone after thrombolysis and angioplasty therapy of acute

myocardial infarction. The TAMI Study Groups. Circulation 1989;80:245–53.

37. Kan G, Visser CA, Lie KI, et al. Early two-dimensional echocardiographic measurement of left ventricular ejection fraction in acute myocardial infarction. Eur Heart J 1984;5:210–17.

38. Picard MH, Wilkins GT, Gillam LD, et al. Immediate regional endocardial surface expansion following coronary occlusion in the canine left ventricle: disproportionate effects of anterior versus inferior ischemia. Am Heart J 1991;121:753–62.

39. McClements BM, Weyman AE, Newell JB, et al. Echocardiographic determinants of left ventricular ejection fraction after acute myocardial infarction. Am Heart J 2000;140:284–90.

40. Peels KH, Visser CA, Dambrink JH, et al. Left ventricular wall motion score as an early predictor of left ventricular dilation and mortality after first anterior infarction treated with thrombolysis. The CATS Investigators Group. Am J Cardiol 1996;77:1149–54.

41. Picard MH, Wilkins GT, Ray PA, et al. Natural history of left ventricular size and function after acute myocardial infarction: assessment and prediction by echocardiographic endocardial surface mapping. Circulation 1990;82:484–94.

42. Popovic AD, Neskovic AN, Marinkovic J, et al. Acute and long-term effects of thrombolysis after anterior wall acute myocardial infarction with serial assessment of infarct expansion and late ventricular remodeling. Am J Cardiol 1996;77:446–50.

43. Popovic AD, Neskovic AN, Babic R, et al. Independent impact of thrombolytic therapy and vessel patency on left ventricular dilation after myocardial infarction: serial echocardiographic follow-up. Circulation 1994;90:800–7.

44. Ito H, Tomooka T, Sakai N, et al. Lack of myocardial reperfusion immediately after successful thrombolysis. Circulation 1992;85:1699–705.

45. Bolognese L, Antoniucci D, Rovai D, et al. Myocardial contrast echocardiography versus dobutamine echocardiography for predicting functional recovery after acute myocardial infarction treated with primary coronary angioplasty. J Am Coll Cardiol 1996;28:1677–83.

46. Czitrom D, Karila-Cohen D, Brochet E, et al. Acute assessment of microvascular perfusion patterns by myocardial contrast echocardiography during myocardial infarction: relation to timing and extent of functional recovery. Heart 1999;81:12–6.

47. Bolli R. Myocardial "stunning" in man. Circulation 1992;86:1671–91.

48. Munk K, Andersen NH, Terkelsen CJ, et al. Global left ventricular longitudinal systolic strain for early risk assessment in patients with acute myocardial infarction treated with primary percutaneous intervention. J Am Soc Echocardiogr 2012;25(6):644–51.

49. Lang RM, Badano LP, Mor-Avi V, et al. Recommendations for cardiac chamber quantification by echocardiography in adults: an update from the American Society of Echocardiography and the European Association of Cardiovascular Imaging. J Am Soc Echocardiogr 2015;28(1):1–39.

50. Levine RA, Thomas JD. Insights into the physiologic significance of the mitral inflow velocity pattern. J Am Coll Cardiol 1989;14:1718–20.

51. Nagueh S, Appleton C, Gillebert T, et al. Recommendations for the evaluation of left ventricular diastolic function by echocardiography. Eur J Echocardiogr 2009;10:165–93.

52. Fujii J, Yazaki Y, Sawada H, et al. Noninvasive assessment of left and right ventricular filling in myocardial infarction with a two-dimensional Doppler echocardiographic method. J Am Coll Cardiol 1985;5:1155–60.

53. Little WC, Ohno M, Kitzman DW, et al. Determination of left ventricular chamber stiffness from the time for deceleration of early left ventricular filling. Circulation 1995;92:1933–9.

54. Popovic AD, Neskovic AN, Marinkovic J, et al. Serial assessment of left ventricular chamber stiffness after acute myocardial infarction. Am J Cardiol 1996;77:361–4.

55. Otasevic P, Neskovic AN, Popovic Z, et al. Short early filling deceleration time on day one after acute myocardial infarction is associated with short- and long-term left ventricular remodeling. Heart 2001;85:527–32.

56. Hillis GS, Moller JE, Pellikka PA, et al. Noninvasive estimation of left ventricular filling pressure by E/e' is a powerful predictor of survival after acute myocardial infarction. J Am Coll Cardiol 2004;43:360–7.

57. Mojsilovic A, Popovic M, Neskovic AN, et al. The wavelet image extension option for analysis and classification of infarcted myocardial tissue. IEEE Trans Biomed Eng 1997;44(9):856–66.

58. Soto JR, Beller GA. Clinical benefit of noninvasive viability studies of patients with severe ischemic left ventricular dysfunction. Clin Cardiol 2001;24:428–34.

59. Braunwald E, Kloner RA. The stunned myocardium: prolonged, postischemic ventricular dysfunction. Circulation 1982;66:1146–9.

60. Neskovic AN, Mojsilovic A, Jovanovic T, et al. Myocardial tissue characterization after acute myocardial infarction using wavelet image decomposition: a novel approach for the detection of myocardial viability in the early postinfarction period. Circulation 1998;98(7):634–41.

61. Pierard LA, De Landsheere CM, Berthe C, et al. Identification of viable myocardium by echocardiography during dobutamine infusion in patients with myocardial infarction after thrombolytic therapy: comparison with positron emission tomography. J Am Coll Cardiol 1990;15:1021–31.

62. Salustri A, Elhendy A, Garyfallydis P, et al. Prediction of recovery of ventricular dysfunction after first acute myocardial infarction using low-dose dobutamine echocardiography. Am J Cardiol 1994;74:853–66.

63. van Loon RB, Veen G, Kamp O, et al. Left ventricular remodeling after acute myocardial infarction: the influence of viability and revascularization—an echocardiographic substudy of the VIAMI-trial. Trials 2014;18(15):329.

64. Kaul S. Response of dysfunctional myocardium to dobutamine. The eyes see what the mind knows! J Am Coll Cardiol 1996;27:1608–11.

65. Bolognese L, Buonamici P, Cerisano G, et al. Early dobutamine echocardiography predicts improvement in regional and global left ventricular function after reperfused acute myocardial infarction without residual stenosis of the infarct related artery. Am Heart J 2000;139:153–63.

66. Nijland F, Kamp O, Verhost PM, et al. Myocardial viability: impact on left ventricular dilation after acute myocardial infarction. Heart 2002;87:17–22.

67. Bolognese L, Cerisano G, Buonamici P, et al. Influence of infarctzone viability on left ventricular remodeling after acute myocardial infarction. Circulation 1997;96:3353–9.

68. Cimino S, Canali E, Petronilli V, et al. Global and regional longitudinal strain assessed by two-dimensional speckle tracking echocardiography identifies early myocardial dysfunction and transmural extent of myocardial scar in patients with acute ST elevation myocardial infarction and relatively preserved LV function. Eur Heart J Cardiovasc Imaging 2013;14(8):805–11.

69. Orii M, Hirata K, Tanimoto T, et al. Two-dimensional speckle tracking echocardiography for the prediction of reversible myocardial dysfunction after acute myocardial infarction: comparison with magnetic resonance imaging. Echocardiography 2015;32(5):768–78.

70. Altiok E, Tiemann S, Becker M, et al. Myocardial deformation imaging by two-dimensional speckle-tracking echocardiography for prediction of global and segmental functional changes after acute myocardial infarction: a comparison with late gadolinium enhancement cardiac magnetic resonance. J Am Soc Echocardiogr 2014;27(3):249–57.

71. Visser CA, Lie KI, Kan G, et al. Detection and quantification of acute, isolated myocardial infarction by two-dimensional echocardiography. Am J Cardiol 1981;47:1020–5.

72. Nishimura RA, Reeder GS, Miller FA, et al. Prognostic value of predischarge 2-dimensional echocardiogram after acute myocardial infarction. Am J Cardiol 1984;53:429–32.

73. Sabia P, Abbott RD, Afrookteh A, et al. Importance of two-dimensional echocardiographic assessment of left ventricular systolic function in patients presenting to the emergency room with cardiac-related symptoms. Circulation 1991;84:1615–24.

74. Neskovic AN, Otasevic P, Bojic M, et al. Association of Killip class on admission and left ventricular dilatation after myocardial infarction: a closer look into an old clinical classification. Am Heart J 1999;137(2):361–7.

75. Hammermeister KE, DeRouen TA, Dodge HT. Variables predictive of survival in patients with coronary disease: selection by univariate and multivariate analyses from clinical, electrocardiographic, exercise, arteriographic, and quantitative angiographic evaluations. Circulation 1979;59:421–30.

76. White HD, Norris RM, Brown MA, et al. Left ventricular systolic volume as the major determinant of survival after recovery from myocardial infarction. Circulation 1987;76:44–51.

77. Neskovic AN, Marinkovic J, Bojic M, et al. Predictors of left ventricular thrombus formation and disappearance after anterior wall myocardial infarction. Eur Heart J 1998;19(6):908–16.

78. Eaton LW, Weiss JL, Bulkley BH, et al. Regional cardiac dilatation after acute myocardial infarction. N Engl J Med 1979;300:57–62.

79. Schuster EH, Bulkley BH. Expansion of transmural myocardial infarction: a pathophysiologic factor in cardiac rupture. Circulation 1979;60:1532–8.

80. Picard MH, Wilkins GT, Gillam LD, et al. Immediate regional endocardial surface expansion following coronary occlusion in the canine left ventricle: disproportionate effects of anterior versus inferior ischemia. Am Heart J 1991;121:653–762.

81. Mannaerts HF, van der Heide JA, Kamp O, et al. Early identification of left ventricular remodelling after myocardial infarction, assessed by transthoracic 3D echocardiography. Eur Heart J 2004;25(8):680–7.

82. Horowitz RS, Morganroth J. Immediate detection of early high risk patients with acute myocardial infarction using two-dimensional echocardiographic evaluation of left ventricular regional wall motion abnormalities. Am Heart J 1982;103:814–22.

83. Sabia P, Abbott RD, Afrookteh A, et al. Importance of two-dimensional echocardiographic assessment of left ventricular systolic function in patients presenting to the emergency room with cardiac-related symptoms. Circulation 1991;84:1615–24.

84. Nishimura RA, Reeder GS, Miller FA, et al. Prognostic value of predischarge 2-dimensional echocardiogram after acute myocardial infarction. Am J Cardiol 1984;53:429–32.

85. Sabia P, Afrookteh A, Touchstone DA, et al. Value of regional wall motion abnormality in the emergency room diagnosis of acute myocardial infarction. A prospective study using two-dimensional echocardiography. Circulation 1991;84(Suppl I):I85–92.

86. Gibson RS, Bishop HL, Stamm RB, et al. Value of early two-dimensional echocardiography in patients with acute myocardial infarction. Am J Cardiol 1982;49:1110–9.

87. Feinberg MS, Schwammenthal E, Shlizerman L, et al. Prognostic significance of mild mitral regurgitation by color Doppler echocardiography in acute myocardial infarction. Am J Cardiol 2000;86:903–7.

88. Bolognese L, Parodi G, Carrabba N, et al. Impact of microvascular dysfunction on left ventricular remodeling and long-term clinical outcome after primary coronary angioplasty for acute myocardial infarction. Circulation 2004;109:1121–6.

89. Sakuma T, Hayashi Y, Sumii K, et al. Prediction of short- and intermediate-term prognoses of patients with acute myocardial infarction using myocardial contrast echocardiography one day after recanalization. J Am Coll Cardiol 1998;32:890–7.

90. Khumri TM, Nayyar S, Idupulapati M, et al. Usefulness of myocardial contrast echocardiography in predicting late mortality in patients with anterior wall acute myocardial infarction. Am J Cardiol 2006;98:1150–5.

91. Poulsen SH, Jensen SE, Gøtzhe O, et al. Evaluation and prognostic significance of left ventricular diastolic function assessed by Doppler echocardiography in the early phase of a first acute myocardial infarction. Eur Heart J 1997;18:1882–9.

92. Nijland F, Kamp O, Karreman AJ, et al. Prognostic implications of restrictive left ventricular filling in acute myocardial infarction: a serial Doppler echocardiographic study. J Am Coll Cardiol 1997;30:1618–24.

93. Cerisano G, Bolognese L, Carrabba N, et al. Doppler derived mitral deceleration time: an early strong predictor of left ventricular remodeling after reperfused anterior acute myocardial infarction. Circulation 1999;99:224–9.

94. Cerisano G, Bolognese L, Buonamici P, et al. Prognostic implications of restrictive left ventricular filling in reperfused anterior acute myocardial infarction. J Am Coll Cardiol 2001;37:793–9.

95. Moller JE, Hillis GS, Oh JK, et al. Left atrial volume: a powerful predictor of survival after acute myocardial infarction. Circulation 2003;107:2207–12.

96. Ersbøll M, Andersen MJ, Valeur N, et al. Early diastolic strain rate in relation to systolic and diastolic function and prognosis in acute myocardial infarction: a two-dimensional speckle-tracking study. Eur Heart J 2014;35(10):648–56.

97. Ersbøll M, Valeur N, Mogensen UM, et al. Prediction of all-cause mortality and heart failure admissions from global left ventricular longitudinal strain in patients with acute myocardial infarction and preserved left ventricular ejection fraction. J Am Coll Cardiol 2013;61(23):2365–73.

98. Ersbøll M, Valeur N, Mogensen UM, et al. Relationship between left ventricular longitudinal deformation and clinical heart failure during admission for acute myocardial infarction: a two-dimensional speckle-tracking study. J Am Soc Echocardiogr 2012;25(12):1280–9.

99. D'Andrea A, Cocchia R, Caso P, et al. Global longitudinal speckle tracking strain is predictive of left ventricular remodeling after coronary angioplasty in patients with recent non-ST elevation myocardial infarction. Int J Cardiol 2011;153(2):185–91.

100. Lacalzada J, de la Rosa A, Izquierdo MM, et al. Left ventricular global longitudinal systolic strain predicts adverse remodeling and subsequent cardiac events in patients with acute myocardial infarction treated with primary percutaneous coronary intervention. Int J Cardiovasc Imaging 2015;31(3):575–84.

101. Bolognese L, Neskovic AN, Parodi G, et al. Left ventricular remodeling after primary coronary angioplasty: patterns of left ventricular dilation and long-term prognostic implications. Circulation 2002;106:2351–7.

Echocardiography in complications of acute myocardial infarction

3

Aleksandar N. Neskovic, Predrag M. Milicevic, and Michael H. Picard

Key Points

- Echocardiography is an ideal noninvasive test to detect mechanical complications of acute myocardial infarction, such as papillary muscle rupture, myocardial free-wall rupture, pseudoaneurysm, and ventricular septal rupture.
- Echocardiography can accurately detect the cause of a new systolic murmur and/or hemodynamic instability in patients with acute myocardial infarction.
- The unique features of echocardiography, its portability and availability, allow examination of the critically ill at the bedside anywhere in the hospital.

For decades, two-dimensional and Doppler echocardiography have had crucial roles in the detection and assessment of complications of acute myocardial infarction (Table 3.1), allowing collection of all necessary information at the bedside. Some of these complications present with overt clinical manifestations (e.g., mechanical complications), whereas others may occur silently (e.g., infarct expansion, thrombi). In both situations, information obtained by echocardiography is often of key importance for decision-making.

It appears that timely reperfusion by either thrombolysis or primary percutaneous coronary intervention (PCI) has resulted in decline of the incidence of mechanical complications of acute myocardial infarction (Table 3.1) to less than 1%.[1] The reported incidence in a large group of patients treated with primary PCI was 0.52% for free left ventricular (LV) wall rupture with tamponade, 0.26% for papillary muscle rupture, and 0.17% for ventricular septal rupture.[1] Mechanical complications usually occur during the first 2 weeks after acute myocardial infarction in *two peaks*: in the first 24 hours and after 3–5 days. The majority of these patients require an urgent mechanical intervention (cardiac surgery or transcatheter device) because medical treatment offers a dismal result. Good logistics and professional trust between cardiologist and cardiac surgeon are important to improve this unfavorable patient outcome.

TABLE 3.1 Complications of Acute Myocardial Infarction That May Be Detected and Assessed by Use of Echocardiography

1. Acute mitral regurgitation
   - Papillary muscle dysfunction
   - Papillary muscle rupture*
2. Ventricular septal rupture*
3. Free-wall rupture* and pseudoaneurysm*
4. Infarct expansion, aneurysm, and left ventricular remodeling
5. Left ventricular thrombi
6. Right ventricular infarction
7. Pericardial effusion

* Denotes mechanical complications.

DOI: 10.1201/9781003245407-3

ACUTE MITRAL REGURGITATION

Evaluation of a new systolic murmur on physical examination in patients with acute myocardial infarction may be challenging. The main goal is to distinguish between acute mitral regurgitation and ventricular septal rupture or, less frequently, acute tricuspid regurgitation (in right ventricular infarction). This distinction can be easily made with use of bedside echocardiography.

Acute mitral regurgitation in a postinfarction patient may occur because of *ischemic dysfunction* of the papillary muscles and underlying LV wall (papillary muscle region dyssynergy), *partial papillary muscle rupture*, or *complete papillary muscle rupture*. Two-dimensional echocardiographic imaging can offer clues to the cause, and Doppler techniques can be used to assess severity of the regurgitation. An accurate diagnosis strongly influences patient management: papillary muscle dysfunction could be stabilized medically, whereas papillary muscle rupture requires emergent cardiac surgery.

From the echocardiographic point of view, *papillary muscle dysfunction* can be detected when maximal systolic position of one or both mitral leaflets is displaced toward the LV apex and above the mitral annulus level (tenting)[2] (Figure 3.1) (V3.1A, V3.1B). Color Doppler typically reveals a centrally oriented turbulent regurgitant jet, although it may be eccentric in some cases because of more pronounced displacement of one of the leaflets (asymmetric tenting). It appears that in addition to ischemic systolic dysfunction of papillary muscles, other mechanisms may play a role in impaired mitral leaflet coaptation, such as LV dilation (especially changes in LV shape toward increased sphericity), mitral annulus dilation, and associated wall motion abnormality of the LV wall underlying the papillary muscle[3,4] (V3.2A, V3.2B). This secondary or functional mitral regurgitation occurs when loss of contractility of the papillary muscles is also associated with abnormal wall motion of the underlying myocardium and segments adjacent to the insertion of papillary muscles.[5]

On two-dimensional echocardiography, *complete papillary muscle transection* typically presents as flail motion of one or both mitral leaflets, with an attached echogenic mass that is moving freely during cardiac cycle, prolapses into the left atrium in systole, and moves back into the left ventricle in diastole (V3.3, V3.29, V10.5A, V10.5B). The attached mass represents the freely ruptured papillary muscle (V14.2A, V14.2B, V14.2C). In the case of *incomplete rupture*, a portion of the papillary muscle is connected by chordal apparatus to the flail leaflets (Figure 3.2) (V3.4A, V3.4B). Color Doppler may reveal different mitral regurgitation jet shapes and directions, and although regurgitation is always severe, it can be difficult to demonstrate its severity with Doppler owing to tachycardia and high left atrial pressure. The large regurgitant orifice often results in regurgitation that is more laminar than turbulent, of lower velocity, and thus more difficult to delineate on color Doppler. Two-dimensional imaging of the freely moving echogenic mass attached to flail

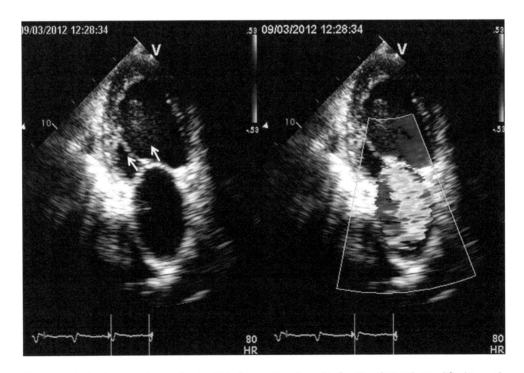

FIGURE 3.1   Papillary muscle dysfunction in a patient with inferoposterolateral infarction (V3.1B). Modified transthoracic apical long-axis view shows that maximal systolic position of both mitral leaflets is displaced toward the left ventricular apex (arrows) and above the mitral annulus level (tenting) (left panel). Corresponding color Doppler image denotes central turbulent jet of moderate mitral regurgitation (right panel).

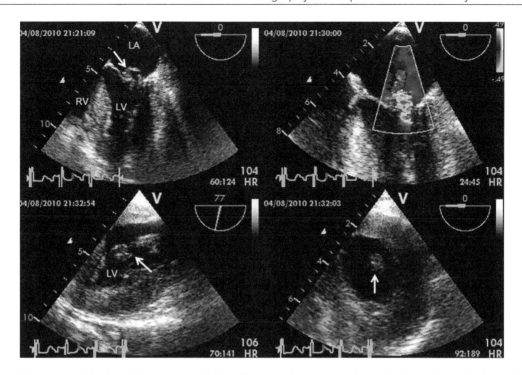

FIGURE 3.2 Partial rupture of the head of posteromedial papillary muscle. Transesophageal echocardiography (V3.4B). Four-chamber view shows the prolapse of the posterior mitral leaflet, with a head of papillary muscle attached (arrow) (upper left panel). The corresponding color Doppler image shows significant mitral regurgitation with a wide vena contracta (upper right panel). Transgastric two-chamber view shows a partial rupture (arrow) of the posteromedial papillary muscle (lower left panel). Transgastric short-axis view shows hypermobile mass (arrow), representing a head of the posteromedial papillary muscle (right lower panel). LA: left atrium; LV: left ventricle; RV: right ventricle.

leaflet(s) remains a key echocardiographic finding for making the diagnosis.

Because of the dual blood supply from the left anterior descending and circumflex coronary arteries, the antero-lateral papillary muscle is less frequently transmurally infarcted as compared with single-vessel—supplied posteromedial papillary muscle.[6] Importantly, in contrast to ventricular septal rupture, which more often occurs in patients with large infarctions, papillary muscle rupture usually complicates small infarcts.

Even mild mitral regurgitation detected within the first 48 hours of admission in patients with acute myocardial infarction is linked to increased 1-year all-cause mortality.[7] Except for patients with acute severe regurgitation, the reason for this remains unclear. Although early mitral regurgitation after infarction is mild to moderate in most patients, it is associated with features recognized as markers of poor prognosis, such as large infarcts, high initial end-systolic volume, and older age.[4] On the other hand, comparison of sequential changes of end-diastolic and end-systolic volumes during 1-year follow-up revealed no significant difference in the pattern of LV dilation between patients with and without early mitral regurgitation.[8,9] It seems, therefore, that increased risk and higher mortality in patients with early mitral regurgitation after myocardial infarction are consequences of more severe LV damage and extent of coronary artery disease, rather than the effects of chronic mitral regurgitation on LV volume.

VENTRICULAR SEPTAL RUPTURE

Ventricular septal rupture in a patient with acute myocardial infarction usually presents as a new holosystolic murmur (V21.4A, V21.4B, V21.4C, V21.4D). Using *multiple standard and modified* echocardiographic views, the septal defect can be visualized by two-dimensional echocardiography in 46–100% of cases.[10,11] The site of the rupture is often localized at the border of the dyssynergic zone.[11] Systolic bulging of the ventricular septum toward the right ventricular cavity may be an indirect sign of septal rupture. Acquired defects caused by myocardial necrosis are of irregular shape (V3.5) and complex three-dimensional form. A rupture may create serpiginous tunnels through the septal wall, with entry points at different levels at the left and right sides of the septum and cannot always be detected by a single two-dimensional echocardiographic image plane. The defects can also be multiple and small ("Swiss cheese" defect) (Figure 3.3) (V3.6A, V3.6B).

Detection of the ventricular septal defect in a region with normal wall motion strongly suggests congenital origin. This may help to avoid confusion that may arise in individuals with congenital ventricular septal defect and recent myocardial infarction (V3.7).

Doppler techniques greatly improve diagnostic accuracy of echocardiography in detection of septal rupture.[11,12]

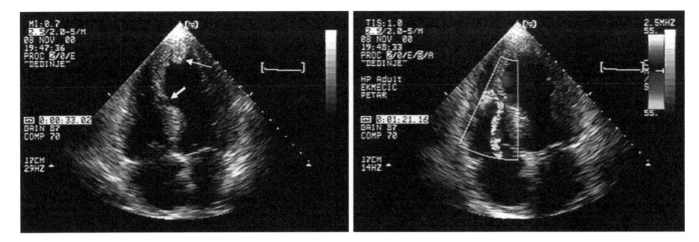

FIGURE 3.3 Ventricular septal rupture. Transthoracic apical four-chamber view. Irregular discontinuity in the midportion of the interventricular septum in a patient with anterior infarction, suggesting possible rupture site (short arrow). In the apex, there is a highly mobile round mass (long arrow), suggesting thrombus of high embolic potential (V3.6A). Color Doppler shows multiple turbulent jets of abnormal flow across the rupture site from left to right ventricle. Note that mobile thrombus is not visible in this frame (V3.6B).

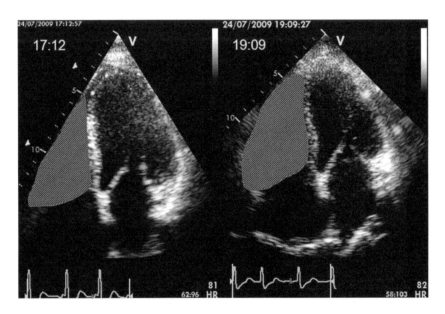

FIGURE 3.4 Rapid deterioration of right ventricular function after ventricular septal rupture. The ventricular septal rupture was diagnosed in the coronary care unit, and the cardiac surgery center was contacted for urgent patient referral. Note the significant enlargement of the right ventricular cavity (dashed area) in relative comparison to the left ventricular size, which developed during 2 hours of waiting for transfer to the cardiac surgery center, indicating worsening hemodynamics and failing right ventricle (V3.10A). Left panel: initial echocardiogram. Right panel: echocardiogram performed 2 hours later.

Color Doppler or pulsed-wave Doppler mapping may reveal *systolic turbulent flow* across the ventricular septum (V3.8A, V3.8B, V14.1A, V14.1B) or on the right ventricular side of the septum, suggesting the presence of a communication even in the case of visually "preserved" continuity of the septum by two-dimensional scan. Scanning in different off-axis planes is often needed to visualize the defect (V3.9).

The maximal width of the turbulent jet on color Doppler may be used to assess the size of the defect, because the results correlate well with intraoperative and autopsy findings.[11]

In patients with ventricular septal rupture, right ventricular function is crucial for maintaining hemodynamic stability[13,14] (Figure 3.4) (V3.10A). The presence of right-to-left shunt in diastole indicates severe right ventricular dysfunction and is associated with high mortality.[10,11,13] Defect of the basal septum caused by inferior infarcts tends to have a worse prognosis than apical defects in anterior infarcts and are typically larger in size.[13]

Continuous-wave Doppler can also be used for the assessment of interventricular pressure gradient and estimation of the right ventricular systolic pressure: the lower the transventricular gradient, the more severe the hemodynamic compromise[11] (V3.10B).

FREE-WALL RUPTURE AND PSEUDOANEURYSM

Free-wall rupture

Acute rupture of the LV free wall (V3.11) typically leads to abrupt cardiac tamponade, electromechanical dissociation, and sudden death, usually before any diagnostic procedure can be performed.[15] Thus, antemortem diagnosis is rare.[16] However, free-wall rupture does not always result in immediate fatal outcome. Patients may survive an acute myocardial wall rupture event if it is constrained by pericardial adhesions or thrombosis at the rupture site (V3.30A, V3.30B). Indeed, up to 40% of ruptures may evolve over hours or even days, representing *subacute* forms of free-wall rupture.[17,18] During this period, patients may be without symptoms and clinically stable. A subacute rupture (Figure 3.5) (V3.12A, V3.12B, V3.12C, V3.12D, V3.12E) is characterized by the presence of moderate to severe pericardial effusion and hypotension of various degrees of severity, with or without signs of tamponade.[17]

Free-wall rupture may occur *early* (within 48 hours) or *late* in the course of infarction (V3.13). Because mortality is extremely high, a *high index of clinical suspicion* may lead to interventions to prevent the rupture and/or significantly reduce mortality when it does occur. Hence, some clinical characteristics are associated with increased risk of the rupture, including first transmural infarction in elderly patients, delayed hospital admission, delayed or late reperfusion, single vessel disease with poor collateral circulation, prolonged and recurrent chest pain, acute episodes of arterial hypertension, persistent ST-segment elevation, infarct expansion, and infarct extension.[15–19]

Echocardiography reveals pericardial effusion in the hemodynamically unstable patient with segmental wall motion abnormality due to myocardial infarction, and echocardiographic signs of tamponade (see Chapter 8). Rarely, the free-wall defect at the rupture site can be visualized, and flow across the defect toward the pericardial space can be detected by Doppler (V14.3A, V14.3B). Successful use of intravenous contrast echocardiography to exclude or to identify myocardial rupture has been documented.[20] In patients with suspected subacute rupture, administration of a contrast agent can be useful to demonstrate active communication into the pericardium.[21] In addition, it has been shown that three-dimensional echocardiography may provide incremental morphologic information in patients with myocardial rupture.[22]

Successful surgical management of patients with LV rupture has been reported in case reports and small series,[23,24] but the overall mortality remains extremely high. For subacute cases, after prompt initial medical stabilization, surgery should also be considered.

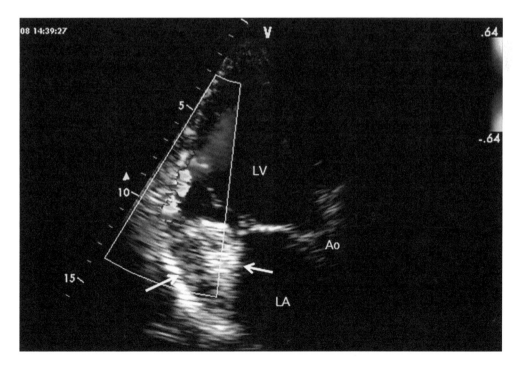

FIGURE 3.5 Subacute ventricular free-wall rupture. Transthoracic apical long-axis view. Note hyperechogenic zone at the level of the posterior mitral annulus (arrows), representing pericardial hematoma. A systolic turbulent jet denotes the site of the free-wall rupture. This was confirmed by transesophageal echocardiography (V3.12A, V3.12E) and intraoperative findings. Ao: aorta; LA: left atrium; LV: left ventricle.

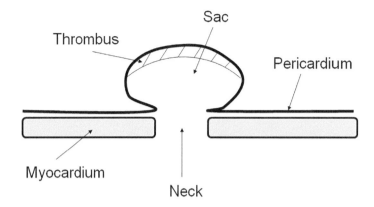

FIGURE 3.6 Schematic illustration of the pseudoaneurysm. Note the narrow neck. The wall of the pseudoaneurysmal sac consists of pericardium and laminar thrombus.

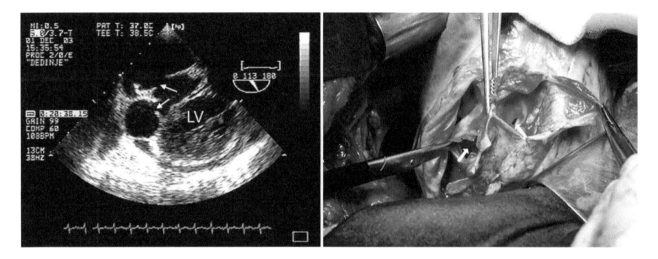

FIGURE 3.7 Double pseudoaneurysm. Transesophageal echocardiography. Modified longitudinal two-chamber view. Discontinuity of the inferoposterior myocardial wall at two separate places (arrows), with two narrow-neck aneurysmal sacs, indicating double pseudoaneurysm formation (left panel) (V3.14A, V3.14B). Intraoperative findings: double myocardial rupture (arrows). LV: left ventricle.[28]

Pseudoaneurysm

As mentioned earlier, patients may survive an acute myocardial wall rupture if it is contained by pericardial adhesions and thrombus, resulting in *pseudoaneurysm* formation.[25–27] In contrast to true aneurysm, pseudoaneurysm communicates with the LV cavity by a narrow neck (rupture site), the diameter of which is typically, although not always (V3.31A, V3.31B, V3.31C), at least half that of the maximal diameter of the pseudoaneurysmal sac.[26] Through this communication, bidirectional blood flow can be identified by color Doppler during the cardiac cycle. At the margins of the neck, sharp discontinuity of the myocardium can be noted, indicating the absence of a myocardial layer in the pseudoaneurysmal sac (Figure 3.6). The wall of the pseudoaneurysm typically is composed of pericardium and clot.[26] Because pseudoaneurysm requires *urgent surgical*

repair (Figure 3.7) (V3.14A, V3.14B) for prevention of spontaneous rupture, which occurs with high incidence,[27,28] it should be promptly distinguished from the true aneurysm[26] (Table 3.2). Differential diagnosis in less typical cases might be challenging (V3.31C). Whereas true aneurysms have a more benign natural history, pseudoaneurysms have a high incidence of rupture.

TABLE 3.2 Echocardiographic Features That May Be Helpful in Differentiation of a Pseudoaneurysm from a True Aneurysm

	PSEUDOANEURYSM	*TRUE ANEURYSM*
Neck	Narrow	Broad
Wall	Pericardium	Myocardium, often thin
Margins	Abrupt myocardial discontinuity	Continuity of myocardial wall

INFARCT EXPANSION, ANEURYSM FORMATION, AND LEFT VENTRICULAR REMODELING

Infarct expansion

Infarct expansion is defined as *acute dilation and thinning* of the area of infarction that cannot be explained by additional myocardial necrosis.[29] It occurs within the first 24 hours after large transmural, mainly anterior infarcts.[30] Patients with infarct expansion have a complicated postinfarction course: heart failure, aneurysm, and myocardial rupture are likely to occur.[31–33] Infarct expansion is associated with an early mortality as high as 50%[34] and has an unfavorable impact on late prognosis.[32,35]

Infarct expansion can be recognized by echocardiographic evidence of distortion of LV topography as a consequence of elongation of the noncontractile region, causing disproportionate dilation of the infarcted segment, which leads to increase in the percentage of the LV surface area occupied by necrotic myocardium.[34,36]

Early echocardiographic studies demonstrated that one-third of patients with myocardial infarction showed infarct expansion during the first few days after admission[34,35] and that it is associated with late ventricular dilation.[32] Echocardiographic endocardial surface mapping allows for accurate assessment of infarct expansion and LV dilation.[30,37] Because infarct expansion most frequently occurs in patients with anterior and apical infarcts, serial measurements of the length of the dyssynergic LV endocardium (infarct perimeter) and total LV perimeter in apical four- and two-chamber views allow detection of subtle changes in the infarcted segment[38] (Figure 3.8).

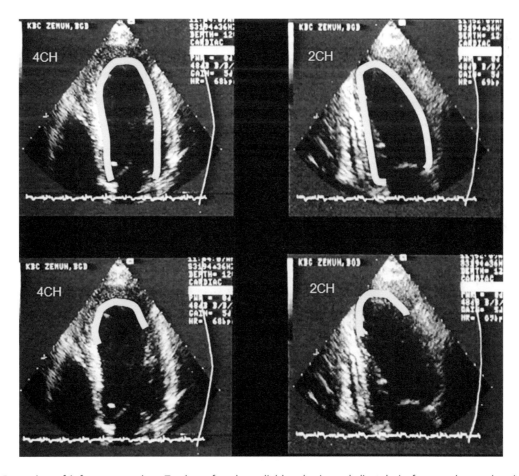

FIGURE 3.8 Detection of infarct expansion. Tracing of endocardial border in end-diastole in four- and two-chamber views. First, total left ventricular endocardial length was traced and measured in four-chamber and two-chamber (upper left and right panels) views *(total left ventricular perimeter*—yellow line). Then the length of left ventricular endocardium with wall motion abnormalities (hypokinesia, akinesia, dyskinesia) was measured *(infarct perimeter*—yellow line) in the same frames (lower left and right panels). Total and infarct perimeters were averaged, and mean perimeters were used for calculations. The ratio of two perimeters represents *infarct percentage. Infarct expansion* is defined as (1) the increase of infarct percentage and total perimeter >5% on days 2 and 3 in either view, or (2) initial infarct percentage >50%, with an increase in total perimeter >5% on day 2 or 3. 4CH: four-chamber view; 2CH: two-chamber view.[38]

Left ventricular aneurysm

LV aneurysm can be detected in 20–40% of patients after acute myocardial infarction.[39] Aneurysm formation is closely related to infarct expansion[31,32,34,35]; consequently, the myocardium in the aneurysmal wall is thin, with gradual transition (V3.15A, V3.15B) toward the normal myocardial wall at the borders of the aneurysmatic sac (V3.16).

Echocardiographic diagnosis of LV aneurysm is made if segmental dyskinesis in systole is associated with abnormal segmental geometry in diastole (Figure 3.9) (V3.17, V3.18, V3.19, V3.20). Aneurysm, as well as the time of its formation, strongly influences the prognosis. Early aneurysm formation was associated with a 1-year mortality rate of 80%, as compared with a 25% mortality rate in those who developed aneurysms later in the course of infarction.[39] Because of stagnant blood flow (smoke sign), LV thrombi can often be seen in the aneurysm (Figure 3.10) (V3.21).

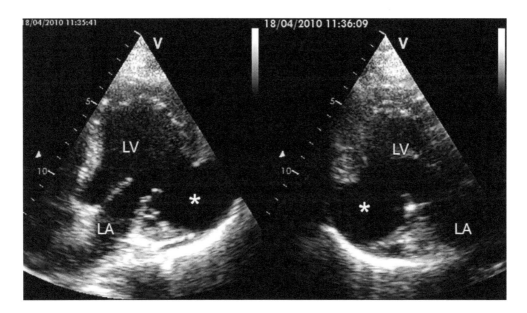

FIGURE 3.9   True aneurysm of the inferoposterolateral wall. Off-axis transthoracic apical four-chamber view showing a large aneurysm (*) of the basal segment of the lateral wall (left panel). Modified apical long-axis view showing a large aneurysm (*) of the basal segment of the inferoposterior wall (right panel) (V3.17). Note the abnormal geometry of the left ventricle. LA: left atrium; LV: left ventricle.

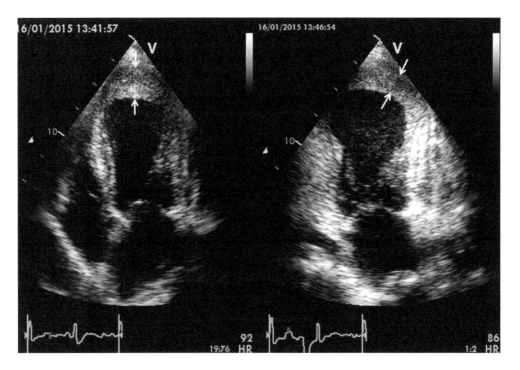

FIGURE 3.10   True apical aneurysm with thrombus. Transthoracic apical four-chamber view (left panel) and two-chamber view (right panel) showing a large left ventricular apical aneurysm filled with a large thrombus (arrows) (V3.21).

Left ventricular remodeling

Infarct expansion is a key event in the initiation of the *LV remodeling* process. This process consists of progressive LV dilation and hypertrophy of noninfarcted segments, leading to changes in LV shape and function over months and years after infarction.[40] The *time and magnitude* of LV remodeling may be assessed by serial echocardiographic evaluation of LV volumes and shape.[41,42]

Although LV remodeling may be prevented or halted by reperfusion therapy,[41] one-third of postinfarction patients may show LV dilation despite successful reopening of the infarct-related artery.[42] The remodeling process is heterogeneous, and it may be early, late, or progressive; however, in contrast to LV dilation itself, the specific pattern of dilation does not independently affect clinical outcome.[41] Finally, LV remodeling can be predicted by simple demographic and echocardiographic variables.[42–44] High initial LV volumes and wall motion score index are strong predictors of long-term LV dilation.[41–44]

LEFT VENTRICULAR THROMBI

The incidence of LV thrombosis is high after acute myocardial infarction.[45,46] Interestingly, in the current era of rapid reperfusion by primary PCI, the rate of thrombus formation appears to be similar to that reported in the past and not different from patients currently treated conservatively or with thrombolysis.[47] The majority of thrombi occur in the LV apex in patients with large anterior infarcts with impaired LV systolic function (V3.22). However, thrombi are not present in all large infarctions. They can also be found in small apical infarcts with preserved global systolic function, as well as after inferior infarcts.[46] These facts indicate the *complex* nature of the process of LV thrombosis, suggesting that factors other than infarct size and site may be involved.

Two-dimensional echocardiography is highly accurate in detection of LV thrombi, with a sensitivity of 92–95% and a specificity of 86–88%.[48,49] The detection of thrombus is operator dependent, and the success rate is higher if meticulous scanning is done with use of both standardized and nonstandardized angulated views. Particular efforts should be made to obtain the best possible visualization of the entire LV apex (V1.3A, V1.3B). The use of contrast agents greatly improves LV thrombus detection rate (V13.10). The incidence of LV thrombi in anterior infarctions detected by echocardiography is 28–57%,[45,46,49,50] which approaches the incidence reported in autopsy studies of 20–60%.[51]

After infarction, thrombus, when present, is located in the dyssynergic zone and typically appears as an echogenic mass with a contour distinct from the endocardial border. However, it may be difficult to see a clear demarcation line between the thrombus and underlying myocardium. To distinguish thrombus from the artifacts seen in the apex, it is helpful to demonstrate the suspected mass in at least two different echocardiographic views.

Transesophageal echocardiography may not be useful in detection of apical thrombi because the true LV apex can often be missed as a result of *foreshortening* of the LV cavity in longitudinal views. Deep transgastric views may be required to adequately visualize the LV apex.

Frequent echocardiographic examinations are essential to determine the exact incidence of LV thrombosis, particularly in the first week after infarction.[50] Thrombi may appear very early, in the first hours in the course of infarction.[50] In the early phase of formation, they may come out as unclear, cloudy, mobile echoes before they change their morphology and develop the characteristic clotlike appearance.[50] Fresh thrombi tend to have acoustic properties similar to adjacent myocardium (V3.24), in contrast to old, organized thrombi (V3.32A, V3.32B), which may look bright and more echogenic.

Thrombi may be of various sizes, ranging from very small, hardly detectable echoes to huge masses that can almost obliterate the LV cavity. Also, thrombi can be of various shapes. Laminated, non-protruding thrombi (V3.21, V13.7) without mobile parts have low embolic potential, in contrast to prominent, globular masses that protrude into the LV cavity (V3.23) and have either independent mobility (V3.6A, V13.9, V3.33) or mobile particles (V3.24) on their surface (Figure 3.11).

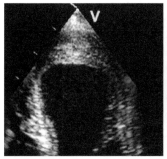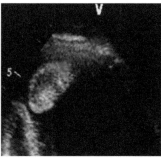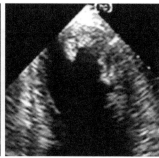

FIGURE 3.11 Various appearances of left ventricular thrombi. Laminated, nonprotruding, nonmobile thrombus, which packs the left ventricular apex with low embolic potential (left panel) (V3.21). Protruding, slightly mobile thrombus in a dyskinetic apex, with certain embolic potential (middle panel) (V3.23). Highly mobile, irregularly shaped, "fresh" thrombi in an apex and over the distal part of the anterior wall, with high embolic potential (right panel) (V3.24).

There are *several clinical implications of LV thrombosis* after acute myocardial infarction, and prediction of thrombus formation and resolution may influence patient management. First, *higher mortality* has been reported in patients with LV thrombi, especially when they develop within the first 48 hours.[52,53] Early thrombus formation should be expected in patients with large infarcts, more severe LV dysfunction, more extensive coronary artery disease, and failed infarct-related artery reperfusion.[50] Interestingly, one study reported lower early morbidity and mortality and improvement of functional class after 1 year in patients with mural thrombus after infarction[54]; this favorable impact was explained by the process of inflammation, healing, and thrombus fibrosis, providing mechanical support and reconstruction of the myocardial wall thickness that may limit wall stress (V3.21), infarct expansion, and remodeling. The second clinical implication is related to thrombus *embolic potential*.[55,56] The majority of systemic embolic episodes occur within 12 weeks after the acute event.[46] Hyperkinesis of the segments of the LV wall adjacent to thrombus was reported to be associated with increased embolic risk.[55]

High initial end-systolic volume is a predictor of thrombus formation.[50] If the initial echocardiogram reveals a large end-systolic volume, a high index of suspicion may warrant a repeat echocardiographic examination in order to not miss LV thrombosis.

LV thrombi can disappear either spontaneously or after anticoagulation (V3.25A, V3.25B). Thrombus disappearance may be associated with embolic events or may occur without any clinically detectable symptom or sign.[50] The reported rate of thrombus resolution ranges from 20 to 71%,[45,46,50,57–59] and it is more likely to occur in patients without LV dyskinesis at the end of the healing phase.[50]

RIGHT VENTRICULAR INFARCTION

Right ventricular infarction occurs in 30–50% of cases with inferoposterior infarction of the left ventricle, as the consequence of proximal occlusion of the right coronary artery.[60] Although it is not considered a mechanical complication, patients with acute inferior myocardial infarction and right ventricular involvement are at increased risk of death, shock, and arrhythmias.[61] This complicated course appears to be related to dysfunction of the right ventricle itself rather than to the extent of LV myocardial damage. Isolated right ventricular infarctions are rare.

Accurate diagnosis is essential because proper management (which includes reperfusion therapy, careful volume loading, inotropic support, and maintenance of atrioventricular synchrony) should be initiated promptly to prevent severe hemodynamic compromise.[62]

Echocardiography has high sensitivity (82%) and specificity (93%) for the detection of right ventricular infarction.[63,64] Two-dimensional examination reveals various degrees of *right ventricular dyssynergy and/or right ventricular dilation* (V3.26A, V3.26B, V3.27A, V3.27B) *associated with dyssynergy of the inferoposterior LV wall*.[63–65] In more than half of the cases, McConnell sign, which is regularly seen in acute pulmonary embolism, can be found[66] (see Chapter 7, V7.3, V7.4A). Echocardiographic images of the right ventricle in right ventricular infarction are quite often indistinguishable from those seen in acute pulmonary embolism (V3.28, V7.3, V7.4A). Other echocardiographic signs that might often be present include paradoxical motion of the ventricular septum[60] and early opening of the pulmonary valve because of increased right-sided filling pressures.[67]

In the majority of cases, spontaneous complete recovery of right ventricular systolic function occurs within several weeks, even without reperfusion.[62,68]

Echocardiography may also be helpful in detection of rare right ventricular free-wall rupture or right ventricular papillary muscle rupture, which may occur after right ventricular infarction.[60,64]

In up to one-third of cases, *significant tricuspid regurgitation* can be detected. It may be the result of papillary muscle dysfunction, right ventricular dilation, or even papillary muscle rupture. It is associated with increased in-hospital mortality.[69] Similar to right ventricular dilation and dyssynergy, tricuspid regurgitation typically resolves with time.[70] When a patent foramen ovale is present in this setting, right-to-left shunting can be detected by Doppler or contrast echocardiography because of increased right atrial pressure.[71]

PERICARDIAL EFFUSION

The reported incidence of pericardial effusion in the acute phase of myocardial infarction ranges from 5.6 to 37%, depending on the techniques used for its detection (M-mode and two-dimensional echocardiography) and the time of the examination after the onset of infarction.[72,73] Pericardial effusion is associated with larger infarcts, anterior infarcts, more extensive wall motion abnormalities, congestive heart failure, severe LV dysfunction, and female gender.[73,74] Other types of pericardial involvement in myocardial infarction include free-wall rupture (see earlier) with tamponade (see Chapter 8) and late Dressler's syndrome. Of note, in patients with acute myocardial infarction, iatrogenic hemopericardium with or without tamponade may rarely complicate primary PCI or temporary pacemaker insertion.

Postinfarction pericardial effusion is usually mild and asymptomatic and has little clinical significance.[72–74] However, confusion may arise when pericardial friction rub is misinterpreted as cardiac murmur, when chest pain caused by pericarditis is present, and/or when electrocardiographic changes mimic ongoing myocardial ischemia. In addition, the presence of pericardial effusion in patients with acute myocardial infarction should always alert a clinician to possible "silent" subacute free-wall rupture (see earlier).[18,19] Also, the possibility of acute aortic dissection with bleeding into the pericardial space should always be considered (see Chapter 6).

Two-dimensional echocardiography is an accurate method for the semiquantitative assessment of the quantity and

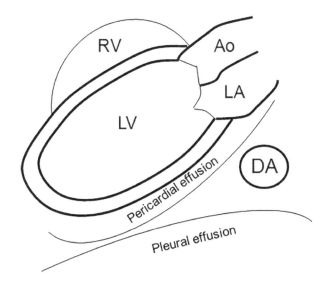

FIGURE 3.12 Distinction between pericardial and pleural effusion. The marker is the descending aorta (DA). Pericardial fluid is located anterior to the descending aorta in the long-axis parasternal view, whereas the left pleural effusion is located posteriorly. Ao: ascending aorta; LA: left atrium; LV: left ventricle; RV: right ventricle.

distribution of pericardial fluid. An echo-free space around the heart due to pericardial effusion should be *differentiated from the pericardial fat pad*; the latter is usually located anteriorly, in front of the right ventricular free wall, does not extend beyond the atrioventricular sulcus, and typically is not accompanied by posterior effusion. Also, *distinction from pleural effusion* can be made using the descending thoracic aorta as a marker: pericardial fluid appears anterior to the descending aorta in the parasternal long-axis view, whereas the left pleural effusion is located posterolateral to the descending aorta (Figure 3.12).

LIST OF VIDEOS

https://routledgetextbooks.com/textbooks/9781032157009/chapter-3.php

VIDEO 3.1A Acute ischemic mitral regurgitation (1/2): Left panel: apical four-chamber view showing akinesis of the lateral wall and hypokinetic septum and apex. Note slightly asymmetric tenting of the mitral valve as a consequence of papillary muscle dysfunction and tethering of both mitral leaflets. Right panel: color Doppler showing functional mitral regurgitation that appears to be moderately severe (see also Video 3.1B).

VIDEO 3.1B Acute ischemic mitral regurgitation (2/2): Left panel: modified apical long-axis view showing akinesis of the posterior wall with slightly asymmetric tenting of the mitral valve caused by a slightly more evident tethering of the posterior mitral leaflet. Right panel: color Doppler showing severe functional mitral regurgitation (see also Video 3.1A).

VIDEO 3.2A Papillary muscle dysfunction (1/2): Transthoracic apical long-axis view showing that maximal systolic position of both mitral leaflets is displaced toward the left ventricular apex and above the mitral annulus level (tenting). Note dyskinesis of the underlying posterior wall and tethering of the leaflets throughout the cardiac cycle, resulting in functional mitral regurgitation (see also Video 3.2B).

VIDEO 3.2B Papillary muscle dysfunction (2/2): Transthoracic apical long-axis view showing functional mitral regurgitation resulting from papillary muscle dysfunction (see also Video 3.2A).

VIDEO 3.3 Complete posteromedial papillary muscle rupture: Upper left panel: transthoracic off-axis apical four-chamber view showing a flail of the anterior mitral leaflet. Upper right panel: modified apical two-chamber view showing a flail of the anterior mitral leaflet with a hypermobile mass attached to it, representing ruptured papillary muscle. Lower left panel: apical two-chamber view showing a flail of the anterior mitral leaflet with a hypermobile mass attached to it, representing ruptured papillary muscle. Note akinesis of the inferior wall. Lower right panel: color Doppler showing mitral regurgitation. Although regurgitation is severe, assessment of its severity with Doppler is often difficult because of tachycardia, high left atrial pressure, and large regurgitant orifice.

VIDEO 3.4A Partial papillary muscle rupture (1/2): Transthoracic echocardiography of a patient with suspected partial rupture of the papillary muscle. Upper left panel: modified apical four-chamber view showing hypermobile, irregularly shaped mass in lower third of the left ventricular cavity, below the bulk of the posteromedial papillary muscle. Also note akinesis of the inferior septum. Upper right panel: modified apical long-axis view showing the same hypermobile, irregularly shaped mass in vicinity of the posterior mitral leaflet. Lower left panel: modified apical long-axis view showing the same hypermobile, irregularly shaped mass that appears to be part of the papillary muscle. Note that, at least in one cardiac cycle, the flail of the posterior leaflet appears to be present, but because of poor quality of images, it cannot be confirmed. Also note the akinesis of the basal half of the posterior wall with hypercontractility of other segments of the left ventricle. Lower right panel: color Doppler apical long-axis view showing the presence of eccentric mitral regurgitation that cannot be truly appreciated but appears to be at least moderately severe (relatively large proximal isovelocity surface area) (see also Video 3.4B).

VIDEO 3.4B Partial papillary muscle rupture (2/2): Transesophageal echocardiography of a patient with suspected partial rupture of the papillary muscle. Upper left panel: transesophageal four-chamber view showing the prolapse of the posterior mitral leaflet. Upper right panel: color Doppler four-chamber view showing significant mitral regurgitation with a large proximal isovelocity surface area and wide vena contracta. Lower left panel: transgastric two-chamber view clearly showing a partial rupture of the posteromedial papillary muscle. Also note akinesis of the basal segment of the inferior wall. Lower right panel: transgastric short-axis view showing hypermobile mass (a head of the posteromedial papillary muscle) (see also Video 3.4A).

VIDEO 3.5   Ventricular septal rupture in a patient with anterior myocardial infarction: A 76-year-old woman presented to the emergency department with a history of chest pain lasting for the previous 7 days. On the day of presentation, she felt severe chest pain lasting for up to 10 minutes, followed by lightheadedness. On physical examination, a loud systolic murmur was heard in the region of the left ventricular (LV) apex. Upper left panel: color Doppler apical four-chamber view showing a turbulence in the apical region of the right ventricle, close to the interventricular septum. Note the akinesis of the distal half of the interventricular septum and apex and hypercontractility of noninfarcted segments of the left ventricle. Also note the normal size of the right ventricle, indicating recent onset of the rupture. Upper right panel: modified apical long-axis showing systolic turbulent jet across the apical segment of interventricular septum and in the apical region of the right ventricle. Lower left panel: modified parasternal short-axis view at the level of LV apex showing the rupture in the apical segment of interventricular septum. Note the thinning of the myocardium in the vicinity of the rupture site. Lower right panel: modified color Doppler parasternal short-axis view at the level of LV apex showing the presence of turbulence jet at the site of the rupture.

VIDEO 3.6A   Multiple postinfarction ventricular septal defects (1/2): In an apical four-chamber view, irregular discontinuity in the midportion of the interventricular septum in a patient with anterior infarction, suggesting possible multiple rupture sites ("Swiss cheese" defect). Note several mobile masses (thrombi) in the left ventricular cavity (see also Video 3.6B).

VIDEO 3.6B   Multiple postinfarction ventricular septal defects (2/2): Color Doppler in the apical four-chamber view shows several turbulent jets of abnormal flow across the rupture site from the left to the right ventricle (see also Video 3.6A)

VIDEO 3.7   Congenital ventricular septal defect in a patient with chest pain and a systolic murmur: A 57-year-old man with multiple risk factors for coronary artery disease presented in the emergency department with chest pain and dyspnea. The electrocardiogram (ECG) showed nonspecific repolarization abnormalities. On physical examination, a harsh systolic murmur was heard along the left sternal border and at the apex. Emergency echocardiography was performed to check for suspected acute mitral regurgitation or ventricular septal defect in a patient with suspected acute coronary syndrome. In the transthoracic apical four-chamber view (left panel) and parasternal short-axis view (right panel), a defect of the apical portion of the septum was detected, with regular borders and shape and, most important, located in the region of normally contracting myocardium. Detection of the ventricular septal defect in the region with normal wall motion strongly suggests congenital origin. Because the initial and repeated serum troponin values were normal and serial ECGs unchanged, the patient was discharged and scheduled for further testing for coronary artery disease.

VIDEO 3.8A   Ventricular septal rupture after delayed reperfusion (1/2): A 73-year-old woman was admitted to the coronary care unit because of acute anterior ST-segment elevation myocardial infarction with a chest pain onset 11 hours before the admission. Primary percutaneous coronary intervention of the left anterior descending artery was performed, with implantation of one drug-eluting stent. Transthoracic parasternal long-axis view with color Doppler performed at admission showed akinesis of the interventricular septum along with only a trace of aortic and mitral regurgitation. Note the hypercontractility of the posterior wall (see also Video 3.8B).

VIDEO 3.8B   Ventricular septal rupture after delayed reperfusion (2/2): On the second day of hospitalization because of anterior ST-segment elevation myocardial infarction (see also Video 3.8A), the patient experienced a new episode of chest pain, followed by hemodynamic deterioration. Repeated echocardiographic examination performed after hemodynamic deterioration revealed the rupture (shown here) of the apical segment of the interventricular septum with left-to-right shunt.

VIDEO 3.9   Ventricular septal rupture and ischemic mitral regurgitation in a patient with inferior myocardial infarction: A 53-year-old construction worker was brought to the emergency department after severe chest pain followed by syncope. He was also complaining of heartburn and nausea lasting for 2 days that he treated with over-the-counter medication, but without relief. During those 2 days he continued to work. On physical examination, a loud systolic murmur over the apex of the heart and along the left sternal border was heard. Upper left panel: apical four-chamber view showing akinesis of the basal septum (RCA territory) and the basal two-thirds of the lateral wall. Upper right panel: color Doppler apical four-chamber view showing ischemic mitral regurgitation. Lower left panel: scanning of the left ventricle from the apical four-chamber view to visualize the presence of ventricular septal rupture. Lower right panel: modified apical four-chamber view with color Doppler showing the turbulence at the site of the rupture across the septum, directed toward the right ventricular cavity. This case illustrates the value of echo in the differential diagnosis of a systolic murmur in the setting of acute myocardial infarction.

VIDEO 3.10A   Rapid deterioration of right ventricular function in a patient with ventricular septal rupture (1/2): The ventricular septal rupture was diagnosed in the coronary care unit, and the cardiac surgery center was contacted for urgent patient referral. Note the significant dilation of the right ventricular cavity (right panel vs. left panel) within 2 hours of waiting for transfer to cardiac surgery center, indicating worsening hemodynamics and failing right ventricle (see also Video 3.10B).

VIDEO 3.10B   Rapid deterioration of right ventricular function in a patient with ventricular septal rupture (2/2): Transthoracic subcostal view. Note the suspected rupture site at the midportion of the septum (upper left panel), where a turbulent jet across the septum directed toward the right ventricular cavity can be seen (upper right panel). Continuous-wave Doppler across the rupture site revealed left-to-right shunt with systolic gradient between ventricles of 73 mmHg (lower left panel). Because systolic pressure simultaneously measured on the patient's arm was 120 mmHg, the estimated right ventricular systolic pressure was approximately 53 mmHg, indicating right ventricular strain. The similar estimated value of right ventricular systolic pressure was obtained by measuring the velocity of tricuspid regurgitation jet (approximately 48 mmHg) (lower right panel) (see also Video 3.10A).

VIDEO 3.11   Free-wall rupture in a patient with anterior myocardial infarction: A 68-year-old man was admitted to the coronary care unit because of cardiogenic shock. His electrocardiogram showed Q-waves in the leads V2–V4 along with ST-segment elevation. Emergency transthoracic echocardiography was performed. Upper left panel: off-axis apical four-chamber view showing akinesis of the left ventricular (LV) apex and spontaneous echo contrast in the LV cavity. Note that myocardium in the apical region is thin. Also note the presence of the pericardial fluid and organized free-floating mass (hematoma) around the right ventricle and LV apex. Upper right panel: subcostal five-chamber view showing the presence of pericardial effusion and large hematoma compressing the right ventricular free wall (impending tamponade). Lower left panel: subcostal short-axis view showing dilation of the inferior vena cava with a lack of collapsibility during inspiration. Lower right panel: pulsed-wave Doppler in the region of the LV apex showing systolic flow through a barely visible free-wall rupture. Pericardiocentesis was attempted, but the patient died as a result of cardiac tamponade.

VIDEO 3.12A   Subacute free-wall rupture (1/5): A 66-year-old man with an acute inferolateral ST-segment elevation myocardial infarction and noncomplicated intrahospital clinical course was referred to echocardiography on the third postinfarction day for the evaluation of a new systolic murmur. Transthoracic echocardiography in the apical long-axis view revealed significant functional mitral regurgitation, which was identified as a cause of the murmur. However, a hyperechogenic zone was identified at the level of the posterior mitral annulus and a turbulent jet of uncertain origin (see Video 3.12B). Also, in a subcostal view, a large hematoma was detected in the pericardial sac (see Video 3.12C), without echocardiographic signs of impending tamponade. Subacute free-wall rupture was suspected, but the communication between the left ventricular cavity and pericardial sac could not be confirmed by transthoracic examination. Transesophageal echocardiography in a modified transgastric short-axis view revealed a thin aneurysmatic inferolateral wall (see Video 3.12D), with a turbulent jet (see Video 3.12E), originating from the border of the akinetic zone and directed toward the pericardial space. The patient underwent urgent cardiac surgery, and intraoperative findings confirmed that the rupture site was blocked by pericardial hematoma. The rupture was successfully repaired.

VIDEO 3.12B   Subacute free-wall rupture (2/5): A 66-year-old man with an acute inferolateral ST-segment elevation myocardial infarction and noncomplicated intrahospital clinical course was referred to echocardiography on the third postinfarction day for the evaluation of a new systolic murmur. Transthoracic echocardiography in the apical long-axis view revealed significant functional mitral regurgitation, which was identified as a cause of the murmur (see Video 3.12A). However, a hyperechogenic zone was identified at the level of the posterior mitral annulus and a turbulent jet of uncertain origin (shown here). Also, in a subcostal view, a large hematoma was detected in the pericardial sac (see Video 3.12C), without echocardiographic signs of impending tamponade. Subacute free-wall rupture was suspected, but the communication between the left ventricular cavity and pericardial sac could not be confirmed by transthoracic examination. Transesophageal echocardiography in a modified transgastric short-axis view revealed a thin aneurysmatic inferolateral wall (see Video 3.12D), with a turbulent jet (see Video 3.12E), originating from the border of the akinetic zone and directed toward the pericardial space. The patient underwent urgent cardiac surgery, and intraoperative findings confirmed that the rupture site was blocked by pericardial hematoma. The rupture was successfully repaired.

VIDEO 3.12C   Subacute free-wall rupture (3/5): A 66-year-old man with an acute inferolateral ST-segment elevation myocardial infarction and noncomplicated intrahospital clinical course was referred to echocardiography on the third postinfarction day for the evaluation of a new systolic murmur. Transthoracic echocardiography in the apical long-axis view revealed significant functional mitral regurgitation, which was identified as a cause of the murmur (see Video 3.12A). However, a hyperechogenic zone was identified at the level of the posterior mitral annulus and a turbulent jet of uncertain origin (see Video 3.12B). Also, in a subcostal view, a large hematoma was detected in the pericardial sac (shown here), without echocardiographic signs of impending tamponade. Subacute free-wall rupture was suspected, but the communication between the left ventricular cavity and pericardial sac could not be confirmed by transthoracic examination. Transesophageal echocardiography in a modified transgastric short-axis view revealed a thin aneurysmatic inferolateral wall (see Video 3.12D), with a turbulent jet (see Video 3.12E), originating from the border of the akinetic zone and directed toward the pericardial space. The patient underwent urgent cardiac surgery, and intraoperative findings confirmed that the rupture site was blocked by pericardial hematoma. The rupture was successfully repaired.

VIDEO 3.12D   Subacute free-wall rupture (4/5): A 66-year-old man with an acute inferolateral ST-segment elevation myocardial infarction and noncomplicated intrahospital clinical course was referred to echocardiography on the third postinfarction day for the evaluation of a new systolic murmur. Transthoracic echocardiography in the apical long-axis view revealed significant functional mitral regurgitation, which was identified as a cause of the murmur (see Video 3.12A). However, a hyperechogenic zone was identified at the level of the posterior mitral annulus and a turbulent jet of uncertain origin (see Video 3.12B). Also, in a subcostal view, a large hematoma was detected in the pericardial sac (see Video 3.12C), without echocardiographic signs of impending tamponade. Subacute free-wall rupture was suspected, but the communication between the left ventricular cavity and pericardial sac could not be confirmed by transthoracic examination. Transesophageal echocardiography in a modified transgastric short-axis view revealed a thin aneurysmatic inferolateral wall (shown here), with a turbulent jet (Video 3.12E), originating from the border of the akinetic zone and directed toward the pericardial space. The patient underwent urgent cardiac surgery, and intraoperative findings confirmed that the rupture site was blocked by pericardial hematoma. The rupture was successfully repaired.

VIDEO 3.12E   Subacute free-wall rupture (5/5): A 66-year-old man with an acute inferolateral ST-segment elevation myocardial infarction and noncomplicated intrahospital clinical course was referred to echocardiography on the third postinfarction day for the evaluation of a new systolic murmur. Transthoracic echocardiography in the apical long-axis view revealed significant functional mitral regurgitation, which was identified as a cause of the murmur (see Video 3.12A). However, a hyperechogenic zone was identified at the level of the posterior mitral annulus and a turbulent jet of uncertain origin (see Video 3.12B). Also, in a subcostal view, a large hematoma was detected in the pericardial sac (see Video 3.12C), without echocardiographic signs of impending tamponade. Subacute free-wall rupture was suspected, but the communication between the left ventricular cavity and pericardial sac could not be confirmed by transthoracic examination. Transesophageal echocardiography in a modified transgastric short-axis view revealed a thin aneurysmatic inferolateral wall (see Video 3.12D), with a turbulent jet (shown here), originating from the border of the akinetic zone and directed toward the pericardial space. The patient underwent urgent cardiac surgery, and intraoperative findings confirmed that the rupture site was blocked by pericardial hematoma. The rupture was successfully repaired.

VIDEO 3.13   Free-wall rupture in a patient with recent acute myocardial infarction and cardiac tamponade: A 71-year-old woman presented to the emergency department (ED) with chest pain lasting for 3 days and extreme fatigue. On physical examination she was hypotensive (85/50 mmHg), with distended neck veins and muffled heart sounds. Emergency transthoracic echocardiography revealed akinesis of the anterior septum and distal half of the anterior wall and dyskinesis of the left ventricular apex. Also, a large pericardial effusion with echocardiographic signs of impending cardiac tamponade was seen. Upper left panel: apical long-axis view showing akinesis of the anterior septum, dyskinetic apex, and the dense circular pericardial effusion. Upper right panel: apical four-chamber view showing akinesis of the distal half of the septum and dyskinesis of the apex, along with a circular pericardial effusion. Note the right atrial systolic collapse as a sign of impending tamponade. Lower left panel: parasternal long-axis view showing circular pericardial effusion with occasional right ventricular diastolic collapse. Lower right panel: pulsed-wave Doppler of the left ventricular outflow tract showing marked variation of flow during respiration. The patient died after cardiac arrest in the ED, despite intensive resuscitation attempts, including pericardiocentesis. The autopsy revealed a large hemothorax and a recent infarction of the anterior myocardial wall and the apex, with numerous small perforations through the large necrotic zone.

VIDEO 3.14A   Double left ventricular pseudoaneurysm (1/2): Transesophageal echocardiography, modified longitudinal two-chamber view. Discontinuity of the inferoposterior myocardial wall at two separate places, with two narrow-neck aneurysmal sacs, indicating pseudoaneurysm formation. Interestingly, the patient reported that he had had myocardial infarction 6 months before the actual presentation. In the meantime, he had undergone three exercise stress tests for the assessment of the recurrent chest pain. Echocardiography was not performed before the actual presentation (see also Video 3.14B). The patient underwent urgent surgical repair of two pseudoaneurysms (for the intraoperative findings, see Figure 3.7 in the book).

VIDEO 3.14B   Double left ventricular pseudoaneurysm (2/2): Color Doppler transesophageal echocardiography, modified longitudinal two-chamber view. Note two turbulent jets at two separate places of discontinuity of the inferoposterior myocardial wall, indicating flow through two separate pseudoaneurysmal necks (see also Video 3.14A). The patient underwent urgent surgical repair of two pseudoaneurysms (for the intraoperative findings, see Figure 3.7 in the book).

VIDEO 3.15A   Left ventricular apical aneurysm (1/2): Transthoracic apical four-chamber view in a patient who presented in the emergency department with recurrent episodes of chest pain in the previous 3 days. He had a history of an old anterior myocardial infarction 1 year before. Note a large apical aneurysm with the additional saccular dilation in the apical segment of the lateral wall. To exclude pseudoaneurysm, cardiac multislice computed tomography was performed (see also Video 3.15B).

VIDEO 3.15B   Left ventricular apical aneurysm (2/2): Cardiac multislice computed tomography in a patient with suspected pseudoaneurysm showing large apical aneurysm with additional saccular

dilation of the apical segment of the lateral wall with preserved continuity of the myocardium. There were no signs of a contained rupture of the left ventricle (see also Video 3.15A).

VIDEO 3.16   Aneurysm of the left ventricular inferior wall: Transthoracic apical two-chamber view showing aneurysm of the basal segment of the inferior wall. Note the abnormal segmental geometry of the inferior wall in both systole and diastole.

VIDEO 3.17   Aneurysm of the left ventricular inferoposterolateral wall: Left panel: off-axis transthoracic apical four-chamber view showing a large aneurysm of the basal segment of the lateral wall. Right panel: modified apical long-axis view showing a large aneurysm of the basal segment of the inferoposterior wall. Note the abnormal segmental geometry of the inferior wall in both systole and diastole.

VIDEO 3.18   Left ventricular apical aneurysm: Three-dimensional transthoracic echocardiogram showing large apical left ventricular aneurysm. *(Video provided by LB.)*

VIDEO 3.19   Left ventricular apical aneurysm—three-dimensional transthoracic echocardiography reconstruction: Reconstruction of large left ventricular apical aneurysm with three-dimensional transthoracic echocardiography. Note dyskinesis of the left ventricular apex in systole. *(Video provided by LB.)*

VIDEO 3.20   Left ventricular inferoposterior aneurysm: Two-dimensional (left panels) and three-dimensional (right panel) transthoracic echocardiograms showing inferoposterior left ventricular (LV) aneurysm. Owing to poor global LV function and refractory heart failure, a left ventricular assist device was implanted. *(Video provided by AH.)*

VIDEO 3.21   Large left ventricular apical aneurysm with thrombus: Transthoracic echocardiogram showing large left ventricular apical aneurysm (note apical dyskinesia) packed with a large thrombus. Note the spontaneous echo contrast ("smoke sign") in the left ventricular cavity. Left panel: apical four-chamber view. Right panel: apical two-chamber view.

VIDEO 3.22   Left ventricular apical thrombus: Two-dimensional (left panels) and three-dimensional (right panel) transthoracic echocardiograms showing a ball-like thrombus in the left ventricular apex with significant embolic potential. *(Video provided by LB.)*

VIDEO 3.23   Prominent left ventricular thrombus: Transthoracic four-chamber view. Note a large protruding thrombus in the dyskinetic left ventricular apex.

VIDEO 3.24   Mobile left ventricular thrombus: Transthoracic two-chamber view. Note a highly mobile thrombus in the akinetic left ventricular apex and also highly mobile thrombotic masses over the akinetic anterior wall.

VIDEO 3.25A   Left and right ventricular thrombus in a patient with acute anterolateral myocardial infarction (1/2): A 54-year-old woman with a history of previous inferoposterior myocardial infarction was admitted to the coronary care unit because of acute anterolateral ST-segment elevation myocardial infarction that was treated with primary percutaneous coronary intervention of the left anterior descending artery. Four days later, transthoracic echocardiography revealed a large thrombus in the left ventricular (LV) apex, along with a smaller, oval thrombus entangled in the right ventricular trabecular network (lower right panel). Note severely reduced global LV function as a result of the large functional infarct size (inferior scar plus actual anterior necrosis). The only regions with preserved contractility are the basal and mid segments of the lateral wall and the basal anterior wall. The right ventricle also appears dilated with hypokinetic free wall. After echo examination, the patient started to take oral anticoagulants along with dual-antiplatelet therapy. Approximately 1½ months later, an echo examination was repeated (see Video 3.25B). Upper left panel: modified apical four-chamber view. Upper right panel: apical two-chamber view. Lower left panel: apical long-axis view. Lower right panel: modified apical four-chamber view showing apical region of both left and right ventricle.

VIDEO 3.25B Left and right ventricular thrombus in a patient with acute anterolateral myocardial infarction (2/2): Repeated echo examination after 1½ months of taking oral anticoagulant and dual-antiplatelet therapy for left and right ventricular thrombi. The examination revealed no significant change in global and regional left and right ventricular function, but both left and right ventricular thrombi vanished. A small aberrant chord can be seen in the left ventricular apex (see also Video 3.25A).

VIDEO 3.26A Right ventricular infarction with hypotension (1/2): A 73-year-old woman with chest pain and electrocardiographic signs of acute inferior ST-segment elevation myocardial infarction was brought by ambulance to the emergency department. Her blood pressure was 95/65 mmHg, and heart rate was 94 bpm. Emergency echocardiography revealed akinesis of the inferior wall (shown here) with preserved global left ventricular function. The basal (inferior) septum was akinetic and the right ventricle was hypokinetic and dilated (see Video 3.26B), because of proximal right coronary artery occlusion and right ventricular infarction. She responded well to intravenous fluid administration and underwent successful primary percutaneous coronary intervention of the proximally occluded dominant right coronary artery.

VIDEO 3.26B Right ventricular infarction with hypotension (2/2): A 73-year-old woman with chest pain and electrocardiographic signs of acute inferior ST-segment elevation myocardial infarction was brought by ambulance to the emergency department. Her blood pressure was 95/65 mmHg, and heart rate was 94 bpm. Emergency echocardiography revealed akinesis of the inferior wall (see Video 3.26A) with preserved global left ventricular function. The basal (inferior) septum was akinetic and the right ventricle was hypokinetic and dilated (shown here) because of proximal right coronary artery occlusion and right ventricular infarction. She responded well to intravenous fluid administration and underwent successful primary percutaneous coronary intervention of the proximally occluded dominant right coronary artery.

VIDEO 3.27A Right ventricular infarction with cardiogenic shock (1/2): A 55-year-old man was admitted to the coronary care unit in cardiogenic shock which complicated acute inferior ST-segment elevation myocardial infarction. Emergency echocardiography revealed inferior wall akinesis with excellent global left ventricular function (shown here), but with marked right ventricular dilation and akinetic right ventricular free wall, with preserved contractility of the right ventricular apex (McConnell's sign) (see Video 3.27B). The patient underwent primary percutaneous coronary intervention of the proximally occluded, huge, dominant right coronary artery with institution of the intra-aortic balloon pump. He was discharged from the hospital after 9 days with recovered right ventricular function.

VIDEO 3.27B Right ventricular infarction with cardiogenic shock (2/2): A 55-year-old man was admitted to the coronary care unit in cardiogenic shock which complicated acute inferior ST-segment elevation myocardial infarction. Emergency echocardiography revealed inferior wall akinesis with excellent global left ventricular function (see Video 3.27A), but with marked right ventricular dilation and akinetic right ventricular free wall, with preserved contractility of the right ventricular apex (McConnell's sign) (shown here). The patient underwent primary percutaneous coronary intervention of the proximally occluded, huge, dominant right coronary artery, with institution of the intra-aortic balloon pump. He was discharged from the hospital after 9 days with recovered right ventricular function.

VIDEO 3.28 Right ventricular infarction: Upper left panel: apical four-chamber view showing dyskinesis of the basal septum, gross dilation of the right ventricle along with akinesis of the right ventricular free wall, and hypercontractility of the apical segment (McConnell's sign). Upper right panel: parasternal short-axis view at the level of the papillary muscles showing dyskinesis of the inferior wall and the inferior septum, flattening of the interventricular septum, and the right ventricular dilation. Lower left panel: parasternal long-axis view showing dyskinesis of the basal segment of the posterior wall, right ventricular dilation, and akinesis of the right ventricular free wall. Lower right panel: apical two-chamber view showing akinesis of the basal half of the inferior wall. Of note, all echocardiographic features described here may be found in acute pulmonary embolism, except inferior wall asynergy, indicating coronary artery disease.

VIDEO 3.29 Papillary muscle rupture. Transthoracic parasternal long-axis view showing mass attached to the flail posterior mitral leaflet, freely moving from left ventricle to left atrium during cardiac cycle, representing part of ruptured posteromedial papillary muscle. *(Video provided by MP.)*

VIDEO 3.30A Free-wall myocardial rupture sealed by the clot (1/2). The patient presented in the emergency room in shock, after successful CPR performed in the ambulance, during transportation from home, where he experienced severe acute chest pain. In a subcostal view, a huge echodense space around the heart was detected, suggesting hemopericardium with tamponade, indicated by almost complete obliteration of the right ventricular cavity during diastole (left panel), and dilated, noncollapsable vena cava inferior (right panel). See also Video 3.30B.

VIDEO 3.30B Free-wall myocardial rupture sealed by the clot (2/2). In a patient with suspected hemopericardium and tamponade (see Video 30.3A), in a apical long-axis view akinetic inferoposterior wall with suspected site of ventricular rupture (discontinuation of the myocardium and pathologic flow) was seen, temporarily sealed by the clot. Patient underwent emergent cardiac surgery where ventricular rupture of the inferoposterior wall was found and fixed.

VIDEO 3.31A   Pseudoaneurysm of the inferoposterior wall (1/3). A patient complaining of episodes of anginal pain that were occurring frequently during the period of 2 months following acute inferoposterolateral infarction. Transthoracic two-chamber view revealed huge pseudoaneurysm of the inferoposterior wall, with abrupt discontinuation of the inferoposterior myocardium, unusually broad neck and thrombus covering pericardial sac (lower left panel). The same can be noticed in apical long-axis view (lower right panel) and modified short-axis view (upper right panel), where pleural effusion can also be seen. In apical four-chamber view, akinesis of the lateral wall can be appreciated (upper left panel). *(Video provided by IV and IS.)*

VIDEO 3.31B   A patient with postinfarction angina—2 months prior to detection of pseudoaneurysm (2/3). Transthoracic echocardiogram recorded 2 months prior to the detection of pseudoaneurysm shown on Video 3.31A, at the time of the occurrence of acute inferoposterior myocardial infarction. Note akinesis of the inferoposterior wall (lower left and right panels, and upper right panel), as well as akinetic lateral wall (upper left panel). Note the absence of the pseudoaneurysm shown on Video 3.31A, recorded 2 months later. *(Video provided by IV and PMM.)*

VIDEO 3.31C   A patient with postinfarction angina—one month prior to detection of pseudoaneurysm (3/3). Transthoracic echocardiogram recorded 1 month prior to the detection of pseudoaneurysm shown on Video 3.31A, in a patient with frequent postinfarction anginal pain. Note the aneurysmal distorsion of the inferoposterior wall (lower left and right panels, and upper right panel), which appears thinner compered to one month before (see Video 3.31B), as well as akinetic lateral wall (upper left panel). Note that inferoposterior myocardium is thin but still intact. Note the spot in the middle of the inferior wall on the left lower panel, which might be the site of the future myocardial rupture resulting in pseudoaneurysm formation (see Video 3.31A). *(Video provided by SM.)*

VIDEO 3.32A   Multiple old left ventricular thrombi in ischemic cardiomyopathy (1/2). Transthoracic apical four-chamber view showing large partially organized echogenic masses in the apical part of the left ventricular cavity attached to apical part of the septum and lateral wall. Note small, mobile part on the top of the mass attached to lateral wall (see also Video 3.32B). Note the poor global left ventricular function. *(Video provided by DK.)*

VIDEO 3.32B   Multiple old left ventricular thrombi in ischemic cardiomyopathy (2/2). Transthoracic apical long-axis view showing large partially organized echogenic masses in the apical part of the left ventricular cavity attached to apical part of the septum and posterolateral wall (see also Video 3.32A). Note the poor global left ventricular function. *(Video provided by DK.)*

VIDEO 3.33   Highly mobile left ventricular thrombus in ischemic cardiomyopathy. Transthoracic four-chamber view showing large, highly mobile left ventricular thrombus with high embolic potential. *(Video provided by DK.)*

REFERENCES

1. French JK, Hellkamp AS, Armstrong PW, et al. Mechanical complications after percutaneous coronary intervention in ST-elevation myocardial infarction (from APEX-AMI). Am J Cardiol 2010;105:59–63.
2. Lancellotti P, Price S, Edvardsen T, et al. The use of echocardiography in acute cardiovascular care: recommendations of the European Association of Cardiovascular Imaging and the Acute Cardiovascular Care Association. Eur Heart J Cardiovasc Imaging 2015;16(2):119–46.
3. Kono T, Sabbah HN, Rosman H, et al. Mechanism of functional mitral regurgitation during acute myocardial ischemia. J Am Coll Cardiol 1992;19:1101–5.
4. Neskovic AN, Marinkovic J, Bojic M, et al. Early predictors of mitral regurgitation after acute myocardial infarction. Am J Cardiol 1999;84:329–32.
5. Mittal AK, Langston M, Cohn KE, et al. Combined papillary muscle and left ventricular wall dysfunction as a cause of mitral regurgitation. Circulation 1971;44:174–180.
6. Nishimura RA, Schaff HV, Shub C, et al. Papillary muscle rupture complicating acute myocardial infarction: analysis of 17 patients. Am J Cardiol 1983;51:373–7.
7. Feinberg MS, Schwammenthal E, Shlizerman L, et al. Prognostic significance of mild mitral regurgitation by color Doppler echocardiography in acute myocardial infarction. Am J Cardiol 2000;86:903–7.
8. Neskovic AN, Marinkovic J, Bojic M, et al. Early mitral regurgitation after acute myocardial infarction does not contribute to subsequent left ventricular remodeling. Clin Cardiol 1999;22:91–4.
9. Guy TS 4th, Moainie SL, Gorman JH 3rd, et al. Prevention of ischemic mitral regurgitation does not influence the outcome of remodeling after posterolateral myocardial infarction. J Am Coll Cardiol 2004;43:377–83.
10. Harrison MR, MacPhail B, Gurley JC, et al. Usefulness of color Doppler flow imaging to distinguish ventricular septal defect from acute mitral regurgitation complicating acute myocardial infarction. Am J Cardiol 1989;64:697–701.
11. Helmcke F, Mahan EF III, Nanda NC, et al. Two-dimensional echocardiography and Doppler color flow mapping in the diagnosis and prognosis of ventricular septal rupture. Circulation 1990;81:1775–83.
12. Panadis IP, Mintz GS, Goel I, et al. Acquired ventricular septal defect after myocardial infarction: detection by combined two-dimensional and Doppler echocardiography. Am Heart J 1986;111:427–9
13. Moore CA, Nygaard TW, Kaiser DL, et al. Postinfarction ventricular septal rupture: the importance of location and right ventricular function in determining survival. Circulation 1986;74:45–55.
14. Radford MJ, Johnson RA, Daggett WM, et al. Ventricular septal rupture: a review of clinical and physiologic features and an analysis of survival. Circulation 1981;64:545–53.
15. Raitt MH, Kraft CD, Gardner CJ, et al. Subacute ventricular free wall rupture complicating myocardial infarction. Am Heart J 1993;126:946–55.
16. Oliva PB, Hammill SC, Edwards WD, et al. Cardiac rupture, a clinically predictable complication of acute myocardial infarction: report of 70 cases with clinicopathologic correlations. J Am Coll Cardiol 1993;22:720–6.
17. Figueras J, Cortadellas J, Soler-Soler J. Left ventricular free wall rupture: clinical presentation and management. Heart 2000;83:499–504.

18. Lopez-Sendon J, Gonzalez A, Lopez de Sa E, et al. Diagnosis of subacute ventricular wall rupture after acute myocardial infarction: sensitivity and specificity of clinical, hemodynamic and echocardiographic criteria. J Am Coll Cardiol 1992;19:1145–53.

19. Figueras J, Curos A, Cortadellas J, et al. Relevance of electrocardiographic findings, heart failure, and infarct site in assessing risk and timing of left ventricular free wall rupture during acute myocardial infarction. Am J Cardiol 1995;76:543–7.

20. Mittle S, Makaryus AN, Mangion J. Role of contrast echocardiography in the assessment of myocardial rupture. Echocardiography 2003;20:77–81.

21. Garcia-Fernandez MA, Macchioli RO, Moreno PM, et al. Use of contrast echocardiography in the diagnosis of subacute myocardial rupture after myocardial infarction. J Am Soc Echocardiogr 2001;14:945–7.

22. Puri T, Liu Z, Doddamani S, et al. Three-dimensional echocardiography of post-myocardial infarction cardiac rupture. Echocardiography 2004;21:279–84.

23. Zoffoli G, Battaglia F, Venturini A, et al. A novel approach to ventricular rupture: clinical needs and surgical technique. Ann Thorac Surg 2012;93(3):1002–3.

24. Flajsig I, Castells y Cuch E, Mayosky AA, et al. Surgical treatment of left ventricular free wall rupture after myocardial infarction: case series. Croat Med J 2002;43(6):643–8.

25. Frances C, Romero A, Grady D. Left ventricular pseudoaneurysm. J Am Coll Cardiol 1998;32:557–61.

26. Brown SL, Gropler RJ, Harris KM. Distinguishing left ventricular aneurysm from pseudoaneurysm. Chest 1997;111:1403–9.

27. Yeo TC, Malouf JF, Oh JK, et al. Clinical profile and outcome in 52 patients with cardiac pseudoaneurysm. Ann Intern Med 1998;128:299–305.

28. Milojevic P, Neskovic V, Vukovic M, et al. Surgical repair of the leaking double postinfarction left ventricular pseudoaneurysm. J Thorac Cardiovasc Surg 2004;128(5):765–7.

29. Hutchins GM, Bulkley BH. Infarct expansion versus extension: two different complications of acute myocardial infarction. Am J Cardiol 1978;41:1127–1132.

30. Picard MH, Wilkins GT, Ray PA, et al. Natural history of left ventricular size and function after acute myocardial infarction: assessment and prediction by echocardiographic endocardial surface mapping. Circulation 1990;82:484–94.

31. Schuster EH, Bulkley BH. Expansion of transmural infarction: a pathologic factor in cardiac rupture. Circulation 1979;60:1532–8.

32. Erlebacher JA, Weiss JL, Eaton LW, et al. Late effects of acute infarct dilation on heart size: a two-dimensional echocardiographic study. Am J Cardiol 1982;49:1120–6.

33. Popovic AD, Thomas JD. Detecting and preventing ventricular remodeling after MI. Cleve Clin J Med 1997;64:319–25.

34. Eaton LW, Weiss JL, Bulkley BH, et al. Regional cardiac dilatation after acute myocardial infarction. N Engl J Med 1979;300:57–62.

35. Erlebacher JA, Weiss JL, Weisfeldt ML, et al. Early dilation of the infarcted segment in acute transmural myocardial infarction: role of infarct expansion in acute left ventricular enlargement. J Am Coll Cardiol 1984;4:201–8.

36. Weiss JL, Marino PN, Shapiro EP. Myocardial infarct expansion: recognition, significance and pathology. Am J Cardiol 1991;68:35D–40D.

37. Picard MH, Wilkins GT, Ray P, et al. Long-term effects of acute thrombolytic therapy on ventricular size and function. Am Heart J 1993;126:1–10.

38. Popovic AD, Neskovic AN, Marinkovic J, et al. Acute and long-term effects of thrombolysis after anterior wall acute myocardial infarction with serial assessment of infarct expansion and late ventricular remodeling. Am J Cardiol 1996;77:446–50.

39. Visser CA, Kan G, Meltzer RS, et al. Incidence, timing and prognostic value of left ventricular aneurysm formation after myocardial infarction: a prospective, serial echocardiographic study of 158 patients. Am J Cardiol 1986;57:729–32.

40. McKay RG, Pfeffer MA, Pasternak RC, et al. Left ventricular remodeling after myocardial infarction: a corollary to infarct expansion. Circulation 1986;74:693–702.

41. Popovic AD, Neskovic AN, Babic R, et al. Independent impact of thrombolytic therapy and vessel patency on left ventricular dilation after myocardial infarction: serial echocardiographic follow-up. Circulation 1994;90:800–7.

42. Bolognese L, Neskovic AN, Parodi G, et al. Left ventricular remodeling after primary coronary angioplasty: patterns of left ventricular dilation and long-term prognostic implications. Circulation. 2002;106:2351–7.

43. Giannuzzi P, Temporelli PL, Bosimini E, et al. Heterogeneity of left ventricular remodeling after myocardial infarction: results of the Gruppo Italiano per lo Studio della Sopravvivenza nell'Infarto Miocardio-3 Echo Substudy. Am Heart J 2001;141:131–8.

44. Bolognese L, Cerisano G. Early predictors of left ventricular remodeling after acute myocardial infarction. Am Heart J 1999;138:S79–83.

45. Asinger RW, Mikell FL, Elsperger J, et al. Incidence of left ventricular thrombosis after acute transmural myocardial infarction: serial evaluation by two-dimensional echocardiography. N Engl J Med 1981;305:297–302.

46. Weinreich DJ, Burke JF, Pauletto FJ. Left ventricular mural thrombi complicating acute myocardial infarction: long-term follow-up with serial echocardiography. Ann Intern Med 1984;100:789–94.

47. Osherov AB, Borovik-Raz M, Aronson D, et al. Incidence of early left ventricular thrombus after acute anterior wall myocardial infarction in the primary coronary intervention era. Am Heart J 2009;157(6):1074–80.

48. Stratton JR, Lighty GW Jr, Pearlman AS, et al. Detection of left ventricular thrombus by two-dimensional echocardiography: sensitivity, specificity, and causes of uncertainty. Circulation 1982;66:156–66.

49. Visser CA, Kan G, David GK, et al. Two-dimensional echocardiography in the diagnosis of left ventricular thrombus: a prospective study of 67 patients with anatomic validation. Chest 1983;83:228–32.

50. Neskovic AN, Marinkovic J, Bojic M, et al. Predictors of left ventricular thrombus formation and disappearance after anterior wall myocardial infarction. Eur Heart J 1998;19:908–16.

51. Hilden T, Inversen K, Raaschon F, et al. Anticoagulants in acute myocardial infarction. Lancet 1961;2:327–31.

52. Vecchio C, Chiarella F, Lupi G, et al. Left ventricular thrombus in anterior acute myocardial infarction after thrombolysis. A GISSI-2 connected study. Circulation 1991;84:512–19.

53. Spirito P, Belloti P, Chiarella F, et al. Prognostic significance and natural history of left ventricular thrombi in patients with acute anterior myocardial infarction: a twodimensional echocardiographic study. Circulation 1985;72:774–80.

54. Nihoyannopoulos P, Smith GC, Maseri A, et al. The natural history of left ventricular thrombus in myocardial infarction: a rationale in support of masterly inactivity. J Am Coll Cardiol 1989;14:903–11.

55. Jugdutt BI, Sivaram CA. Prospective two-dimensional echocardiographic evaluation of left ventricular thrombus and embolism after acute myocardial infarction. J Am Coll Cardiol 1989;13:554–64.

56. Kupper AJ, Verheught FW, Peels CH, et al. Left ventricular thrombus incidence and behavior studied by serial two-dimensional echocardiography in acute anterior myocardial

infarction, ventricular wall motion, systemic embolism and oral anticoagulation. J Am Coll Cardiol 1989;13:1514–20.

57. Eigler N, Maurer G, Shah PK. Effect of early systemic thrombolytic therapy on left ventricular mural thrombus formation in acute myocardial infarction. Am J Cardiol 1984;54:261–3.

58. Visser CA, Kan G, Meltzer RS, et al. Long-term follow-up of left ventricular thrombus after acute myocardial infarction: a two-dimensional echocardiographic study in 96 patients. Chest 1984;86:532–6.

59. Stratton JR, Nemanich JW, Johannessen KA, et al. Fate of left ventricular thrombi in patients with remote myocardial infarction or idiopathic cardiomyopathy. Circulation 1988;78:1388–93.

60. Setaro JF, Cabin HS. Right ventricular infarction. Cardiol Clin 1992;10:69–90.

61. Mehta SR, Eikelboom JW, Natarajan MK, et al. Impact of right ventricular involvement on mortality and morbidity in patients with inferior myocardial infarction. J Am Coll Cardiol 2001;37:37–43.

62. Haji SA, Movahed A. Right ventricular infarction—diagnosis and treatment. Clin Cardiol 2000;23:473–82.

63. Bellamy GR, Rasmussen HH, Nasser FN, et al. Value of two dimensional echocardiography, electrocardiography and clinicalsigns in detecting right ventricular infarction. Am Heart J 1986;112:304–9.

64. Kozakova M, Palombo C, Distante A. Right ventricular infarction: the role of echocardiography. Echocardiography 2001;18:701–7.

65. D'Arcy B, Nanda NC. Two-dimensional echocardiographic features of right ventricular infarction. Circulation 1982;65:167–73.

66. Casazza F, Bongarzoni A, Capozi A, Agostoni O. Regional right ventricular dysfunction in acute pulmonary embolism and right ventricular infarction. Eur J Echocardiogr 2005; 6(1):11–4.

67. Legrand V, Rigo P. Premature opening of the pulmonary valve in right ventricular infarction. Acta Cardiol 1982;37:227–31.

68. Ketikoglou DG, Karvounis HI, Papadopoulos CE, et al. Echocardiographic evaluation of spontaneous recovery of right ventricular systolic and diastolic function in patients with acute right ventricular infarction associated with posterior wall left ventricular infarction. Am J Cardiol 2004;93:911–3.

69. Daubert JC, Langella B, Besson C, et al. Etude prospective des critères diagnostiques et pronostiques de l'atteinte ventriculaire droite à la phase aiguë des infarctus infero-postérieurs. Arch Mal Coeur 1983;76:991–1003.

70. Descaves C, Daubert J, Langella B, et al. L'insuffisance tricuspidienne des infarctus du myocarde biventriculaire. Arch Mal Coeur 1985;78:1287–98.

71. Rietveld AP, Merrman L, Essed CE, et al. Right to left shunt with severe hypoxemia, at the atrial level in a patient with hemodynamically important right ventricular infarction. J Am Coll Cardiol 1983;2:776–9.

72. Galve E, Garcia-Del-Castillo H, Evangelista A, et al. Pericardial effusion in the course of myocardial infarction: incidence, natural history, and clinical relevance. Circulation 1986;73:294–9.

73. Otasevic P, Neskovic AN, Bojic M, et al. Pericardial effusion after thrombolysis for acute myocardial infarction: an echocardiographic 1-year follow-up study. Cardiology 1997;88:544–7.

74. Correale E, Maggioni AP, Romano S, et al. Comparison of frequency, diagnostic and prognostic significance of pericardial involvement in acute myocardial infarction treated with and without thrombolytics. Am J Cardiol 1993;71:1377–81.

Echocardiography in acute heart failure and cardiogenic shock

4

Sean P. Murphy and Michael H. Picard

Key Points

- The value of echocardiography in acute heart failure and cardiogenic shock includes its use for efficiently diagnosing cause, guiding management, quantifying response to therapy, and assessing prognosis, which may result in improved outcome.
- The incidence of cardiogenic shock after myocardial infarction (MI) remains relatively unchanged, and it is still a major cause of death in patients hospitalized with acute MI.
- The role of echo in cardiogenic shock is at least twofold. First, it is used early after presentation to assist in the rapid diagnosis of the cause of shock; second, it is used later to assess the response or effect of treatment.
- The most common cause of post-MI cardiogenic shock is severe left ventricular (LV) dysfunction, but other causes include mechanical complications of MI and right ventricular (RV) infarction.
- Early assessment of the severity of mitral regurgitation (MR) and the left ventricular ejection fraction (LVEF) are strong predictors of prognosis in patients with heart failure and those with cardiogenic shock.

ECHOCARDIOGRAPHY IN ACUTE HEART FAILURE

Heart failure (HF) is a clinical syndrome in which structural or functional abnormalities of the heart result in elevated intracardiac pressures and/or inadequate cardiac output at rest or during exercise.[1] Approximately 1–2% of the adult population in developed countries has HF, with the prevalence rising to ≥10% among persons 70 years of age or older.[2]

Echocardiography provides value on multiple levels ranging from use in those with early symptoms to use in those with advanced end-stage HF, including in diagnosis, etiologic classification, assessment of response to therapy, guidance of advanced treatments, and identification of prognosis. The echocardiogram can be *tailored to the need*—be it a complete initial diagnostic assessment with a fully equipped machine or a quick check of left ventricular ejection fraction (LVEF) with a handheld device. Its use can assist in *appropriate triage* to medical therapy or advanced treatments such as cardiac resynchronization therapy or mechanical circulatory support (MCS) devices. Thus, it has an important role in determining who to treat, how to treat, and when to treat.

Acute HF may arise de novo and present acutely, as in the case of acute myocardial infarction (MI), acute valvular

TABLE 4.1 Echocardiographic Assessment Checklist in Acute Heart Failure

- Regional and global left ventricular function
- Regional and global right ventricular function
- Left ventricular diastolic function
- Valvular structure and function
- Aorta
- Pericardial pathology
- Preload
- Pulmonary pressures
- Cardiac output
- Space-occupying lesions

disease, myocarditis (V4.1), or toxic effects of chemotherapy (V4.2A and V4.2B). More commonly, however, a chronic HF condition may decompensate suddenly (V4.3). Use of echocardiography *early at presentation* in patients with suspected acute HF improves disease identification and results in more efficient triage to appropriate medical care.[3] Echocardiography provides immediate information about cardiac anatomy (e.g., volumes, geometry, and mass) and function (e.g., left ventricular [LV] function and wall motion, valvular function, right ventricular (RV) function, pulmonary artery pressure, and pericardial physiology) (Table 4.1).[4–11]

Echocardiography can *classify patients with acute HF* into three groups according to whether the LVEF is reduced (≤40%), mildly reduced (41–49%) or preserved (≥50%).[12] Heart failure with reduced ejection fraction (HFrEF) results from impaired LV systolic function accompanied by adverse cardiac remodeling, in which the LV cavity size dilates over time. Heart failure with preserved ejection fraction (HFpEF) is a more heterogenous disorder with cardiac and extracardiac organ system involvement, with varying contributions from diastolic dysfunction (impaired LV relaxation and/or reduced LV filling), right ventricular dysfunction, pulmonary vascular disease, left atrial myopathy, arterial stiffness, skeletal muscle dysfunction and impaired peripheral oxygen extraction.[13]

EF is a universal measure of *global LV function* that has prognostic importance and guides various treatments.[14] The recommended two-dimensional echocardiographic method for this measurement is the *biplane method of discs*[15] (Figure 4.1). The accuracy of this method is dependent on detection of endocardial borders. The use of an ultrasound enhancing agent (also known as echocardiographic contrast) to better delineate such borders is recommended when image quality is suboptimal (i.e., where <80% of the endocardial border is adequately visualized). In addition, more routine use of echocardiographic contrast in patients admitted with acute HF may reduce downstream testing and healthcare costs and lead to shorter length of hospital stay.[16] Methods of calculating EF from linear dimensions may result in inaccuracies, particularly in patients with regional LV dysfunction, because in such patients the function in any one plane may underestimate or overestimate the global function. *Visual assessment* of EF should be used as an adjunct or an internal check that the calculated value is in the correct range.[17] In addition to assessment of global LVEF, it is important to evaluate regional LV systolic function including

adequate visualization of the LV apex where akinesis may predispose to LV thrombus formation.

LVEF is not an index of contractility because it depends on volumes, preload, afterload (V4.4A and V4.4B), heart rate, and valvular function. It is not the same as stroke volume. In fact, in a patient with HFrEF, stroke volume may be maintained by LV dilation, whereas it may be reduced in patients with HFpEF and concentric LV hypertrophy. EF will also be preserved, and forward stroke volume will be reduced in patients with significant mitral or aortic regurgitation. Thus, EF must be interpreted in its clinical context.

In patients with acute HF, the *assessment of RV size and function* is important in order to determine if the source of symptoms is an RV, an LV, or a biventricular problem. For example, conditions that primarily affect the right side of the heart, such as pulmonary embolus (Chapter 7), RV MI (Chapter 3), pulmonary hypertension, or decompensated pulmonary disease, may cause symptoms that are similar to HFrEF. Although biomarkers such as brain natriuretic peptide (BNP) quickly identify that the heart is the cause of dyspnea, they are not able to localize whether the RV or LV is to blame, nor can they determine if the EF is reduced or preserved. Owing to the geometry of the RV and the fact that its inflow portion, apex, and outflow tract cannot all be imaged in any single two-dimensional plane, RV function quantitation is more complex than LV function quantitation. Current echocardiographic measures include fractional area change and measures of longitudinal myocardial excursion such as tricuspid annular plane systolic excursion (TAPSE), peak tricuspid annular velocity (s'), and RV free-wall global longitudinal strain.[8] There is increasing interest in metrics that account for RV afterload when describing RV function, referred to as indices reflecting "RV—pulmonary artery (PA) coupling," such as the TAPSE/PA systolic pressure (PASP) ratio[18] (Figure 4.2) The segmental and global RV longitudinal strain can be measured by speckle tracking and is considered a more sensitive marker of systolic function than echocardiographic measures that rely on changes in the RV volume.[19]

In patients with acute HF, *the valves should be evaluated* by Doppler echocardiography to quantify degrees of regurgitation or stenosis, because either can be a cause of HF symptoms. Mitral and tricuspid regurgitation can be classified as primary (i.e., a disease of the valve apparatus) or secondary (i.e., a disease of the atrium or ventricle). The latter also known as functional regurgitation is commonly present in patients with acute HF as ventricular dilation and dysfunction leads to leaflet tethering and imbalance between opening and closing forces on the valve. Careful evaluation of the etiology and severity of valvular regurgitation should be performed. In certain patients with severe secondary mitral regurgitation (MR) despite medical optimization, the structure of the mitral valve and its apparatus should be assessed so that suitability for new percutaneous treatments (see Chapter 22) such as transcatheter edge-to-edge repair (TEER) can be determined.[20] The tricuspid valve regurgitant peak velocity, coupled with measurement of inferior vena cava (IVC) diameter and its response during respiration, provides estimates of PASP and central venous

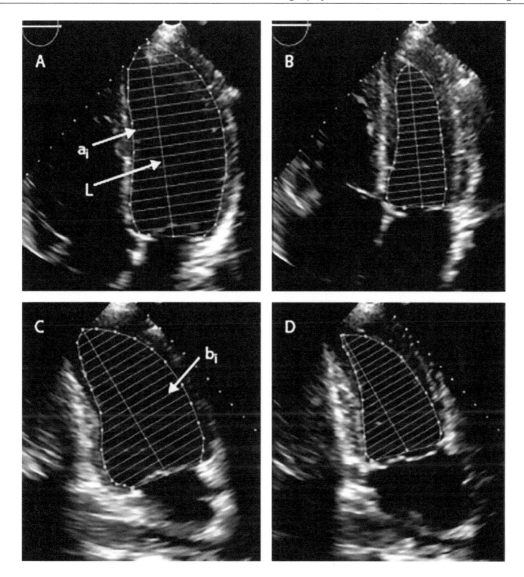

FIGURE 4.1 Determination of left ventricular (LV) volumes from transthoracic echocardiogram. The biplane method of discs is used to measure the left ventricular end-diastolic volume (EDV) and end-systolic volume (ESV) with subsequent calculation of the ejection fraction (EF). In each image the endocardial border is traced to depict the LV cavity. A series of discs of equal height (length (L)/20) are then constructed from the traced area. The dimensions of each disc from the apical four-chamber (ai) and two-chamber (bi) views are used to calculate the volume of each disc, and then the total volume is calculated as a summation of all disc volumes. In this case, the EDV is 177 mL, the ESV is 54 mL, and the derived EF is 70%. (A) Apical four-chamber end-diastolic frame. (B) Apical four-chamber end-systolic frame. (C) Apical two-chamber end-diastolic frame. (D) Apical two-chamber end-systolic frame.

pressure (CVP).[8,21] Pericardial diseases and pericardial effusions may be associated with acute HF or may mimic acute HF symptoms. Cardiac tamponade should be considered in the differential diagnosis when appropriate (Chapter 8).

The *diagnosis of HFpEF is more difficult* than the diagnosis of HFrEF as there is no widely accepted consensus on how to define it, with various society and clinical trial criteria.[22] Potential non-cardiac causes of the patient's symptoms such as anemia or chronic lung disease must first be discounted.[4,5] Usually, patients with HFpEF do not have a dilated heart, and many have an increase in LV wall thickness and left atrial (LA) size (Figure 4.3).

There is no single echocardiographic parameter that is sufficiently accurate and reproducible to be used in isolation to make a diagnosis of LV diastolic dysfunction, with current guidelines recommending a multiparametric approach to establish the diagnosis.[23] Therefore, a comprehensive echocardiographic examination incorporating all relevant two-dimensional and Doppler echocardiographic data is necessary. This should include the evaluation of both structural (LV hypertrophy, LA dilation) and functional abnormalities. Quantification of transmitral valve and mitral annular velocities allows for the assessment of LV diastolic filling and function. Specifically, the different patterns of LV relaxation abnormalities and impairment of LV filling can be categorized based on the ratio of early (E) and late (A) transmitral velocities, E deceleration time, and mitral annular early diastolic velocity (e′). A normal e′ is very unusual in a patient with HF,

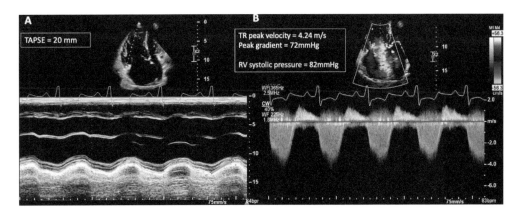

FIGURE 4.2 A patient with significant pulmonary hypertension and severe tricuspid regurgitation. (A) TAPSE was measured at 20 mm using M-mode echocardiography. (B) Peak systolic velocity of the tricuspid regurgitation jet was 4.24 m/sec using continuous-wave Doppler, corresponding to an estimated pulmonary artery systolic pressure of 82 mmHg when accounting for right atrial pressure. In this case, the TAPSE/PASP ratio is 20/82 = 0.24, which is consistent with abnormal RV-PA coupling and has been associated with worse prognosis.

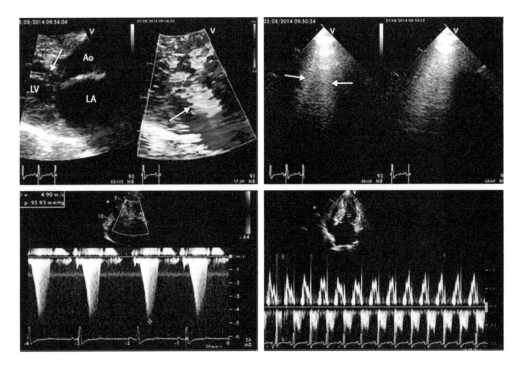

FIGURE 4.3 A 24-year-old female patient was admitted to the coronary care unit because of hypotensive pulmonary edema (blood pressure 85/55 mmHg) associated with harsh systolic cardiac murmur on auscultation. Lung ultrasound revealed multiple bilateral B-lines (lung comets) reflective of extravascular lung water resulting from decompensated hypertrophic cardiomyopathy (arrows, upper right panel). A marked septal hypertrophy was present (V4.10), along with systolic anterior motion (SAM) of the anterior mitral valve leaflet (upper left panel, arrow) causing a very high left ventricular outflow tract gradient of 95 mmHg (lower left panel). In addition, the SAM leads to altered mitral valve leaflet coaptation and significant mitral regurgitation (upper left panel). Also note pseudonormal filling pattern (lower right panel), as indicated by changes of transmitral inflow pattern from normal to impaired relaxation during forced respiration as a result of dyspnea, which may be considered as a Valsalva maneuver equivalent in this case. Instead of diuretics, this patient with hypertrophic obstructive cardiomyopathy was cautiously treated with intravenous beta-blockers, and as blood pressure rose and heart rate slowed down, her condition improved. Ao: aorta; LA: left atrium; LV: left ventricle.

(Images and video provided by IS.)

except in constrictive pericarditis where the septal e′ velocity is normal or increased. In addition to delayed relaxation and pseudonormal or restrictive transmitral filling patterns, echocardiographic evidence of LV diastolic dysfunction may consist of a reduced e′ (septal e′ velocity <7 cm/s or lateral e′ velocity <10 cm/s), an increased E/e′ ratio (>14), TR peak velocity >2.8 m/s and left atrial volume index >34 mL/m². [23] The E/e′ ratio typically correlates with LV filling pressure in chronic HF but *may not* correlate with filling pressures in acute decompensated HF.[24]

The use of echocardiography is recommended by most guidelines for the management of patients with suspected congestive HF. Data derived from echocardiography also are useful in *assessing prognosis* in patients with HF. The presence and degrees of LV hypertrophy, dilatation, diastolic dysfunction, and pulmonary hypertension, as determined by echocardiography, have been shown, in addition to LVEF, to have predictive value in patients with HF.[25–28] Speckle-tracking echocardiography allows for measurement of LV global longitudinal strain[29] and LA strain,[30] both of which are prognostic markers in acute HF independent of LVEF.

In the vasodilator–heart failure trials (V-HeFT I and V-HeFT II), baseline clinical variables were not helpful in predicting the HF patients who would experience an improvement in LV function. However, changes in LVEF were a strong predictor of mortality.[26]

Pulmonary hypertension, as estimated by the velocity of tricuspid regurgitation, is also associated with adverse outcome in HF patients. Although the degree of LV dysfunction is not independently predictive of pulmonary artery pressure, independent echocardiographic predictors of pulmonary artery pressure include mitral valve E deceleration time and the effective regurgitant orifice area of secondary MR.[27] A restrictive LV filling pattern (E deceleration time <150 ms) is a powerful predictor of mortality and need for advanced therapies such as heart transplantation.[28]

RV dysfunction may be an indicator of impending decompensation or poor prognosis in HF patients. It may develop via various mechanisms: it may arise as a consequence of pulmonary venous congestion and an increase in pulmonary arterial pressure secondary to LV failure, or it may be caused by the primary cardiomyopathic process involving the right ventricle[31] (V4.3). RV size and function have important prognostic value. Symptoms and LVEF have been shown to be worse in patients with biventricular dysfunction (V4.11A, V4.11B) than in those with LV dysfunction alone.[32] In addition, patients with ischemic cardiomyopathy and severely depressed LVEF have increased 2-year mortality when they have worse RV function.[33] A low TAPSE/PASP ratio (<0.35), reflecting impaired RV-PA coupling, is associated with in-hospital and 1-year mortality in cardiac intensive care unit patients.[34] RV peak systolic strain and its improvement after medical therapy of advanced decompensated HF are also markers of prognosis.[35]

ECHOCARDIOGRAPHY IN CARDIOGENIC SHOCK

Cardiogenic shock (CS) may be defined as a state in which an abnormality of cardiac structure or function results in inadequate cardiac output with clinical and biochemical evidence of end-organ hypoperfusion. Hemodynamic definitions are variable, although patients with CS typically have persistent hypotension (systolic blood pressure [SBP] <90 mmHg for >30 minutes, or requiring catecholamines to maintain SBP >90 mmHg) with severe reduction in the cardiac index (<1.8 L/min/m^2 without support or <2.0 to 2.2 L/min/m^2 with support) and adequate or elevated ventricular filling pressure.[36] The severity of cardiogenic shock can be graded according to the Society for Cardiovascular Angiography and Interventions (SCAI) SHOCK classification system, which allocates patients as Stage A ("at risk"), Stage B ("beginning"), Stage C ("classic"), Stage D ("deteriorating"), or Stage E ("extremis").[37] The SCAI SHOCK classification has been validated to correlate with mortality in patients both with and without acute myocardial infarction cardiogenic shock (AMI-CS), and has been recently updated with further gradations of severity within each stage.[38]

Despite advances in pharmacologic, mechanical, and reperfusion strategies, the mortality rate of CS remains high with contemporary registry data reporting in-hospital mortality rates of ~40% in AMI-CS and ~25% in CS related to advanced HF.[39,40] This syndrome remains a challenge, and the prudent use of echocardiography can assist in managing these patients and in reducing the unacceptably high mortality.

In patients with CS complicating acute MI, there is often concern regarding performing a left ventriculogram at the time of coronary angiography because a contrast load can adversely affect hemodynamics and further impair renal function. Only 44% of all patients who underwent coronary angiography had an LV angiogram in the "*Sh*ould we emergently revascularize *o*ccluded *c*oronaries for cardiogenic shoc*k*?" (SHOCK) trial. Echocardiographic assessments of LV function and degree of MR are generally a reliable substitute for a left ventriculogram in the setting of acute CS.[41]

Echocardiography is a valuable tool in the assessment and management of the patient with suspected or confirmed cardiogenic shock. *Early use of echocardiography* allows for rapid diagnosis of the cause of shock, timely recognition of patients in whom early implementation of mechanical circulatory support (MCS) or surgical intervention may be necessary (e.g., ruptured papillary muscle or ventricular septal rupture) and facilitates monitoring the response or effect of treatment. It has been established that echocardiography and specific features of cardiac structure or function early in the course of CS can provide prognostic value.[42] For example, higher SCAI SHOCK classification and in-hospital mortality have been associated with LVEF <40%, stroke volume index <35 mL/m^2 and medial E/e′ >15 after multivariable adjustment.[43]

Echocardiography provides incremental diagnostic information for diagnosing or excluding CS. CS can be readily excluded if there is normal or hyperkinetic ventricular function in the absence of valvular heart disease. In addition, intravascular volume status can be assessed using 2D echocardiography by measuring IVC diameter and percent IVC collapse with sniff (caval index),[44] although IVC collapsibility index by 3D echocardiography is a newer method that more accurately correlates with CVP.[45]

Establishing the cause of cardiogenic shock

Transthoracic echocardiography (TTE) can be used acutely in the evaluation of the patient with symptoms of acute HF or cardiogenic shock that is suspected due to acute MI, through recognition of LV regional wall motion abnormalities in a coronary distribution. Moreover, in the patient with left bundle branch block or other ECG abnormalities that may obscure the classic ECG findings in MI, the echocardiogram can be used to establish the diagnosis of significant LV dysfunction as the cause of shock.

Although the most common cause of post-MI CS is severe LV systolic dysfunction from a *large area of ischemic myocardial dysfunction* (V4.5), one must also consider *other causes of shock*. In an international registry of CS, as many as 15% of those with post-MI CS were found to have a cause other than LV dysfunction. Mechanical causes such as acute MR or ventricular septal rupture were found in 8% and isolated RV shock in 2%, and 5% of the patients had concurrent conditions contributing to the development of shock, including severe valve disease, hypovolemia, or sepsis.[46] These data suggest that clinical evaluation alone is not accurate enough to establish the cause of shock in all post-MI patients. In addition, this registry found that it took a much longer time to make the diagnosis of a mechanical cause of shock, with a median time from MI

onset to shock diagnosis of 24 hours. This was a significantly longer time than in patients with primary LV failure (8 hours). While the current incidence of mechanical complications of acute MI has decreased to 0.27% compared to 1.7% in the pre-reperfusion era, such patients have a high mortality rate of at least 40%.[47] Echocardiography plays a valuable role in the prompt recognition of this critical diagnosis so that timely implementation of mechanical circulatory support (MCS) as a bridge to corrective surgery can be instituted (Chapter 15) before the development of irreversible end-organ damage.

TTE provides a *rapid bedside assessment of wall motion and global LV function*. The most common echocardiographic findings early in the course of CS are those of a dilated hypocontractile left ventricle (Figure 4.4) (V4.3) (V4.6). In those with prior infarctions, the entire ventricle may show diffuse hypokinesis or akinesis (V4.7). In those with shock caused by an extensive first MI, a more regional pattern of wall motion reflecting the coronary distribution will be present. In those with a significant infarction but patency of one or both of the other coronary arteries, a zone of hyperkinesis may be identified in the early stages of MI. This is a compensatory response to the falling stroke volume. In contrast, if this early compensatory hyperkinesis is not noted, there is increased likelihood that significant coronary artery disease exists in these other territories.[48] In addition to LV dysfunction, RV involvement may or may not be present. Studies of

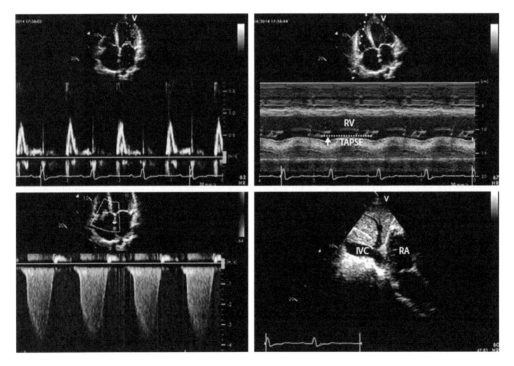

FIGURE 4.4   In a patient with severe acute heart failure leading to cardiogenic shock with severe biventricular systolic dysfunction (V4.3 and V4.6), the restrictive transmitral flow pattern indicates high left ventricular filling pressures (upper left panel), and the velocity of tricuspid regurgitation jet indicates high right heart systolic pressures (of around 70 mmHg) (lower left panel). TAPSE of 8 mm confirms poor right ventricular function (upper right panel), and the non-collapsible inferior vena cava indicates congestion (lower right panel) (V4.3). IVC: inferior vena cava; RA: right atrium; RV: right ventricle; TAPSE: tricuspid annular plane systolic excursion.

(Images and video provided by PMM.)

HF patients suggest that those with biventricular involvement have a poorer outcome.[49,50]

MR is commonly present in the enlarged hypokinetic heart. With LV enlargement, the papillary muscles become displaced from their usual relationship to the mitral valve (MV) leaflets and annulus. This apical displacement results in a tethering of the leaflets and incomplete closure of the valve (Figure 4.5) (V4.8A and V4.8B) (V4.9). Quantification by color Doppler may be more challenging when the heart rate is increased, limiting the period of systole available for Doppler detection of regurgitation. Moreover, as the pressure difference between the left ventricle and the left atrium decreases as the LV dP/dt decreases and LA pressure rises, the MR velocity may be lower and more difficult to detect. For those in sinus rhythm, a *restrictive* transmitral velocity filling pattern is often detected by pulse-wave Doppler, reflecting the decreased LV compliance and elevated LA pressures. Numerous studies in HF patients have identified this as a marker of adverse outcome.[51]

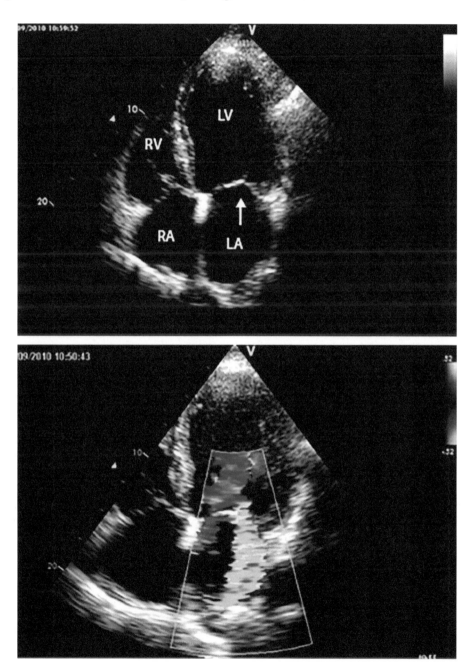

FIGURE 4.5   Significant functional mitral regurgitation. Apical four-chamber view of a transthoracic echocardiogram displays dilated left ventricle (upper panel) with severely reduced left ventricular function in a patient with acute decompensated heart failure caused by dilated cardiomyopathy (V4.8A). Because of the left ventricular dilation, there is apical displacement (arrow) of the mitral valve leaflet tips (incomplete mitral leaflet closure) resulting in abnormal coaptation of the leaflets and severe mitral regurgitation (lower panel) (V4.8B). LA: left atrium; LV: left ventricle; RA: right atrium; RV: right ventricle.

(Images and videos provided by RV.)

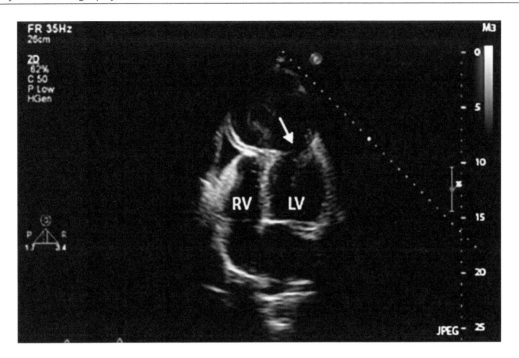

FIGURE 4.6   Apical four-chamber view of a transthoracic echocardiogram from a 70-year-old man who developed recurrent chest pain and shock 3 days after presenting with myocardial infarction. An apical pseudoaneurysm due to cardiac rupture was identified as the cause of shock. The arrow shows the narrow neck or communication of the pseudoaneurysm with the left ventricle. LV: left ventricle; RV: right ventricle.

TABLE 4.2   Common Abnormalities Seen in Patients Presenting with Cardiogenic Shock

Extensive left ventricular dysfunction
Right ventricular dysfunction/dilation
Papillary muscle rupture
Ventricular septal rupture
Left ventricular free-wall rupture
Pseudoaneurysm formation
Aortic dissection

TTE is uniquely suited to identify the cause of shock from a *mechanical complication* (Chapter 3) after MI (Figure 4.6). A knowledge of the risk factors for post-MI mechanical complications is important to increase one's level of suspicion for these abnormalities. The risk factors include older age, female gender, first MI, hypertension, delayed recognition of infarction, and continued physical activity after MI.[47] In the shock patient with a cause other than extensive LV dysfunction to explain the condition, it is not unusual for the LV to be small and hyperkinetic. Thus, even if the image quality on TTE is inadequate to identify a papillary muscle rupture or ventricular septal rupture, the presence of a small, hyperkinetic LV in the setting of shock should raise the suspicion of a mechanical complication. Another clue to the presence of a mechanical complication is a hyperdynamic LV combined with a low LV outflow tract velocity time integral or reduced aortic leaflet opening. Table 4.2 shows the most common abnormalities seen in patients presenting with CS. Each of them has findings on the echocardiogram that should discriminate it from the others.

Although TTE is typically the first imaging tool used in the early assessment of CS, transesophageal echocardiography (TEE) can be safely used by experienced operators. Careful attention to the type and degree of medications used for sedation and their potential for exacerbating the altered hemodynamic state is critical. *Important indications for TEE* are when (1) the TTE is of inadequate quality to visualize cardiac structures, (2) the clinician has a high index of suspicion for a mechanical complication and it is not identified by TTE, or (3) the degree of hemodynamic instability is unexplained, as in a patient with a small region of abnormal LV wall motion but CS, or a patient who remains in shock despite aggressive treatment, including reperfusion and revascularization. With a current focus on acute MI treatment strategies that include primary percutaneous coronary interventions but may not include LV angiography, one must remember that such revascularization procedures will not reverse the effects of a papillary muscle transection or ventricular septal rupture that occurred before the intervention. Thus, TEE may be a critical adjunct in the patient with persistent hemodynamic compromise despite an open infarct-related artery.

Studies have suggested that *handheld echocardiographic devices* (HUDs) (Chapter 18) can add to the clinical assessment in patients presenting with HF and thus even those with shock. Because traditional bedside examination to assess volume status (including the jugular venous pressure [JVP], peripheral edema, and ascites) has poor sensitivity[52,53] and significant interobserver and intraobserver variability, the addition of point-of-care imaging with these small ultrasound devices may have a role.[54] Most therapeutic interventions in acute decompensated HF target optimization of cardiac output and volume status. Therefore, an HUD may provide accurate bedside evaluation of the LVEF and volume status (Chapter 19) in patients with decompensated HF and thus help guide therapy.[54]

Role of early echocardiography as a prognostic tool

The SHOCK trial was an international, multicenter, randomized trial of acute treatment in CS. The trial demonstrated a 6-month and 1-year survival benefit for patients who received early emergency revascularization compared with initial medical stabilization.[55,56] Two-dimensional echocardiograms were performed on entry into the trial and thus offer a unique opportunity to assess the value of echocardiography and clarify the pathophysiology of this disease.

In the SHOCK trial, the mean LVEF of the 175 early echocardiograms was 30 ± 11.5% (the median LVEF was 28%), demonstrating that there is a wide range of systolic function in patients with CS. This LVEF was usually measured while patients were on inotropic and/or intra-aortic balloon pump (IABP) support.[57] The LVEF, however, was similar in the acute phase of CS and 2 weeks later. At least mild MR was found in 39% of the patients.[42]

The significant univariate predictors of 1-year survival were LVEF, LV end-diastolic volume, LV end-systolic volume, and the severity of MR. For example, regardless of the treatment arm, patients with less than mild MR on the entry echocardiogram had a 58% 1-year survival compared with a 31% 1-year survival for those with mild or worse MR. Those with an LVEF of less than 28% had a 24% 1-year survival compared with a 56% 1-year survival for those with LVEF greater than or equal to 28%. Multivariate analysis showed that both LVEF and MR provided independent prognostic information. Regardless of the treatment arm, an important survival difference was noted for those with 0 to 1+ MR and an LVEF greater than or equal to 28% on presentation with shock (70% 1-year survival) compared with patients with 2+ to 4+ MR and LVEF of less than 28% (10% 1-year survival).[42]

An important finding of this study is that the prognostic features on the echocardiogram early in the course of CS (LVEF and MR) are the same as for less complicated MI except that the cutoff point or threshold value may differ.[58–60]

As would be expected, the extent and severity of regional dysfunction, the end-diastolic volume, the end-systolic volume, and the sphericity of the LV all influenced the LVEF. The degree of MR on this early echocardiogram was related to factors that influenced mitral leaflet geometry, especially the LV end-diastolic volume.[42]

Because severe MR is a marker of worse coronary artery disease and worse prognosis, the presence of MR should be specifically evaluated and sought as a marker of high risk. Other echocardiographic risk markers for in-hospital mortality in patients admitted to the cardiac intensive care unit include stroke volume index <35 mL/m^2 and mitral E/e′ >15.[43]

Role of echocardiography in triage and management of mechanical circulatory support devices

Temporary MCS can be considered to stabilize those acutely ill patients with CS who demonstrate inadequate tissue perfusion despite therapy with mechanical ventilation, reperfusion, and inotropic pharmacologic agents. A range of temporary MCS devices are available, with device selection dependent on whether isolated LV, RV, or biventricular support is necessary and whether support for respiratory failure is also required. Temporary MCS options include the intra-aortic balloon pump (IABP), percutaneous RV or LV assist devices (LVADs), and extracorporeal membrane oxygenation (ECMO). Temporary MCS is theoretically appealing to interrupt the vicious spiral of ischemia, hypotension, and myocardial dysfunction. It allows for recovery of stunned and hibernating myocardium and reversal of neurohormonal derangements.[57] Typically, the goal of early temporary MCS is to bridge the patient to myocardial recovery, surgical revascularization, or more permanent heart replacement therapy such as durable surgical LVAD or heart transplant.

Echocardiography is an essential tool in identifying patients for triage to MCS and plays a critical role in management after device implementation (Chapter 15). Uses of echocardiography includes *assessing appropriateness* for certain temporary MCS devices (such as a small LV cavity or the presence of an LV thrombus that would preclude use of percutaneous LVADs, or severe aortic regurgitation that would preclude use of IABP), excluding *device complications* in patients with worsening cardiopulmonary status (e.g., aortic dissection, aortic and MV insufficiency, thrombus, and cardiac tamponade), confirming *proper position* of the cannulae, assessing *effects of pump speeds* on RV and LV volume, evaluating the *need for an LV venting strategy* in patients on ECMO, and determining the *timing and degree of ventricular recovery*.[61,62]

In a study of 16 patients, *dobutamine stress echocardiography* was used to assess myocardial recovery in patients supported with LVADs (>30 days). Those with improved cardiac index, LV dP/dt, and LVEF and decreased LV end-diastolic dimension had a favorable outcome.[63]

Other studies on MCS patients have shown that echocardiographic parameters predictive of recovery include LVEF ≥45%, LV end-diastolic diameter ≤55 mm, and a relative wall thickness ≥0.38, as well as the pattern of aortic valve opening in response to changes in the degree of LVAD support or with exercise.[62,64] Aortic valve opening, in this situation, measures the ability of the left ventricle to generate sufficient force and output to support the circulation. In another study, mitral annular plane systolic excursion was found to reflect LV systolic and diastolic function in critically ill patients with shock and added to the predictive value for 28-day mortality.[65] This finding suggests that annular tissue velocities and myocardial strain may be of value. A protocol for MCS weaning using TEE monitoring has been described.[66]

Role of later echocardiography to assess response to therapy

For patients who have recovered from their shock syndrome, echocardiography can be of value later in their hospital course. First, this later assessment of cardiac structure and function can determine whether there has been a significant improvement compared with that at initial presentation. This includes assessment of LVEF, regional LV wall motion (as a marker of infarct size), MR, RV systolic pressure, and markers of LV remodeling, such as LV size, volume, and sphericity.[67,68]

This later echocardiogram *can assist management* in several ways. For example, the presence of decreased LV systolic function and significant regional LV dysfunction in patients with persistent severe HF despite maximal medical therapy may prompt the following: (1) consideration of revascularization in those who have not had such therapy, (2) consideration of a more complete revascularization in those who have undergone an early intervention on a culprit lesion, (3) need for implantable cardiac defibrillator, (4) consideration of long-term MCS, and (5) consideration of cardiac transplant.[69] On the other hand, the presence of a persistent decrease in functional capacity despite echocardiographic evidence of a significant improvement in LV function might suggest that the patient's clinical status is the result of other problems such as MR, deconditioning, another valve disease, or concomitant lung disease. In patients with persistent severe secondary MR despite medical optimization, echocardiography is important to identify the mechanism of MR and understand the MV anatomy so that it can be determined whether transcatheter MV intervention or surgery is necessary or feasible.

The use of transcatheter edge-to-edge repair (TEER) techniques have gained a significant role in the management of patients with secondary MR. However, certain patient or anatomic factors that may lead to risk for development of mitral stenosis, inadequate reduction in MR, inability to perform TEER or procedural futility must be assessed as part of the decision-making process for the procedure. Important MV features assessed include a short or restricted posterior mitral valve leaflet, size of the coaptation gap, severely calcified or fibrotic valve leaflets, clefts or mitral stenosis.[20] In such patients with secondary MR, understanding the "proportionality" of MR severity in comparison to the extent of LV dilation is important; patients with MR that is "disproportionately" worse than the degree of LV enlargement may be expected to derive greater benefit from TEER, although further research is necessary to better understand patient selection.[70]

A careful quantitation of the *regional LV wall motion* on this later echocardiogram and comparison to one performed earlier in the course of the disease can help identify areas of stunned myocardium that may have recovered. In addition, if there is any question about the suitability of a particular patient for late revascularization, the use of *dobutamine echocardiography* can identify those patients with viable myocardium and significant coronary artery disease.[71]

SUMMARY

Echocardiography has several roles in patients with acute HF and CS. First, early echocardiography can *assist in the prompt diagnosis* of the cause of symptoms. This can lead to appropriate therapy. Second, the echocardiogram can assist in *assessing prognosis*. Identification of high- and low-risk groups on the basis of echocardiographic parameters offers the potential for *more tailored therapy* for individuals early in the course of disease. Lastly, echocardiography can assist in assessing *response to therapy* and identifying *other causes* of the symptoms.

LIST OF VIDEOS

https://routledgetextbooks.com/textbooks/9781032157009/chapter-4.php

VIDEO 4.1   Acute heart failure presumably caused by myocarditis: A 35-year-old man with no previous history of heart disease had undergone outpatient treatment for interstitial pneumonia 3 weeks before hospital admission because of rapid onset of severe dyspnea and fatigue. In the emergency department, physical examination revealed distended jugular veins, basal lung rales, and an S₃ gallop. Transthoracic echocardiography from apical views (upper left video, four-chamber; upper right video, two-chamber; lower left video, long-axis) revealed severe global hypocontractility of the left ventricle with severely reduced global systolic function (reverberation artifact can be noted in all views). There was a restrictive transmitral flow pattern (high E-wave, short DT, absent A-wave) suggesting high left ventricular (LV) filling pressures (lower right panel). After 2 weeks of intensive heart failure therapy, clinical improvement was achieved but without significant recovery of LV function. The patient was considered a heart transplant candidate. *(Video provided by PMM.)*

VIDEO 4.2A   Acute heart failure induced by cardiotoxic effects of chemotherapy (1/2): A 42-year-old woman was admitted to the intensive care unit because of severe dyspnea and cough. Twenty days before, she had received the first cycle of a chemotherapy protocol for nasal rhabdomyosarcoma, including etoposide and doxorubicin. She had no history of heart disease. Transthoracic parasternal long-axis view showed a dilated left ventricle with severe global systolic dysfunction (estimated ejection fraction of 25%) with some regional differences in contractility. Note hypercontractility of the posterior wall as opposed to the akinetic septum. After 10 days of treatment with angiotensin-converting enzyme (ACE) inhibitors, diuretics, and beta-blockers, dramatic improvement of global left ventricular function was noted (see Video 4.2B). *(Video provided by MMP.)*

VIDEO 4.2B   Acute heart failure induced by cardiotoxic effects of chemotherapy (2/2): Transthoracic parasternal long-axis view showing dramatic global left ventricular function improvement after 10 days of treatment with angiotensin-converting enzyme (ACE) inhibitors, diuretics, and beta-blockers in a patient with acute heart failure after cardiotoxic chemotherapy (see Video 4.2A). *(Video provided by MMP.)*

VIDEO 4.3   Acute decompensated heart failure caused by biventricular dysfunction: Transthoracic apical four-chamber (upper left video), apical two-chamber (upper right), apical long-axis (lower left), and parasternal short-axis (lower right) views showing severe global left ventricular systolic dysfunction with slightly better contractility of the basal lateral and basal posterior walls. Note severely hypokinetic ventricular free wall (upper left). Note the dilation of all heart chambers (see Figure 4.4 in the book). *(Video provided by PMM.)*

VIDEO 4.4A   Post–mitral valve repair acute heart failure (1/2): A 56-year-old man underwent mitral valve repair for chordal rupture for flail posterior mitral leaflet and severe mitral regurgitation. Preoperative transthoracic apical four-chamber view demonstrates posterior mitral leaflet flail as a result of chordal rupture and relatively good global left ventricular (LV) function. Note that the left ventricle was dilated (measured end-diastolic diameter was 70 mm, and end-systolic diameter was 51 mm). A few hours after successful mitral valve repair, in the cardiothoracic intensive care unit, low cardiac output syndrome developed. Echocardiography revealed dramatic deterioration of global LV function (see Video 4.4B) caused by acute increase of afterload after surgical correction of severe mitral regurgitation. *(Video provided by ANN.)*

VIDEO 4.4B   Post–mitral valve repair acute heart failure (2/2): A 56-year-old man underwent mitral valve repair for chordal rupture for posterior mitral leaflet and severe mitral regurgitation. A few hours after successful mitral valve repair, in the cardiothoracic intensive care unit, a low cardiac output syndrome developed. Echocardiography revealed dramatic deterioration of global left ventricular (LV) function (shown here), resulting from acute increase of afterload after surgical correction of severe mitral regurgitation. Preoperative study revealed relatively good global LV function (see Video 4.4A). *(Video provided by ANN.)*

VIDEO 4.5   Impending cardiogenic shock after recent extensive anterior myocardial infarction (MI): A 74-year-old woman was transferred from a regional center to a tertiary healthcare facility due to worsening heart failure after a recent anterior MI. Because of late presentation at the regional center (48 hours after the onset of pain), she did not receive reperfusion therapy. On admission she was hypotensive and cold, with slightly altered mental status and no signs of pulmonary or peripheral congestion. Transthoracic echocardiography revealed akinesis of the septum, apex, and distal part of the lateral wall (upper left video, four-chamber view), akinesis of the distal two-thirds of the anterior wall and hypokinesis of the inferior wall (upper right video, two-chamber view), akinesis of the anterior septum and apex (lower left video, apical long-axis view), and hypercontractility of the basal half of the lateral wall and posterior wall of

the left ventricle. The lower right panel shows estimation of cardiac output by measurement of left ventricular outflow tract (LVOT) diameter and LVOT VTI, which revealed an extremely low value of 2.5 L/min. *(Video provided by PMM.)*

VIDEO 4.6   Acute decompensated heart failure caused by biventricular dysfunction: Transthoracic apical four-chamber views show severe global left ventricular systolic dysfunction with slightly better contractility of basal lateral wall and dilated severely hypokinetic right ventricle. *(Video provided by PMM.)*

VIDEO 4.7   Cardiogenic shock after reinfarction: Apical four-chamber view of transthoracic echocardiogram from a patient with two prior myocardial infarctions who developed cardiogenic shock after another MI. Severely depressed left ventricular function with a degree of regional variability (lateral wall worse than septal wall). Right ventricular systolic function is at the lower limits of normal.

VIDEO 4.8A   Significant functional mitral regurgitation (1/2): Apical four-chamber view of a transthoracic echocardiogram displays dilated left ventricle with severely reduced left ventricular function in a patient with acute decompensated heart failure from dilated cardiomyopathy. Because of the left ventricular dilation, there is an apical displacement ("tenting") of the mitral valve leaflet tips (incomplete mitral leaflet closure), resulting in abnormal coaptation of the leaflets and severe functional mitral regurgitation (see Video 4.8B). *(Video provided by RV.)*

VIDEO 4.8B   Significant functional mitral regurgitation (2/2): Color Doppler transthoracic echocardiography (TTE) in apical four-chamber view showing a severe functional mitral regurgitation caused by left ventricular (LV) dilation and apical displacement ("tenting") of the mitral valve leaflet tips (incomplete mitral leaflet closure) (see Video 4.8A) resulting in abnormal coaptation of the leaflets in systole. *(Video provided by RV.)*

VIDEO 4.9   Significant functional mitral regurgitation in cardiogenic shock: Significant functional mitral regurgitation noted in apical four-chamber view of a transthoracic echocardiogram. The left ventricle is dilated and exhibits significantly reduced left ventricular (LV) function. Because of the LV dilation, there is apical displacement of the mitral valve leaflet tips (incomplete mitral leaflet closure) resulting in a reduction in the normal coaptation of the leaflets and severe mitral regurgitation.

VIDEO 4.10   Acute diastolic heart failure in a patient with hypertrophic obstructive cardiomyopathy: A 24-year-old female patient was admitted to the coronary care unit because of hypotensive (blood pressure 85/55 mmHg) pulmonary edema associated with a harsh systolic cardiac murmur on auscultation. Lung ultrasound revealed multiple bilateral B-lines (lung comets) reflective of extravascular lung water. This quad screen of different transthoracic echocardiography (TTE) views shows marked septal hypertrophy with supernormal global systolic function. Note systolic anterior motion (SAM) of the anterior mitral valve leaflet causing a very high left ventricular outflow tract gradient of 95 mmHg, associated with significant mitral regurgitation (see Figure 4.3 in the book). The transmitral filling pattern was pseudonormal, as indicated by changes in transmitral inflow pattern from normal to impaired relaxation during forced respiration as a result of dyspnea, which may be considered a Valsalva maneuver equivalent in this case (Figure 4.3 in the book). Instead of diuretics, the patient was cautiously treated with intravenous beta-blockers, and as blood pressure rose and heart rate slowed down, the patient improved. *(Video provided by IS.)*

VIDEO 4.11A   Acute myocarditis with acute heart failure (1/2). Transthoracic echocardiogram in a young lady with severe dyspnea, tachypnea, and hypotension after viral infection revealed severe biventricular dysfunction with massive intracavitary thrombosis of both ventricles (see also Video 4.11B). *(Video provided by GK.)*

VIDEO 4.11B   Acute myocarditis with acute heart failure (2/2). In modified transthoracic four-chamber view massive LV thrombosis is even better appreciated (see also Video 4.11A). *(Video provided by GK.)* Hypotension after viral infection revealed severe biventricular dysfunction with massive intracavitary thrombosis of both ventricles. *(Video provided by GK.)*

REFERENCES

1. McDonagh TA, Metra M, Adamo M, et al. 2021 ESC guidelines for the diagnosis and treatment of acute and chronic heart failure. *Eur Heart J.* 2021;42(36):3599–3726.
2. Mosterd A, Hoes AW. Clinical epidemiology of heart failure. *Heart.* 2007;93(9):1137–1146.
3. Francis CM, Caruana L, Kearney P, et al. Open access echocardiography in management of heart failure in the community. *BMJ.* 1995;310(6980):634–636.
4. Borlaug BA, Paulus WJ. Heart failure with preserved ejection fraction: pathophysiology, diagnosis, and treatment. *Eur Heart J.* 2011;32(6):670–679.
5. Paulus WJ, Tschöpe C, Sanderson JE, et al. How to diagnose diastolic heart failure: a consensus statement on the diagnosis of heart failure with normal left ventricular ejection fraction by the Heart Failure and Echocardiography Associations of the European Society of Cardiology. *Eur Heart J.* 2007;28(20):2539–2550.
6. Marwick TH, Raman SV, Carrió I, et al. Recent developments in heart failure imaging. *JACC Cardiovasc Imaging.* 2010;3(4):429–439.
7. Paterson DI, OMeara E, Chow BJ, et al. Recent advances in cardiac imaging for patients with heart failure. *Curr Opin Cardiol.* 2011;26(2):132–143.
8. Rudski LG, Lai WW, Afilalo J, et al. Guidelines for the echocardiographic assessment of the right heart in adults: a report from the American Society of Echocardiography endorsed by the European Association of Echocardiography, a registered branch of the European Society of Cardiology, and the Canadian Society of Echocardiography. *J Am Soc Echocardiogr.* 2010;23(7):685–713; quiz 786–688.
9. Dokainish H, Nguyen JS, Bobek J, et al. Assessment of the American Society of Echocardiography-European Association of Echocardiography guidelines for diastolic function in patients with depressed ejection fraction: an echocardiographic and invasive haemodynamic study. *Eur J Echocardiogr.* 2011;12(11):857–864.
10. Kirkpatrick JN, Vannan MA, Narula J, et al. Echocardiography in heart failure: applications, utility, and new horizons. *J Am Coll Cardiol.* 2007;50(5):381–396.
11. Nagueh SF, Bhatt R, Vivo RP, et al. Echocardiographic evaluation of hemodynamics in patients with decompensated systolic heart failure. *Circ Cardiovasc Imaging.* 2011;4(3):220–227.
12. Bozkurt B, Coats AJS, Tsutsui H, et al. Universal definition and classification of heart failure: a report of the Heart Failure Society of America, Heart Failure Association of the European Society of Cardiology, Japanese Heart Failure Society and Writing Committee of the Universal Definition of Heart Failure. *J Card Fail.* 2021;27(4):387–413.
13. Ho JE, Redfield MM, Lewis GD, et al. Deliberating the diagnostic dilemma of heart failure with preserved ejection fraction. *Circulation.* 2020;142(18):1770–1780.
14. Curtis JP, Sokol SI, Wang Y, et al. The association of left ventricular ejection fraction, mortality, and cause of death in stable outpatients with heart failure. *J Am Coll Cardiol.* 2003;42(4):736–742.
15. McMurray JJ, Adamopoulos S, Anker SD, et al. ESC Guidelines for the diagnosis and treatment of acute and chronic heart failure 2012: the Task Force for the Diagnosis and Treatment of Acute and Chronic Heart Failure 2012 of the European Society of Cardiology. Developed in collaboration with the Heart Failure Association (HFA) of the ESC. *Eur Heart J.* 2012;33(14):1787–1847.
16. Lee KC, Liu S, Callahan P, et al. Routine use of contrast on admission transthoracic echocardiography for heart failure reduces the rate of repeat echocardiography during index admission. *J Am Soc Echocardiogr.* 2021;34(12):1253–1261.e1254.
17. Lang RM, Bierig M, Devereux RB, et al. Recommendations for chamber quantification. *Eur J Echocardiogr.* 2006;7(2):79–108.
18. Guazzi M, Bandera F, Pelissero G, et al. Tricuspid annular plane systolic excursion and pulmonary arterial systolic pressure relationship in heart failure: an index of right ventricular contractile function and prognosis. *Am J Physiol Heart Circ Physiol.* 2013;305(9):H1373–1381.
19. Longobardo L, Suma V, Jain R, et al. Role of two-dimensional speckle-tracking echocardiography strain in the assessment of right ventricular systolic function and comparison with conventional parameters. *J Am Soc Echocardiogr.* 2017;30(10):937–946.e936.
20. Lim DS, Herrmann HC, Grayburn P, et al. Consensus document on non-suitability for transcatheter mitral valve repair by edge-to-edge therapy. *Structural Heart.* 2021;5(3):227–233.
21. Tsutsui RS, Borowski A, Tang WH, et al. Precision of echocardiographic estimates of right atrial pressure in patients with acute decompensated heart failure. *J Am Soc Echocardiogr.* 2014;27(10):1072–1078.e1072.
22. Ho JE, Zern EK, Wooster L, et al. Differential clinical profiles, exercise responses, and outcomes associated with existing HFpEF definitions. *Circulation.* 2019;140(5):353–365.
23. Nagueh SF, Smiseth OA, Appleton CP, et al. Recommendations for the evaluation of left ventricular diastolic function by echocardiography: an update from the American Society of Echocardiography and the European Association of Cardiovascular Imaging. *J Am Soc Echocardiogr.* 2016;29(4):277–314.
24. Mullens W, Borowski AG, Curtin RJ, et al. Tissue Doppler imaging in the estimation of intracardiac filling pressure in decompensated patients with advanced systolic heart failure. *Circulation.* 2009;119(1):62–70.

25. Stevenson WG, Stevenson LW, Middlekauff HR, et al. Sudden death prevention in patients with advanced ventricular dysfunction. *Circulation.* 1993;88(6):2953–2961.

26. Cintron G, Johnson G, Francis G, et al. Prognostic significance of serial changes in left ventricular ejection fraction in patients with congestive heart failure. The V-HeFT VA Cooperative Studies Group. *Circulation.* 1993;87(6 Suppl):Vi17–23.

27. Enriquez-Sarano M, Rossi A, Seward JB, et al. Determinants of pulmonary hypertension in left ventricular dysfunction. *J Am Coll Cardiol.* 1997;29(1):153–159.

28. Pinamonti B, Di Lenarda A, Sinagra G, et al. Restrictive left ventricular filling pattern in dilated cardiomyopathy assessed by Doppler echocardiography: clinical, echocardiographic and hemodynamic correlations and prognostic implications. Heart Muscle Disease Study Group. *J Am Coll Cardiol.* 1993;22(3):808–815.

29. Park JJ, Park JB, Park JH, et al. Global longitudinal strain to predict mortality in patients with acute heart failure. *J Am Coll Cardiol.* 2018;71(18):1947–1957.

30. Park JH, Hwang IC, Park JJ, et al. Prognostic power of left atrial strain in patients with acute heart failure. *Eur Heart J Cardiovasc Imaging.* 2021;22(2):210–219.

31. Voelkel NF, Quaife RA, Leinwand LA, et al. Right ventricular function and failure: report of a National Heart, Lung, and Blood Institute working group on cellular and molecular mechanisms of right heart failure. *Circulation.* 2006;114(17):1883–1891.

32. La Vecchia L, Paccanaro M, Bonanno C, et al. Left ventricular versus biventricular dysfunction in idiopathic dilated cardiomyopathy. *Am J Cardiol.* 1999;83(1):120–122, a129.

33. Polak JF, Holman BL, Wynne J, et al. Right ventricular ejection fraction: an indicator of increased mortality in patients with congestive heart failure associated with coronary artery disease. *J Am Coll Cardiol.* 1983;2(2):217–224.

34. Jentzer JC, Anavekar NS, Reddy YNV, et al. Right ventricular pulmonary artery coupling and mortality in cardiac intensive care unit patients. *J Am Heart Assoc.* 2021;10(7):e019015.

35. Verhaert D, Mullens W, Borowski A, et al. Right ventricular response to intensive medical therapy in advanced decompensated heart failure. *Circ Heart Fail.* 2010;3(3):340–346.

36. van Diepen S, Katz JN, Albert NM, et al. Contemporary management of cardiogenic shock: a scientific statement from the American Heart Association. *Circulation.* 2017;136(16):e232–e268.

37. Baran DA, Grines CL, Bailey S, et al. SCAI clinical expert consensus statement on the classification of cardiogenic shock: this document was endorsed by the American College of Cardiology (ACC), the American Heart Association (AHA), the Society of Critical Care Medicine (SCCM), and the Society of Thoracic Surgeons (STS) in April 2019. *Catheter Cardiovasc Interv.* 2019;94(1):29–37.

38. Naidu Srihari S, Baran David A, Jentzer Jacob C, et al. SCAI SHOCK stage classification expert consensus update: a review and incorporation of validation studies. *J Am Coll Cardiol.* 2022;79(9):933–946.

39. Hunziker L, Radovanovic D, Jeger R, et al. Twenty-year trends in the incidence and outcome of cardiogenic shock in AMIS plus registry. *Circ Cardiovasc Interv.* 2019;12(4):e007293.

40. Hernandez-Montfort J, Sinha SS, Thayer KL, et al. Clinical outcomes associated with acute mechanical circulatory support utilization in heart failure related cardiogenic shock. *Circ Heart Fail.* 2021;14(5):e007924.

41. Berkowitz MJ, Picard MH, Harkness S, et al. Echocardiographic and angiographic correlations in patients with cardiogenic shock secondary to acute myocardial infarction. *Am J Cardiol.* 2006;98(8):1004–1008.

42. Picard MH, Davidoff R, Sleeper LA, et al. Echocardiographic predictors of survival and response to early revascularization in cardiogenic shock. *Circulation.* 2003;107(2):279–284.

43. Jentzer Jacob C, Wiley Brandon M, Anavekar Nandan S, et al. Noninvasive hemodynamic assessment of shock severity and mortality risk prediction in the cardiac intensive care unit. *JACC Cardiovasc Imaging.* 2021;14(2):321–332.

44. Klein T, Ramani GV. Assessment and management of cardiogenic shock in the emergency department. *Cardiol Clin.* 2012;30(4):651–664.

45. Huguet R, Fard D, d'Humieres T, et al. Three-dimensional inferior vena cava for assessing central venous pressure in patients with cardiogenic shock. *J Am Soc Echocardiogr.* 2018;31(9):1034–1043.

46. Hochman JS, Boland J, Sleeper LA, et al. Current spectrum of cardiogenic shock and effect of early revascularization on mortality. Results of an international registry. SHOCK Registry Investigators. *Circulation.* 1995;91(3):873–881.

47. Damluji AA, van Diepen S, Katz JN, et al. Mechanical complications of acute myocardial infarction: a scientific statement from the American Heart Association. *Circulation.* 2021;144(2):e16–e35.

48. Stamm RB, Gibson RS, Bishop HL, et al. Echocardiographic detection of infarct-localized asynergy and remote asynergy during acute myocardial infarction: correlation with the extent of angiographic coronary disease. *Circulation.* 1983;67(1):233–244.

49. Mendes LA, Picard MH, Sleeper LA, et al. Cardiogenic shock: predictors of outcome based on right and left ventricular size and function at presentation. *Coron Artery Dis.* 2005;16(4):209–215.

50. Mendes LA, Dec GW, Picard MH, et al. Right ventricular dysfunction: an independent predictor of adverse outcome in patients with myocarditis. *Am Heart J.* 1994;128(2):301–307.

51. Hansen A, Haass M, Zugck C, et al. Prognostic value of Doppler echocardiographic mitral inflow patterns: implications for risk stratification in patients with chronic congestive heart failure. *J Am Coll Cardiol.* 2001;37(4):1049–1055.

52. Shah MG, Cho S, Atwood JE, et al. Peripheral edema due to heart disease: diagnosis and outcome. *Clin Cardiol.* 2006;29(1):31–35.

53. Stevenson LW, Perloff JK. The limited reliability of physical signs for estimating hemodynamics in chronic heart failure. *JAMA.* 1989;261(6):884–888.

54. Goonewardena SN, Spencer KT. Handcarried echocardiography to assess hemodynamics in acute decompensated heart failure. *Curr Heart Fail Rep.* 2010;7(4):219–227.

55. Hochman JS, Sleeper LA, Webb JG, et al. Early revascularization in acute myocardial infarction complicated by cardiogenic shock. SHOCK Investigators. Should we emergently revascularize occluded coronaries for cardiogenic shock. *N Engl J Med.* 1999;341(9):625–634.

56. Hochman JS, Sleeper LA, White HD, et al. One-year survival following early revascularization for cardiogenic shock. *JAMA.* 2001;285(2):190–192.

57. Reynolds HR, Hochman JS. Cardiogenic shock: current concepts and improving outcomes. *Circulation.* 2008;117(5):686–697.

58. Feinberg MS, Schwammenthal E, Shlizerman L, et al. Prognostic significance of mild mitral regurgitation by color Doppler echocardiography in acute myocardial infarction. *Am J Cardiol.* 2000;86(9):903–907.

59. Moss AJ, The Multicenter Postinfarction Research Group. Risk stratification and survival after myocardial infarction. *N Engl J Med.* 1983;309(6):331–336.

60. Volpi A, De Vita C, Franzosi MG, et al. Determinants of 6-month mortality in survivors of myocardial infarction after thrombolysis. Results of the GISSI-2 data base. The Ad hoc Working Group of the Gruppo Italiano per lo Studio della Sopravvivenza nell'Infarto Miocardico (GISSI)-2 Data Base. *Circulation*. 1993;88(2):416–429.

61. Scalia GM, McCarthy PM, Savage RM, et al. Clinical utility of echocardiography in the management of implantable ventricular assist devices. *J Am Soc Echocardiogr*. 2000;13(8):754–763.

62. Estep JD, Stainback RF, Little SH, et al. The role of echocardiography and other imaging modalities in patients with left ventricular assist devices. *JACC Cardiovasc Imaging*. 2010;3(10):1049–1064.

63. Khan T, Delgado RM, Radovancevic B, et al. Dobutamine stress echocardiography predicts myocardial improvement in patients supported by left ventricular assist devices (LVADs): hemodynamic and histologic evidence of improvement before LVAD explantation. *J Heart Lung Transplant*. 2003;22(2):137–146.

64. Firstenberg MS, Orsinelli DA. ECMO and ECHO: the evolving role of quantitative echocardiography in the management of patients requiring extracorporeal membrane oxygenation. *J Am Soc Echocardiogr*. 2012;25(6):641–643.

65. Bergenzaun L, Ohlin H, Gudmundsson P, et al. Mitral annular plane systolic excursion (MAPSE) in shock: a valuable echocardiographic parameter in intensive care patients. *Cardiovasc Ultrasound*. 2013;11:16.

66. Cavarocchi NC, Pitcher HT, Yang Q, et al. Weaning of extracorporeal membrane oxygenation using continuous hemodynamic transesophageal echocardiography. *J Thorac Cardiovasc Surg*. 2013;146(6):1474–1479.

67. Picard MH, Wilkins GT, Ray PA, et al. Natural history of left ventricular size and function after acute myocardial infarction. Assessment and prediction by echocardiographic endocardial surface mapping. *Circulation*. 1990;82(2):484–494.

68. Mendes LA, Picard MH, Dec GW, et al. Ventricular remodeling in active myocarditis. Myocarditis treatment trial. *Am Heart J*. 1999;138(2 Pt 1):303–308.

69. Rose EA, Gelijns AC, Moskowitz AJ, et al. Long-term use of a left ventricular assist device for end-stage heart failure. *N Engl J Med*. 2001;345(20):1435–1443.

70. Grayburn Paul A, Sannino A, Packer M. Proportionate and disproportionate functional mitral regurgitation. *JACC Cardiovasc Imaging*. 2019;12(2):353–362.

71. Nijland F, Kamp O, Verhorst PM, et al. In-hospital and long-term prognostic value of viable myocardium detected by dobutamine echocardiography early after acute myocardial infarction and its relation to indicators of left ventricular systolic dysfunction. *Am J Cardiol*. 2001;88(9):949–955.

Echocardiography and focus cardiac ultrasound in cardiac arrest

5

Hatem Soliman-Aboumarie, Christopher Shirley,
Gregory M. Scalia, and Henry Skinner

Key Points

- Ultrasound examination of the heart, either echocardiography or focus cardiac ultrasound (FoCUS), is incorporated in Advanced Cardiac Life Support (ACLS) algorithms to identify reversible causes of cardiac arrest.
- Coronary thrombosis, pulmonary embolism, cardiac tamponade, hypovolemia, and tension pneumothorax are treatable and reversible causes of cardiac arrest that can be readily diagnosed by cardiac ultrasound examination (CUS).
- CUS can be used to assess the efficacy of chest compressions during cardiopulmonary resuscitation (CPR).
- Image acquisition in cardiac arrest is challenging and the examination should be performed by experienced operators.
- Proper training and teamwork are essential to enable clinical integration of CUS findings while minimizing interruption in chest compressions during CPR.
- Focused transesophageal echocardiography can also be used in cardiac arrest settings and may often be required for reaching a definite diagnosis.

Cardiac arrest represents the pinnacle of clinical challenges. It justifiably provokes a sense of urgency and drama for the attending staff. Many cardiac arrest situations occur suddenly, without warning or obvious precipitant. On discovery of a patient in cardiac arrest, the process of emergency resuscitation begins, with a view to restoring cardiac output and systemic oxygenation, diagnosing the underlying cause, and correcting any reversible contributing factors. Early identification of the cause of arrest may increase the likelihood of survival. Ultrasound examination of the heart is an invaluable diagnostic aid during cardiac arrest (see Box 5.1).

Patients with out-of-hospital cardiac arrest, usually brought in by ambulance and paramedics under full cardiopulmonary resuscitation (CPR), typically have prolonged resuscitation times before reaching the arrest team. These patients frequently are severely hypoxic and acidotic, especially if inadequate bystander CPR was undertaken. In these cases, cardiac ultrasound examination (CUS) is often of limited value because of agonal cardiac function at this late stage.

Cardiac arrests that occur in the hospital are often (although not always) witnessed and in some cases may be predicted. Indeed, in many situations, CUS is called for when a patient is severely hypotensive before full cardiac arrest. It is

BOX 5.1

The terms FoCUS, POCUS, and echocardiography are often used interchangeably. For the purpose of this chapter, it may be useful to think of these in distinct terms.

POCUS (point-of-care ultrasound) denotes the application of an ultrasound scan of any degree of complexity that is delivered at the point of care (such as the patient's bedside) and outside of a specialist sonography department setting.

FoCUS (focus cardiac ultrasound) is a scan that uses defined and limited views, to rapidly answer only targeted and very specific clinical questions often in a binary way (see Chapter 19). For example, during a cardiac arrest, time is critically limited and a full diagnostic echo study is not feasible.

Echocardiography is an assessment beyond the scope of FoCUS, performed by the operator fully trained in echocardiography (see Chapters 1 and 19).

CUS (cardiac ultrasound examination) denotes either echocardiography or FoCUS, as appropriate. In this chapter, CUS is essentially the same as POCUS.

in these situations that emergency CUS is probably of most use. Resuscitation times tend to be shorter, and acidosis has not become so profound, improving the chances of a successful outcome.

The major international resuscitation societies have incorporated cardiac ultrasound examination (CUS) in ACLS algorithms to identify treatable and reversible causes. Image acquisition during cardiac arrest is challenging. Therefore, proper training and understanding of the importance of team dynamics and human factors are essential to enable clinical integration of CUS while minimizing interruption in chest compressions. This chapter will provide to the reader a primer for clinical integration of CUS during cardiac arrest and peri-arrest situations while highlighting the importance of training, team dynamics, and human factors for effective resuscitation teamwork. The special role and potential added value of focused transesophageal echocardiography (TEE) in this scenario is also considered. Finally, the recognition that it is important to interpret the information obtained from CUS within the clinical context is discussed.

THE ROLE OF CARDIAC ULTRASOUND EXAMINATION

Cardiac arrest is the cessation of cardiac circulation. It is either unheralded (for example, in out-of-hospital cardiac arrest), or could be the final common pathway in critically ill patients who deteriorate and exceed their physiological reserve. Out-of-hospital cardiac arrest carries a high mortality. In Europe, only 8% of patients who suffered out-of-hospital cardiac arrest left hospital alive.[1] In the UK, up to 0.2% of patients admitted to hospital suffer a cardiac arrest. According to the National Cardiac Arrest Audit, the initial rhythm was pulseless electrical activity (PEA) in just over half of the patients, with asystole in 20% and just under 20% was shockable rhythm; the remainder is unknown. A quarter of those treated survived to hospital discharge.[2] Priorities for the resuscitation team include oxygenating the heart and brain though effective cardiopulmonary resuscitation (CPR), identifying shockable rhythms, and eliciting the cause of the cardiac arrest. CUS can help to rule in (and direct treatment) or rule out (if possible) some of the *reversible causes of cardiac arrest*, the so-called Hs and Ts. Of relevance to CUS are hypovolemia, tamponade, thrombo-embolism (pulmonary and coronary), and tension pneumothorax.

In the last decade, ACLS algorithms advised that CUS may be considered as an adjunct to patient evaluation provided it does not interfere with standard CPR protocols; an example of such a scenario will be discussed later in this chapter.[3,4] There is a *potential for conflict* when different team members try and execute their respective responsibilities (sometimes encroaching on each other's space and time), and *the team leader* may need to reiterate the defined and limited role of CUS in this scenario. To this end, CUS needs to be deliberate and to be performed during the period of pulse check and for no longer than 10 seconds.

Cardiac arrest situations typically involve many staff members gathered around the patient, including medical doctors, nurses, and technicians. The atmosphere is usually hectic, and the situation is often cramped and strained. Typically, there will be an operator at the head of the patient managing the airway with oxygenation and ventilation, an operator on one side of the patient undertaking external chest compressions and an operator at the arms obtaining intravenous access and administering drugs. By the time CUS has been called for, the resuscitation process has usually been going on for some time. It is important that the resuscitation team does not become preoccupied by getting good ultrasound images at the expense of recommencing effective chest compressions. Transthoracic windows are often suboptimal during an arrest, and it is desirable that CUS is performed by an experienced sonographer.

In the current era of point-of-care ultrasound examinations with handheld ultrasound devices (HUDs), emergency-focused imaging of the abdomen and chest is becoming routine. FoCUS (see Chapter 19) will quickly *rule in* or *rule out* the "big four"—cardiac tamponade, left ventricular dysfunction, right ventricular dysfunction, and hypovolemia. In addition, emergency procedures such as pericardiocentesis may be guided by using HUDs. Comprehensive transthoracic echocardiography may then be pursued for complex or subtle findings beyond the scope of FoCUS, such as regional wall motion abnormalities or signs of aortic dissection. The *subcostal window is preferred* as it is feasible in supine patients and least likely to interfere with chest compressions (V5.1A, V5.1B, V19.7). The apical windows may be obscured by

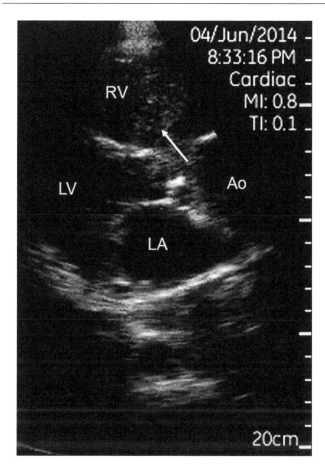

FIGURE 5.1 The parasternal long-axis (PLAX) view obtained with a handheld imaging device (HUD) in a patient with cardiac arrest showing the communication (arrow) between the enlarged right ventricle and the ruptured aortic root, presumably caused by trauma during cardiopulmonary resuscitation (V5.2). Ao: aorta; LA: left atrium; LV: left ventricle; RV: right ventricle.

(Image and video provided by IS.)

defibrillation pads. Pleural and parasternal windows may also be utilized but only within the time constraints (Figure 5.1) (V5.2). Practitioners should be mindful not to contaminate the area of chest compression with residual ultrasound gel.

Importantly, comprehensive echocardiography should always be performed after initial stabilization after a severe hypotensive episode or in cardiac arrest survivors to look for causes detectable by ultrasound (Table 5.1). Particular findings related to specific diseases and conditions are discussed in detail in respective chapters in this book.

Cases that begin with profound hypotension or with frank electromechanical dissociation (EMD) will evolve with time, along with increasing hypoxia and acidosis, to ventricular fibrillation and, of course, if not corrected, to asystole.

Finally, *medicolegal considerations* are also relevant to CUS during resuscitation. The digital record of the ultrasound examination represents a time-coded recording of the resuscitation process and the interventions that may be undertaken (e.g., pericardiocentesis, defibrillation). The CUS report should preferably include a chronology of the events for future reference.

TABLE 5.1   Causes of Cardiac Arrest and Hemodynamic Collapse Detectable by Cardiac Ultrasound Examination

Electromechanical dissociation and severe hypotension
Cardiac tamponade
Left ventricular abnormalities
    Severe global left ventricular dysfunction
        Dilated cardiomyopathy
        Acute myocarditis
    Regional left ventricular dysfunction
        Coronary artery disease
        Acute myocarditis
        Sarcoidosis
        Intracranial hemorrhage or trauma
Right ventricular dysfunction
        Acute pulmonary embolism
        Arrhythmogenic right ventricular dysplasia
Takotsubo "stress" cardiomyopathy
Hypertrophic cardiomyopathy
Severe hypovolemia
Valvular heart disease (native, prosthetic valves)
Aortic dissection
Rare causes
    Cardiac amyloidosis
    Cardiac tumors
Miscellaneous conditions
    Air embolism

Arrhythmic cardiac arrest
Asystole (end-stage cardiac arrest)
Ventricular arrhythmias

Furthermore, cardiac arrest may be the result of some misadventure, accident, or violent trauma, and thus, the data from CUS may become part of subsequent investigations and review.

CONFIRMING HEART CONTRACTILITY

Although confirming cardiac arrest seems straightforward for some practitioners by palpating central pulses or obtaining a blood pressure measurement, around 45% of healthcare professionals reported not being able to accurately assess central pulses during cardiac arrest.[5] In PEA, electrical cardiac activity is present yet without detectable mechanical effect (no palpable pulse). PEA is the presenting rhythm in roughly 50% of cardiac arrests within hospital.[2,6] On the other hand, asystole is identified by the lack of electrical activity and mechanical cardiac contractions. Such non-shockable rhythms are known to have poorer prognosis.[6] Studies have shown that 10–35% of patients with PEA cardiac arrest have demonstrable cardiac contraction on point of care echocardiographic assessment.[7] Therefore, emergency CUS could be pivotal in differentiating true PEA from pseudo PEA (patients with demonstrable cardiac contraction on CUS despite no palpable central pulses). Moreover, demonstrating ventricular contractility has the potential to diagnose a shockable rhythm when the electrocardiogram is not optimal.

IDENTIFYING REVERSIBLE CAUSES

Identifying and treating reversible causes of cardiac arrest is essential to achieve return of spontaneous circulation (ROSC) and CUS, through rapid identification and directed management, can potentially improve patient outcome.[8] Coronary thrombosis, pulmonary embolism (PE), cardiac tamponade, hypovolemia, and tension pneumothorax are reversible causes that can be readily diagnosed by CUS. Acute myocardial ischemia and massive pulmonary embolism are the leading causes of cardiac arrest.

Coronary thrombosis and ventricular failure

Coronary thrombosis is a major cause of cardiac arrest in the western countries (see Chapters 2 and 3). Echocardiographic assessment of regional wall motion abnormalities (RWMA) can suggest the presence of acute myocardial ischemia (V5.3A, V5.3B, V5.3C). However, RWMA are neither 100% specific nor sensitive for coronary thrombosis.[5] Left ventricular free-wall rupture (Figure 5.2) was found in 0.8% to 6.2% of patients after acute myocardial infarction and is frequently deadly due to cardiac tamponade.[5] The finding of severe global left ventricular dysfunction should direct the resuscitation process toward inotrope administration (V5.4).

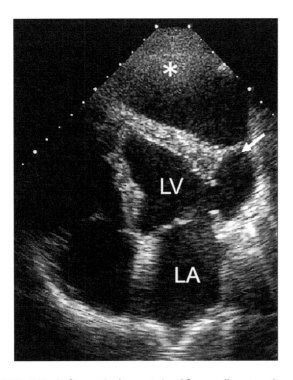

FIGURE 5.2   Left ventricular contained free-wall rupture (arrow) with large pseudoaneurysm (*) causing cardiac arrest. LA: left atrium; LV: left ventricle.

Pulmonary embolism

Echocardiography is recommended to assess PE in patients who are hemodynamically unstable and not fit for transfer for a computed tomography scan (Table 5.2). However, it should not be used as a single rule-out test due to its low negative predictive value (40–50%).[9] The hallmark of echocardiographic findings in massive PE is the presence of dilated right ventricle (RV) mainly due to elevated pulmonary artery pressures from the increase in pulmonary vascular resistance (Figure 5.3) (V5.5A, V5.5B, V5.5C). However, RV dilatation detected by CUS during cardiac arrest should not be interpreted as an exclusive sign of acute pulmonary embolism since other conditions which could lead to RV dilatation need to be taken in consideration (pulmonary hypertension, RV infarction, arrhythmogenic right ventricular cardiomyopathy, tension pneumothorax, chronic cor pulmonale, and prolonged CPR itself).

ESC guidelines for management of suspected PE in patients with hemodynamic instability suggest transthoracic echocardiography as the first line investigation.[9] The guidelines state that if signs of RV pressure overload are seen and computed tomographic pulmonary angiography (CTPA) is not readily available/feasible, then treatment of suspected PE is justified. In the absence of signs of RV dysfunction, PE becomes unlikely to be the cause of the hemodynamic instability. Therefore, RV dilatation is considered a sensitive but not specific echocardiographic finding in the *diagnosis* of PE. It is paramount to integrate these findings within the clinical context (see Chapter 7).

Cardiac tamponade

This is a potentially life-threatening complication that could develop after trauma, cardiac surgery, acute myocardial infarction (AMI), acute or chronic heart failure (HF), pericarditis, rheumatological disease, and interventional cardiological procedures. The subcostal view is usually the best window to provide a quick assessment of pericardial effusion (Table 5.3). This view is also used to guide pericardiocentesis if needed (V21.5A, V21.5B, V21.5C). Although cardiac tamponade is a clinical diagnosis, CUS is the method of choice to identify a pericardial effusion (V19.5, V19.5.1) and assess its hemodynamic consequences (Figure 5.4) (V5.6, V19.6, V19.6.1); its pathophysiology depends primarily on the speed of accumulation of fluid rather than on the absolute volume of fluid (see also Chapter 8).

Hypovolemia

Hypovolemia is among the commonest causes of PEA cardiac arrest.[12] Typically, resuscitation of hypotensive patients requires the administration of fluids to increase the circulating volume. The left ventricle is small and vigorous in function (V5.7, V19.4, V19.4.1). In some cases, cavity obliteration and left ventricular outflow tract obstruction are present. The right ventricle is also

TABLE 5.2   Key Echocardiographic Findings in Patients with Pulmonary Embolism[10]

ECHOCARDIOGRAPHIC FEATURES OF PULMONARY EMBOLISM	PITFALLS
• Increased RV dimensions in PLAX/A4CH	Seen in around 25% of PEs, check for other causes
• McConnell's sign (akinetic free wall with hyperdynamic apex)	Poor sensitivity (20%), potentially high specificity
• Flattening of the interventricular septum	High sensitivity (81%), low specificity (41%)
• Distended non-collapsing IVC	Check for other causes
• Direct clot visualization in the RA, RV, RVOT, or PA	Clot rarely seen
• RV dysfunction (e.g., TAPSE <16 mm)	Non-specific and may aid in prognostication
• Mid-systolic notching of the pulmonary artery systolic waveform on PW Doppler	Low sensitivity (25%), high specificity (>90%)
• 60/60 sign (pulmonary artery acceleration time <60 ms, RVSP <60 mmHg).	

Abbreviations: A4CH, apical four-chamber view; IVC, inferior vena cava; PA, pulmonary artery; PE, pulmonary embolism; PLAX, parasternal long-axis view; PW, pulsed wave; RA, right atrium; RV, right ventricle; RVOT, right ventricular outflow tract; RVSP, right ventricular systolic pressure; TAPSE, tricuspid annular plane systolic excursion.

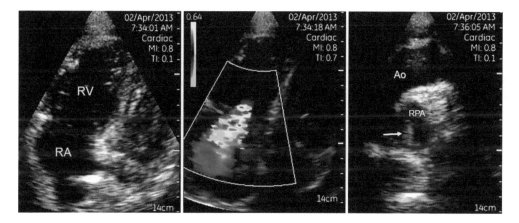

FIGURE 5.3   Focused cardiac ultrasound (FoCUS) after successful resuscitation of patient with sudden cardiac arrest in the emergency department. Cardiac ultrasound examination performed with a handheld ultrasound device revealed, in off-axis four-chamber view, dilated and akinetic right ventricle (left panel) (V5.5A), and significant tricuspid regurgitation (middle panel) (V5.5B). Suprasternal view demonstrates mobile hyperechogenic mass (arrow) consistent with thrombus within the lumen of the right pulmonary artery (right panel) (V5.5C). Note that the diagnosis of massive pulmonary embolism as a cause of cardiac arrest was made in 2 minutes and thrombolytic therapy immediately started. The patient survived the acute episode. Ao: aorta; RA: right atrium; RPA: right pulmonary artery; RV: right ventricle.

(Images and videos provided by RV.)

TABLE 5.3   Key Echocardiographic Findings in Patients with Cardiac Tamponade[11]

ECHOCARDIOGRAPHIC FEATURES OF CARDIAC TAMPONADE	PITFALLS
• RV dilation with interventricular septum shift (and consequent LV underfilling) • Large amount of pericardial effusion with heart movement within the pericardial space (the "swinging heart") • Early diastolic RV collapse (the most specific sign) • Systolic right atrial wall invagination (for more than one-third of the cardiac cycle) • Respiratory transvalvular Doppler variation (in spontaneous breathing patients): transmitral E-wave increases >25% on expiration and reduces on inspiration—the opposite happens for RV inflow (for patients with mechanical ventilation these phasic changes are reversed) • Dilated IVC without collapsibility during inspiration (which has low specificity especially in mechanically ventilated patients)	• Early after cardiac surgery, cardiac tamponade may not present with the classical clinical and echocardiographic features and can present with a localized rather than global pericardial effusion. • Extracardiac factors, such as a massive pleural effusion, tension pneumothorax, or lung hyperinflation due to positive pressure ventilation, can mimic tamponade physiology. CUS combined with LUS can confirm such a diagnosis and prevent an unnecessary pericardiocentesis.

Abbreviations: CUS, cardiac ultrasound examination; IVC, inferior vena cava; LV, left ventricle; LUS, lung ultrasound; RV, right ventricle.

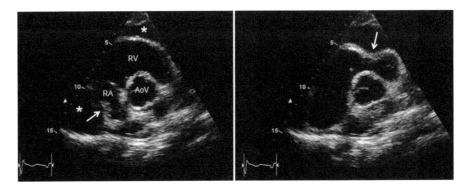

FIGURE 5.4 Transthoracic echocardiography (TTE) short-axis view of the base of the heart reveals large pericardial effusion (*) with right atrial systolic (arrow, left panel) and right ventricular diastolic (arrow, right panel) collapse, indicating tamponade physiology (V5.6). The patient underwent emergent pericardiocentesis. AoV: aortic valve; RA: right atrium; RV: right ventricle.

(Images and video provided by BAP.)

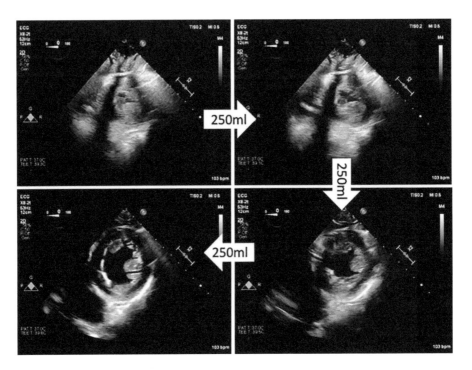

FIGURE 5.5 Hypovolemia detected by transesophageal echocardiography. The hallmark of hypovolemia is a small LV internal diameter, papillary muscles kissing, and pseudohypertrophy. The images obtained by TEE show how the hypovolemia is corrected with consecutive fluid challenges of 250 mL of saline (V5.9A, V5.9B, V5.9C, V5.9D). Note gradual increase in LV internal diameter.

small and dynamic. The right atrium is underfilled and the inferior vena cava is collapsed or collapsible (V5.8).

Echocardiography has an important role in the prediction of preload responsiveness, which is defined by an increase in the stroke volume by 15% or more after an intravenous bolus of fluid of 300 mL over 10–15 minutes. It has been shown that 40–70% of cases of shock will respond to volume expansion. The increase in LV internal diameter can closely be tracked by CUS in response to fluid challenges (Figure 5.5) (V5.9A, V5.9B, V5.9C, V5.9D).

Static and dynamic indices exist for the assessment of preload responsiveness. Table 5.4 summarizes cardiac ultrasound signs of hypovolemia and Table 5.5 summarizes echocardiographic preload responsiveness indices.

Tension pneumothorax

Tension pneumothorax is an important reversible cause of cardiac arrest and around 5% of major trauma patients were found to have tension pneumothorax in one study.[13] The diagnosis of pneumothorax relies on combining clinical assessment with imaging and chest radiography has lower sensitivity than

TABLE 5.4 Cardiac Ultrasound Signs of Hypovolemia[10]

PARAMETER	FINDING SUGGESTIVE OF HYPOVOLEMIA	PITFALLS
LV cavity size and function	Small, hyperkinetic LV with end-systolic cavity obliteration	Inotropic support, severe valvular regurgitation, LV hypertrophy
LV end-diastolic area	<5.5 cm^2/m^2 BSA	Inotropic support, severe valvular regurgitation, LV hypertrophy
IVC size and inspiratory collapse	>10 mm collapse on inspiration	Requires spontaneously breathing patient in sinus rhythm
IVC size and expiratory collapse	Variable	Requires mechanically ventilated patient in sinus rhythm

Abbreviations: BSA, body surface area; IVC, inferior vena cava; LV, left ventricle.

TABLE 5.5 Echocardiographic Dynamic Indices of Preload Responsiveness[10]

PARAMETER	FINDING SUGGESTIVE OF PRELOAD RESPONSIVENESS	PITFALLS
SVC collapsibility index	>36%	Passively mechanically ventilated; sinus rhythm
IVC distensibility index	>18%	Passively mechanically ventilated; sinus rhythm
LV ejection fraction	LVOT V$_{max}$ variability >12%	

Abbreviations: IVC, inferior vena cava; LV, left ventricle; LVOT V$_{max}$, left ventricular outflow tract maximal velocity; SVC, superior vena cava.

ultrasound for the diagnosis of pneumothorax; lung ultrasound (LUS) has a sensitivity of 95% for the detection of pneumothorax in the critically ill patients.[14]

The presence of pleural sliding can unequivocally exclude a pneumothorax at the area of scanning.[15] Loss of pleural sliding on two-dimensional scan with the appearance of the stratosphere sign on M-mode, the presence of A-lines, loss of B-lines with the loss of lung pulse, and the presence of lung point increase the diagnostic yield of LUS in diagnosing pneumothorax by increasing the sensitivity and specificity. The lung point (the transition zone between an area of pleural sliding and an area with no pleural sliding) is the most specific sign for pneumothorax and it has 100% specificity for pneumothorax (V2.16).

Moreover, the assessment of pneumothorax is especially pertinent in peri-arrest situations as the assessment of pleural sliding relies on the presence of tidal lung ventilation; therefore, it will be lost during cardiopulmonary arrest or one-sided main stem bronchial intubation even in the absence of pneumothorax.

POCUS PULSE CHECK

Manual pulse checks could be unreliable even in experienced hands and can lead to unnecessary initiation of chest compressions when pulse is present; conversely, it could lead to delays in commencing chest compressions in true cardiac arrest. Most contemporary literature have so far focused on using POCUS

to detect reversible causes of cardiac arrest and to assess for cardiac standstill. However, during CPR, challenges can arise which may lead to difficulty in obtaining standard cardiac views especially in obese patients and due to ongoing air insufflation in the stomach from bag-mask ventilation. A novel use of POCUS is to detect central pulsations (carotid or femoral arteries) during cardiac arrest to differentiate between true loss of pulse due to cardiac arrest from loss of pulse due to very poor cardiac output states.[16] True loss of pulsatility is confirmed by a no-flow state in both central artery and vein, and both will be easily compressible while applying pressure of the ultrasound transducer on the skin. Conversely, the presence of non-compressible central artery with visible pulsations rules out true cardiac arrest and can be seen in very low cardiac output states.

FOCUSED TRANSESOPHAGEAL ECHOCARDIOGRAPHY DURING CARDIAC ARREST

As seen in the following table, the teamwork during cardiac arrest needs to facilitate effective CPR and concurrently identify the cause of the arrest so that treatment can be tailored in the most appropriate and efficient way. Echocardiography (or FoCUS) has a key role in the latter but has been associated in some studies with increases in CPR pauses if not implemented optimally.[17,18] The reasons focused TEE is becoming

TABLE 5.6   Transesophageal versus Transthoracic Echocardiography during Cardiac Arrest

PARAMETER	FOCUSED TEE	TTE
Ergonomics and equipment	• The echocardiographer can stand out of the way at the head-end of the patient. • Requires endotracheal intubation. • More cumbersome. • Requires expertise in TEE.	• Sonographer may be crowded in with other team members when space is a premium. • Expertise and equipment more readily available. • Equipment is smaller, possibly even handheld. • Does not require intubation.
Safety	• Risk of esophageal injury.	• Safe.
CPR	• Probe remains *in situ* during chest compressions and pulse check and provides a continuous rather than intermittent assessment of cardiac function. • Pulse/rhythm check pauses may be shorter. • Clear role in cannula placement while establishing a patient on percutaneous ECMO-CPR. • Can guide the effectiveness of CPR by assessing opening of the aortic valve during compressions;[19] this is especially valuable in patients who do not have invasive arterial pressure monitoring in place.	• Reliant on the window of 10 seconds pause for pulse check during CPR in order to achieve images. • May extend CPR "hands off" time.
US windows	• Not affected by positive pressure ventilation and PEEP.	• Transthoracic windows are adversely affected by positive pressure ventilation and PEEP, the presence of air in the stomach, the presence of intercostal and subcostal chest drains (after chest surgery), defibrillation pads, or automated compression device. • Patients likely to be supine (with associated challenges of suboptimal views).
Identifying the cause of cardiac arrest	• TEE is more sensitive than TTE to diagnose certain pathologies known to cause cardiac arrest (e.g., aortic dissection, ruptured papillary muscle, isolated atrial tamponade). In a pooled study the cause of arrest was identified in 41%.[20]	

Abbreviations: CPR, cardiopulmonary resuscitation; ECMO, extracorporeal membrane oxygenation; PEEP, positive end-expiratory pressure; TEE, transesophageal echocardiography; TTE, transthoracic echocardiography; US, ultrasound.

established as a very useful adjunct in the peri-arrest environment is outlined in Table 5.6. Of note, TEE probes are resistant to defibrillation voltages (although the probe should not be touched during the actual shock).

The focused TEE views acquired during the peri-arrest period are limited to those views required to

1. make a diagnoses of the causing pathology (mid-esophageal four-chamber and long-axis views, ascending aortic short-axis view, transgastric short-axis views);
2. assess efficacy of CPR (mid-esophageal long-axis view); and
3. facilitate placement of percutaneous extracorporeal membrane oxygenation (ECMO) cannulae (mid-esophageal bicaval view and descending aortic short-axis views).

Despite these potential advantages the evidence for focused TEE in cardiac arrest resuscitation remains of low certainty and studies are affected by a high risk of bias.[20]

TEE itself is associated with serious injury in 1:800 cases.[21] It is possible that when the probe is inserted under a high-pressure peri-arrest environment, injury is more likely to occur, but it is the authors' view that the risk-benefit balance is still favorable in this scenario. Prior to focused TEE, it is imperative that the patient has a definitive airway in situ. Transgastric views should be performed with utmost caution during chest compressions and certainly any probe flexion should be avoided. Focused TEE should only be performed by clinicians who are trained to do so. Several training models now exist for training or accreditation in focused TEE. The minimum number recommended to achieve proficiency in transthoracic FoCUS is 50[22]; similar numbers would apply to focused TEE, but fewer numbers would be required with prior FoCUS experience or if training is supplemented by high fidelity TEE simulators.

PROGNOSTICATION IN CARDIAC ARREST

Cardiac activity generates cardiac output and circulation. In the peri-arrest environment cardiac activity represents a spectrum (V5.10A, V5.10B, V5.10C, V5.10D). Intuitively, cardiac arrests with evidence of organized intrinsic mechanical activity should be associated with better prognosis and outcomes. Not surprisingly, the presence of sonographically identified cardiac kinetic motion in emergency department was associated with ROSC.[23] Breitkreutz's landmark pre-hospital resuscitation study in 2010 concluded that the presence of coordinated cardiac activity was associated with increased survival.[24] At least ten more studies, including two meta-analyses, have reported similar findings; the latter estimated the overall pooled odds ratio for ROSC in the presence of cardiac motion during CPR to be between 4.35 (p < 0.00001) in patients with PEA[25] and 12.4 (p < 0.001) in all types of arrest.[26] The main criticism of cardiac arrest studies investigating association between echocardiographic parameters and outcome are a lack of a consistent definition of "cardiac activity." Studies are often not blinded and lack consistent timing points regarding performing CUS. Some studies include any cardiac motion (as a prognostic factor) whereas others require motion to be organized insofar as activity would have to *change the dimensions of the ventricle* rather than just be agonal twitching. The inter-rater reliability of FoCUS during cardiac arrest remains uncertain. Furthermore, when interpreting cardiac motion (or lack of), the clinical context is very important; for example, lack of cardiac motion in the presence of hypothermia or after cardioplegia has an entirely different outlook than cardiac arrest after major trauma. In common with many cardiac arrest outcome studies, there is also a survival bias.

Reynolds on behalf of the Advanced Life Support Task Force of the International Liaison Committee on Resuscitation conducted a systematic review in 2020.[27] Reynolds reported that most studies displayed a high risk of bias from prognostic factor and outcome measures and lacked adjustment for other prognostic factors. Ultimately, heterogeneity of studies and risk of bias precluded meta-analyses. Reynolds concluded the evidence for using POCUS as a prognostic tool for clinical outcomes during cardiac arrest is of very low certainty.

POCUS seems to have better specificity than sensitivity to diagnose the etiology of cardiac arrest. The 2020 international consensus task force on CPR and emergency cardiovascular care science expressed caution against overinterpreting the finding of right-ventricular dilation in isolation to diagnose massive pulmonary embolism as this finding is common after a few minutes of CPR regardless of the etiology and seem to occur as blood is shifted from systemic circulation to the right heart along the pressure gradient.[27] They reiterated the evidence supporting the use of POCUS as a prognostic tool during cardiac arrest *is uniformly of very low certainty*. They also found the inter-rater reliability of POCUS during cardiac arrest to be uncertain.

CUS is very useful to diagnose the etiology of cardiac arrest but again studies are hampered by risk of bias and low certainly of evidence. The etiology in itself has important prognostic value, as tamponade in particular is associated with better outcomes. No single CUS finding has sufficient sensitivity to be used as sole criteria to terminate resuscitation. CUS findings should be interpreted in light of these limitations and considered as a diagnostic and prognostic adjunct. The presence of cardiac activity is clearly an encouraging sign although *its absence is not a reason in itself to discontinue.*

Focused TEE studies are emerging to show better outcomes with pseudo (as opposed to true) PEA. Other studies report poor outcomes with certain conditions and better outcomes in the absence of "causative" findings. Nevertheless, similar concerns regarding low quality and potential for bias means reserving judgement in this modality for now.

TEAM DYNAMICS AND HUMAN FACTORS OF THE APPLICATION OF ULTRASOUND IN CARDIAC ARREST MANAGEMENT

In addition to the clinical challenges already discussed in this chapter, cardiac arrests present the responding clinicians with additional "non-clinical" challenges due to various factors. They represent highly stressed and often emotive situations in which teams of people who do not regularly work together must make time critical judgements and carry out actions with potentially life-and-death consequences. The environment is often suboptimal with constraints on the following:

• Space
• Patient position
• Lighting and noise levels
• Availability and quality of clinical information and patient history

In such situations, the efficacy of the responding team can be greatly influenced by several factors that have become known as human factors, and they include the following:

• Team leadership/membership skills
• Communication
• Decision-making
• Situational awareness

A breakdown or failure in any one of these factors could lead quickly to adverse patient outcomes. As already discussed, the inclusion of POCUS into cardiac arrest management protocols aims to assist decision-making by assisting with the identification of causality and the effectiveness of treatment actions. However, without careful consideration of the effect on the other human factors, this can have a detrimental effect. To illustrate this point, it may be useful to picture the scene in the Box 5.2.

BOX 5.2

Resuscitation is ongoing on a 65-year-old man, who has been suffering acute deterioration following a recent STEMI. The underlying rhythm has been on the non-shockable side of the algorithm throughout and the reversible causes of cardiac arrest have been considered clinically, but no definitive cause has been identified. At the next pulse check pause, FoCUS has been requested. The resuscitation team leader calls for CPR to pause for the 10 seconds pulse check, and the sonographer moves in to place the probe in the subcostal position. As this is a new and relatively uncommon occurrence in the hospital, the entire team is watching the screen and an image appears after approximately 6 seconds. The team leader then recognizes that nobody has looked at the ECG or carried out a pulse check and asks for this to be done. The sonographer optimizes the image and starts to record at 8 seconds.

Team leader to sonographer: *"Are you done? Have you got the image?"*
Sonographer: *"Just a couple more seconds . . ."*
(10, 11, 12 s)
Team leader to resus team member: *"Is there a pulse?"*
Team member: *"There is no pulse." (13, 14 s)*
Sonographer: *"Okay I have an image saved." (15 s)*
Team leader: *"What is the rhythm?" (16, 17 s)*
Team member: *"Still non-shockable." (18, 19 s)*
Team leader: *"Restart CPR please." (20, 21 s)*

TOTAL HANDS-OFF TIME = 21 seconds

As you can see the implementation and inclusion of FoCUS in this example led to a total hands-off time from CPR of 21 seconds—more than double the recommended time for CPR to pause for a rhythm check. While in real life it is quite possible to imagine the event to unfold exactly as described in Box 5.2, this is precisely what we need to avoid. This outcome is cautioned by several studies who noted similar prolonged CPR pauses and warn that such pauses are inevitable.[17,18] Others argue, however, that this can be achieved in a protocol compliant way if FoCUS-assisted CPR is planned, communicated, and carried out effectively by suitably trained personnel.[5] As a consequence, several courses now teach both the technical and non-technical skills required to achieve this.

Achieving FoCUS-assisted CPR in an algorithm-compliant manner

In the example in Box 5.2, there are a number of factors that led to the breach of the 10-second window available for the rhythm check pause in CPR:

- The team leader did not brief the team and plan the actions of key team members prior to the pause in CPR.
- The sonographer was not already in position and the probe was not in place when CPR was paused.
- The team became distracted by the inclusion of a new technique with which they were unfamiliar.
- The sonographer, team leader, and team members lost situational awareness.

To achieve a successful and compliant POCUS within the limited 10 second timeframe the entire resuscitation team must act in a coordinated and planned manner (V5.11, audiovisual). The whole team must be familiar with the process of including POCUS into cardiac arrest management and this requires training together. The team leader must plan and coordinate the rhythm checks well in advance of the pause in CPR to ensure everyone is in place knows their role, and is ready before CPR is ceased. The sonographer requires *training in the technical skills required to achieve POCUS images in the limited timeframe*, and in *effectively communicating with the team leader*. The sonographer should not attempt to "live report" on the images in the 10 seconds available but should instead *concentrate on recording and optimizing the image*, later withdrawing to review the recorded images under better conditions while allowing the resuscitation team to continue. When the *team work in this coordinated manner*, all of these things will happen simultaneously, and situational awareness will be retained. When reporting findings back to the team leader, the sonographer should give a structured report that answers all of the specific targeted questions with either confirmation, exclusion, or that the views cannot confirm or exclude for each clinical question. In particular, where views are not sufficient to exclude a cause this should also be relayed to the team leader; *remember that "not seen" is not the same as "not there."*

SUMMARY

Cardiac arrest remains a devastating condition; outcomes have improved but remain poor despite advances in resuscitation and rescue therapy. CUS may have an important role in the management of cardiac arrest insofar that it can help diagnose treatable and reversible conditions. Furthermore, it provides important information regarding underlying cardiac function—organized contractility with a reduction in chamber size may be associated with improved outcomes. It can also help establish if cardiac output is present in patients in whom it is difficult to detect central pulses. Finally, it can assess the efficacy of chest compressions during CPR. It is important that the desire to acquire this information does not interfere with effective CPR. Well-rehearsed protocols with attention to human factors, in particular leadership and communication, can ensure CUS can be performed in a timely fashion without incurring pauses >10 seconds between chest compressions. Focused TEE may be considered in preference to transthoracic CUS if it is readily available, the expertise in probe insertion and image acquisition exists and transthoracic windows are poor. More studies are needed in CUS and focused TEE in peri-arrest practice to demonstrate better outcomes and provide stronger evidence to guide treatment and cessation thereof.

The following additional videos related to this chapter (see Table 5.1) are available in the online resources: V5.12, V5.13, V5.14A, V5.14B, V5.15A, V5.15B, V5.16A, V5.16B, V5.17, V5.18A, V5.18B, V5.18C.

LIST OF VIDEOS

https://routledgetextbooks.com/textbooks/9781032157009/chapter-5.php

VIDEO 5.1A   Focused cardiac ultrasound (FoCUS) with a handheld imaging device (HUD) in a patient with pulseless electrical activity (1/2): Imaging from the subcostal window does not significantly interfere with resuscitation procedures (shown here), but it should be done during brief interruptions (see Video 5.1B) of chest compressions to provide the information on potential underlying cause of cardiac arrest or to assess the success of resuscitation efforts. *(Video provided by IS.)*

VIDEO 5.1B   Focused cardiac ultrasound (FoCUS) with a handheld imaging device (HUD) in a patient with pulseless electrical activity (2/2): Although imaging from the subcostal window does not significantly interfere with resuscitation procedures (see Video 5.1A), it should be done during brief interruptions (shown here) of chest compressions to provide the information on potential underlying cause of cardiac arrest or to assess the success of resuscitation efforts. *(Video provided by IS.)*

VIDEO 5.2   Rupture of the aortic root during cardiopulmonary resuscitation (CPR): The parasternal long-axis view obtained with a handheld ultrasound device in a patient with cardiac arrest showing the communication between the enlarged right ventricle and the ruptured aortic root presumably caused by trauma during CPR. *(Video provided by IS.)*

VIDEO 5.3A   Focused cardiac ultrasound (FoCUS) during cardiopulmonary resuscitation (CPR) (1/3): The patient was brought to the emergency department by friends in cardiac arrest, which lasted 20 minutes. Severe chest pain occurred before cardiac arrest. CPR was started, but the patient did not respond. FoCUS revealed cardiac standstill in the parasternal short-axis (SAX) view (shown here) and no signs of aortic dissection from suprasternal view (see Video 5.3B). CPR was continued, and after 10 minutes, central pulse was established. Follow-up FoCUS showed fair global cardiac function in the apical two-chamber view (see Video 5.3C) with inferoposterior akinesis, indicating inferoposterior acute myocardial infarction as the most likely cause of the arrest—which was confirmed later in the coronary care unit. Although cardiac function recovered, the patient died a few days later from brain death and multiorgan failure. *(Video provided by RV.)*

VIDEO 5.3B   Focused cardiac ultrasound (FoCUS) during cardiopulmonary resuscitation (CPR) (2/3): The patient was brought to the emergency department by friends in cardiac arrest, which lasted 20 minutes. Severe chest pain occurred before cardiac arrest. CPR was started, but the patient did not respond. FoCUS revealed cardiac standstill in the parasternal short-axis (SAX) view (see Video 5.3A), and no signs of aortic dissection from suprasternal view (shown here). CPR was continued, and after 10 minutes central pulse was established. Follow-up FoCUS showed fair global cardiac function (see Video 5.3C) in the apical two-chamber view with inferoposterior akinesis, indicating inferoposterior acute myocardial infarction as the most likely cause of the arrest—which was confirmed later in the coronary care unit. Although cardiac function recovered, the patient died a few days later from brain death and multiorgan failure. *(Video provided by RV.)*

VIDEO 5.3C   Focused cardiac ultrasound (FoCUS) during cardiopulmonary resuscitation (CPR) (3/3): The patient was brought to the emergency department by friends in cardiac arrest, which lasted 20 minutes. Severe chest pain occurred before cardiac arrest. CPR was started, but the patient did not respond. FoCUS revealed cardiac standstill in the parasternal short-axis (SAX) view (see Video 5.3A), and no signs of aortic dissection from suprasternal view (see Video 5.3B). CPR was continued, and after 10 minutes central pulse was established. Follow-up FoCUS showed fair global cardiac function (shown here) in the apical two-chamber view with inferoposterior akinesis, indicating inferoposterior acute myocardial infarction as the most likely cause of the arrest—which was confirmed later in the coronary care unit. Although cardiac function recovered, the patient died a few days later from brain death and multiorgan failure. *(Video provided by RV.)*

VIDEO 5.4   Transthoracic emergency echocardiography in a patient with imminent cardiogenic shock: Images obtained from multiple views demonstrate severe left ventricular systolic dysfunction (both upper and bottom left panels) along with pleural effusion (bottom right panel). *(Video provided by IS.)*

VIDEO 5.5A   Acute massive pulmonary embolism detected with focused cardiac ultrasound (FoCUS) (1/3): After successful resuscitation of a patient with sudden cardiac arrest in the emergency department, cardiac ultrasound examination performed with a handheld ultrasound device revealed, in off-axis four-chamber view, dilated right ventricle with free-wall akinesia (shown here) and significant tricuspid regurgitation (see Video 5.5B). Suprasternal view demonstrates mobile, hyperechogenic mass consistent with thrombus within the lumen of the right pulmonary artery (see Video 5.5C). The diagnosis of massive pulmonary embolism as a cause of cardiac arrest was made in 2 minutes, and thrombolytic therapy immediately started. The patient survived the acute episode. *(Video provided by IS.)*

VIDEO 5.5B Acute massive pulmonary embolism detected with focused cardiac ultrasound (FoCUS) (2/3): After successful resuscitation of a patient with sudden cardiac arrest in the emergency department, cardiac ultrasound examination performed with a handheld ultrasound device revealed, in off-axis four-chamber view, dilated right ventricle with free-wall akinesia (see Video 5.5A) and significant tricuspid regurgitation (shown here). Suprasternal view demonstrates mobile, hyperechogenic mass consistent with thrombus within the lumen of the right pulmonary artery (see Video 5.5C). The diagnosis of massive pulmonary embolism as a cause of cardiac arrest was made in 2 minutes, and thrombolytic therapy immediately started. The patient survived the acute episode. *(Video provided by IS.)*

VIDEO 5.5C Acute massive pulmonary embolism detected with focused cardiac ultrasound (FoCUS) (3/3): After successful resuscitation of patient with sudden cardiac arrest in the emergency department, cardiac ultrasound examination performed with a handheld ultrasound device revealed, in off-axis four-chamber view, dilated right ventricle with free-wall akinesia (see Video 5.5A) and significant tricuspid regurgitation (see Video 5.5B). Suprasternal view demonstrates mobile, hyperechogenic mass consistent with thrombus within the lumen of the right pulmonary artery (shown here). The diagnosis of massive pulmonary embolism as a cause of cardiac arrest was made in 2 minutes, and thrombolytic therapy immediately started. The patient survived the acute episode. *(Video provided by IS.)*

VIDEO 5.6 Cardiac tamponade: Transthoracic echocardiography (TTE) short-axis view of the base of the heart reveals a large pericardial effusion with RV diastolic and RA systolic collapse, indicating tamponade physiology. The patient underwent emergent pericardiocentesis. *(Video provided by BAP.)*

VIDEO 5.7 Hypovolemia: In a patient on mechanical ventilation in the intensive care unit with intracerebral hemorrhage and episodes of profound bradycardia, transthoracic echocardiography (TTE) from different views revealed small, hyperdynamic left and right ventricles with almost complete cavity obliteration (left panels and upper right panel). Subcostal view reveals collapsible inferior vena cava during respiration. *(Video provided by IS.)*

VIDEO 5.8 Hypovolemia: Subcostal view reveals narrow and completely collapsible inferior vena cava (IVC) in a septic patient with hypotension, indicating hypovolemia. IVC <1.2 cm has 100% specificity for right atrial pressure of <10 mmHg (but low sensitivity). *(Video provided by IS.)*

VIDEO 5.9A Correction of hypovolemia with consecutive fluid challenge (1/4). The hallmark of hypovolemia is a small LV internal diameter, papillary muscles kissing, and pseudohypertrophy. This video and Videos 5.9B, 5.9C, and 5.9D show how hypovolemia is corrected with consecutive fluid challenges. Note increase in LV size on TEE (transgastric short-axis view) with consecutive fluid loading.

VIDEO 5.9B Correction of hypovolemia with consecutive fluid challenge (2/4). The hallmark of hypovolemia is a small LV internal diameter, papillary muscles kissing, and pseudohypertrophy. Videos 5.9A, 5.9C, and 5.9D and this video show how hypovolemia is corrected with consecutive fluid challenges. Note increase in LV size on TEE (transgastric short-axis view) with consecutive fluid loading.

VIDEO 5.9C Correction of hypovolemia with consecutive fluid challenge (3/4). The hallmark of hypovolemia is a small LV internal diameter, papillary muscles kissing, and pseudohypertrophy. Videos 5.9A, 5.9B, and 5.9D and this video show how hypovolemia is corrected with consecutive fluid challenges. Note increase in LV size on TEE (transgastric short-axis view) with consecutive fluid loading.

VIDEO 5.9D Correction of hypovolemia with consecutive fluid challenge (4/4). The hallmark of hypovolemia is a small LV internal diameter, papillary muscles kissing, and pseudohypertrophy. Videos 5.9A, 5.9B, 5.9C, and this video show how hypovolemia is corrected with consecutive fluid challenges. Note increase in LV size on TEE (transgastric short-axis view) with consecutive fluid loading.

VIDEO 5.10A Cardiac activity after recovery from cardioplegia-induced cardiac arrest in cardiac theatre (1/4). Please note asystole (shown here); true pulseless electrical activity (PFA), with agonal disorganized activity without any change in ventricular size (see Video 5.10B); pseudo PEA, organized activity but without ejection (see Video 5.10C), likely to have better prognosis than true PEA; return of spontaneous circulation (ROSC), with evident more forceful contraction (see Video 5.10D).

VIDEO 5.10B Cardiac activity after recovery from cardioplegia-induced cardiac arrest in cardiac theatre (2/4). True pulseless electrical activity (PEA), with agonal disorganized activity without any change in ventricular size (shown here); asystole (see Video 5.10A); pseudo PEA, organized activity but without ejection (see Video 5.10C), likely to have better prognosis than true PEA; return of spontaneous circulation (ROSC), with evident more forceful contraction (see Video 5.10D).

VIDEO 5.10C Cardiac activity after recovery from cardioplegia-induced cardiac arrest in cardiac theatre (3/4). Pseudo PEA, organized activity but without ejection (shown here), likely to have better prognosis than true PEA; asystole (see Video 5.10A); true pulseless electrical activity (PEA), with agonal disorganized activity without any change in ventricular size (see Video 5.10B; return of spontaneous circulation (ROSC), with evident more forceful contraction (see Video 5.10D).

VIDEO 5.10D Cardiac activity after recovery from cardioplegia-induced cardiac arrest in cardiac theatre (4/4). Return of spontaneous circulation (ROSC), with evident more forceful contraction (shown here); asystole (see Video 5.10A); pulseless electrical activity (PEA), with agonal disorganized activity without any change in ventricular size (see Video 5.10B); pseudo PEA, organized activity but without ejection (see Video 5.10C), likely to have better prognosis than true PEA.

VIDEO 5.11 Implementation of cardiac ultrasound examination (CUS) during CPR in Advance Cardiac Life Support (ACLS) compliant manner and proper communication within resuscitation team (audiovisual). Video shows CPR in real-time frame with proper use of CUS. Appropriate planning, communication, and training enables CUS to be conducted within the 10-second window of a rhythm check successfully, along with strategies for, when it is appropriate, to abandon the scan in order to prevent the CPR pause being prolonged, or to enable other treatments (such as defibrillation) when necessary.

VIDEO 5.12 Effusive-constrictive pericarditis: Transthoracic echocardiography (an off-axis apical four-chamber view) showing large fibrin strands within pericardial effusion in a patient with effusive-constrictive pericarditis. *(Video provided by IS.)*

VIDEO 5.13 Pericardiocentesis in a patient with cardiac tamponade ("swinging heart"): Microbubble appearance within the pericardial space after agitated saline (or contrast) injection confirms intrapericardial position of the needle. *(Video provided by IS.)*

VIDEO 5.14A Takotsubo cardiomyopathy (1/2): Typical "apical ballooning" in apical four-chamber view in a woman with chest pain resembling acute myocardial infarction and collapse. This pattern of wall motion abnormality does not completely fit with presumed distribution of coronary artery territories and more likely indicates Takotsubo cardiomyopathy than acute myocardial infarction. Complete recovery of left ventricular function was noted 10 days later (see also Video 5.14B). *(Video provided by BP.)*

VIDEO 5.14B Takotsubo cardiomyopathy (2/2): Typical "apical ballooning" in apical two-chamber view in a woman with chest pain resembling acute myocardial infarction and collapse. This pattern of wall motion abnormality does not completely fit with presumed distribution of coronary artery territories and more likely indicates Takotsubo cardiomyopathy than acute myocardial infarction. Complete recovery of left ventricular function was noted 10 days later (see also Video 5.14A). *(Video provided by BP.)*

VIDEO 5.15A Hypertrophic obstructive cardiomyopathy (1/2): Transthoracic echocardiography (TTE) parasternal long-axis view reveals asymmetric septal hypertrophy of the left ventricle, with systolic anterior motion of the mitral leaflets and left ventricular outflow tract (LVOT) obstruction. This appearance is consistent with hypertrophic obstructive cardiomyopathy. Color Doppler revealed turbulence in the LVOT caused by dynamic obstruction and some degree of mitral regurgitation (see Video 5.15B). The peak gradient in the LVOT is measured as 110 mmHg. *(Video provided by MSt.)*

VIDEO 5.15B Hypertrophic obstructive cardiomyopathy (2/2): Transthoracic echocardiography (TTE) parasternal long-axis view reveals asymmetric septal hypertrophy of the left ventricle, with systolic anterior motion of the mitral leaflets and left ventricular outflow tract (LVOT) obstruction. This appearance is consistent with hypertrophic obstructive cardiomyopathy. Color Doppler revealed turbulence in the LVOT caused by dynamic obstruction and some degree of mitral regurgitation (shown here). The peak gradient in the LVOT is measured as 110 mmHg (see also Video 5.15A). *(Video provided by MSt.)*

VIDEO 5.16A Cardiac amyloidosis (1/2): In a severely hypotensive patient with irregular cardiac rhythm (atrial fibrillation), transthoracic echocardiography (TTE) in parasternal long-axis view revealed concentric left ventricular thickening with characteristic "granular speckling" myocardial texture. Note thickened valves, enlarged left atrium, and minimal pericardial fluid. These are echo features of cardiac amyloidosis. In the two-chamber view (see Video 5.16B), hypertrophy and characteristic texture of papillary muscles can also be noted. *(Video provided by MMP.)*

VIDEO 5.16B Cardiac amyloidosis (2/2): In a severely hypotensive patient with irregular cardiac rhythm (atrial fibrillation), transthoracic echocardiography (TTE) in apical two-chamber view revealed hypertrophy and characteristic "granular speckling" texture of papillary muscles and left ventricular walls. These are echo features of cardiac amyloidosis (see also Video 5.16A). *(Video provided by MMP.)*

VIDEO 5.17 Dilated cardiomyopathy: In different transthoracic echocardiography (TTE) views, note the dilated cardiac chambers with severely depressed global left ventricular and right ventricular systolic function. *(Video provided by PMM.)*

VIDEO 5.18A Arrhythmogenic right ventricular cardiomyopathy (1/3): Transthoracic echocardiography (TTE) showing typical features of arrhythmogenic right ventricular (RV) dysplasia and cardiomyopathy—RV dilation in parasternal long-axis view (shown here), accompanied by RV free-wall akinesis and hyperechogenic area in the apical four-chamber view (see Video 5.18B), and RV free-wall systolic bulging best seen from the subcostal view (see Video 5.18C). *(Video provided by IS.)*

VIDEO 5.18B Arrhythmogenic right ventricular cardiomyopathy (2/3): Transthoracic echocardiography (TTE) showing typical features of arrhythmogenic right ventricular (RV) dysplasia and cardiomyopathy—RV dilation and free-wall akinesis and hyperechogenic area in the apical four-chamber view (see also Videos 5.18A and 5.18C). *(Video provided by IS.)*

VIDEO 5.18C Arrhythmogenic right ventricular cardiomyopathy (3/3): Transthoracic echocardiography (TTE) showing typical features of arrhythmogenic right ventricular (RV) dysplasia and cardiomyopathy—RV dilation and free-wall systolic bulging best seen from the subcostal view (see also Videos 5.18A and 5.18B). *(Video provided by IS.)*

REFERENCES

1. Gräsner JT, Wnent J, Herlitz J, et al. Survival after out-of-hospital cardiac arrest in Europe—results of the EuReCa TWO study. Resuscitation 2020;148:218–226.
2. https://ncaa.icnarc.org/
3. Soar J, Callaway CW, Aibiki M, et al. Part 4: advanced life support: 2015 international consensus on cardiopulmonary resuscitation and emergency cardiovascular care science with treatment recommendations. Resuscitation 2015;95:e71–e120.
4. Link M, Berkow LC, Kudenchuk PJ, et al. 2015 American Heart Association guidelines update for cardiopulmonary resuscitation and emergency cardiovascular care; part 7: adult advanced cardiovascular life support. Circulation 2015;132:S444–S464.

5. Price S, Uddin S, Quinn T. Echocardiography in cardiac arrest. Curr Opin Crit Care 2010;16:211–215.
6. Bergum, D, Skjeflo GW, Nordseth T, et al. ECG patterns in early pulseless electrical activity: associations with aetiology and survival of in-hospital cardiac arrest. Resuscitation 2016;104:34–39.
7. Gaspari R, Weekes A, Adhikari S, et al. Emergency department point-of-care ultrasound in out-of-hospital and in-ED cardiac arrest. Resuscitation 2016;109:33–39.
8. Chen N, Callaway CW, Guyette FX, et al. Pittsburgh Post-Cardiac Arrest Service: arrest etiology among patients resuscitated from cardiac arrest. Resuscitation 2018;130:33–40.
9. Konstantinides SV, Meyer G, Becattini C, et al. 2019 ESC Guidelines for the diagnosis and management of acute pulmonary embolism developed in collaboration with the European Respiratory Society (ERS): the Task Force for the diagnosis and management of acute pulmonary embolism of the European Society of Cardiology (ESC). Eur Heart J 2020;41:543–603.
10. Zafiropoulos A, Asrress K, Redwood S, et al. Critical care echo rounds: echo in cardiac arrest. Echo Res Pract 2014;1:15–21.
11. Soliman-Aboumarie H, Pastore MC, Galiatsou E, et al. Echocardiography in the intensive care unit: an essential tool for diagnosis, monitoring and guiding clinical decision-making. Physiol Int 2022;14:1–15.
12. Hughes S, McQuillan PJ. Sequential recall of causes of electromechanical dissociation (EMD). Resuscitation 1998;37:51.
13. Coats TJ, Wilson AW, Xeropotamous N. Pre-hospital management of patients with severe thoracic injury. Injury 1995;26:581–585.
14. Lichtenstein DA, Menu Y. A bedside ultrasound sign ruling out pneumothorax in the critically ill. Lung sliding. Chest 1995;108:1345–1348.
15. Volpicelli G. Sonographic diagnosis of pneumothorax. Intensive Care Med 2011;37:224.
16. Simard RD, Unger AG, Betz M, et al. The POCUS pulse check: a case series on a novel method for determining the presence of a pulse using point-of-care ultrasound. J Emerg Med 2019;56:674–679.
17. Huis In't Veld MA, Allison MG, Bostick DS, et al. Ultrasound use during cardiopulmonary resuscitation is associated with delays in chest compressions. Resuscitation 2017;119:95–98.
18. Clattenburg EJ, Wroe P, Brown S, et al. Point-of-care ultrasound use in patients with cardiac arrest is associated prolonged cardiopulmonary resuscitation pauses: a prospective cohort study. Resuscitation 2018;122:65–68.
19. Catena E, Ottolina D, Fossali T, et al. Association between left ventricular outflow tract opening and successful resuscitation after cardiac arrest. Resuscitation 2019;138:8–14.
20. Hussein L, Rehman MA, Jelic T, et al. Transoesophageal echocardiography in cardiac arrest: a systematic review. Resuscitation 2021;168:167–175.
21. Ramalingam G, Choi SW, Agarwal S, et al. Complications related to peri-operative transoesophageal echocardiography—a one-year prospective national audit by the Association of Cardiothoracic Anaesthesia and Critical Care. Anaesthesia 2020;75:21–26.
22. Neskovic AN, Skinner H, Susanna Price S, et al. Focus cardiac ultrasound core curriculum and core syllabus of the European Association of Cardiovascular Imaging. Eur Heart J Cardiovasc Imaging 2018;19:475–481.
23. Salen P, Melniker L, Chooljian C, et al. Does the presence or absence of sonographically identified cardiac activity predict resuscitation outcomes of cardiac arrest patients? Am J Emerg Med 2005;23:459–462.
24. Breitkreutz R, Price S, Steiger HV, et al. Focused echocardiographic evaluation in life support and peri-resuscitation of emergency patients: a prospective trial. Resuscitation 2010;81:1527–1533.
25. Wu C, Zheng Z, Jiang L, et al. The predictive value of bedside ultrasound to restore spontaneous circulation in patients with pulseless electrical activity: a systematic review and meta-analysis. PLoS One 2018;13:e0191636.
26. Kedan I, Ciozda W, Palatinus JA, et al. Prognostic value of point-of-care ultrasound during cardiac arrest: a systematic review. Cardiovasc Ultrasound 2020;18:1.
27. Reynolds JC, Issa MS, Nicholson T, et al. Prognostication with point-of-care echocardiography during cardiac arrest: a systematic review. Resuscitation. 2020;152:56–68.

Echocardiography in acute aortic dissection

6

Tomasz Baron and Frank A. Flachskampf

Key Points

- The most important clue to diagnosis of aortic dissection is to keep its possibility in mind in all patients with chest pain or shock.
- The presence of (new) aortic regurgitation or pericardial effusion on transthoracic echo in a patient with chest pain should raise the "red flag" of possible type A dissection, even if a dissection flap is not immediately detectable.
- A significant blood pressure rise caused by discomfort or gagging during transesophageal echocardiography (TEE) must be avoided.
- Although diagnosis of dissection in the descending aorta is accomplished most easily with TEE, both false-positive and false-negative findings occur in the ascending aorta. Use additional computed tomography or magnetic resonance imaging if the diagnosis is not evident.

CLINICAL AND PATHOPHYSIOLOGICAL BACKGROUND

Aortic dissection occurs when aortic intramural hemorrhage or bleeding into the aortic wall leads to separation of the aortic intima from the adventitia, creating the dissection membrane or flap. It is more frequent in men than in women. The most frequently associated diseases are arterial hypertension, Marfan's syndrome, bicuspid aortic valve, and chest trauma, but aortic dissection can occur spontaneously in nonhypertensive patients. An association with late pregnancy has also been noted.

The ascending aorta is affected in 60% of cases, and the thoracic descending aorta immediately distal to the takeoff of the left subclavian artery in 30% of cases. Based on the segments of the aorta involved in the dissection (Figure 6.1), two classifications are traditionally used: Stanford and DeBakey (Table 6.1). Other classifications also exist.[1,2]

Ascending aortic dissection is an *extraordinarily lethal* disease, with a mortality rate of up to 1–2% per hour in the first 48 hours if untreated. Death ensues by aortic rupture into the pericardial space or into the mediastinum. Other severe complications are torrential aortic regurgitation and propagation of dissection into the carotid arteries with subsequent stroke, or into the coronary arteries with subsequent myocardial infarction. Dissection of the ascending aorta (that is, DeBakey I or II or Stanford A) therefore mandates immediate surgery, and its rapid diagnosis is of the utmost importance. Elevated blood pressure should be lowered and intravenous beta-blockers administered, if blood pressure allows this, to reduce the rate of aortic pressure rise in systole.

In comparison, descending aortic dissection carries a lower risk, mainly of rupture or of organ ischemia, such as

DOI: 10.1201/9781003245407-6

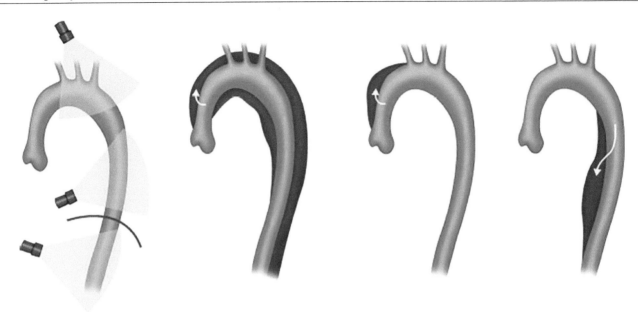

FIGURE 6.1 Transthoracic echocardiographic examination allows visualization of different parts of the aorta from multiple acoustic windows (left panel), but leaves multiple "blind spots" and thus the possibility to miss important pathology. Starting from the parasternal long-axis view, probe orientation in suprasternal, apical two-chamber, and subcostal views is shown in a clockwise direction. Classification of aortic dissection: DeBakey type I (Stanford A) (middle left panel), in which blood penetrates the intima layer in the ascending aorta and extends distally toward the aortic arch and descending aorta; DeBakey type II (Stanford A) (middle right panel), in which dissection is confined to the ascending aorta; DeBakey type III (Stanford B) (right panel), in which dissection originates in the descending aorta.

(Artwork provided by SUP.)

TABLE 6.1 Classification of Aortic Dissection (See Figure 6.1)

	Ascending aorta	*Aortic arch*	*Descending aorta*
DeBakey I	Yes	Yes	Yes
DeBakey II	Yes	No	No
DeBakey III	No	No	Yes
Stanford A	Yes	Possible	Possible
Stanford B	No	No	Yes

renal or enteral ischemia. Dissection of the descending aorta is therefore primarily treated medically by blood pressure control and supportive measures, with endovascular stent treatment or surgery in case of organ damage or ongoing aortic dilatation.

Aortic dissection manifests predominantly with severe chest pain, which often changes localization during propagation of the dissection. Other signs include dyspnea caused by aortic regurgitation or intrapericardial bleeding, organ or limb ischemia, side difference of arterial pulses, syncope, and shock. Given the enormous morbidity and mortality, especially of ascending aortic dissection, time is of the essence in diagnosis. Unfortunately, the main problem with the diagnosis of aortic dissection is the *low index of suspicion*. Once the possibility is kept in mind, it is usually not very difficult to establish the diagnosis.

ECHOCARDIOGRAPHIC SIGNS OF ACUTE AORTIC DISSECTION

Features of the dissected aorta

The classic and pathognomonic sign of aortic dissection is the *dissection membrane or flap*, a thin mobile membrane attached to the wall of the aorta, which separates the true from the false lumen. The membrane is very pliable and changes its shape during the cardiac cycle (Figure 6.2) (V6.1, V6.2, V6.3, V6.4, V6.5, and V6.6). Blood pressure and velocity in the *true lumen* are higher than in the *false lumen*, and therefore, the flap has a *convexity toward the false lumen during systole* (Figure 6.3) (V6.7). Most frequently, the false lumen is larger than the true lumen. If the blood velocity in the false lumen is low, spontaneous echo contrast or thrombosis may occur (Figure 6.4) (V6.8). Frequently on color Doppler, no or only sparse flow signals are seen in the false lumen, whereas there is color-coded systolic flow in the true lumen (Figure 6.5) (V6.9). This may help during the examination to identify an intraluminal structure as a dissection membrane. The communication sites between true and false lumen are often multiple and are designated *entry and re-entry sites*, with pulsatile flow from one lumen to the other, visualized by color Doppler. Typically, entry sites show systolic flow from the true lumen into the false lumen,

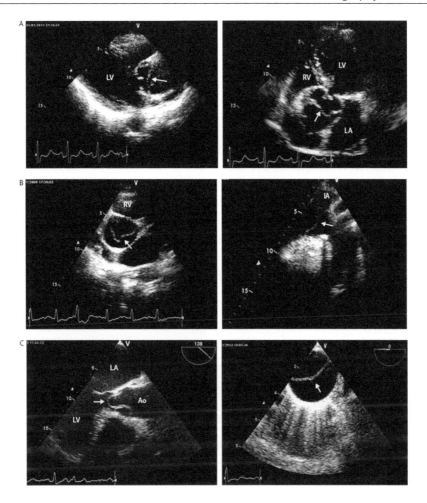

FIGURE 6.2 Dissection membrane (flap) seen from different views (arrows): (A) Transthoracic echocardiography (TTE) parasternal long-axis view of the aortic root (left panel) (V6.1); TTE apical five-chamber view of the proximal aorta (right panel) (V6.2). (B) TTE parasternal cranial short-axis view of the aortic root (left panel) (V6.3); TTE suprasternal view of the aortic arch (right panel) (V6.4). (C) Transesophageal echocardiography (TEE) long-axis view of the ascending aorta (left panel) (V6.5); TEE short-axis view of the descending aorta (right panel) (V6.6). Ao: aorta; IA: innominate artery; LA: left atrium; LV: left ventricle; RV: right ventricle.

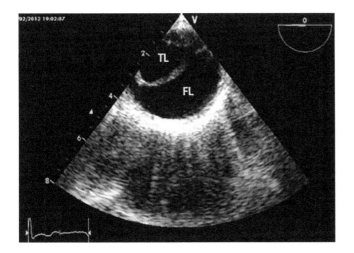

FIGURE 6.3 Transesophageal echocardiography short-axis view of descending aorta showing intimal flap separating true lumen (TL) from false lumen (FL). Note that the false lumen is larger than the true lumen and that the flap has a convexity toward the false lumen during systole (V6.7).

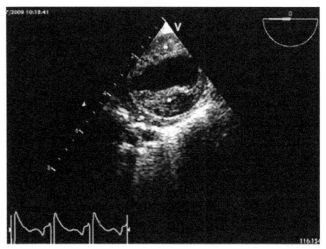

FIGURE 6.4 Transesophageal echocardiography short-axis view of descending aorta showing thrombosis (*) of the false lumen (V6.8).

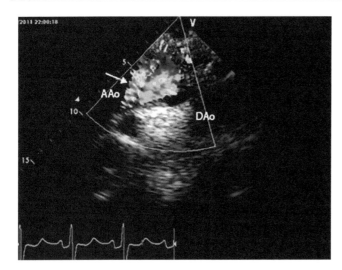

FIGURE 6.5 Color Doppler showing brisk (red/yellow) systolic flow (arrow) in the true lumen in the aortic arch and slower, opposite-direction flow in the false lumen (blue) (V6.9). AAo: ascending aorta; DAo: descending aorta.

followed by reverse flow in diastole (V6.10). Some authors, on the basis of cases with no apparent entry and no false lumen flow, describe "noncommunicating dissection" as a distinct disease type, similar to but more extensive than intramural hematoma (see later). The diameter of the aorta is mostly, but *not necessarily*, increased over 4 cm. Periaortic echolucent areas represent either free mediastinal fluid or pleural fluid.

The heart in acute ascending aortic dissection

The following three cardiac structures or events may be acutely affected by dissection of the ascending aorta (Table 6.2):

1. The *aortic valve*. Very frequently, aortic regurgitation accompanies dissection. The following mechanisms may lead to regurgitation[3]:
   - Presence of a bicuspid aortic valve, which is associated with an increased risk of aortic dissection.
   - Aortic root dilatation with central aortic regurgitation.
   - Interference of the dissection flap with diastolic closure of the aortic cusps (V6.11). The flap prolapses into the left ventricle in diastole, leading to massive regurgitation (Figure 6.6) (V6.12A and V6.12B). In this case, the valve itself is not damaged and does not necessarily have to be replaced at surgery.
2. *Pericardial effusion*. This represents bleeding into the pericardial space. It is frequent in dissection of the ascending aorta, and fatal hemorrhage with pericardial tamponade (V6.13) is a frequent immediate cause of death in aortic dissection.

TABLE 6.2   Cardiac Abnormalities Associated with or Suggestive of Aortic Dissection

- Bicuspid aortic valve
- Hypertensive heart disease
- Hypertensive aortic dilation
- Marfan's syndrome (aortic dilation with effacement of the sinotubular junction ridge, central aortic regurgitation, and mitral valve prolapse)
- Pericardial effusion
- Aortic regurgitation
- Inferior hypokinesia or akinesia

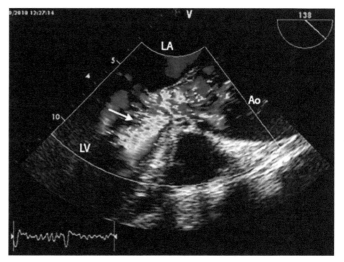

FIGURE 6.6 Color Doppler transesophageal echocardiography showing massive aortic regurgitation (turbulent jet, arrow) caused by interference of the dissection flap with diastolic closure of the aortic cusps (V6.12A and V6.12B). Ao: aorta; LA: left atrium; LV: left ventricle.

3. Obstruction or dissection of *coronary vessels*, mostly the right coronary artery, with consequent myocardial infarction or ischemia (V6.14A and V6.14B), which may be waxing and waning.

GOALS AND STRATEGY OF ECHOCARDIOGRAPHY IN AORTIC DISSECTION

Only a *few segments of the thoracic aorta are seen on transthoracic echo* (Figure 6.1). The first few centimeters of the ascending aorta are usually seen on the parasternal or apical long-axis view (V6.15), apical five-chamber view (V6.2, V6.16), and parasternal cranial short-axis view (V6.3). The descending aorta is seen in cross-section in the parasternal long-axis view and the apical views close to the left atrium and in the subcostal view (V6.17). The images of the aorta in these views often are of limited quality, although in most cases of dissection considerable dilation of the aorta is detected, and often the flap can also be seen (V6.18). However, *the presence of more than minimal aortic regurgitation and/ or of a pericardial effusion in a patient with chest pain or other suggestive symptoms outlined should immediately suggest aortic dissection* to the examiner. Suprasternal images should be attempted, although in elderly individuals they are often of low quality (V6.19 and V6.20). Left heart contrast can help in detecting dissection from this window. *In most cases, transesophageal echocardiography (TEE) or computed tomography should be performed to delineate the type and complications of dissection or to exclude the disease altogether.* In rare cases, with excellent image quality and clear visibility of aortic valve, aortic root, and dissection flap by transthoracic echo, the patient may be sent to surgery without TEE, which still can be performed in the operating room if new questions arise. TEE, because of its discomfort, necessitates *vigorous control of blood pressure* by sedation or anesthesia and/or antihypertensive medication; cases of aortic rupture during TEE in aortic dissection have been described. Food intake within the last hours is not an absolute contraindication to TEE in this particular circumstance; vomiting and aspiration, however, should be anticipated, and in unstable patients, tracheal intubation before TEE may be wise.

In the setting of acute aortic dissection, echocardiography must answer the following questions:

1. *Presence and extent of a dissection membrane; in particular, is the ascending aorta involved?* This is the most critical question, because it determines whether the patient should be sent to surgery immediately or not.
2. *Is the aortic annulus massively dilated, is there severe aortic regurgitation, and is the aortic valve bicuspid?* The answers to these questions, as well as whether the dissection begins in the aortic root or higher, may modify the surgical strategy with regard to aortic valve replacement.
3. *Is the dissection membrane in close proximity to the coronary ostia?* The right coronary ostium especially may be blocked by the membrane, or the dissection may propagate into the right coronary artery.

Other questions are of interest but not of vital importance, and answering them should not prolong the examination unduly. The location and configuration of true and false lumina, as well as entry and re-entry sites, usually are not critical for surgery. However, in a few cases the entry may be more distal than the beginning of the flap. This would suggest *retrograde dissection*, which may influence surgical strategy to resect the primary entry tear. A large *pericardial effusion* predicts imminent tamponade by free rupture into the pericardial space, hence adding to the urgency. The same is true of the detection of *periaortic fluid*. The *supra-aortic vessels* should, in any circumstance, be inspected intraoperatively for dissection.

TRANSESOPHAGEAL ECHOCARDIOGRAPHY IN AORTIC DISSECTION

With TEE, the ascending aorta can be seen *almost completely* in the midesophageal long-axis view of the left ventricle at approximately 120–150°, by pulling the instrument gently up from the lower esophageal position used for the ventricles and mitral valve to a higher midesophageal position (V6.21A and V6.21B). The corresponding ascending aorta short-axis views, at approximately 30–70°, after withdrawal of the instrument from an aortic valve short-axis view, are important to confirm visualization of structures in the long-axis view, but one should be aware that *because of tracheal and left main bronchus interference*, the short-axis views do not reach as far upward toward the aortic arch as the long-axis view does. The short-axis view a few millimeters cranial to the aortic leaflets shows the left main ostium at approximately 2–3 o'clock; the right coronary ostium, at approximately 6 o'clock, is less well seen and often better found by going to a long-axis view, in which the takeoff of the right coronary artery away from the transducer can regularly be seen. In elderly patients, immediately distal to the ostium of the right coronary artery there is frequently an atherosclerotic plaque of the aortic wall, which is a predilection site for the attachment of the dissection membrane.

Apart from visualizing the dissection membrane as unequivocally as possible, one should note the morphology of the aortic valve, the mechanism of regurgitation, the pericardial effusion, and the thickness of the aortic walls. A rapid look at left and right ventricular function and the mitral valve should also be part of the examination. For examination of the descending aorta, the probe should be positioned as distally as the thoracic descending aorta can be visualized, and then slowly pulled back, preferentially in the 0° horizontal plane, using other planes for confirmation if pathologic structures are seen. Aortic diameter, presence of a flap, entry and re-entry sites, wall thickening suggesting intramural hematoma, and periaortic fluid should be noted. An increase in distance between probe (esophagus) and aorta may indicate intramural or periaortic hematoma. At the takeoff of the left subclavian artery, the distal arch is visualized. By slow retraction of the probe, most of the arch can be inspected, with the anterior or superior aortic wall close to the transducer and the inner curvature of the arch away from the transducer. Involvement of the carotid arteries in a dissection can be much better ascertained by direct transcutaneous ultrasound examination of the carotid arteries than by TEE.

PITFALLS AND PROBLEMS

The dissection membrane usually is unmistakable and can be brought into view very clearly by TEE, separating a zone of high and one of low flow by color Doppler. However, a *small section of the distal ascending aorta and parts of the aortic arch frequently escape visualization by TEE.* In rare cases, DeBakey type II dissections may hide in this region. False-positive findings of intra-aortic structures also occur more frequently in the ascending aorta owing to reverberation and other *artifacts*, such as from right-sided Swan-Ganz catheters or pacemakers. Structures and color-coded flow at exactly double the distance from the transducer of other structures and flows, moving in parallel with each other, should be suspected of being reverberation artifacts. In the descending aorta, reverberation can create the image of a *"double-barrel" aorta*, with color Doppler flow signals in a "second" aorta distal and parallel to the true aorta.

No matter how experienced the examiner, not every diagnosis of aortic dissection or intramural hematoma (see later) can confidently be made by TEE alone, and computed tomography or magnetic resonance imaging should be performed if serious doubts remain.

DIFFERENTIAL DIAGNOSIS

The similarity in presentation to *myocardial infarction*, which typically is treated by fibrinolysis or percutaneous coronary intervention, warrants an aggressive effort to confirm or refute the diagnosis, because both therapies are contraindicated in dissection, and surgical repair is urgent in ascending aortic dissection. The problem is compounded by the fact that ascending aortic dissection itself may lead to myocardial infarction or myocardial ischemia (V6.14A and V6.14B), including electrocardiographic changes and troponin elevation. In this case, misdiagnosis of aortic dissection as primary myocardial ischemia is almost the rule. In practice, in the patient with severe chest pain, unclear shock, or unclear neurologic deficit, dissection should be ruled out by TEE or computed tomography if there is a reasonable suspicion that dissection might be the underlying cause. Severe pulmonary embolism in rare cases may enter the differential diagnosis. Usually, pulmonary embolism causes far less pain and far more dyspnea than dissection does. The echo quickly reveals whether there is striking right ventricular enlargement and hypokinesia, which would strongly argue against aortic dissection.

INTRAMURAL HEMATOMA AND PENETRATING AORTIC ULCER

Intramural hematoma (V6.22) is a variant and an early form of aortic dissection, often coexisting with or progressing to typical dissection (Figure 6.7) (V6.23A, V6.23B, and V6.23C). Therapeutically, it is managed in the same way as classic dissection, depending on involvement of the ascending aorta (V6.24A, V6.24B, V6.24C, V6.25A, and V6.25B).

Pericardial effusion may be present. Intramural hematoma is more frequent (or more frequently detected) in the descending than in the ascending aorta. The diagnostic criteria are the absence of an intimal flap, an aortic wall thickness over 5 mm, and/or an echolucent zone in the aortic wall. Unfortunately, an echolucent zone is not always present, and considerable wall thickening may occur because of atherosclerosis itself. Hence, the diagnosis of pure intramural hematoma is not easy, and magnetic resonance imaging or computed tomography should be considered in cases of suspicious aortic wall thickening.

Another variant is a *penetrating aortic ulcer*, which develops as a result of an erosion of the atheromatous plaque into the aortic media (V6.26 and V6.27). Clinical presentation and imaging findings depend on how deeply into the aortic wall the plaque erosion penetrates, ranging from intramural hematoma to saccular aneurysm, pseudoaneurysm, and rarely, aortic wall rupture.

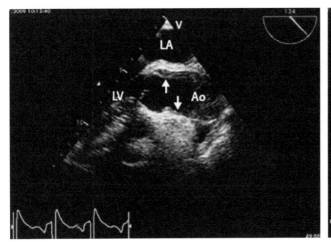 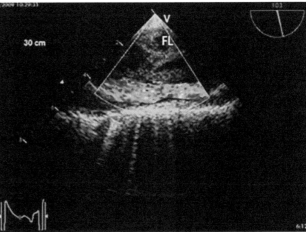

FIGURE 6.7 Coexisting intramural hematoma of the ascending aorta and complex dissection of the descending aorta. Transesophageal echocardiography long-axis view showing thickened wall (arrows) of the ascending aorta consistent with intramural hematoma (left panel) (V6.23A). At the same time, complex aortic dissection can be noted in the descending aorta (right panel) (V6.23B). Ao: aorta; FL: false lumen; LA: left atrium; LV: left ventricle.

IS ECHO SUFFICIENT TO SEND THE PATIENT TO SURGERY FOR AORTIC DISSECTION?

As always with echocardiography, the diagnostic quality is decisively influenced by the skills of the examiner. Several comparative studies, however, have clearly shown that in experienced hands TEE is considerably superior to transthoracic imaging and practically as good as computed tomography or magnetic resonance imaging for detection of dissection. However, there are cases in which this technique is not conclusive, and another modality should be sought.[4,5]

LIST OF VIDEOS

https://routledgetextbooks.com/textbooks/9781032157009/chapter-6.php

VIDEO 6.1   Intimal flap: Transthoracic parasternal long-axis view showing dissection flap in the dilated aortic root, just above the aortic valve.

VIDEO 6.2   Intimal flap: Transthoracic apical five-chamber view showing a dissection flap in the dilated aortic root.

VIDEO 6.3   Intimal flap: Transthoracic parasternal cranial short-axis view showing a dissection flap in the dilated aortic root just above the aortic valve plane. Note that imaging was difficult because of the patient's unstable condition.

VIDEO 6.4   Intimal flap: Transthoracic suprasternal view showing a dissection flap in the aortic arch extending into the innominate artery.

VIDEO 6.5   Intimal flap: Transesophageal echocardiography showing intimal flap in the proximal aorta that interferes with the diastolic closure of the aortic cusps.

VIDEO 6.6   Intimal flap and false versus true lumen: Transesophageal echocardiography short-axis view of the descending aorta showing an intimal flap that separates true (above the flap) from false lumen (below the flap). Note that the flap has a convexity toward the false lumen during systole.

VIDEO 6.7   Intimal flap and false versus true lumen: Transesophageal echocardiography short-axis view of descending aorta showing an intimal flap that separates true from false lumen. Most frequently, the false lumen is larger than the true lumen and the flap has a convexity toward the false lumen during systole.

VIDEO 6.8   Thrombosis of the false lumen: Transesophageal echocardiography short-axis view of descending aorta showing thrombosis of the false lumen.

VIDEO 6.9   True versus false lumen (color Doppler): Color Doppler showing brisk (red/yellow) systolic flow in the true lumen in the aortic arch, and slower, opposite-direction flow in the false lumen (blue).

VIDEO 6.10   Communications between true and false lumina: Transesophageal short-axis view showing two small communications by color Doppler between true (left) and false (right) lumina, with flow into the false lumen in systole and some backflow in diastole.

VIDEO 6.11   Intimal flap interference with aortic valve closure: Transesophageal long-axis view of the aortic valve and ascending aorta showing interference of the intimal flap with diastolic closure of the aortic cusps. Note mobile flap changing configuration during the cardiac cycle and prolapsing in diastole through the aortic valve into the left ventricular outflow tract. This is one of the possible mechanisms of aortic regurgitation caused by aortic dissection.

VIDEO 6.12A   Intimal flap causing aortic regurgitation (1/2): Transesophageal echocardiography showing interference of the dissection flap with diastolic closure of the aortic cusps. The flap prolapses into the left ventricular outflow tract in diastole, leading to massive aortic regurgitation (see Video 6.12B).

VIDEO 6.12B   Intimal flap causing aortic regurgitation (2/2): Color Doppler transesophageal echocardiography showing massive aortic regurgitation caused by interference of the dissection flap with diastolic closure of the aortic cusps (see also Video 6.12A).

VIDEO 6.13   Proximal aortic dissection causing hematopericard: Transthoracic echocardiography showing large pericardial effusion in a patient with proximal aortic dissection that represents bleeding into the pericardial space. Note the large mass inside the effusion, consistent with hematoma. Fatal hemorrhage with pericardial tamponade is frequent in dissection of the ascending aorta.

VIDEO 6.14A   Acute myocardial infarction associated with acute aortic dissection (1/2): Transthoracic apical long-axis view showing a hypokinetic inferoposterior left ventricular wall, better appreciated in parasternal short-axis view (see Video 6.14B) and an intimal flap in the proximal aorta. The patient was admitted to the emergency department with severe chest pain radiating to the back and ST-segment elevation in the inferior electrocardiographic leads. He was immediately referred to the cardiac surgery center, where coronary angiography (which revealed obstruction of the ostium of the right coronary artery by the intimal flap) and emergent surgery were performed. *(Video provided by PMM.)*

VIDEO 6.14B   Acute myocardial infarction associated with acute aortic dissection (2/2): Transthoracic parasternal short-axis view showing akinesis of the inferoposterior left ventricular (LV) wall.

The asynergy of the posterior LV wall can be appreciated also in apical long-axis view, in which the intimal flap in the proximal aorta can be seen (see Video 6.14A). The patient was admitted to the emergency department with severe chest pain radiating to the back and ST-segment elevation in the inferior electrocardiographic leads. He was immediately referred to cardiac surgery center, where coronary angiography (which revealed obstruction of the ostium of the right coronary artery by the intimal flap) and emergent surgery were performed. *(Video provided by PMM.)*

VIDEO 6.15   Intimal flap: Transthoracic parasternal long-axis view showing an intimal flap in the aortic root.

VIDEO 6.16   Intimal flap: Modified transthoracic five-chamber view was used for better visualization of an intimal flap in the proximal aorta.

VIDEO 6.17   Intimal flap: Subcostal view clearly showing an intimal flap in the descending aorta.

VIDEO 6.18   Intimal flap: Subcostal short-axis view of the base of the heart showing an intimal flap in the aortic root. This view may be useful in case of poor parasternal and apical echocardiographic windows.

VIDEO 6.19   Intimal flap: In elderly individuals, the suprasternal images of the aortic arch are often of poor quality. In this case, the presence of an intimal flap just opposite to the great vessels of the aortic arch is suspected. The diagnosis was confirmed by transesophageal echocardiography. *(Video provided by IS.)*

VIDEO 6.20   Intimal flap: Rarely in the elderly, excellent image from suprasternal window can be obtained, allowing easy detection of an intimal flap in the ascending aorta and the arch. *(Video provided by IS.)*

VIDEO 6.21A   Intimal flap causing aortic regurgitation (1/2): Transesophageal echocardiography showing intimal flap in the proximal aorta. The flap interferes with diastolic closure of the aortic cusps. Note the prolapse of one of the cusps, leading to massive aortic regurgitation (see Video 6.21B).

VIDEO 6.21B   Intimal flap causing aortic regurgitation (2/2): Color Doppler transesophageal echocardiography showing massive aortic regurgitation caused by interference of the dissection flap with diastolic closure of the aortic cusps and prolapse of one of the cusps (see also Video 6.21A).

VIDEO 6.22   Intramural hematoma: Transesophageal long-axis view showing intramural hematoma of the anterior wall of the ascending aorta.

VIDEO 6.23A   Coexisting intramural hematoma of the ascending aorta and complex dissection in the descending aorta (1/3): Transesophageal long-axis view revealed thickened aortic wall of the ascending aorta consistent with intramural hematoma. At the same time, complex aortic dissection can be noted in the descending aorta (see Videos 6.23B and 6.23C).

VIDEO 6.23B   Coexisting intramural hematoma of the ascending aorta and complex dissection in the descending aorta (2/3): Coexisting intramural hematoma of the ascending aorta and complex dissection of the descending aorta. Transesophageal echocardiography at longitudinal (shown here) and short-axis (see Video 6.23C) views of the descending aorta revealed complex aortic dissection. At the same time, intramural hematoma of the ascending aorta can be noted (see Video 6.23A).

VIDEO 6.23C   Coexisting intramural hematoma of the ascending aorta and complex dissection in the descending aorta (3/3): Transesophageal echocardiography at longitudinal (see Video 6.23B) and short-axis (shown here) views of the descending aorta revealed complex aortic dissection. At the same time, intramural hematoma of the ascending aorta can be noted (see Video 6.23A).

VIDEO 6.24A   Initially overlooked intramural hematoma (1/3): Modified transthoracic parasternal long-axis view showing intramural hematoma of the proximal aorta in a patient with chest pain and normal electrocardiogram. A night before in the emergency department the diagnosis had been overlooked (see Video 6.24B). The thickened aortic wall is better appreciated in the short-axis view (see Video 6.24C). *(Video provided by PMM.)*

VIDEO 6.24B   Initially overlooked intramural hematoma (2/3): In this standard parasternal view, the diagnosis of the aortic intramural hematoma can be easily missed in the emergency department, which in fact had happened. The next morning, the diagnosis was made in modified parasternal long-axis view, which allowed better visualization of the ascending aorta (see Video 6.24A). The thickened aortic wall is even better appreciated in the short-axis view (see Video 6.24C). *(Video provided by PMM.)*

VIDEO 6.24C   Initially overlooked intramural hematoma (3/3): Transthoracic short-axis view of the ascending aorta showing the thickened aortic wall, consistent with intramural hematoma (see also Video 6.24A). *(Video provided by PMM.)*

VIDEO 6.25A   Intramural hematoma (1/2): Transesophageal echocardiography showing intramural hematoma in the wall of the proximal aorta. Note that the hematoma does not interfere with the aortic annulus or cusps, and color Doppler reveals no significant aortic regurgitation (see Video 6.25B).

VIDEO 6.25B   Intramural hematoma (2/2): Color Doppler transesophageal echocardiography showing no significant aortic regurgitation in the patient with intramural hematoma of the proximal aorta. The hematoma does not interfere with the aortic annulus or cusps (see Video 6.25A).

VIDEO 6.26   Penetrating aortic ulcer: This transesophageal echocardiography longitudinal view of the descending aorta shows a deep ulcer-like defect of the aortic wall, filled with thrombus (hematoma). Note that there is no intimal flap. *(Video provided by JS.)*

VIDEO 6.27   Penetrating aortic ulcer: Three-dimensional transesophageal echocardiography showing penetrating ulcer of the descending aorta (right panel). *(Video provided by JS.)*

REFERENCES

1. Hiratzka LF, Bakris GL, Beckman JA, et al. 2010 ACCF/AHA/AATS/ACR/ASA/SCA/SCAI/SIR/STS/SVM guidelines for the diagnosis and management of patients with thoracic aortic disease. A report of the American College of Cardiology Foundation/American Heart Association Task Force on Practice Guidelines, American Association for Thoracic Surgery, American College of Radiology, American Stroke Association, Society of Cardiovascular Anesthesiologists, Society for Cardiovascular Angiography and Interventions, Society of Interventional Radiology, Society of Thoracic Surgeons, and Society for Vascular Medicine. J Am Coll Cardiol 2010; 55:e27–129.

2. Evangelista A, Flachskampf FA, Erbel R, et al. Echocardiography in aortic diseases: EAE recommendations for clinical practice. Eur J Echocardiogr 2010; 11(8):645–58. Erratum in: Eur J Echocardiogr 2011; 12:642.

3. Movsowitz HD, Levine RA, Hilgenberg AD, et al. Transesophageal echocardiographic description of the mechanisms of aortic regurgitation in acute type A aortic dissection: implications for aortic valve repair. J Am Coll Cardiol 2000; 36:884–90.

4. Goldstein SA, Evangelista A, Abbara S, et al. Multimodality imaging of diseases of the thoracic aorta in adults: from the American Society of Echocardiography and the European Association of Cardiovascular Imaging: endorsed by the Society of Cardiovascular Computed Tomography and Society for Cardiovascular Magnetic Resonance. J Am Soc Echocardiogr 2015; 28(2):119–82.

5. Erbel R, Aboyans V, Boileau C, et al. 2014 ESC guidelines on the diagnosis and treatment of aortic diseases: document covering acute and chronic aortic diseases of the thoracic and abdominal aorta of the adult. The Task Force for the Diagnosis and Treatment of Aortic Diseases of the European Society of Cardiology (ESC). Eur Heart J 2014; 35(41):2873–926.

Echocardiography in acute pulmonary embolism

7

Piotr Pruszczyk, Katarzyna Kurnicka, and Adam Torbicki

Key Points

- The hemodynamic consequences of acute pulmonary embolism (PE) can be detected by echocardiography.
- Normal right ventricular morphology and function make acute PE highly unlikely as a cause of hemodynamic instability.
- Echocardiographic signs of right ventricular overload (McConnell's sign and 60/60 sign) are indirect signs suggestive of intermediate- or high-risk acute PE, but could also result from other causes.
- Thrombi in the pulmonary artery and the right side of the heart (direct signs of PE) are rarely detected by transthoracic echocardiography, but nevertheless indicate high mortality risk.
- Transesophageal echocardiography can frequently detect thrombi in the proximal parts of the pulmonary arteries in patients with significant acute PE.
- Echocardiographic signs of right ventricular dysfunction indicate worse prognosis in normotensive acute PE patients.
- Patent foramen ovale is associated with worse prognosis in patients with acute PE.
- Ultrasonographic detection of deep venous thrombosis supports the diagnosis of PE in a patient with clinically suspected acute PE.

Acute pulmonary embolism (PE) remains one of the major causes of in-hospital mortality. According to the current guidelines, an optimal management of acute PE depends on adequate *risk assessment* of PE-related early death, which should be done in all PE patients.[1] Patients with *high-risk PE* are defined by the presence of at least one of the following clinical criteria at presentation: cardiac arrest, or cardiogenic obstructive shock, or systolic blood pressure <90 mmHg or its drop >40 mmHg (lasting longer than 15 minutes and not caused by new-onset arrhythmia, hypovolemia, or sepsis) with the presence or right ventricular (RV) dysfunction detected by imaging modalities. Approximately 5% of all PE patients present as a high-risk PE. Early PE-related fatality in high-risk PE exceeds 15%,[1] with most deaths occurring during the first hours after admission. Therefore, urgent

primary reperfusion mostly systemic thrombolysis is recommended as treatment of choice.[1] In hemodynamically unstable patients, urgent bedside transthoracic echocardiography (TTE) is the first imagining method for the initial assessment of a mechanism of hemodynamic collapse and is very important for guiding further management. Importantly, if immediate computed tomography pulmonary angiography (CTPA) is not feasible, bedside transthoracic echocardiography (TTE) is an acceptable alternative to reach the diagnosis and even to start a life-saving therapy.[2,3] It can provide evidence of acute pulmonary hypertension and RV dysfunction. Moreover, direct echocardiographic signs of acute PE can be detected, such as thrombi in the right heart and/or pulmonary artery or "in transit" right heart thrombi can be detected, that reinforce PE diagnosis. In a highly unstable

DOI: 10.1201/9781003245407-7

patient with suspected PE, echocardiographic evidence of RV dysfunction is sufficient to prompt immediate reperfusion without further testing. However, visualization of pulmonary thromboemboli, preferably by CTPA, is indicated whenever possible. Bedside compression venous ultrasound or TEE can be considered to reinforce indications for primary reperfusion when direct confirmation of PE by CTPA is not feasible.

Importantly, in hemodynamically stable patients with suspected PE (non-high-risk PE), echocardiography is not recommended as a diagnostic modality; however, it provides important information regarding differential diagnosis and prognosis. This chapter provides information that should help to optimize the use of echocardiography in emergency assessment of patients with suspected or confirmed PE.

INDIRECT ECHOCARDIOGRAPHIC SIGNS IN SUSPECTED PE

Echocardiographic signs of right ventricular overload

The hemodynamic consequences of PE can be detected by echocardiography. They depend not only on the degree of thrombotic load in pulmonary arteries but also on individual cardiopulmonary reserve. Therefore, in a young patient without pre-existing cardiopulmonary disorders, even total occlusion of one pulmonary artery may not alter RV morphology and function, whereas in a patient with low cardiopulmonary reserve, even a smaller thromboembolic burden can result in acute cor pulmonale with

systemic hypotension or even shock. However, it can be reasonably expected that PE will cause acute RV pressure overload when obstruction of pulmonary vascular bed exceeds 30–50%. Due to complex RV geometry, there is no individual echocardiographic parameter that provides fast and reliable information on RV size or function. This is why echocardiographic criteria for the diagnosis of PE differed across studies. Importantly, preserved RV function on TTE does not exclude PE.

Acutely increased systolic and filling pressures result in *dilation of the right ventricle, right atrium*, and *inferior vena cava* (IVC). Of note, although quite obvious in severe obstruction of pulmonary arteries, in less severe cases, RV enlargement can be more subtle and more difficult to detect. The *interventricular septum may be flattened or even bulge* into the left ventricle (D-shaped septum)[4,5] (Figure 7.1) (V7.1). Thus, in an acute setting, with the pericardium limiting cardiac enlargement, the underfilled left ventricle becomes compressed and distorted by an expanding right ventricle. The presence of RV pressure overload can be diagnosed by measuring *peak velocity of the jet of tricuspid regurgitation*.[6] In addition, assessment of *pulmonary ejection pattern* can reveal abnormalities highly suggestive of proximal obstruction of pulmonary arteries.[7] However, although suggestive, none of these signs is fully diagnostic for PE.

Several studies have assessed sensitivity and specificity of the diagnosis of PE using various sets of echocardiographic criteria reflecting RV dysfunction. According to French authors who studied 132 patients with suspected PE, the combined criteria, including tricuspid regurgitant flow peak velocity greater than 2.5 m/s and enlarged right ventricle would have sensitivity of 93% and specificity of 81% for the diagnosis of PE.[6] This study excluded patients with a history of cardiac or pulmonary diseases, in whom signs of RV overload are often present and might adversely affect specificity of the suggested echocardiographic criteria.

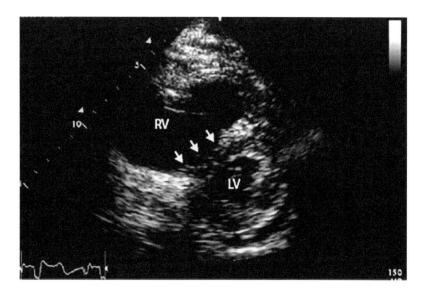

FIGURE 7.1   Parasternal short-axis view of a patient with acute pulmonary embolism showing flattening of the interventricular septum (D-shaped left ventricle, arrows) resulting from right ventricular pressure overload. Right ventricular enlargement can also be seen (V7.1). LV: left ventricle; RV: right ventricle.

(Image and video provided by IS.)

An Italian group studying 117 consecutive, nonselected patients with suspected PE reported an even higher specificity (87%) but a lower sensitivity (51%) of echocardiographic diagnosis of PE.[8] When clinical, echocardiographic, and venous ultrasonographic evaluation was integrated, overall sensitivity increased to 89%, but specificity fell to 74%, which was lower than with echocardiographic evaluation alone.

Importantly, it was shown that the clinical impact of echocardiographic signs of RV overload for the diagnosis of PE was highly influenced by the clinical probability of this disease.[9] Coexistence of at least two of three signs (RV hypokinesis, RV dilation, and systolic velocity of tricuspid valve regurgitation >2.5 m/s) was analyzed, and for a pretest clinical probability of 10%, 50%, or 90%, the post-test probability of PE was 38%, 85%, or 98%, respectively.[9]

The assessment of the *diameter of the IVC during the respiratory cycle* can also be useful in the diagnosis and assessment of acute PE.[10] When defined as inspiratory change in the IVC diameter of less than 40% of its maximum expiratory value, decreased inferior vena cava collapsibility index

(IVCCI) was reported in majority of patients with PE presenting with RV dilation (V7.2).

On the other hand, *signs of RV dysfunction may also be found in the absence of acute PE* but resulting from concomitant cardiac or respiratory disease. Hence, RV overload was found in 8.7% of patients with adult respiratory distress syndrome (ARDS)[11] (V7.24A, V7.24B, V7.24C). Also, RV myocardial infarction can lead to RV enlargement and hypokinesis, dilation of tricuspid annulus and severe tricuspid regurgitation, and often distention of the IVC without respiratory changes.[12] (see Chapter 3, V3.28.) Echocardiographic data summarized in Table 7.1 may be helpful in the differentiation of RV enlargement.

Although signs of RV pressure overload in an appropriate clinical setting are highly suggestive of acute PE, they are not fully reliable. It is very important to remember that *false-positive diagnoses* may potentially lead to an unnecessary thrombolysis with all its inherent risks. Therefore, definitive confirmation of PE before thrombolysis initiation, whenever possible and feasible, is the optimal strategy.

TABLE 7.1 Echocardiographic Signs Useful in the Differentiation of Causes of Right Ventricular Dilation

	MAXIMAL TRICUSPID PEAK SYSTOLIC GRADIENT	ACCELERATION TIME OF RV EJECTION	INFERIOR VENA CAVA	OTHER
Acute RV overload in acute PE	30–60 mmHg	<80 ms, frequently <60 ms with midsystolic notch	>20 mm, noncollapsing at inspiration	Hypokinesis of RV free wall, preserved contractility of its apical segments (McConnell's sign), TAPSE ≤16 mm
Chronic thromboembolic pulmonary hypertension	Frequently >60 mmHg	<80 ms, frequently <60 ms with midsystolic notch	>20 mm, noncollapsing at inspiration	Signs of RV hypertrophy; diastolic thickness of RV free wall >6 mm
PH due to CLD	Usually <80 mmHg	<80 ms infrequently with notch	>20 mm, collapsing at inspiration	Signs of RV hypertrophy; diastolic thickness of RV free wall >6 mm
RV infarction	Mostly <30 mmHg	>100 ms	>20 mm, noncollapsing at inspiration	Coexisting regional asynergy of inferior or posterior LV wall; McConnell's sign possible
Isolated tricuspid regurgitation	Mostly <30 mmHg	>100 ms	>20 mm, noncollapsing at inspiration	Preserved contractility of both ventricles
LV dysfunction; mitral valve disease	Mostly <60 mmHg, but may be higher	<100 ms, rarely midsystolic notch	>20 mm, noncollapsing at inspiration	Advanced LV systolic dysfunction or mitral valve pathology
Intracardiac shunts (early stage)	Mostly <60 mmHg	Normal or only slightly shortened <100 ms; signs of increased pulmonary cardiac output	Frequently normal	Signs of intracardiac shunts
Eisenmenger's syndrome	Mostly >60 mmHg	Relatively less shortened than in other pathologies with similar level of pulmonary arterial hypertension	Frequently normal	RV hypertrophy; intracardiac shunt usually with low pressure gradients

Abbreviations: CLD, chronic lung disease; LV, left ventricular; PH, pulmonary hypertension; PE, pulmonary embolism; RV, right ventricular.

More specific echocardiographic signs of pulmonary embolism

More specific echocardiographic signs of acute PE have been defined. The presence of *hypokinesis of the RV free wall with preserved contractility of its apical segment (McConnell's sign)* has been suggested as a useful tool to differentiate between acute pressure overload caused by PE and other diseases leading to RV strain (Figure 7.2) (V7.3).[13] McConnell's sign showed a specificity of 94% with a sensitivity of 77% in a retrospective analysis of 85 patients. Although the pathophysiology of

this phenomenon has not been clearly defined yet, successful treatment of PE led to the recovery of RV regional function (Figure 7.3) (V7.4A and V7.4B). However, patients with RV infarction may also have a similar pattern of RV dysfunction[12] (see Chapter 3, V3.28), and additional echocardiographic signs of pressure overload may be needed to differentiate between PE and RV infarction.

Doppler echocardiography can also provide signs that appear to be more specifically linked to PE. Characteristic *disturbances of the flow velocity curve of RV ejection* were observed in patients with hemodynamically significant PE. Because pressure waves reflected from centrally located

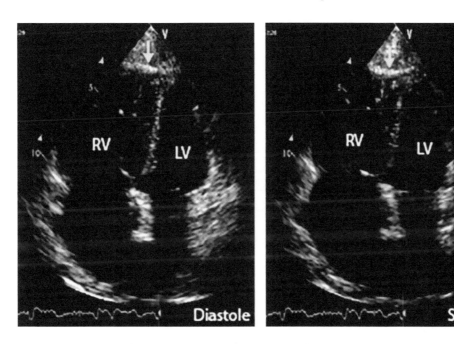

FIGURE 7.2   McConnell's sign. Apical four-chamber view of a patient with acute pulmonary embolism showing marked right ventricular dilation with free-wall hypokinesis and preserved contractility of the apical segment (V7.3). LV: left ventricle; RV: right ventricle.

(Images and video provided by IS.)

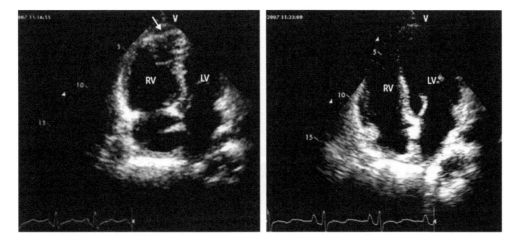

FIGURE 7.3   Right ventricular dilation with free-wall akinesia and relative apical sparing (arrow) seen at admission in a patient with acute pulmonary embolism (McConnell's sign, left panel, V7.4A) completely waned after thrombolytic therapy. Note normal right ventricular dimension and function recovery on the third hospital day (right panel, V7.4B). LV: left ventricle; RV: right ventricle.

(Images and videos provided by ANN.)

pulmonary arterial masses interfere with pulmonary ejection, this results in a markedly *shortened acceleration time (AcT)* and midsystolic deceleration *(mid-systolic notch)*, both measured by pulsed-wave Doppler in the RV outflow tract (Figure 7.4). AcT can be very short in patients with central PE even in cases with only slightly increased RV systolic pressure. Coexistence of AcT of pulmonary ejection below 60 ms measured in the RV outflow tract and of tricuspid valve peak systolic gradient less than 60 mmHg

(60/60 sign) is highly suggestive of PE (Figure 7.5). In a retrospective observation of 86 patients with various causes of pulmonary hypertension, this 60/60 sign was 94% specific, with a sensitivity of 48% for the diagnosis of PE.[14] In a prospective study of 100 consecutive patients with clinically suspected PE, the clinical value of both McConnell's sign and the 60/60 sign was assessed.[7] Importantly, this group consisted of unselected patients and included subjects with various coexisting cardiopulmonary diseases. PE

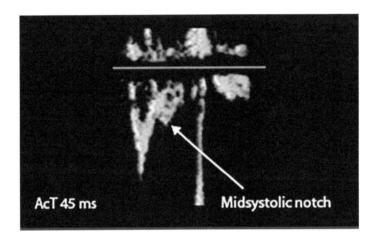

FIGURE 7.4   Disturbed pulmonary ejection assessed with pulsed-wave Doppler in right ventricular outflow tract. Markedly shortened acceleration time (AcT) of 45 ms with midsystolic notch (arrow) in a patient with massive pulmonary embolism.

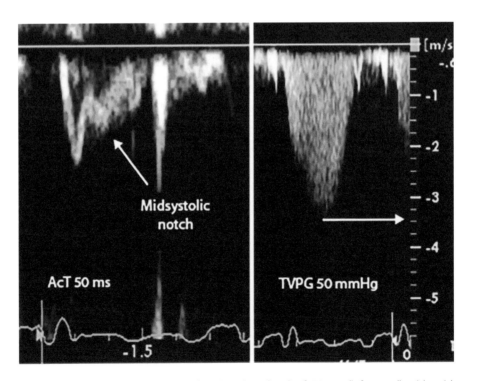

FIGURE 7.5   The 60/60 sign. Shortened pulmonary acceleration time (AcT) of 50 ms (left panel) with midsystolic notch but only moderately elevated tricuspid valve peak systolic gradient (TVPG) of 50 mmHg (right panel).

(Images provided by IS.)

was confirmed by reference tests in 67% of patients, and the reported sensitivity and specificity in diagnosis of PE were 25% and 94% for the 60/60 sign and 19% and 100% for McConnell's sign. When combined, the two signs were 94% specific and 36% sensitive in diagnosis of PE. In our opinion, if McConnell's or the 60/60 sign is detected, even in a patient without clinical suspicion for PE and with a potential explanation for hemodynamic instability or dyspnea, PE still should be strongly suspected and suitable diagnostic work-up should be undertaken. The major limitation of both McConnell's and the 60/60 signs is limited sensitivity. Therefore, their absence or even lack of any echocardiographic signs of RV overload cannot exclude PE. While hemodynamically stable patients with no echocardiographic RV dysfunction belong to a low-risk PE population, this is true only if adequate anticoagulation is promptly introduced to prevent recurrence.

In some patients with suspected acute PE, echocardiography may detect an increased RV wall thickness, or tricuspid insufficiency jet velocity beyond values compatible with acute RV pressure overload (>3.8 m/s, or a tricuspid valve peak systolic gradient >60 mmHg).[15] In these cases, chronic thromboembolic (or other) pulmonary hypertension (PH) should be considered in the differential diagnosis.

An echocardiographic pattern of acute PE has been described in a single-center analysis of 511 consecutive patients with PE confirmed by CTPA. It showed RV enlargement, RV free-wall hypokinesis, and interventricular septal flattening were present in 27.4%, 26.6%, and 18.4% of patients, respectively.[5] Tricuspid regurgitation peak systolic gradient >30 mmHg and pulmonary ejection acceleration time <80 ms were measured in 46.6% and 37.2% of patients, respectively. RV dysfunction diagnosed when echocardiography showed RV free-wall hypokinesis, and the RV to LV end-diastolic ratio was >0.9 in the four-chamber apical view was found in only 20.0% of these unselected consecutive PE patients. Notably, typical echocardiographic signs for acute PE – the McConnell sign, 60/60 sign, and right heart thrombus – were found in 19.8%, 12.9%, 1.8% of subjects, respectively. However, importantly, all 16 high-risk PE patients presented at least one of aforementioned typical echocardiographic signs. This confirms the diagnostic value of TTE in hemodynamically unstable PE patients.[5]

DIRECT ECHOCARDIOGRAPHIC SIGNS IN SUSPECTED PULMONARY EMBOLISM: VISUALIZATION OF RIGHT HEART AND PULMONARY ARTERY THROMBI

PE can be definitively confirmed only by direct visualization of thromboemboli inside pulmonary arteries. It is generally accepted that "in-transit" thrombi found in right heart chambers (Figure 7.6) (V7.5A, V7.5B, V7.5C, V7.5D, V7.5E, V7.6A and V7.6B) in patients with suspected PE also prove the disease. Moreover, detection of thrombi in the peripheral venous system (see the following figure) in a patient with clinically suspected PE discloses a potential source of emboli, justifies initiation of treatment, and confirms PE diagnosis when clinical symptoms are present.[1] Documentation of venous thrombi may be especially helpful for therapeutic decisions in patients in whom echocardiographic signs of RV overload are equivocal.

Pulmonary artery thrombi

TTE infrequently allows visualization of pulmonary artery thromboemboli. However, the *pulmonary trunk and the initial segments of pulmonary arteries* can be assessed from the subcostal approach or from a modified short-axis parasternal view (Figure 7.7) (V7.7, V7.8). Mobile right-heart thrombi are detected by TTE or transesophageal echocardiography (TEE), or by CTPA, in less than 4% of unselected patients with PE.[16–18] Their prevalence may reach 18% among PE patients in the intensive care setting.[19] The suprasternal window may enable visualization of the right pulmonary artery, and it has been reported to be useful for thrombus detection (Figure 7.8) (V7.9, V7.10, and V7.11). Although we encourage the use of all these approaches in a patient with suspected acute PE, the chance of unequivocal visualization of pulmonary arterial thrombus is rather low.

Transesophageal echocardiography (TEE) improves visualization not only of heart structures but also of the great vessels *including the proximal segments of pulmonary arteries*. After the first report by Nixdorff et al., who detected pulmonary artery thrombus during TEE[20] many case reports and short series have been published indicating the clinical value of TEE in the prompt confirmation of PE.[21–23] Later, more systematic studies were performed to assess clinical value of TEE in suspected PE.[24,25] High specificity of TEE diagnosis can be expected only when unequivocally visualized *intrapulmonary masses with distinct borders and different echodensity* from the vascular wall are reported as thromboemboli (Figure 7.9) (V7.12, V7.17B, V7.18, V7.19, V7.20, V7.21, V7.25). The echocardiographic diagnosis of thrombi should always be attempted with the understanding that the result of TEE can serve as a justification for aggressive treatment, including thrombolysis or even embolectomy. Therefore, at the beginning of the learning curve, special care should be taken not to overdiagnose PE. Limited sensitivity of TEE for PE results from the imaging windows restricted to central pulmonary arteries. In the early studies, the left pulmonary artery was considered inaccessible for TEE evaluation because much of it was shielded from the ultrasound beam by the left main bronchus. Selection criteria of patients for TEE strongly influence its sensitivity. In our laboratory only patients with RV overload at TTE undergo TEE to search for thrombi. Thus, in a group of 113 patients with clinical suspicion of PE presenting with RV overload, TEE reached

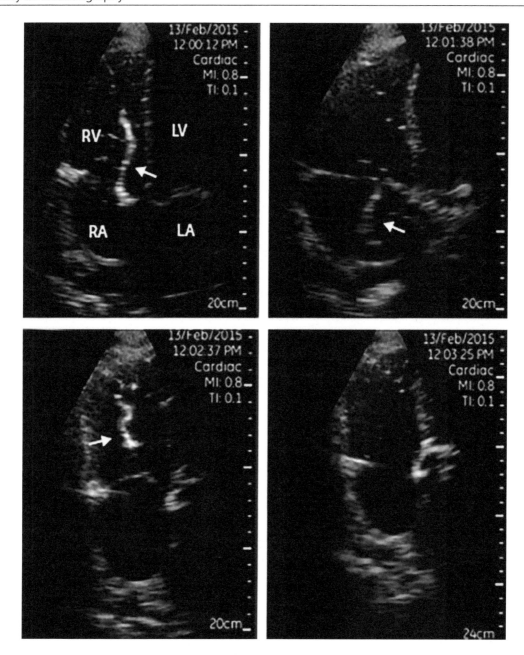

FIGURE 7.6 Acute pulmonary embolism with right heart thrombi "in transit" imaged with a handheld ultrasound device. A large wormlike thrombus (arrow) freely moving from the right atrium to the right ventricle and microbubbles from vigorous fluid resuscitation are visible in upper left panel (V7.5A). Smaller thrombi (arrows) floating in the right atrium (upper right panel, V7.5B) and also in dilated right ventricle (bottom left panel, V7.5C and V7.5D) were observed shortly after the first mass disappeared. All thrombi left the right heart in approximately 3 minutes (bottom right panel, V7.5E). LA: left atrium; LV: left ventricle; RA: right atrium; RV: right ventricle.

(Images and videos provided by MMP.)

a sensitivity of 80% with a specificity of 97.4%.[25] However, sensitivity would be probably much lower in an unselected group of patients, which would include many patients with PE limited to smaller and more distal thrombi. The experience level of the echocardiographic team may also influence the diagnostic value of TEE; the practice of routine evaluation of pulmonary arteries in patients undergoing TEE for other indications might lead to improved diagnostic performance in patients with suspected PE.

TEE performed in patients with suspected high-risk PE, in our opinion, is a safe bedside method. The diagnosis of PE has been established by TEE even in patients with shock or during cardiopulmonary resuscitation.[26] Pulmonary arteries can be evaluated within a few minutes, and the procedure can be stopped after the first thrombus is unequivocally detected. Direct visualization of intrapulmonary thrombi may be of special importance in patients with suspected high-risk PE and coexisting relative contraindication

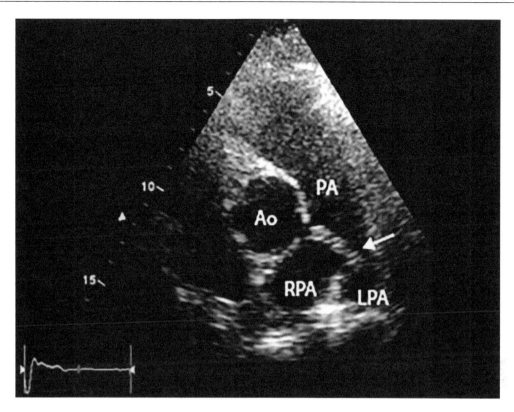

FIGURE 7.7   A large mobile thrombus bouncing at the pulmonary artery bifurcation (arrow) and protruding into the left pulmonary artery (V7.7). Ao: aorta; LPA: left pulmonary artery; PA: pulmonary artery; RPA: right pulmonary artery.

(Image and video provided by BAP.)

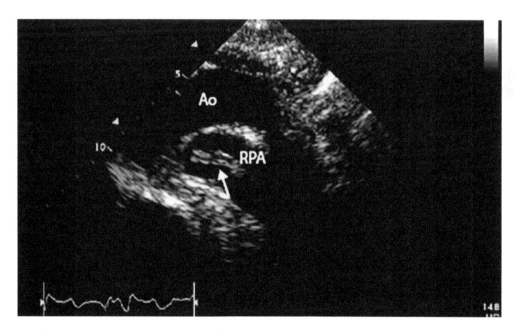

FIGURE 7.8   A wormlike thrombus (arrow) in the right pulmonary artery (RPA), as seen from the suprasternal window (V7.9). Ao: aorta.

(Image and video provided by VC.)

for thrombolysis. However, visualization of high-degree thrombotic obstruction of pulmonary arteries or saddle PE per se is not always an indication for aggressive treatment; patient management should be primarily guided by actual clinical status. Due to high availability of CTPA, the role of TEE for the diagnosis of PE is currently limited mostly to hemodynamically compromised patients when CTPA is not feasible.

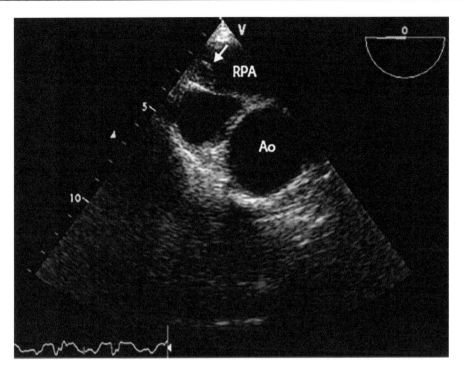

FIGURE 7.9   Transesophageal echocardiogram in a patient with suspected pulmonary embolism showing a thrombus (arrow) in the right pulmonary artery (RPA) (V7.12). Ao: aorta.

(Image provided by VC.)

Right heart thrombi

Echocardiography may detect thrombi in the right heart chambers. Mobile right-heart thrombi (RHT) are detected by TTE or transesophageal echocardiography, or by CTPA, in less than 4% of unselected patients with PE.[16–18] Their prevalence may reach 18% among PE patients in the intensive care setting.[19] Mobile RHT essentially confirm the diagnosis of PE and are associated with high early mortality especially in patients with RV dysfunction.[18,27–29] Usually thrombi are found in the right atrium and frequently present as highly mobile structures, sometimes prolapsing during diastole into the right ventricle. Their snake-like appearance and coexistence with deep vein thrombosis often suggest a venous origin (Figure 7.10) (V7.13A, V7.13B, V7.6A, V7.6B). Almost invariably RHT occur in patients with dilatation and systolic dysfunction of the right ventricle usually caused of earlier embolic episodes. Sluggish flow enables even non-anchored large thrombi to remain for some time within the right heart chambers. In some cases, right heart thrombus can be lodged in patent foramen ovale (PFO) and even protrude into the left atrium (Figure 7.11) (V7.16, V13.25) when dislodgement of left-sided part of protruding thrombus may cause peripheral embolization, including stroke. The possibility of myxoma or extracardiac tumor extending into the right atrium via the inferior or superior vena cava should always be considered before the final decision regarding therapy is made (V7.14, V7.15).

Although right heart thrombus confirms the diagnosis of PE, the optimal therapy has not been defined and treatment selection is still a subject of ongoing debate. Current guidelines on

PE management underscore that the *presence* right heart thrombi should be considered a potentially life-threatening condition.[1] Interestingly, a meta-analysis showed that 99 of 593 patients with echocardiography-detectable RHT died (16.7% [95% CI, 13.8–19.9]) compared with 639 of 14,627 without RHT (4.4% [95% CI, 4.0–4.7]). RHT had a significant association with short-term all-cause mortality in all patients (OR, 3.0 [95% CI, 2.2 to 4.1]; I(2) = 20%) and with PE-related death (OR: 4.8 [95% CI, 2.0–11.3]; I(2) = 76%). In patients diagnosed with acute PE, concomitant RHT were significantly associated with an increased risk of death within 30 days of PE diagnosis[28] The Right Heart Thrombi European Registry (RiHTER) with data on 138 patients with right heart thrombi indicate that hemodynamic instability and not characteristics of the thrombi is the strongest predictor of outcome; neither thrombus size nor shape influenced the prognosis. However, PE-related 30-day mortality exceeded 40% in high-risk patients with PE and reached 16% in intermediate-risk PE, and no PE-related death was observed in patients with low-risk PE.[27] Of note, the mortality rate of 16% in intermediate-risk PE with RHT was higher than usually reported in normotensive PE patients with RV dysfunction.[27] Thus, we believe that prognosis in patients with RHT is predominantly related to hemodynamic consequences of PE and not to thrombus characteristics.

At the moment, it is difficult to propose evidence-based recommendations regarding management of these patients. Although some studies suggested that thrombolytic therapy was associated with an improved survival rate when compared with either anticoagulation therapy or surgery, potential therapeutic benefits of thrombolysis in stable patients with RHT

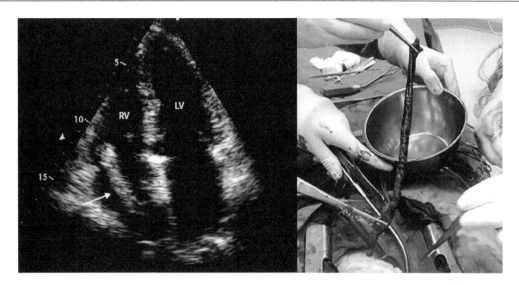

FIGURE 7.10 Apical four-chamber view showing a large serpiginous thrombus (arrow) in the right atrium extending to the right ventricle (RV) across the tricuspid valve (left panel; V7.13A and V7.13B). Also note that RV does not appear dilated, which may indicate that massive pulmonary embolism has not occurred yet. The same thrombus as seen intraoperatively, during emergency surgical thrombectomy (right panel).

(Images and videos provided by IS.)

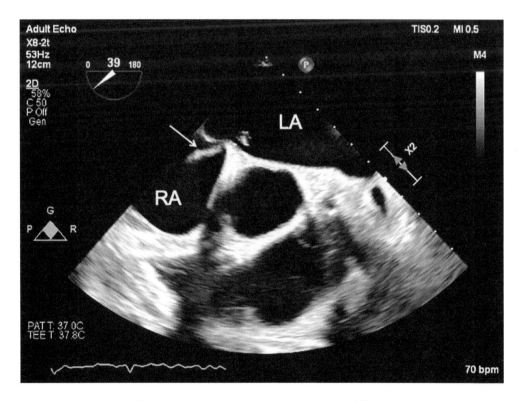

FIGURE 7.11 Transesophageal echocardiography showing a large thrombus (arrows) floating in the right atrium (RA) and protruding in the left atrium (LA) through a patent foramen ovale (V7.16).

remain controversial.[1] Thrombolysis may be risky and should be avoided in stable patients because of the risk of systemic embolism and embolic stroke if right atrial thrombus extends through the PFO into the left atrium (Figure 7.11) (V7.16) or in cases of thrombus dislodgement with recurrent PE. Left-sided

protrusion of a thrombus through the PFO is not always easy to exclude without TEE. Surgical treatment is attractive also when the clinical context and/or appearance of the right heart mass on echocardiography suggests a nonthrombotic origin. Moreover, our data suggest that hemodynamically stable PE patients with right heart thrombi have a fair prognosis, and anticoagulation seems to be sufficient. However, apart from echocardiographic findings, the clinical condition of the patient is crucial for decision-making, and in the presence of life-threatening hypotension or shock, thrombolysis should not be delayed if surgery is not immediately available (V18.18A, V18.18B, V18.18C, V18.18D).

ADDITIONAL DIAGNOSTIC WORK-UP AND STRATEGIES

Venous ultrasound

PE is one of the clinical presentations of venous thromboembolism (VTE). In the majority of cases, PE originates from deep vein thrombosis (DVT) in lower limbs or pelvis, and unfrequently in upper limbs (mostly following venous catheterization). *Compression venous ultrasound (VUS)* has a well-established value in the diagnosis of patients with suspected DVT, and nowadays, lower-limb compression VUS has largely replaced venography for diagnosing DVT. VUS has a sensitivity >90% and a specificity of approximately 95% for proximal symptomatic DVT.[30, 31] Importantly, VUS is highly specific and totally noninvasive and can be performed at the bedside, and simplified protocols limited to groin and popliteal vessels are rapid to perform and easy to learn.[32] Point-of-care ultrasound

(POCUS), bedside ultrasound examination performed by the clinician, has been increasingly used for detection of DVT in the urgent and critical care setting and it has shown excellent diagnostic accuracy for acute proximal DVT when performed by well-trained users.[32]

In a recent meta-analysis, the prevalence of ultrasound-detectable concomitant DVT in PE patients reached 55%, and this may be an underestimation as venous clots may embolize entirely.[33,34] *Detection of proximal DVT in a patient with suspected PE virtually confirms the diagnosis and fully justifies anticoagulation.*[1,35] However, patients with suspected PE and confirmed DVT by VUS should undergo risk assessment for PE severity and the risk of early death.

Confirmation of DVT with compression VUS is particularly rewarding in patients who have RV pressure overload but also a potential alternative cause, such as chronic obstructive pulmonary disease (COPD). Also, in an unstable patient with RV pressure overload, documentation of a thrombus in proximal veins makes the decision to start thrombolytic treatment without further delay much easier.

"Integrated ultrasound" approach

Echocardiography, especially TEE, allows direct visualization of thromboemboli in the proximal parts of pulmonary arteries (Figure 7.12) (V7.18, V7.19, V7.20, V7.21). TTE can detect in-transit thrombi on their way to pulmonary circulation. In addition, compression VUS of the peripheral venous system can

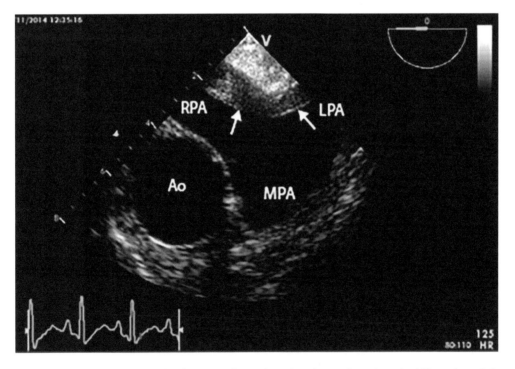

FIGURE 7.12   Transesophageal echocardiography showing a large thrombus (arrows) stuck at the bifurcation of the main pulmonary artery and protruding into both branches. Note the dilation of the main pulmonary artery and their branches (V7.18). Ao: aorta; LPA: left pulmonary artery; MPA: main pulmonary artery; RPA: right pulmonary artery.

(Image and video provided by VC.)

find sources of emboli and confirm venous thromboembolic disease. Therefore, the extension of standard TTE to TEE and to compression VUS (and, most likely, lung ultrasound, see Chapter 20) increases the diagnostic impact of the ultrasound examination. This integrated ultrasound approach can be performed by a single echocardiographer using a single machine equipped with three probes (transthoracic, transesophageal, and vascular), at the bedside of an unstable patient.

In our opinion, integrated ultrasound represents major progress in the emergency diagnosis and management of suspected PE. Clearly, *this approach is useful for confirming but not excluding* venous thromboembolic disease. If this integrated ultrasound fails to document intravascular or intracardiac thrombi, further diagnostic procedures are warranted.

Suggested diagnostic strategy for severely hemodynamically compromised patients with suspected pulmonary embolism

According to current European Society of Cardiology (ESC) guidelines, in patients with unexplained hypotension or shock, emergency bedside echocardiography is indicated.[1] Preserved RV morphology and function make high-risk PE highly unlikely; hence, alternative causes of hemodynamic instability should be considered. In patients with clinically suspected high-risk PE with RV strain, the presence of more specific echocardiographic signs (McConnell's sign, 60/60 sign) practically confirms the diagnosis and may justify even primary revascularization, including thrombolysis. However, signs of RV overload may result from other causes, such as COPD (V19.9, V19.9.1), pneumonia, and ARDS (V7.24A, V7.24B, V7.24C). Evidence of RV hypertrophy may be helpful in the differential diagnosis between acute and chronic RV pressure overload. Rarely, TTE may solve the problem by visualization of thromboemboli in the right heart chambers or proximal parts of pulmonary arteries (V7.23A, V7.23B, V7.23C). Otherwise, bedside confirmation of intrapulmonary thrombi with TEE is an option, especially useful in unstable patients with relative contraindications for thrombolysis (V7.22A, V7.22B). Importantly, VUS performed according to a simplified protocol focusing on the groin and popliteal region may promptly and definitely confirm VTE, making decisions to start the treatment much easier. In most cases, however, after stabilization of the patient, CTPA, lung scan, or (rarely) pulmonary angiography should be performed to definitely confirm PE.

Alternative diagnoses

Echocardiography can detect alternative causes of acute hemodynamic instability, dyspnea, shock, or chest pain, including left ventricular (LV) systolic dysfunction, cardiac tamponade, aortic dissection, and infective endocarditis. Of note, patients with ARDS can have echocardiographic findings quite similar

to those seen in acute pulmonary embolism (V7.24A, V7.24B, V7.24C).

Importantly, normal RV function was present at TTE in one-third of consecutive 511 patients with PE.[5] It is worth mentioning that TTE revealed also other abnormalities potentially explaining patient's signs and symptoms (significant valvular lesions such as at least moderate aortic stenosis, reduced left ventricular ejection fraction) in almost 10% of stable patients with PE without RV dysfunction or any typical for PE echocardiographic findings. Thus, in 70% of subjects with PE, TTE may provide no clues for PE, or even approximately 10% of them may show potentially deceiving comorbidities, which could falsely redirect the diagnostic process and make the proper diagnosis of PE more difficult or even overlooked.[5]

A typical case is that of "cryptogenic stroke" (see Chapter 13), which may in fact result from right-to-left shunting of blood containing venous clots that were originally in transit to pulmonary arteries but on their way paradoxically embolized to the left atrium and systemic circulation through a PFO.[1,36,37]

ECHOCARDIOGRAPHY IN CONFIRMED PULMONARY EMBOLISM

Echocardiography has been found to be useful not only in the diagnosis of suspected PE, but also in the *assessment of prognosis in patients with proven PE.*[1]

Normotensive patients with acute PE include not only those with a benign clinical course, but also patients with an increased risk of PE-related mortality. Whereas the former may be candidates for a short hospital stay or even ambulatory treatment, the latter may require close monitoring and, in some cases, aggressive therapy, including thrombolysis, especially when hemodynamic deterioration occurs.[1] As mentioned earlier, RV dysfunction on echocardiography is found in approximately 20–25% of unselected patients with acute PE.[5] Systematic reviews and meta-analyses have suggested that RV dysfunction on echocardiography is associated with an increased risk of short-term mortality in patients who appear hemodynamically stable at presentation,[38,39] but its overall positive predictive value for PE-related death was low (<10%).[38] This weakness is partly related to the fact that echocardiographic parameters have been proven to be difficult to standardize.[38,40] Moreover, since heterogeneous definitions for RV dysfunction for risk stratification have been used, there are no universally accepted prognostic echocardiographic criteria. Nevertheless, echocardiographic evaluation of the RV morphology and function is widely recognized as a valuable tool for the prognostic assessment of normotensive patients with acute PE in clinical practice.

There is a large set of echocardiographic parameters used to stratify the early risk of patients with PE. However, the American Heart Association arbitrarily proposed that RV dysfunction should be diagnosed when the *RV-to-LV end-diastolic ratio* (RV/LV) measured by echocardiography or tomography exceeds 0.9.[41] Indeed, an increased an RV/LV diameter ratio and a decreased *tricuspid annular plane systolic excursion* (TAPSE) are the findings for which an association with unfavorable prognosis has most frequently been reported.[40] A decreased TAPSE has been reported to be a significant predictor of outcome in patients with PE. Analysis of 782 normotensive patients with PE who underwent echocardiography in a multicenter study showed that those with TAPSE of ≤16 cm at the time of PE diagnosis were more likely to die from any cause, including PE, during follow-up. In an external validation cohort of 1,326 patients with acute PE enrolled in the international multicenter Registro Informatizado de la Enfermedad TromboEmbólica (RIETE), a TAPSE of ≤16 mm remained a significant predictor of all-cause mortality and PE-specific mortality.[42] In multivariable analysis of 411 consecutive PE patients normotensive at admission showed that among various evaluated echocardiographic parameters, TAPSE was the only independent echocardiographic predictor of outcome. Importantly, TAPSE was superior to other echocardiographic prognostic parameters, including RV/LV ratio.[40] Thus, among normotensive patients, TAPSE ≤16 mm identified subjects at increased risk of complicated clinical course (30-day PE-related death or rescue thrombolysis occurred in 20.9% of them), whereas TAPSE >20 mm can be used for identification of a very-low-risk group.[40]

Recently, a large European multicenter prospective cohort study including 490 normotensive PE patients managed according to the current ESC guidelines provided a proposal of the optimal definition of RV dysfunction for prognostic assessment.[36] A multivariable analysis identified systemic systolic blood pressure, RV/LV, and TAPSE to be independent predictors of PE-related mortality, hemodynamic collapse, or rescue thrombolysis within the first 30 days. Importantly, a combined RV dysfunction criterion (TAPSE <16 mm and RV/LV ratio >1) was present in 12% of patients and showed a positive predictive value of 23.3% with a high negative predictive value of 95.6% for adverse outcomes (HR 6.5; 95% CI 3.2–13.3; p < 0.0001). It seems that RV dysfunction on echocardiography defined by RV/LV ratio >1, in combination with TAPSE <16 mm, identifies among normotensive PE patients subjects with an increased risk of 30-day adverse outcome, including PE-related mortality. This echocardiographic definition of RV dysfunction may be helpful in better defining intermediate high-risk PE.[36]

In line with decreased TAPSE (TAPSE ≤16 mm), decreased peak systolic velocity of tricuspid annulus derived from Doppler tissue imaging and strain (S' <9.5 m/s) may also be detected in patients with acute PE, although reported sensitivity is low.[1]

Finally, patients with evidence of both RV dysfunction and elevated troponin levels should be classified into an intermediate high-risk category. Close monitoring is recommended in these cases to permit early detection of hemodynamic deterioration and the need for initiation of rescue reperfusion therapy.

Of note, RV dysfunction assessed by echocardiography, CTPA and increased troponin are associated with short-term death in patients with acute PE appraised as at low risk for death based on clinical scores.[37] Therefore, RV dysfunction assessment should be considered also in low-risk patients according to ESC guidelines to improve selection of patients that may be candidates for outpatient management or short hospital stay.

PARADOXICAL EMBOLIZATION AND PATENT FORAMEN OVALE

Paradoxical embolization has been observed in patients with acute PE with coexisting PFO. PFO is present in 20–30% of the general population and is generally accepted as a risk factor for ischemic stroke or peripheral embolism (see also Chapter 13). The diagnosis is usually made if at least five microbubbles of contrast (5.5% oxypolygelatine solution or agitated saline) injected into a peripheral vein can be seen in the left heart chambers with delay not exceeding three cardiac cycles after opacification of the right atrium (V13.22, V13.23) Elevated right atrial pressure in patients with RV dysfunction secondary to PE predisposes to right-to-left intracardial shunt, which may lead to pronounced hypoxemia.

In addition to RV dysfunction, echocardiography can identify right-to-left shunt through a patent *foramen ovale*, which is associated with increased mortality in patients with acute PE.[28,43] PFO was reported to be a significant predictor of poor outcome in patients with PE. In patients with diagnosed PFO, in-hospital mortality was significantly higher than in those without PFO (33% versus 14%).[43] A patent foramen ovale also increases the risk of ischemic stroke due to paradoxical embolism (V13.24), especially in patients with acute PE resulting in RV dysfunction.[44,45] Peripheral arterial emboli as well as episodes of ischemic stroke were more frequent in patients with right-to-left shunt, contributing to an increased mortality. There was also a trend toward a higher rate of intracranial bleeding in patients with PFO (4.2% versus 1.1%); it appears that even a clinically silent acute ischemic stroke caused by paradoxical embolization across PFO may increase the rate of intracranial hemorrhage if thrombolysis is given.

Silent brain infarctions found at MRI have been reported in patients with PE and PFO.[44,45] Interestingly, acute ischemic strokes occurred in the PFO-positive group, but not in those without PFO. Moreover, all strokes occurred in patients with RV dysfunction and PFO, and none in patients with PFO without RV dysfunction.[45] Recent multicenter study of 361 consecutive patients with symptomatic acute PE showed that stroke occurred more frequently in those patients with PFO (21% vs. 5.5%; relative risk 3.9, 95%; CI 1.6 to 8.7).[46] Unfortunately, although PFO seems to be a marker of increased risk in patients with PE, no evidence supporting specific modifications in standard management is available as yet.

SUMMARY

In the majority of patients with suspected high-risk PE, ultrasound examination that includes standard TTE, extended to compression VUS for proximal DVT and to TEE in patients with RV pressure overload at transthoracic examination, can promptly confirm PE or at least make the diagnosis highly likely. Echocardiography can be performed in the emergency room, intensive care unit, or operating room. Its bedside application makes echocardiography especially attractive in severely compromised patients, who should be diagnosed as quickly as possible, preferably without being transported. Moreover, echo can provide alternative explanations for hemodynamic instability. However, it should be always remembered that RV strain on TTE is only an *indirect sign* of PE, and definitive confirmation is advised. Normal RV function does not exclude PE, but its presence indicates an excellent prognosis with treatment limited to anticoagulation. In contrast, patients with signs of RV dysfunction and overload are at higher risk of in-hospital complications and death, especially when elevated troponin levels or PFO are present.

LIST OF VIDEOS

https://routledgetextbooks.com/textbooks/9781032157009/chapter-7.php

VIDEO 7.1   Flattening of the interventricular septum: Parasternal short-axis view of a patient with acute pulmonary embolism showing flattening of the interventricular septum (D-shaped left ventricle) resulting from right ventricular pressure overload. Right ventricular enlargement can also be seen. *(Video provided by IS.)*

VIDEO 7.2   Dilated, noncollapsible inferior vena cava. The subcostal view of a patient with massive pulmonary embolism showing dilated, noncollapsible inferior vena cava.

VIDEO 7.3   Right ventricular dilation and McConnell's sign: Apical four-chamber view of a patient with acute pulmonary embolism showing marked right ventricular dilation with free-wall hypokinesia and preserved contractility of the apical segment (McConnell's sign). *(Video provided by IS.)*

VIDEO 7.4A   Right ventricular (RV) dilation and McConnell's sign in acute pulmonary embolism before thrombolysis (1/2): RV dilation with free-wall akinesia and relative apical sparing seen at admission in a patient with acute pulmonary embolism (McConnell's sign, shown here) completely waned after thrombolytic therapy (see Video 7.4B). *(Video provided by ANN.)*

VIDEO 7.4B   Recovering of right ventricular (RV) function after thrombolysis (2/2): Note the normal RV dimension and recovered function at the third hospital day after thrombolytic therapy for acute pulmonary embolism (shown here). On initial presentation, RV dilation with free-wall akinesia and relative apical sparing were seen (McConnell's sign, see Video 7.4A). *(Video provided by ANN.)*

VIDEO 7.5A   Acute pulmonary embolism with right heart thrombi "in transit" imaged with a handheld ultrasound device (1/5): A large wormlike thrombus freely moving from the right atrium to the right ventricle and microbubbles from vigorous fluid resuscitation can be appreciated (shown here). Smaller thrombi floating in the right atrium (see Video 7.5B) and also in the dilated right ventricle (see Videos 7.5C and 7.5D) were observed shortly after the first mass disappeared. All thrombi left the right heart in approximately 3 minutes (see Video 7.5E). *(Video provided by MMP.)*

VIDEO 7.5B   Acute pulmonary embolism with right heart thrombi "in transit" imaged with a handheld ultrasound device (2/5): A large wormlike thrombus freely moving from the right atrium to the right ventricle and microbubbles from vigorous fluid resuscitation was appreciated (see Video 7.5A). Smaller thrombi floating in the right atrium (shown here) and also in the dilated right ventricle (see Videos 7.5C and 7.5D) were observed shortly after the first mass disappeared. All thrombi left the right heart in approximately 3 minutes (see Video 7.5E). *(Video provided by MMP.)*

VIDEO 7.5C   Acute pulmonary embolism with right heart thrombi "in transit" imaged with a handheld ultrasound device (3/5): A large wormlike thrombus freely moving from the right atrium to the right ventricle and microbubbles from vigorous fluid resuscitation was appreciated (see Video 7.5A). Smaller thrombi floating in the right atrium (see Video 7.5B) and also in the dilated right ventricle (shown here, see also Video 7.5D) were observed shortly after the first mass disappeared. All thrombi left the right heart in approximately 3 minutes (see Video 7.5E). *(Video provided by MMP.)*

VIDEO 7.5D   Acute pulmonary embolism with right heart thrombi "in transit" imaged with a handheld ultrasound device (4/5): A large wormlike thrombus freely moving from the right atrium to the right ventricle and microbubbles from vigorous fluid resuscitation was appreciated (see Video 7.5A). Another smaller thrombi floating in the right atrium (see Video 7.5B) and also in the dilated right ventricle (shown here, see also Video 7.5C) were observed shortly after the first mass disappeared. All thrombi left the right heart in approximately 3 minutes (see Video 7.5E). *(Video provided by MMP.)*

VIDEO 7.5E   Acute pulmonary embolism with right heart thrombi "in transit" imaged with a handheld ultrasound device (5/5): No visible thrombi in the right heart (shown here) in a patient with acute pulmonary embolism with right heart thrombi in transit imaged with pocket-size imaging device. A large wormlike thrombus freely moving from the right atrium to the right ventricle and microbubbles from vigorous fluid resuscitation was appreciated (see Video 7.5A). Smaller thrombi floating in the right atrium (see Video 7.5B) and also in the dilated right ventricle (see Videos 7.5C and 7.5D) were observed shortly after the first mass disappeared. All thrombi left the right heart in approximately 3 minutes. *(Video provided by MMP.)*

VIDEO 7.6A   Acute pulmonary embolism with hypermobile right heart thrombi (1/2). Transthoracic four-chamber view showing right heart dilatation and a large wormlike thrombus freely moving from the right atrium to the right ventricle during cardiac cycle in a patient with acute massive pulmonary embolism (see also Video 7.6B).

VIDEO 7.6B   Acute pulmonary embolism with hypermobile right heart thrombi (2/2). Subcostal view showing right heart dilatation and a large mobile thrombus in the right atrium in a patient with acute massive pulmonary embolism (see also Video 7.6A).

VIDEO 7.7   Thrombus in the main pulmonary artery: A large mobile thrombus bouncing at the pulmonary artery bifurcation and protruding into the left pulmonary artery. *(Video provided by BAP.)*

VIDEO 7.8   A large mobile thrombus "sitting" at the pulmonary artery bifurcation and protruding into both left and right branch.

VIDEO 7.9   Thrombus in the right pulmonary artery: A wormlike thrombus in the right pulmonary artery, as seen from the suprasternal window. *(Video provided by VC.)*

VIDEO 7.10   Thrombus in the right pulmonary artery: A highly mobile thrombus in the right pulmonary artery, as seen from the suprasternal window. *(Video provided by IS.)*

VIDEO 7.11   Thrombus in the right pulmonary artery: A large wormlike thrombus in the right pulmonary artery, as seen from the suprasternal window. *(Video provided by IS.)*

VIDEO 7.12   Thrombus in the right pulmonary artery: Transesophageal echocardiogram in a patient with suspected pulmonary embolism showing a thrombus in the right pulmonary artery. *(Video provided by VC.)*

VIDEO 7.13A   Thrombus in the right side of the heart (1/2): Apical four-chamber view showing a large serpiginous thrombus in the right atrium extending to the right ventricle across the tricuspid valve. Also note that the right ventricle does not appear dilated, which may indicate that massive pulmonary embolism has not occurred yet (see also Video 7.13B). *(Video provided by IS.)*

VIDEO 7.13B   Thrombus in the right side of the heart (2/2): Subcostal view showing a large snakelike serpiginous thrombus in the right atrium extending to the right ventricle across the tricuspid valve (see also Video 7.13A). *(Video provided by IS.)*

VIDEO 7.14   Mass in the inferior vena cava and right atrium: The subcostal view obtained by handheld imaging device in a patient with gynecologic malignancy showing a large serpiginous mass extending from the inferior vena cava into the right atrium. *(Video provided by IS.)*

VIDEO 7.15   Mass in the inferior vena cava and right atrium. The subcostal view in a patient with clear cell tumor of the kidney showing a large serpiginous mass extending from the inferior vena cava into the right atrium.

VIDEO 7.16   Acute pulmonary embolism—thrombus lodged in the patent foramen ovale. Transesophageal echocardiography showing a large thrombus floating in the right atrium and protruding in the left atrium through a patent foramen ovale in a patient with suspected acute pulmonary embolism.

VIDEO 7.17A   Acute pulmonary embolism—right heart dilation (1/2): Transthoracic four-chamber view showing striking right heart dilation in a patient with suspected acute pulmonary embolism (shown here). Transesophageal echocardiography showed a large round mass obstructing dilated right pulmonary artery, consistent with thrombus (see Video 7.17B). *(Video provided by BP.)*

VIDEO 7.17B   Acute pulmonary embolism—thrombus in the right pulmonary artery (2/2): Transesophageal echocardiography showing a large round mass obstructing dilated right pulmonary artery, consistent with thrombus, in a patient with suspected acute pulmonary embolism (shown here). Striking right heart dilation was noted at transthoracic four-chamber view (see Video 7.17A). *(Video provided by BP.)*

VIDEO 7.18   Thrombus at the bifurcation of the main pulmonary artery: Transesophageal echocardiography showing a large thrombus stuck at the bifurcation of the main pulmonary artery and protruding into both branches. Note the dilation of the main pulmonary artery and their branches. *(Video provided by VC.)*

VIDEO 7.19   Thrombus in the right pulmonary artery: Transesophageal echocardiography showing a large thrombus adherent to the posterior wall of dilated right pulmonary artery with a partially mobile part, causing virtually complete obstruction of the vessel. *(Video provided by VC.)*

VIDEO 7.20   Thrombus in the right pulmonary artery: Transesophageal echocardiography showing a large ball-like thrombus causing almost total obstruction of the lumen of dilated right pulmonary artery. *(Video provided by VC.)*

VIDEO 7.21   Thrombus in the right pulmonary artery: Transesophageal echocardiography showing a large fixed thrombus causing subtotal obstruction of the lumen of dilated right pulmonary artery. *(Video provided by BP.)*

VIDEO 7.22A   Massive pulmonary embolism in a young woman in the postpartum period (1/2): Transesophageal echocardiography showing dilated right ventricle and a large mobile mass in the right ventricular outflow tract (shown here) in a young woman 1 week after delivery. A mass consistent with thrombus stuck in the dilated main pulmonary artery was also detected (see also Video

7.22B). Immediately after diagnosis of acute massive pulmonary embolism was made, the patient was transferred by helicopter to remote cardiac surgery center (300 km), where the patient underwent open-heart surgery with successful pulmonary embolectomy. *(Video provided by AL.)*

VIDEO 7.22B   Massive pulmonary embolism in a young woman in the postpartum period (2/2): Transesophageal echocardiography showing mass consistent with thrombus stuck in the dilated main pulmonary artery. Note the dilated pulmonary artery as compared to diameter of the aorta (see also Video 7.22A). Immediately after diagnosis of acute massive pulmonary embolism was made, the patient was transferred by helicopter to remote cardiac surgery center (300 km), where the patient underwent open-heart surgery with successful pulmonary embolectomy. *(Video provided by AL.)*

VIDEO 7.23A   Diagnosis of massive pulmonary embolism in 2 minutes by focus cardiac ultrasound (FOCUS) (1/3): In a patient presented with shock after successful CPR, FoCUS performed by a handheld ultrasound device revealed a dilated right heart in a four-chamber view. Note the time: 7:34:01. (See also Videos 7.23B and 7.23C.) *(Video provided by IS.)*

VIDEO 7.23B   Diagnosis of massive pulmonary embolism in 2 minutes by focus cardiac ultrasound (FOCUS) (2/3): In a patient presented with shock after successful CPR, FoCUS performed by a handheld ultrasound device revealed a dilated right heart and significant tricuspid insufficiency in a four-chamber view. Note the time: 7:34:18 (see also Videos 7.23A and 7.23C). *(Video provided by IS.)*

VIDEO 7.23C   Diagnosis of massive pulmonary embolism in 2 minutes by focus cardiac ultrasound (FOCUS) (3/3): In a patient presented with shock after successful CPR, FoCUS performed by a handheld ultrasound device revealed a dilated right heart and significant tricuspid insufficiency (see also Videos 7.23A and 7.23B), and a suprasternal view revealed mass in the right pulmonary artery consistent with thrombus. Note the time: 7:35:58. In less than 2 minutes (please note the time indicated on consecutive Videos 7.23A, 7.23B and 7.23C), diagnosis of massive pulmonary embolism was made and thrombolysis (alteplase) was administered *(Video provided by IS.)*

VIDEO 7.24A   Differential diagnosis of the right heart dilation in a patient with dyspnea and tachypnea in the emergency department (1/3): A 46-year-old male presented in the emergency department with severe dyspnea and tachypnea lasting for 7 days, with hypotension (90/70 mmHg), D-dimer 18,000 (norm. <230), CRP 160 (norm. <4), and leukocytosis 14,500. ECG revealed sinus rhythm, 110/min, with S1Q3T3 pattern and RV strain (negative T-waves in V1-V3). FoCUS showed a dilated right ventricle (shown here) with D-shaped left ventricle (see Video 7.24B) and McConnell's sign (see Video 7.24C). Full echocardiography revealed moderate tricuspid regurgitation with TR jet of 3.8 m/s and pulmonary artery flow profile with short acceleration time and midsystolic notching, indicating increased pulmonary artery systolic pressure. All echocardiographic signs, ECG, and laboratory results were highly suggestive for acute pulmonary embolism. However, acute pulmonary embolism was excluded by CTPA. Final diagnosis was adult respiratory distress syndrome. *(Video provided by IS.)*

VIDEO 7.24B   Differential diagnosis of the right heart dilation in a patient with dyspnea and tachypnea in the emergency department (2/3): A 46-year-old male presented in the emergency department with severe dyspnea and tachypnea lasting for 7 days, with hypotension (90/70 mmHg), D-dimer 18,000 (norm. <230), CRP 160 (norm. <4), and leukocytosis 14,500. ECG revealed sinus rhythm, 110/min, with S1Q3T3 pattern and RV strain (negative T-waves in V1-V3). FoCUS showed a dilated right ventricle (see Video 7.24A) with D-shaped left ventricle (shown here) and McConnell's sign (see Video 7.24C). Full echocardiography revealed moderate tricuspid regurgitation with TR jet of 3.8 m/s and pulmonary artery flow profile with short acceleration time and midsystolic notching, indicating increased pulmonary artery systolic pressure. All echocardiographic signs, ECG, and laboratory results were highly suggestive for acute pulmonary embolism. However, acute pulmonary embolism was excluded by CTPA. Final diagnosis was adult respiratory distress syndrome. *(Video provided by IS.)*

VIDEO 7.24C   Differential diagnosis of the right heart dilation in a patient with dyspnea and tachypnea in the emergency department (3/3): A 46-year-old male presented in the emergency department with severe dyspnea and tachypnea lasting for 7 days, with hypotension (90/70 mmHg), D-dimer 18,000 (norm. <230), CRP 160 (norm. <4), and leukocytosis 14,500. ECG revealed sinus rhythm, 110/min, with S1Q3T3 pattern and RV strain (negative T-waves in V1-V3). FoCUS showed a dilated right ventricle (see Video 7.24A) with D-shaped left ventricle (see Video 7.24B) and McConnell's sign (shown here). Full echocardiography revealed moderate tricuspid regurgitation with TR jet of 3.8 m/s and pulmonary artery flow profile with short acceleration time and midsystolic notching, indicating increased pulmonary artery systolic pressure. All echocardiographic signs, ECG, and laboratory results were highly suggestive for acute pulmonary embolism. However, acute pulmonary embolism was excluded by CTPA. Final diagnosis was adult respiratory distress syndrome. *(Video provided by IS.)*

VIDEO 7.25   Thrombus in the right pulmonary artery. At the beginning of the video, showing transesophageal echocardiography in a patient with suspected pulmonary embolism, note the dilated main pulmonary artery; a couple of seconds later, as the transesophageal probe is moving, the right pulmonary artery is reached, showing a large thrombus stuck in its lumen. *(Video provided by VC.)*

REFERENCES

1. Konstantinides SV, Meyer G. The 2019 ESC guidelines on the diagnosis and management of acute pulmonary embolism. Eur Heart J 2019;**40**(42):3453–55.
2. Neskovic AN, Hagendorff A, Lancellotti P, Guarracino F, Varga A, Cosyns B, Flachskampf FA, Popescu BA, Gargani L, Zamorano JL, Badano LP, European Association of Cardiovascular I. Emergency echocardiography: the European Association of Cardiovascular Imaging recommendations. Eur Heart J Cardiovasc Imaging 2013;**14**(1):1–11.
3. Lancellotti P, Price S, Edvardsen T, Cosyns B, Neskovic AN, Dulgheru R, Flachskampf FA, Hassager C, Pasquet A, Gargani L, Galderisi M, Cardim N, Haugaa KH, Ancion A,

Zamorano JL, Donal E, Bueno H, Habib G. The use of echocardiography in acute cardiovascular care: recommendations of the European Association of Cardiovascular Imaging and the Acute Cardiovascular Care Association. Eur Heart J Acute Cardiovasc Care 2015;**4**(1):3–5.

4. Miniati M, Monti S, Pratali L, Di Ricco G, Marini C, Formichi B, Prediletto R, Michelassi C, Di Lorenzo M, Tonelli L, Pistolesi M. Value of transthoracic echocardiography in the diagnosis of pulmonary embolism: results of a prospective study in unselected patients. Am J Med 2001;**110**(7):528–35.

5. Kurnicka K, Lichodziejewska B, Goliszek S, Dzikowska-Diduch O, Zdonczyk O, Kozlowska M, Kostrubiec M, Ciurzynski M, Palczewski P, Grudzka K, Krupa M, Koc M, Pruszczyk P. Echocardiographic pattern of acute pulmonary embolism: analysis of 511 consecutive patients. J Am Soc Echocardiogr 2016;**29**(9):907–13.

6. Nazeyrollas P, Metz D, Jolly D, Maillier B, Jennesseaux C, Maes D, Chabert JP, Chapoutot L, Elaerts J. Use of transthoracic Doppler echocardiography combined with clinical and electrocardiographic data to predict acute pulmonary embolism. Eur Heart J 1996;**17**(5):779–86.

7. Kurzyna M, Torbicki A, Pruszczyk P, Burakowska B, Fijalkowska A, Kober J, Oniszh K, Kuca P, Tomkowski W, Burakowski J, Wawrzynska L. Disturbed right ventricular ejection pattern as a new Doppler echocardiographic sign of acute pulmonary embolism. Am J Cardiol 2002;**90**(5):507–11.

8. Grifoni S, Olivotto I, Cecchini P, Pieralli F, Camaiti A, Santoro G, Pieri A, Toccafondi S, Magazzini S, Berni G, Agnelli G. Utility of an integrated clinical, echocardiographic, and venous ultrasonographic approach for triage of patients with suspected pulmonary embolism. Am J Cardiol 1998;**82**(10):1230–5.

9. Perrier A, Tamm C, Unger PF, Lerch R, Sztajzel J. Diagnostic accuracy of Doppler-echocardiography in unselected patients with suspected pulmonary embolism. Int J Cardiol 1998;**65**(1):101–9.

10. Khemasuwan D, Yingchoncharoen T, Tunsupon P, Kusunose K, Moghekar A, Klein A, Tonelli AR. Right ventricular echocardiographic parameters are associated with mortality after acute pulmonary embolism. J Am Soc Echocardiogr 2015;**28**(3):355–62.

11. Jardin F, Dubourg O, Bourdarias JP. Echocardiographic pattern of acute cor pulmonale. Chest 1997;**111**(1):209–17.

12. Casazza F, Bongarzoni A, Capozi A, Agostoni O. Regional right ventricular dysfunction in acute pulmonary embolism and right ventricular infarction. Eur J Echocardiogr 2005;**6**(1):11–4.

13. McConnell MV, Solomon SD, Rayan ME, Come PC, Goldhaber SZ, Lee RT. Regional right ventricular dysfunction detected by echocardiography in acute pulmonary embolism. Am J Cardiol 1996;**78**(4):469–73.

14. Torbicki A, Kurzyna M, Ciurzynski M, Pruszczyk P, Pacho R, Kuch-Wocial A, Szulc M. Proximal pulmonary emboli modify right ventricular ejection pattern. Eur Respir J 1999;**13**(3):616–21.

15. Guerin L, Couturaud F, Parent F, Revel MP, Gillaizeau F, Planquette B, Pontal D, Guegan M, Simonneau G, Meyer G, Sanchez O. Prevalence of chronic thromboembolic pulmonary hypertension after acute pulmonary embolism. Prevalence of CTEPH after pulmonary embolism. Thromb Haemost 2014;**112**(3):598–605.

16. Casazza F, Becattini C, Guglielmelli E, Floriani I, Morrone V, Caponi C, Pizzorno L, Masotti L, Bongarzoni A, Pignataro L. Prognostic significance of free-floating right heart thromboemboli in acute pulmonary embolism: results from the Italian Pulmonary Embolism Registry. Thromb Haemost 2014;**111**(1):53–7.

17. Mansencal N, Attias D, Caille V, Desperramons J, Guiader J, El Hajjam M, Lacombe P, Abi Nasr I, Jardin F, Vieillard-Baron A, Dubourg O. Computed tomography for the detection of free-floating thrombi in the right heart in acute pulmonary embolism. Eur Radiol 2011;**21**(2):240–5.

18. Torbicki A, Galie N, Covezzoli A, Rossi E, De Rosa M, Goldhaber SZ, Group IS. Right heart thrombi in pulmonary embolism: results from the International Cooperative Pulmonary Embolism Registry. J Am Coll Cardiol 2003;**41**(12):2245–51.

19. Casazza F, Bongarzoni A, Centonze F, Morpurgo M. Prevalence and prognostic significance of right-sided cardiac mobile thrombi in acute massive pulmonary embolism. Am J Cardiol 1997;**79**(10):1433–5.

20. Nixdorff U, Erbel R, Drexler M, Meyer J. Detection of thromboembolus of the right pulmonary artery by transesophageal two-dimensional echocardiography. Am J Cardiol 1988;**61**(6):488–9.

21. Popovic AD, Milovanovic B, Neskovic AN, Pavlovski K, Putnikovic B, Hadzagic I. Detection of massive pulmonary embolism by transesophageal echocardiography. Cardiology 1992;**80**(2):94–9.

22. Pruszczyk P, Torbicki A, Kuch-Wocial A, Chlebus M, Miskiewicz ZC, Jedrusik P. Transoesophageal echocardiography for definitive diagnosis of haemodynamically significant pulmonary embolism. Eur Heart J 1995;**16**(4):534–8.

23. Wittlich N, Erbel R, Eichler A, Schuster S, Jakob H, Iversen S, Oelert H, Meyer J. Detection of central pulmonary artery thromboemboli by transesophageal echocardiography in patients with severe pulmonary embolism. J Am Soc Echocardiogr 1992;**5**(5):515–24.

24. Antakly-Hanon Y, Vieillard-Baron A, Qanadli SD, Fourme T, Lewy P, Jondeau G, Lacombe P, Jardin F, Bourdarias JP, Dubourg O. The value of transesophageal echocardiography for the diagnosis of pulmonary embolism with acute pulmonary heart disease. Arch Mal Coeur Vaiss 1998;**91**(7):843–8.

25. Pruszczyk P, Torbicki A, Kuch-Wocial A, Szulc M, Pacho R. Diagnostic value of transoesophageal echocardiography in suspected haemodynamically significant pulmonary embolism. Heart 2001;**85**(6):628–34.

26. Krivec B, Voga G, Zuran I, Skale R, Pareznik R, Podbregar M, Noc M. Diagnosis and treatment of shock due to massive pulmonary embolism: approach with transesophageal echocardiography and intrapulmonary thrombolysis. Chest 1997;**112**(5):1310–6.

27. Koc M, Kostrubiec M, Elikowski W, Meneveau N, Lankeit M, Grifoni S, Kuch-Wocial A, Petris A, Zaborska B, Stefanovic BS, Hugues T, Torbicki A, Konstantinides S, Pruszczyk P, Ri HI. Outcome of patients with right heart thrombi: the Right Heart Thrombi European Registry. Eur Respir J 2016;**47**(3):869–75.

28. Barrios D, Rosa-Salazar V, Morillo R, Nieto R, Fernandez S, Zamorano JL, Monreal M, Torbicki A, Yusen RD, Jimenez D. Prognostic significance of right heart thrombi in patients with acute symptomatic pulmonary embolism: systematic review and meta-analysis. Chest 2017;**151**(2):409–16.

29. Barrios D, Rosa-Salazar V, Jimenez D, Morillo R, Muriel A, Del Toro J, Lopez-Jimenez L, Farge-Bancel D, Yusen R, Monreal M, investigators R. Right heart thrombi in pulmonary embolism. Eur Respir J 2016;**48**(5):1377–85.

30. Perrier A, Bounameaux H. Ultrasonography of leg veins in patients suspected of having pulmonary embolism. Ann Intern Med 1998;**128**(3):243.

31. Kearon C, Ginsberg JS, Hirsh J. The role of venous ultrasonography in the diagnosis of suspected deep venous thrombosis and pulmonary embolism. Ann Intern Med 1998;**129**(12):1044–9.

32. Barrosse-Antle ME, Patel KH, Kramer JA, Baston CM. Point-of-care ultrasound for bedside diagnosis of lower extremity DVT. Chest 2021;**160**(5):1853–63.

33. Becattini C, Cohen AT, Agnelli G, Howard L, Castejon B, Trujillo-Santos J, Monreal M, Perrier A, Yusen RD, Jimenez D. Risk stratification of patients with acute symptomatic pulmonary embolism based on presence or absence of lower extremity DVT: systematic review and meta-analysis. Chest 2016;**149**(1):192–200.

34. van Langevelde K, Tan M, Sramek A, Huisman MV, de Roos A. Magnetic resonance imaging and computed tomography developments in imaging of venous thromboembolism. J Magn Reson Imaging 2010;**32**(6):1302–12.

35. Le Gal G, Righini M, Sanchez O, Roy PM, Baba-Ahmed M, Perriers A, Bounameaux H. A positive compression ultrasonography of the lower limb veins is highly predictive of pulmonary embolism on computed tomography in suspected patients. Thromb Haemost 2006;**95**(6):963–6.

36. Pruszczyk P, Kurnicka K, Ciurzynski M, Hobohm L, Thielmann A, Sobkowicz B, Sawicka E, Kostrubiec M, Ptaszynska-Kopczynska K, Dzikowska-Diduch O, Lichodziejewska B, Lankeit M. Defining right ventricular dysfunction by echocardiography in normotensive patients with pulmonary embolism. Pol Arch Intern Med 2020;**130**(9):741–7.

37. Becattini C, Maraziti G, Vinson DR, Ng ACC, den Exter PL, Cote B, Vanni S, Doukky R, Khemasuwan D, Weekes AJ, Soares TH, Ozsu S, Polo Friz H, Erol S, Agnelli G, Jimenez D. Right ventricle assessment in patients with pulmonary embolism at low risk for death based on clinical models: an individual patient data meta-analysis. Eur Heart J 2021;**42**(33):3190–9.

38. Coutance G, Cauderlier E, Ehtisham J, Hamon M, Hamon M. The prognostic value of markers of right ventricular dysfunction in pulmonary embolism: a meta-analysis. Crit Care 2011;**15**(2):R103.

39. Sanchez O, Trinquart L, Colombet I, Durieux P, Huisman MV, Chatellier G, Meyer G. Prognostic value of right ventricular dysfunction in patients with haemodynamically stable pulmonary embolism: a systematic review. Eur Heart J 2008;**29**(12):1569–77.

40. Pruszczyk P, Goliszek S, Lichodziejewska B, Kostrubiec M, Ciurzynski M, Kurnicka K, Dzikowska-Diduch O, Palczewski P, Wyzgal A. Prognostic value of echocardiography in normotensive patients with acute pulmonary embolism. JACC Cardiovasc Imaging 2014;**7**(6):553–60.

41. Jaff MR, McMurtry MS, Archer SL, Cushman M, Goldenberg N, Goldhaber SZ, Jenkins JS, Kline JA, Michaels AD, Thistlethwaite P, Vedantham S, White RJ, Zierler BK, American Heart Association Council on Cardiopulmonary CCP, Resuscitation, American Heart Association Council on Peripheral Vascular D, American Heart Association Council on Arteriosclerosis T, Vascular B. Management of massive and submassive pulmonary embolism, iliofemoral deep vein thrombosis, and chronic thromboembolic pulmonary hypertension: a scientific statement from the American Heart Association. Circulation 2011;**123**(16):1788–830.

42. Lobo JL, Holley A, Tapson V, Moores L, Oribe M, Barron M, Otero R, Nauffal D, Valle R, Monreal M, Yusen RD, Jimenez D, Protect, investigators R. Prognostic significance of tricuspid annular displacement in normotensive patients with acute symptomatic pulmonary embolism. J Thromb Haemost 2014;**12**(7):1020–7.

43. Konstantinides S, Geibel A, Kasper W, Olschewski M, Blumel L, Just H. Patent foramen ovale is an important predictor of adverse outcome in patients with major pulmonary embolism. Circulation 1998;**97**(19):1946–51.

44. Doyen D, Castellani M, Moceri P, Chiche O, Lazdunski R, Bertora D, Cerboni P, Chaussade C, Ferrari E. Patent foramen ovale and stroke in intermediate-risk pulmonary embolism. Chest 2014;**146**(4):967–73.

45. Goliszek S, Wisniewska M, Kurnicka K, Lichodziejewska B, Ciurzynski M, Kostrubiec M, Golebiowski M, Babiuch M, Paczynska M, Koc M, Palczewski P, Wyzgal A, Pruszczyk P. Patent foramen ovale increases the risk of acute ischemic stroke in patients with acute pulmonary embolism leading to right ventricular dysfunction. Thromb Res 2014;**134**(5):1052–6.

46. Le Moigne E, Timsit S, Ben Salem D, Didier R, Jobic Y, Paleiron N, Le Mao R, Joseph T, Hoffmann C, Dion A, Rousset J, Le Gal G, Lacut K, Leroyer C, Mottier D, Couturaud F. Patent foramen ovale and ischemic stroke in patients with pulmonary embolism: a prospective cohort study. Ann Intern Med 2019;**170**(11):756–63.

Echocardiography in cardiac tamponade

8

Mauro Pepi, Gloria Tamborini, and Manuela Muratori

Key Points

- Cardiac tamponade is a clinical diagnosis based on elevated systemic venous pressure, tachycardia, dyspnea, and paradoxical arterial pulse.
- Echocardiography allows bedside detection, semiquantitation, and localization of pericardial effusions.
- Echocardiography may reveal *warning signs* that suggest tamponade physiology, including right ventricular (RV) and right atrial (RA) collapse, inferior vena cava plethora, and increased transmitral and aortic flow reduction during inspiration.
- The duration/severity of collapses and respiratory severity of transmitral and transaortic flow changes are directly related to the severity of tamponade.
- Right-sided collapse may be insensitive in RV hypertrophy and high RV intracavitary pressures.
- Localized pericardial effusion or clot may occur after cardiac surgery or percutaneous procedures. These "iatrogenic" effusions may be difficult to explore, and off-axis transthoracic echocardiographic views should be used. In cases with poor or inconclusive transthoracic images, transesophageal echocardiography should always be performed.
- Percutaneous pericardiocentesis guided by echocardiography is an effective and safe procedure.

Cardiac tamponade is a medical emergency and life-threatening condition that requires urgent therapeutic intervention. This chapter covers the role of echocardiography in the detection of pericardial effusion and warning signs of cardiac tamponade and the contribution of ultrasound technique in patient management.

DEFINITION AND PHYSIOLOGY

Cardiac tamponade is defined as significant compression of the heart by accumulation of abnormal pericardial contents (effusion fluids, clots, pus, and gas, separately or in combination). When liquid is injected into the pericardial sac of an experimental animal, intrapericardial and right and left atrial (LA) pressure begins to rise equally; this may occur also in the presence of a small amount of fluid (20–40 mL). If fluid continues to accumulate, each successive diastolic period leads to less blood entering the ventricles. Therefore, as more fluid is added, cardiac stroke volume falls while cardiac output falls less because of compensating tachycardia. The output of both ventricles depends on adequate diastolic filling. Normally, intrapericardial pressure is zero or slightly negative, and the transmural pressure gradient across the myocardium during diastole is positive (the intraventricular pressures are greater than the intrapericardial pressures), thus facilitating ventricular filling. As the chambers become progressively smaller and myocardial diastolic compliance is reduced, cardiac inflow becomes limited, ultimately equalizing mean diastolic and chamber pressures.

DOI: 10.1201/9781003245407-8

A small pericardial effusion can cause clinically significant cardiac tamponade when it accumulates rapidly. Important elements in this process are the *rate of fluid accumulation* relative to pericardial stretch and the effectiveness of compensatory mechanisms. Even in cases of diffuse circumferential effusion, the hemodynamic effects of tamponade are *primarily the result of right heart compression*; the pressures of these thinner chambers equilibrate with rising pericardial pressure before the LA and left ventricular (LV) pressures. With overt tamponade, rising of the pericardial pressure progressively reduces and ultimately intermittently reverses the transmural pressure of first the right and then the left heart chambers. Filling of the heart is therefore maintained by a parallel increase in systemic and pulmonary venous pressures; as compensatory mechanisms (primarily tachycardia) are defeated, cardiac filling decreases, pericardial pressure equilibrates with LV diastolic pressure, and cardiac output decreases critically. Inspiration increases the filling gradient across the right heart but not the left heart; the augmented right ventricular (RV) filling occurs at the expense of reduced filling and stroke output of the left ventricle (Figure 8.1). These mechanisms cause a typical clinical sign of tamponade: pulsus paradoxus (systolic drop in arterial pressure of 10 mmHg or more during normal breathing).[1-5]

CLINICAL SIGNS

Although the clinical condition may markedly vary in patients with cardiac tamponade (mainly as a result of the different causes of the syndrome), three signs are typically associated with cardiac tamponade (Beck's triad): hypotension, jugular venous distention (elevated systemic venous pressure), and pulsus paradoxus. Tachycardia, dyspnea, cough and dysphagia, chest discomfort, oliguria, shock, and unconsciousness may also be present. Beck's triad may be lacking in patients with "medical tamponade" with slowly accumulating pericardial fluid; therefore, the *rate* of pericardial accumulation is critical for the clinical presentation.

Atypical clinical presentation is frequent, especially in the setting of cardiac surgery or percutaneous procedures, and the three signs, in particular pulsus paradoxus, may be absent in several settings: LV dysfunction, regional RA tamponade, positive-pressure ventilation, atrial septal defect, pulmonary arterial obstruction, and severe aortic regurgitation.

ECHOCARDIOGRAPHIC FEATURES OF CARDIAC TAMPONADE

Pericardial effusion appears as an echo-free space between the two layers of the pericardium and is easily demonstrated with echocardiography. When tamponade is suspected, the evaluation of the pericardial sac should be carefully performed through all the echocardiographic windows to quantitate pericardial fluid and distinguish *diffuse circumferential* effusions from *loculated regional* ones. Echocardiography allows discrimination among *small, moderate, and large* effusions and may also detect the association with *pleural effusions*.[6-9] Specifically, the dimension of the pericardial effusion corresponds to the average quantity of pericardial fluid: small (5–10 mm, corresponding to a fluid volume of 50–100 mL),

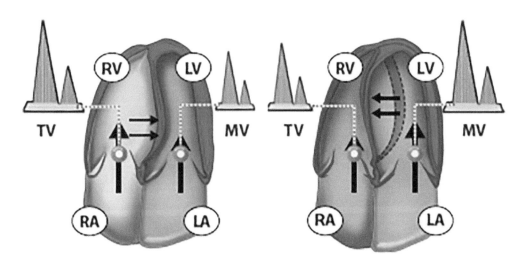

FIGURE 8.1 Schematic representation of exaggerated respiratory changes of ventricular filling in cardiac tamponade and constrictive pericarditis (ventricular interdependence). During inspiration (left panel), an exaggerated increase in right ventricular filling occurs at the expense of diminished left ventricular filling (interventricular septum shifts to the left), which can be appreciated on pulsed Doppler as an increase in tricuspid and decrease in mitral inflow. Expiration is associated with reciprocal changes (right panel). LA: left atrium; LV: left ventricle; MV: mitral valve; RA: right atrium; RV: right ventricle; TV: tricuspid valve.

(Artwork provided by SUP.)

moderate (10–20 mm, corresponding to a fluid volume of 250–500 mL), and severe (>20 mm separation, corresponding to a volume of >500 mL).[10] In this regard, pericardial effusions can be detected and analyzed from different standard but also non standard or modified views (Figures 8.2 and 8.3) (V8.1, V8.2, V8.3).

The assessment of the *character of the fluid by ultrasound is not possible* because serous effusions, hemopericardium, and chylopericardium all appear as similar clear spaces. However, *fibrous strands* are frequently observed in cases of chronic diseases, and *hematomas and clots* may be detected

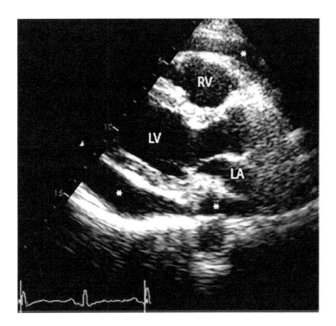

FIGURE 8.2 A large circumferential pericardial effusion (*), as seen from the parasternal long-axis view (V8.1), but without chamber inversions suggestive of tamponade physiology. LA: left atrium; LV: left ventricle; RV: right ventricle.

(Image and video provided by IS.)

as solid masses of granular echoes inside the pericardial sac. Echogenic masses attached to the visceral pericardium may suggest the presence of metastasis.

Excessive cardiac motion up to the "swinging heart" is frequently seen in severe pericardial effusion with chronically accumulated effusion and a minimum of adhesions (V8.4). This movement has been observed in malignancies, chronic tuberculous pericarditis, and benign viral pericarditis.

Echocardiographic and Doppler signs that have been described in cardiac tamponade are listed in Table 8.1. The major criteria that suggest cardiac tamponade on echocardiogram are (1) interventricular septum deviation toward the LV cavity on inspiration, (2) RV diastolic and RA collapse, (3) decrease in transmitral inflow E-wave velocity of more than 25% on inspiration and/or increase in tricuspid inflow E-wave velocity by greater than 40% on inspiration, and (4) inferior vena cava (IVC) dilation without collapse on inspiration.[11,12]

An exaggerated inspiratory expansion of the right ventricle with simultaneous compression of the left ventricle is a nonspecific sign of increased direct interdependence and therefore has a low specificity. *Diastolic collapse of the RA and RV free walls* are accepted signs of cardiac tamponade. This can be evaluated

TABLE 8.1   Echo-Doppler Signs of Cardiac Tamponade

- Exaggerated inspiratory variation of the two ventricles (inspiratory expansion of the right ventricle and simultaneous compression of the left ventricle; reciprocal changes in the expiratory phase)
- Right atrial collapse
- Right ventricular collapse
- Left atrial collapse
- Left ventricular collapse
- Inferior vena cava plethora
- Abnormal increased respiratory variation in transvalvular blood flow velocities (mitral and aortic flow reduction in the inspiratory phase)

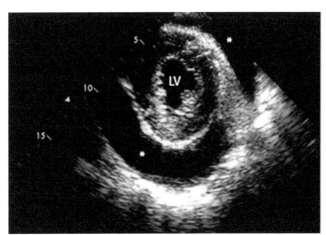
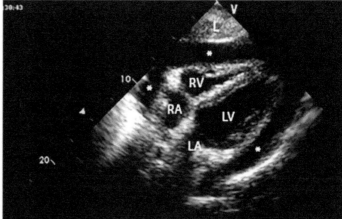

FIGURE 8.3   A large circumferential pericardial effusion surrounding all cardiac chambers (*), as seen from the parasternal short-axis (left panel) (V8.2) and subcostal (right panel) views (V8.3). L: liver; LA: left atrium; LV: left ventricle; RA: right atrium; RV: right ventricle.

(Images and videos provided by IS.)

by both M-mode (Figure 8.4) and two-dimensional echocardiography (Figures 8.5 and 8.6) (V8.5, V8.6). RV collapse is a transient invagination of the RV free wall that occurs in early diastole, whereas RA collapse is a transient invagination of the RA wall that occurs in late diastole and early systole. Timing of these two collapses is related to the *lowest intracavitary pressures* occurring in the two chambers in early (RV) or late (RA) diastole, respectively. These two signs of tamponade may be too sensitive (sensitivity of 50–100% for RA and 48–100% for RV collapse) on the one hand and lack specificity on the other (specificity of 48% for RA and 72% for RV diastolic collapse). Therefore, the *duration of the collapse* should be taken into account. In fact, the duration of collapses is directly related to severity of tamponade (duration of RA inversion/cardiac cycle length >34% has >90% sensitivity and 100% specificity), and it improves the specificity and predictive value of these diagnostic signs.[13–16] With increasing severity, RA collapse tends to begin earlier and RV collapse to extend later in diastole (V8.7, V8.8). Even though these two signs are too sensitive, the *presence of both RA and RV collapse always indicates that the effusion is hemodynamically significant.*

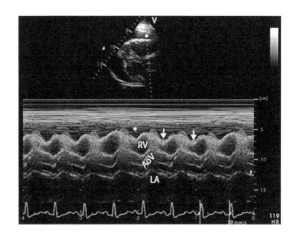

FIGURE 8.4 M-mode recording of the parasternal long-axis view demonstrating right ventricular wall diastolic collapse (arrows) in a patient with cardiac tamponade. Note that right ventricular collapse occurs when aortic valve (AoV) is closed, indicating right ventricular collapse in diastole. *: pericardial effusion; LA: left atrium; RV: right ventricle.

(Image provided by IS.)

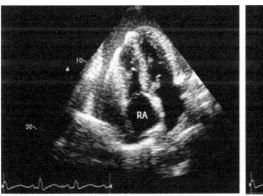 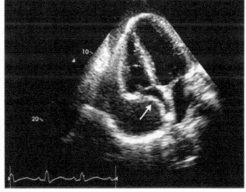

FIGURE 8.5 Apical four-chamber view of a patient with lung adenocarcinoma showing a large circular pericardial effusion (both panels). Note the right atrial systolic collapse (arrow), consistent with cardiac tamponade physiology (right panel) (V8.5). RA: right atrium.

(Images and video provided by IS.)

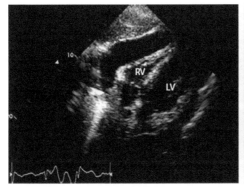 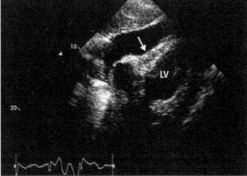

FIGURE 8.6 Early diastolic collapse of the right ventricular free wall (arrow, right panel), consistent with cardiac tamponade, in a hemodynamically unstable patient with large pericardial effusion, as seen from the subcostal view (both panels) (V8.6). LV: left ventricle; RV: right ventricle.

(Images and video provided by IS.)

In an experimental animal study, Leimgruber et al.[17] showed that the earliest appearance of RV diastolic collapse is associated with a 21% reduction in cardiac output at a time when mean aortic pressure is unchanged. Lopez-Sendon et al.,[18] in an open-chest dog model, showed the sequence and characteristics of RA collapse: long before hemodynamic alterations of fully established cardiac tamponade are present, RA compression becomes apparent as a quick inward motion of a small portion of the posterior RA wall, and as the intrapericardial pressure increases, a wider portion of the RA wall presents an abnormal motion. With a further increase in intrapericardial pressure, RA inversion throughout the entire cardiac cycle becomes progressively apparent, and finally the complete distortion of the RA shape and dimensions indicates an extreme situation of cardiac tamponade. These old experimental studies underline the concept that *early echocardiography may detect tamponade physiology* and the hemodynamic significance of pericardial effusion. Tamponade should always be considered as a *continuum of events:* in the early phase of cardiac compression, even minor elevations of intrapericardial pressure produce some effects on ventricular filling, and echocardiographic signs could be present even in the absence of overt clinical tamponade.[19–23] There are few exceptions to the use of right-sided collapse for diagnosing tamponade: RV hypertrophy and high RV intracavitary pressures may prevent the occurrence of these collapses.

LA and LV collapse are *rarely* seen in patients with cardiac tamponade. This is mainly because of local factors. The left ventricle is much thicker and stiffer than the other chambers, and for that reason, it resists collapse. The left atrium is posteriorly positioned, and it is tightly clasped by the pericardium; rarely, in cases with very large effusions, fluid gets behind the left atrium and causes wall collapse. Facilitating factors of LA and LV wall collapse are, therefore, posteriorly loculated effusions and conditions in which pressures in these chambers are relatively low (V14.8A, V14.8B, V14.8C). LV collapse has been described in postoperative effusion.[24]

IVC plethora with reduced inspiratory collapse (Figure 8.7) (V8.9) is another sign of cardiac tamponade.[25] Several studies have shown that dilation, particularly blunted inspiratory variation of the IVC, correlates with increased RA pressure. Therefore, this is a sensitive but nonspecific sign of the

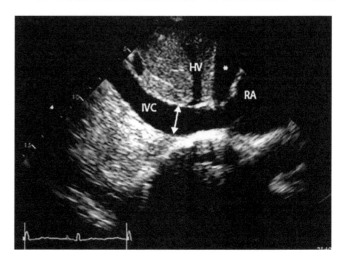

FIGURE 8.7 The subcostal view of a patient with cardiac tamponade showing a dilated noncollapsible inferior vena cava (IVC) and hepatic vein (HV) (V8.9). *: pericardial effusion; RA: right atrium.

(Image and video provided by IS.)

syndrome, which may be seen also in constrictive pericarditis, RV infarction, pulmonary hypertension, and tricuspid regurgitation. Through this method (inspiratory variation during regular respiration), RA pressure can be estimated and classified as normal (6 mmHg in the presence of an inspiratory reduction of the IVC diameter by over 45%), moderately elevated (9 mmHg; 35–45%), or markedly elevated (16 mmHg; <35%).[26]

Cardiac tamponade is associated with an *abnormally increased respiratory variation in transvalvular blood flow velocities.*[27,28] Normally, inspiration causes a minimal increase in systemic venous, tricuspid, and pulmonary valvular blood flow and a corresponding decrease in pulmonary venous, mitral, and aortic flow velocities. Thus, in a normal subject, inspiratory variations in these measurements do not exceed 20%. With cardiac tamponade, ventricular interdependence is exaggerated, and inspiration produces a significant decrease in left-sided filling. Accordingly, mitral and aortic valvular flows are reduced by >25% and a corresponding increase of >40% is observed in right-sided flow velocities. Figure 8.8 demonstrates

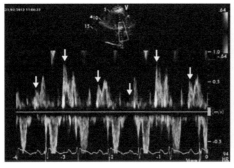 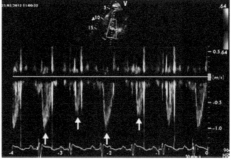

FIGURE 8.8 Pulsed-wave Doppler recordings of the transmitral (left panel) and left ventricular outflow tract (right panel) flows in a patient with cardiac tamponade. Note significant respiratory variations of both flows (arrows) recorded during normal respiration.

(Images provided by IS.)

the usefulness of Doppler echocardiography in the setting of cardiac tamponade. From a technical point of view, it is important to control the positioning of the sample volume during the examination by trying to exclude differences in location during respiration and to use the electrocardiographic cable for respiratory monitoring (several ultrasound devices have this option).

Tamponade physiology may mimic or contribute to acute heart failure symptoms and should be considered in the differential diagnosis as appropriate (V8.17).

PERICARDIAL EFFUSION AND CARDIAC TAMPONADE AFTER CARDIAC SURGERY

Pericardial effusion is not a rare complication of cardiac surgery.[29–33] Although it is generally reversible and not life-threatening, it may sometimes evolve toward cardiac tamponade (see also Chapter 14). The role of echocardiography is extremely important in the diagnosis of cardiac tamponade in the postoperative period because the clinical and imaging presentations could be atypical; therefore, a specific knowledge of this disorder is very useful.[34]

Virtually all pericardial effusions are found by postoperative day 5; effusion peaks on day 10 and resolves within 1 month. In a large, prospective study,[35] pericardial effusion was detected in 64% of cases and was more often associated with coronary artery bypass grafting (75%) than with valve replacement (52%) or other types of surgery (50%). It was small in 68%, moderate in 30%, and large in 2% of cases. *Loculated effusions were more frequent* (58%) than diffuse ones (42%).

The size and site of effusions were related to the type of surgery; in particular, small pericardial effusion was slightly more frequent after valve replacement than after coronary artery bypass grafting. After valve replacement, diffuse fluid accumulations were more frequent (55%) than loculated ones, whereas after coronary artery bypass grafting, loculated effusions were more common (63.5%). In particular, anterior loculated effusions were more common after coronary artery bypass grafting, and posterolateral ones after valve replacement. Interestingly, 6% of the patients had *isolated effusion along the RA wall;* this type of effusion can compress the heart and can be difficult to diagnose in patients with postoperative low output failure. Fifteen of 780 patients had cardiac tamponade; this event was significantly more common after valve replacement than after coronary artery bypass grafting or other types of surgery. All these epidemiologic data are extremely important because the recognition of cardiac tamponade in the early or late postoperative periods is not easy.

Loculated effusions may be difficult to explore, and *off-axis views* should be attempted in cases in which the differential diagnosis with pleural effusion is difficult or in the presence of atypical presentation. In particular, localized pericardial effusion or clot at the level of the RA wall, right ventricle, left ventricle, and left atrium may occur after cardiac surgery and present with unique clinical and echo-Doppler features. Modified apical, subcostal (Figure 8.9) (V8.10), and posterior views are extremely useful in the evaluation of all these isolated effusions; however, in several cases, particularly when transthoracic

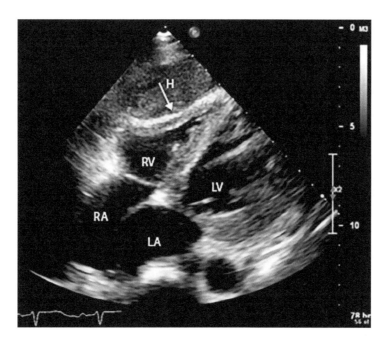

FIGURE 8.9 In this subcostal four-chamber view of a patient who bled after placement of a left ventricular assist device, a large pericardial hematoma (H) compressing (arrow) the right ventricle (RV) is seen (V8.10). LA: left atrium; LV: left ventricle; RA: right atrium.

(Image and video provided by MHP.)

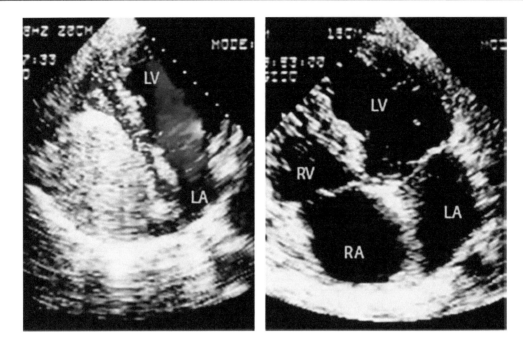

FIGURE 8.10   Apical four-chamber view showing an echodense, voluminous mass (pericardial clot) at the level of the right atrium (left panel). Because of this compression, the right atrial cavity is virtual. After subxiphoid pericardial drainage, the pericardial clot has been completely removed, and the size of the right atrium is normal (right panel). LA: left atrium; LV: left ventricle; RA: right atrium; RV: right ventricle.

echocardiography does not provide complete imaging of the pericardial sac and unstable hemodynamics coexists with suspected cardiac tamponade, transesophageal echocardiography is mandatory (V8.11).[36,37] Figure 8.10 shows an example of detection of pericardial clot compressing the right atrium by transthoracic echocardiography; thrombosis of this loculated pericardial effusion after aortic valve replacement mimicked an RA mass.[38] A transesophageal example of pericardial hematoma compressing the left atrium is shown in Figure 8.11. In both cases, patients were in shock, and emergency echocardiography was requested. Echocardiography allowed rapid diagnosis, and immediate surgical decompression was performed successfully with clinical resolution of shock. These two cases reinforce the concept of the usefulness of echocardiography in unstable patients after cardiac surgery.[39] Russo et al.[34] demonstrated that 9 of 10 patients with cardiac tamponade (10 of 510 consecutive patients evaluated after cardiac surgery) had *atypical* clinical, hemodynamic, and/or echocardiographic findings. The authors found that patients frequently had vague and nonspecific initial symptoms, including general malaise, lethargy, anorexia, and palpitations, whereas dyspnea, chest pain, confusion, diaphoresis, and oliguria occurred later, in general. *Selective chamber compression* was the more frequent cause of atypical clinical and echo presentation. LV and RV compressions and LA and RA compressions have been demonstrated after cardiac surgery. Pericardial clots, particularly at the level of the right chambers, may produce low cardiac output soon after open-heart surgery with hemodynamic signs very similar to constrictive pericarditis; Beppu et al.[37] showed the indispensability of transesophageal echocardiography in these cases (Figure 14.7) (V14.7A,

V14.7B, V14.7C). Several reports confirmed that in tamponade after cardiac surgery caused by loculated regional RA compression, pulsus paradoxus may be absent, whereas regional compression of the left ventricle and tamponade may occur despite normal RA and peripheral venous pressure.

In conclusion, atypical clinical presentation of cardiac tamponade is very frequent after cardiac surgery. In terms of hemodynamic effects, Fowler et al.[40] demonstrated that right-sided cardiac compression has more important effects than does left-sided compression. However, left-sided tamponade still makes a significant contribution to the total hemodynamic picture of cardiac tamponade. Therefore, the echocardiographic search for regional pericardial effusion should be very detailed and precise. Postoperative cardiac tamponade might be suspected in the presence of loculated effusions along the RA and/or along its junction with the superior vena cava, LA or bilateral atrial compression, and RV or LV effusions. In this setting, we investigated the type and frequency of Doppler and echocardiographic findings of cardiac tamponade.[35] We invariably (15 of 15 cases in our series) recorded an inspiratory decrease (>25%) in the velocity of flow through the aortic and mitral valves; five patients had RA collapse, RV collapse, and IVC plethora; eight had two of these signs; and two had one. In four patients, moderate pericardial effusions were associated with one or two echocardiographic signs of cardiac tamponade, but not with clinical evidence of hemodynamic embarrassment or with Doppler signs of tamponade.

Of note, tamponade physiology may be caused not only by clots and loculated pericardial effusions but also by solid tumors (V8.17).

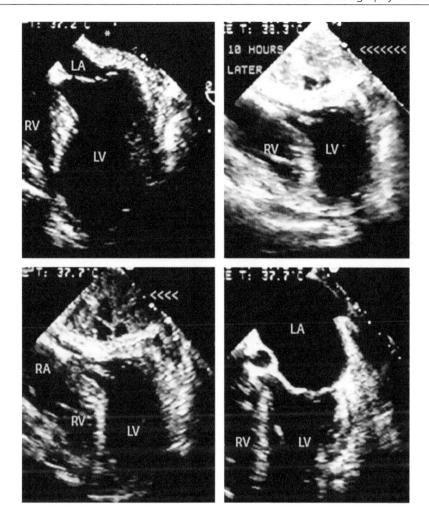

FIGURE 8.11 Transesophageal four-chamber view (top, left panel) in a patient with hemodynamic instability immediately after coronary artery bypass grafting. A moderate pericardial effusion (*) along the left atrium was demonstrated, but the presence of severe left ventricular dysfunction led to the decision to institute the intra-aortic balloon pump, starting the counterpulsation and optimizing the medical therapy. However, a few hours later, transesophageal echocardiography was repeated because of severe cardiogenic shock; this time a large pericardial hematoma compressing the left atrium (arrow) was clearly demonstrated (top right panel and bottom left panel). The patient underwent immediate surgical drainage of the pericardium with resolution of the clinical and hemodynamic instability and normalization of the left atrial cavity size (bottom right panel). LA: left atrium; LV: left ventricle; RA: right atrium; RV: right ventricle.

ECHO-GUIDED PERICARDIOCENTESIS

Early recognition and treatment of patients with suspected tamponade is an important clinical goal. Once tamponade is diagnosed, decompression by a safe, simple, and rapid method is required.

When one is deciding to perform pericardiocentesis, many clinical and echocardiographic factors must be considered.[41] These include the amount and location of the effusion, hemodynamics by echocardiography, sufficient margins of the echo free space (to avoid myocardial laceration), clinical indication and urgency, underlying causes, and bleeding tendency.[42] It can be efficiently performed during cardiopulmonary resuscitation (V21.5A, V21.5B, V21.5C).

As already discussed, it should be always kept in mind that even a small amount of pericardial fluid may cause cardiac tamponade if it accumulates rapidly, as it may happen during percutaneous interventional procedures. Often in these situations not all echocardiographic signs of impending tamponade are present and the decision to perform pericardiocentesis should be guided mainly by actual clinical status (Figure 8.12) (V8.12A, 8.12B).

Aortic dissection is a major contraindication to pericardiocentesis. Relative contraindications include uncorrected coagulopathy, anticoagulant therapy, thrombocytopenia (<50,000), and small, posterior, loculated effusion—the more frequent cause of atypical clinical and echo presentation.[12] The surgical approach, rather than percutaneous pericardiocentesis, is preferred in traumatic hemopericardium (V16.2A), purulent pericarditis (V21.7B), recurrent malignant effusion,

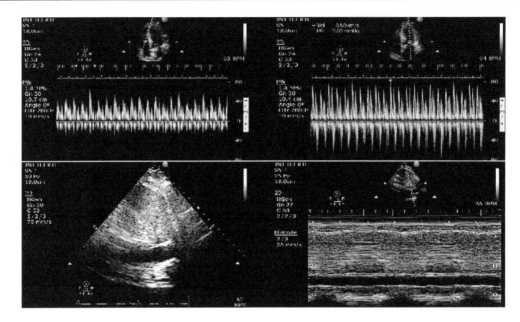

FIGURE 8.12 Left upper panel: Transtricuspid pulsed-wave Doppler signal with nonsignificant respiratory variation in maximal velocities (<40%). Right upper panel: Transmitral pulsed-wave Doppler signal with nonsignificant respiratory variation in maximal velocities (<20%). Left lower panel: Dilated vena cava inferior (22 mm). Right lower panel: M-mode signal through vena cava inferior showing absence of normal respiratory variation in its diameter (V8.12A).

(Images and video provided by IV and PMM.)

loculated effusion in the posterior side of the heart (V14.8A), and a need for pericardial biopsy.[43,44]

Drainage of an acute, effusion-producing cardiac tamponade may be performed by *two alternative techniques:* surgical subxiphoid pericardiotomy and percutaneous pericardiocentesis. Surgical subxiphoid pericardiotomy[45] is performed under either local or general anesthesia, via a midline longitudinal incision from the xiphisternal junction to 6–8 cm below the tip of the xiphoid.

Percutaneous pericardiocentesis has been described in detail by several authors,[46–50] who proposed improvements of the technique, starting from the blind procedure, and passing through echo-guided and contrast echo-guided pericardiocentesis. There are *three approaches* to needle entry during pericardiocentesis: left parasternal, subxiphoid, and left apical.[51] In the *left parasternal approach*, the puncture needle is inserted close to the sternum, usually in the left fifth or sixth intercostal space. This approach is associated with higher risk of pneumothorax than with the subxiphoid approach. In the *subxiphoid approach*, the needle is inserted at an angle between the sternum and left costal margin, directed toward the left shoulder at a 15–30° angle to the skin. This route is extrapleural and avoids the coronary and internal mammary arteries. Irritation of the diaphragm and phrenic nerve may result in bradycardia and shock, and higher procedure-related mortality have been reported with this approach than with others. In the *apical approach*, the puncture needle is inserted into the intercostal space and the entry site is selected avoiding the internal mammary artery and the vascular bundle at the inferior margin of the rib (Figure 8.13).

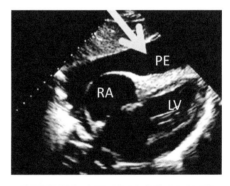
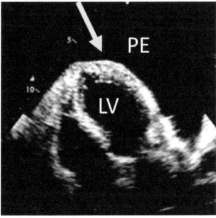

FIGURE 8.13 "Ideal" pericardial effusion characteristics for the subxiphoid (upper panel) and apical (lower panel) pericardiocentesis approach. Direction of yellow arrows indicates ideal direction of needle insertion. LV: left ventricle; PE: pericardial effusion; RA: right atrium.

Callahan et al.[48] emphasized *visualization of the pericardial needle* during their study on *echo-guided pericardiocentesis* with the assistance of *contrast echocardiography*, thus reducing the likelihood of heart puncture. An improvement of ultrasonically guided pericardiocentesis has been proposed by our group,[49] with the specific purpose of facilitating posterior drainage. The Tuohy needle used in this study, thanks to its curved tip, greatly facilitated guidance of the wire and catheter to the posterior pericardial space, so that the standard Seldinger technique was successful not only in massive and diffused effusions, but also in loculated posterior ones. More recently, we compared the combined use of two-dimensional echo monitoring by the described technique with surgical subxiphoid pericardiotomy in the treatment of acute cardiac tamponade caused by pericardial effusion occurring after cardiac surgery.[50] Forty-two patients were included in the study: during the first period, one of the two methods was chosen by the clinical staff, whereas in the second period percutaneous pericardiocentesis was the treatment of choice. Complete drainage of pericardial fluid by percutaneous pericardiocentesis was obtained in 26 of 29 patients (90%). No major complication occurred with the use of the two techniques. In three cases, in the second study period, the minimal amount of fluid or pericardial hematoma indicated surgical approach as the first therapeutic choice; percutaneous pericardiocentesis was unsuccessful in three cases without complications, and surgical drainage was therefore performed. This study suggested that the more invasive technique (subxiphoid surgical pericardiotomy) should be selected in cases in which percutaneous pericardiocentesis is unsuccessful or when the echocardiographic examination discourages a percutaneous approach.

Tsang et al.[51] reported the Mayo Clinic experience in cardiac tamponade caused by cardiac perforation as a complication of cardiac catheterization procedures. Echocardiography-guided pericardiocentesis was safe and effective in rescuing patients from tamponade and reversing hemodynamic instability complicating invasive cardiac-based procedures (Figure 8.14) (V8.13). In this clinical setting and in cardiac tamponade from other causes, they proposed a specific technique based on the two-dimensional characteristics of effusions. Two-dimensional echocardiography allowed the examiner to localize the largest collection of pericardial fluid in closest proximity to the transducer, thereby *identifying the ideal entry site*. The trajectory of the pericardiocentesis needle was defined by transducer angulation. After local infiltration with 1% lidocaine, a polytef-sheathed needle (16–18 gauge) was used for the initial pericardial entry. On reaching the pericardial fluid, the steel core of the needle was immediately withdrawn, leaving only the polytef sheath in the pericardial space. In the presence of hemorrhagic effusion, *injection of a small volume of agitated saline as a contrast* was used for echocardiographic confirmation of the sheath position (Figure 8.15) (V8.14, V8.15, V8.16). After introducing the guidewire into the pericardial space, the sheath was withdrawn,

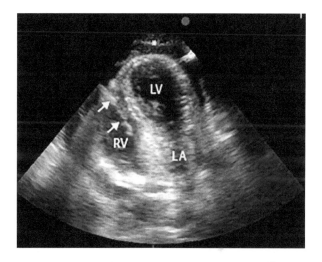

FIGURE 8.14 Transthoracic four-chamber view showing a pacemaker electrode (arrows) in the right heart that went through the right ventricular wall and entered pericardial space (*). Note significant rapidly accumulated pericardial effusion (*) (V8.13). LA: left atrium; LV: left ventricle; RV: right ventricle.

(Image and video provided by LZ.)

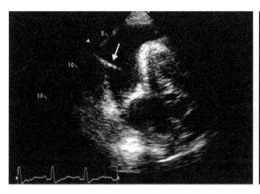 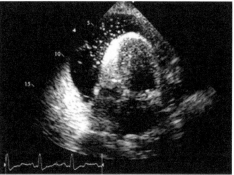

FIGURE 8.15 Echo-guided pericardiocentesis. After the needle reached the pericardial space (arrow in left panel) (V8.14), a small amount of contrast was injected to confirm intrapericardial position of the needle, as indicated by bubble appearance within pericardial effusion (right panel) (V8.15).

(Images and videos provided by IS.)

and a standard dilator and introducer (6–7F) were advanced over the guidewire. A pigtail angiographic catheter (65 cm; 6–7F) was then introduced into the pericardial space. Rescue echo-guided pericardiocentesis by the described technique was the only treatment required for the majority of these patients. Surgical exploration or intervention is indicated when complete control of the bleeding is in question or when hemodynamic stability is not rapidly restored by rescue pericardiocentesis alone.

Many investigators have suggested two-dimensional echocardiography to guide not only the placement of the pericardiocentesis needle, but also biopsy forceps, balloon catheters (pericardioplasty), and other new percutaneous devices.[52,53] Instillation in the pericardial sac of various agents with sclerosing, anti-inflammatory, or cytostatic activity has also been proposed under echocardiographic assistance.

CONCLUSIONS

Echocardiography aids in the detection, localization, and quantitation of pericardial effusion. Various echocardiographic modalities including M-mode, two-dimensional transthoracic, and transesophageal echocardiography are used in assessment and management of cardiac tamponade. Echocardiography is successfully used not only in cases of large and diffuse pericardial effusion and classic clinical presentations but also in patients with atypical clinical presentation and/or loculated pericardial effusion. Echocardiography is useful in guiding and monitoring pericardiocentesis.

It should be emphasized that in everyday clinical practice, cardiac tamponade is a *clinical diagnosis* supported by echocardiographic findings. Most hypotensive and dyspneic patients with large pericardial effusions will also exhibit echocardiographic signs of impending cardiac tamponade. Importantly, not only may echo signs of tamponade be challenging to obtain in an unstable patient, but cardiac tamponade can also occur even in the absence of these signs.

LIST OF VIDEOS

https://routledgetextbooks.com/textbooks/9781032157009/chapter-8.php

VIDEO 8.1   Pericardial effusion in parasternal long-axis view: Transthoracic parasternal long-axis view showing a large circular pericardial effusion, but without chamber inversions suggestive of tamponade physiology. *(Video provided by IS.)*

VIDEO 8.2   Pericardial effusion in parasternal short-axis view: A large circular pericardial effusion surrounding all cardiac chambers can be seen from the parasternal short-axis view. *(Video provided by IS.)*

VIDEO 8.3   Pericardial effusion in subcostal view: A large circular pericardial effusion surrounding all cardiac chambers can be seen from the subcostal view. *(Video provided by IS.)*

VIDEO 8.4   "Swinging heart": Transthoracic echocardiographic apical four-chamber view of a patient with lung carcinoma showing excessive cardiac motion up to the swinging heart; this is frequently seen in severe pericardial effusion with chronically accumulated effusion and a minimum of adhesions. *(Video provided by IS.)*

VIDEO 8.5   Right atrial systolic collapse (cardiac tamponade): Transthoracic echocardiographic apical four-chamber view of a patient with lung adenocarcinoma showing a large circular pericardial effusion. Note the right atrial systolic collapse consistent with cardiac tamponade physiology. *(Video provided by IS.)*

VIDEO 8.6   Right ventricular diastolic collapse (cardiac tamponade): Subcostal four-chamber view of a hemodynamically unstable patient with large pericardial effusion showing an early diastolic collapse of the right ventricular free wall, consistent with cardiac tamponade. *(Video provided by IS.)*

VIDEO 8.7   Large pericardial effusion and right atrial collapse: Transthoracic echocardiographic apical four-chamber view showing large pericardial effusion and discrete right atrial collapse, indicating early tamponade physiology (see also Video 8.8).

VIDEO 8.8   Large pericardial effusion and marked right atrial collapse: Transthoracic echocardiographic apical four-chamber view showing large pericardial effusion and marked and long-lasting right atrial collapse, indicating progression of hemodynamic deterioration and impending tamponade (see also Video 8.7).

VIDEO 8.9   Inferior vena cava plethora: Subcostal view of a patient with cardiac tamponade showing a dilated noncollapsible inferior vena cava and hepatic vein. Note the right atrial collapse. *(Video provided by IS.)*

VIDEO 8.10   Cardiac tamponade caused by hematoma: In this subcostal four-chamber view of a patient who bled after placement of a left ventricular assist device, a large pericardial hematoma compressing the right ventricle is seen. Note the very poor left and right ventricular function. *(Video provided by MHP.)*

VIDEO 8.11   Postoperative hematoma behind the right atrium: Transesophageal echocardiography four-chamber view showing postoperative hematoma behind the right atrium in a patient with a drop in hematocrit and hypotension. *(Video provided by MHP.)*

VIDEO 8.12A   Cardiac tamponade due to rapid accumulation of the small amount of pericardial fluid (1/2). During PCI of the chronic total left circumflex occlusion in a 60-year-old gentleman, a small perforation of obtuse marginal artery was noted. Patient received protamine sulfate and was observed for 30 minutes in the cath lab during which an emergency echo was performed and showed no pericardial effusion. Since patient was hemodynamically stable, without signs of further contrast extravasation on control coronary angiography, he was transferred to the CCU for further monitoring. After 45 minutes patient became diaphoretic and pale, and his blood pressure dropped from 140/95 mmHg to 100/60 mmHg, with stop of diuresis. Repeated emergency echo revealed showing small pericardial effusion (upper panels), with noticeable systolic collapse of the right atrial wall (lower panels), without signs of diastolic collapse of the right ventricular free wall (compare this with echocardiogram recorded prior to PCI shown on Video 8.12B). In addition, there were no significant respiratory variations in transtricuspid or transmitral flow. However, vena cava inferior was dilated (22 mm) with no respiratory variations in size (see Figure 8.12 in the book). Considering these findings and the presence of clinical signs of tamponade physiology aggressive intravenous volume replacement was initiated and patient underwent urgent pericardiocentesis. After removal of 150 mL of hemorrhagic pericardial fluid, hemodynamic stability was achieved, and the patient was transferred to cardiac surgery for further monitoring and possible need for surgical intervention. He had uneventful course during the rest of hospitalization. *(Video provided by IV and PMM.)*

VIDEO 8.12B   Cardiac tamponade due to rapid accumulation of the small amount of pericardial fluid (2/2). Routine echocardiogram performed prior to PCI intervention showing no signs of pericardial effusion (compare this with findings on Video 8.12A recorded after PCI). *(Video provided by IV and PMM.)*

VIDEO 8.13   Cardiac tamponade caused by right ventricular perforation with pacemaker electrode: Transthoracic echocardiography apical four-chamber view showing pacemaker electrode in the right heart that went through the right ventricle wall and entered pericardial space. Note significant pericardial effusion. *(Video provided by LZ.)*

VIDEO 8.14   Echo-guided pericardiocentesis (1/2): After the needle reached the pericardial space (shown here, at 10 o'clock), a small amount of contrast was injected to confirm intrapericardial position of the needle, as indicated by bubble appearance within pericardial effusion (see Video 8.15). *(Video provided by IS.)*

VIDEO 8.15   Echo-guided pericardiocentesis (2/2): After the needle reached the pericardial space (see Video 8.14), a small amount of contrast was injected to confirm intrapericardial position of the needle, as indicated by bubble appearance within pericardial effusion (shown here). Note the "swinging heart." *(Video provided by IS.)*

VIDEO 8.16   Echo-guided pericardiocentesis: An 82-year-old woman was admitted to the hospital for progressive/worsening dyspnea. Transthoracic echocardiography revealed a large circular pericardial effusion, with right atrial collapse (upper left and right panels). Pericardiocentesis was performed via left parasternal approach (the puncture site was determined by echocardiography). Agitate saline was used to confirm needle position in the pericardial space; after injection, note bubble appearance within pericardial effusion (lower right panel; compare with upper right panel). After removal of 400 mL of serohemorrhagic fluid, note an absence of right atrial collapse and a significant reduction of the pericardial effusion (lower left panel). The patient reported immediate relief of symptoms. *(Video provided by VC and ANN.)*

VIDEO 8.17   Acute decompensated heart failure and tamponade caused by external heart compression by mediastinal tumor: A 79-year-old patient with a history of an old anteroseptal myocardial infarction was admitted to the hospital with symptoms and signs of acute decompensated heart failure. Transthoracic apical four-chamber (upper left video), modified apical four-chamber (lower left), apical long-axis (upper right), and modified apical long-axis (lower right) views show very poor global left ventricular function with akinetic and thin septum and apex, indicating ischemic cardiomyopathy. However, an unexpected finding was the mass compressing the right ventricle with cardiac tamponade effect. The mass is best seen in the lower right video and in the lower left video (at the end of the scanning). Because the patient was resistant to maximal heart failure therapy, despite poor left ventricular function and his age he underwent thoracic surgery, and a huge (22 × 9 cm) tumor was removed from his chest. After initial hemodynamic improvement, he died 4 days later from multiorgan failure. *(Video provided by IS.)*

REFERENCES

1. Spodick D. Pericardial disease. In: Braunwald E, Libby P, Zipe DP (eds) Heart Disease, 6th edn. Philadelphia: WB Saunders, 2001:1823–76.
2. Brockington G, Schwartz S, Pandian N. Echocardiography in pericardial diseases. In: Marcus ML, Schelbert HR (eds) Cardiac Imaging: A Companion to Braunwald's Heart Disease. Philadelphia: Saunders, 1991.
3. Spodick DH. Acute cardiac tamponade. N Engl J Med 2003; 349(7):684–90.
4. Reddy PS, Curtiss EI, Uetsky BF. Spectrum of hemodynamic changes in cardiac tamponade. Am J Cardiol 1990; 66(20):1487–91.
5. Saito Y, Donohue A, Attai S, Chandraratna A. The syndrome of cardiac tamponade with "small" pericardial effusion. Echocardiography 2008; 25(3)321–7.
6. Cosyns B, Plein S, Nihoyanopoulos P, et al. On behalf of the European Association of Cardiovascular Imaging (EACVI) and European Society of Cardiology Working Group (ESC WG) on myocardial and pericardial diseases European Association of Cardiovascular Imaging (EACVI) position paper: multimodality imaging in pericardial disease. Eur Heart J Cardiovasc Imaging 2015; 16(1):12–31.
7. Parameswaran R, Goldberg H. Echocardiographic quantitation of pericardial effusion. Chest 1983; 83:767–70.
8. Vazquez de Prada J, Jiang L, Handschumacher M, et al. Quantification of pericardial effusions by three-dimensional echocardiography. J Am Coll Cardiol 1994; 24:254–9.
9. D'Cruz I, Hoffman P. A new cross sectional echocardiographic method for estimating the volume of large pericardial effusions. Br Heart J 1991; 66:448–51.
10. Munt BL, Moss RR, Grewal J. Pericardial disease. In: Otto CM (ed.) The Practice of Clinical Echocardiography, 4th edn. Philadelphia: Saunders/Elsevier, 2011:565–78.
11. Troughton RW, Asher CR, Klein AL. Pericarditis. Lancet 2004; 363(9410):717–27.
12. Maisch B, Seferovic PM, Ristic AD, et al. Guidelines on the diagnosis and management of pericardial diseases of the European Society of Cardiology. Eur Heart J 2004; 25(7):587–610.

13. Singh S, Wann S, Schuchard G, et al. Right ventricular and right atrial collapse in patients with cardiac tamponade—a combined echocardiographic and hemodynamic study. Circulation 1984; 70:966–71.

14. Armstrong W, Schilt B, Helper D, et al. Diastolic collapse of the right ventricle with cardiac tamponade: an echocardiographic study. Circulation 1982; 65:1491–6.

15. Reydel B, Spodick D. Frequency and significance of chamber collapses during cardiac tamponade. Am Heart J 1990; 119:1160–3.

16. Imazio M, Yehuda A. Management of pericardial effusion. Eur Heart J 2013; 34:1186–97.

17. Leimgruber P, Klopfenstein S, Wann S, Brooks H. The hemodynamic derangement associated with right ventricular diastolic collapse in cardiac tamponade: an experimental echocardiographic study. Circulation 1983; 68:612–20.

18. Lopez-Sendon J, Garcia-Fernandez M, Coma-Canella I, et al. Mechanism of right atrial wall compression in pericardial effusion: an experimental echocardiographic study in dogs. J Cardiovasc Ultrasonogr 1988; 7:127–34.

19. Fowler N. Cardiac tamponade. A clinical or an echocardiographic diagnosis? Circulation 1993; 87:1738–41.

20. Eisenberg M, Schiller N. Bayes' theorem and the echocardiographic diagnosis of cardiac tamponade. Am J Cardiol 1991; 68:1242–4.

21. Fowler N. The significance of echocardiographic-Doppler studies in cardiac tamponade. J Am Coll Cardiol 1988; 11:1031–3.

22. Shabetai R. Changing concepts of cardiac tamponade. J Am Coll Cardiol 1988; 12:194–5.

23. Levine M, Lorell B, Diver D, et al. Implications of echocardiographically assisted diagnosis of pericardial tamponade in contemporary medical patients: detection before hemodynamic embarrassment. J Am Coll Cardiol 1991; 17:59–65.

24. Chuttani K, Pandian N, Mohanty PK, et al. Left ventricular diastolic collapse. An echocardiographic sign of regional cardiac tamponade. Circulation 1991; 83:1999–2006.

25. Himelman R, Kircher B, Rockey D, et al. Inferior vena cava plethora with blunted respiratory response: a sensitive echocardiographic sign of cardiac tamponade. J Am Coll Cardiol 1988; 12:1470–7.

26. Pepi M, Tamborini G, Galli C, et al. A new formula for echo-Doppler estimation of right ventricular systolic pressure. J Am Soc Echocardiogr 1994; 7:20–6.

27. Appleton C, Hatle L, Popp R. Cardiac tamponade and pericardial effusion: respiratory variation in transvalvular flow velocities studied by Doppler echocardiography. J Am Coll Cardiol 1988; 11:1020–30.

28. Schutzman J, Obarski T, Pearce G, et al. Comparison of Doppler and two-dimensional echocardiography for assessment of pericardial effusion. Am J Cardiol 1992; 70:1353–7.

29. Miller R, Horneffer P, Gardner T, et al. The epidemiology of the postpericardiotomy syndrome: a common complication of cardiac surgery. Am Heart J 1988; 116:1323–9.

30. Weitzman L, Tinker WP, Kronzon I, et al. The incidence and natural history of pericardial effusion after cardiac surgery—an echocardiographic study. Circulation 1984; 69:506–11.

31. Ofori-Krakie S, Tuberg T, Geha A, et al. Late cardiac tamponade after open heart surgery: incidence, role of anticoagulants in its pathogenesis and its relationship to the postpericardiotomy syndrome. Circulation 1981; 63:1323–8.

32. Bommer W, Follette D, Pollock M, et al. Tamponade in patients undergoing cardiac surgery: a clinical echocardiographic diagnosis. Am Heart J 1995; 130:1216–23.

33. Ikaheimo M, Huikuri H, Airaksinen J, et al. Pericardial effusion after cardiac surgery: incidence, relation to the type of surgery, antithrombotic therapy, and early coronary bypass graft patency. Am Heart J 1988; 116:97–102.

34. Russo A, O'Connor W, Waxman H. Atypical presentations and echocardiographic findings in patients with cardiac tamponade occurring early and late after cardiac surgery. Chest 1993; 104:71–8.

35. Pepi M, Muratori M, Barbier P, et al. Pericardial effusion after cardiac surgery: incidence, site, size, and haemodynamic consequences. Br Heart J 1994; 72:327–31.

36. Saner H, Olson J, Goldenberg I, et al. Isolated right atrial tamponade after open heart surgery: role of echocardiography in diagnosis and management. Cardiology 1995; 86:464–72.

37. Beppu S, Tanaka N, Nakatani S, et al. Pericardial clot after open heart surgery: its specific localization and haemodynamics. Eur Heart J 1993; 14:230–4.

38. Pepi M, Doria E, Fiorentini C. Cardiac tamponade produced by a loculated pericardial hematoma simulating a right atrial mass. Int J Cardiol 1990; 29:383–6.

39. Shanewise J, Cheung A, Aronson S, et al. ASE/SCA guidelines for performing a comprehensive multiplane transesophageal echocardiography examination: recommendations of the American Society of Echocardiography Council for Intraoperative Echocardiography and the Society of Cardiovascular Anesthesiologists Task Force for Certification of Perioperative Transesophageal Echocardiography. Anesth Analg 1999; 89:870–84.

40. Fowler N, Gabel M, Buncher R. Cardiac tamponade: a comparison of right versus left heart compression. J Am Coll Cardiol 1988; 12:187–93.

41. Chandraratna PA, Mohar DS, Sidarous PF. Role of echocardiography in the treatment of cardiac tamponade. Echocardiography 2014; 31(7):899–910.

42. Jung HO. Pericardial effusion and pericardiocentesis: role of echocardiography. Korean Circ J 2012; 42:725–34.

43. Allen KB, Faber LP, Warren WH, et al. Pericardial effusion: subxiphoid pericardiostomy versus percutaneous catheter drainage. Ann Thorac Surg 1999; 67:437–40.

44. Mc Donald J, Meyers B, Guthrie T, et al. Comparison of open subxiphoid pericardial drainage with percutaneous catheter drainage for symptomatic pericardial effusion. Ann Thorac Surg 2003; 76:811–5; discussion 816.

45. Alcan K, Zabetakis P, Marino N, et al. Management of acute cardiac tamponade by subxiphoid pericardiotomy. JAMA 1982; 247:1143–8.

46. Goldberg B, Pollack H. Ultrasonically guided pericardiocentesis. Am J Cardiol 1973; 31:490–3.

47. Stewart J, Gott V. The use of a Seldinger wire technique for pericardiocentesis following cardiac surgery. Ann Thorac Surg 1983; 35:467–8.

48. Callahan J, Seward J, Nishimura R, et al. Two-dimensional echocardiographically guided pericardiocentesis: experience in 117 consecutive patients. Am J Cardiol 1985; 55:476–9.

49. Pepi M, Maltagliati A, Tamborini G, et al. Improvement in ultrasonically guided pericardiocentesis. J Cardiovasc Ultrason 1988; 7:193–6.

50. Susini G, Pepi M, Sisillo E, et al. Percutaneous pericardiocentesis versus subxiphoid pericardiotomy in cardiac tamponade due to postoperative pericardial effusion. J Cardiothorac Vasc Anesth 1993; 7:178–83.

51. Tsang T, Freeman W, Sinak LJ, et al. Echocardiographically guided pericardiocentesis: evolution and state-of-art technique. Mayo Clinic Proc 1998; 73:647–52.

52. Selig M. Percutaneous transcatheter pericardial interventions: aspiration, biopsy, and pericardioplasty. Am Heart J 1993; 125:269–71.

53. Ziskind A, Pearce C, Lemmon C, et al. Percutaneous balloon pericardiotomy for the treatment of cardiac tamponade and large pericardial effusions: description of technique and report of the first 50 cases. J Am Coll Cardiol 1993; 21:1–5.

Echocardiography in acute aortic insufficiency

9

Emily K. Zern and Michael H. Picard

Key Points:

- Acute severe aortic insufficiency (AI) is an uncommon yet life-threatening condition that necessitates prompt recognition and management.
- Acute AI can occur in a variety of clinical conditions affecting the aortic valve or the aortic root, including proximal aortic dissection (type I or type A), endocarditis of the aortic valve, trauma, or deterioration of an aortic prosthetic valve.
- Echocardiography has become an indispensable tool to confirm the presence of aortic insufficiency, assess its severity, and define its etiology.
- In acute AI, the left ventricle size may be normal with a hyperdynamic LVEF. A variety of two-dimensional and color and spectral Doppler echocardiographic assessments can help to determine the size and severity of the aortic regurgitant jet and demonstrate the acute diastolic volume load on the left ventricle.
- Transthoracic and transesophageal echocardiography are crucial in the perioperative management of the patient with acute severe AI.

Acute severe aortic insufficiency (AI) is an uncommon yet life-threatening condition that necessitates prompt recognition and management.[1] The clinical presentation of acute AI, which can range from pulmonary edema to severe cardiogenic shock or cardiac arrest, is in contrast to the presentation of chronic AI, in which compensatory mechanisms exist and clinical signs and symptoms occur much later in the course of disease.[2,3] Fortunately, echocardiography is a widely available noninvasive modality that affords prompt diagnosis and invaluable information for management of these often critically ill patients. Two-dimensional echocardiography and color and spectral Doppler evaluation remain essential components of the echocardiographic examination in these patients. In addition to its role in the initial diagnosis, echocardiography can identify the etiology of the acute AI to guide management decision-making.

PATHOPHYSIOLOGIC MECHANISMS AND CLINICAL PRESENTATION

The clinical presentation of acute severe AI is often dramatic and relates to a sudden volume load placed on a normal left ventricle (LV). The left ventricle then operates on the much steeper portion of a normal end-diastolic pressure–volume relationship curve (Figure 9.1). The inability of the left ventricle to quickly adapt to this rapid increase in volume caused by the regurgitant blood results in a sudden marked increase in left ventricular end-diastolic pressure (LVEDP).[4] As a result, left atrial (LA) pressures also become markedly elevated, resulting in subsequent pulmonary congestion.

DOI: 10.1201/9781003245407-9

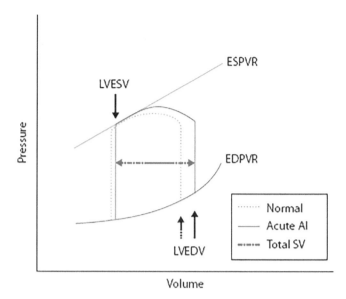

FIGURE 9.1   Left ventricular pressure–volume loop in acute aortic insufficiency. Demonstrating that in acute severe aortic insufficiency the end-diastolic pressure is increased, the end-diastolic pressure-volume relationship is increased, the LV volume can be increased and the total stroke volume is preserved or increased. EDPVR: end-diastolic pressure–volume relationship; ESPVR: end-systolic pressure–volume relationship; LVEDV: left ventricular end-diastolic volume; LVESV: left ventricular end-systolic volume; SV: stroke volume.

These changes are exaggerated in patients with a noncompliant left ventricle at baseline (such as those with left ventricular hypertrophy from hypertension or aortic stenosis), where the left ventricle already has been functioning on a steeper end-diastolic pressure–volume relationship curve.[5] Accordingly, the symptoms of acute AI in these individuals are frequently more striking and result in a more rapid hemodynamic collapse. In extreme cases, LVEDP equilibrates with aortic diastolic pressure. In contrast, the LV end-systolic pressure and the systemic systolic pressure usually exhibit little change.

Compensatory dilation of the left ventricle is limited in acute AI and usually results in a near normal-sized left ventricle.[6] However, LV end-diastolic volume (LVEDV) can increase, depending on the severity of the regurgitation, and results in an increase in total LV stroke volume (SV). Despite this, the effective or forward SV is reduced because a significant portion of this total SV returns to the left ventricle as the regurgitant volume. This is distinct from chronic decompensated AI, in which the left ventricle is dilated, the LVEDV is markedly increased, and the total SV and forward SV are reduced with a reduction in left ventricular ejection fraction (LVEF).[7]

Clinically, patients present with dyspnea, tachycardia, and signs of distal hypoperfusion from peripheral vasoconstriction. There is a paucity of findings on physical examination, in contrast to the classic examination findings commonly found with chronic aortic regurgitation. The pulse pressure is usually normal, with a short aortic diastolic murmur occurring only in early diastole. The diastolic murmur in acute AI may terminate in early diastole due to rapid equalization of LV and aortic pressures. The first heart sound (S₁) is usually soft in severe AI because there is early diastolic closure of the mitral valve. Occasionally, mid-diastolic closure of the mitral valve may be heard (due to a rapid rise in LVEDP from the regurgitant volume load). An Austin Flint murmur (a mid-diastolic low-pitch rumble at the LV apex, often best heard with the patient leaning forward with breath hold after exhalation) and an aortic outflow systolic murmur may also be heard.

ETIOLOGY OF ACUTE AI

Acute AI can be the result of various abnormalities of the aortic valve and/or the aortic root. These conditions include proximal aortic dissection (type I or type A) (Figure 9.2) (V9.1), endocarditis of the aortic valve, prosthetic valve dysfunction, consequence of percutaneous balloon valvuloplasty, or trauma to the aorta or the valve. When acute AI is the result of aortic dissection (see also Chapter 6), proximal aortic dissection may produce valvular insufficiency via incomplete leaflet closure resulting from aortic root dilation, leaflet prolapse, or a dissection flap prolapsing through normal leaflets inhibiting leaflet closure (Figure 9.2) (V9.1).[8]

Endocarditis involving the aortic valve can produce acute AI when leaflet destruction produces leaflet perforation or when normal leaflet coaptation is prevented (Figure 9.3) (V9.2A, V9.2B, V9.2C, V9.5A, V9.5B).

Severe acute AI may also result less commonly after balloon valvuloplasty, from nonpenetrating chest trauma, during

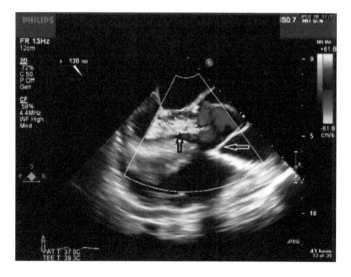

FIGURE 9.2   Severe aortic regurgitation due to ascending aortic dissection. Color Doppler display of acute severe aortic insufficiency on transesophageal echocardiography (black open arrow). This long-axis view of the ascending aorta demonstrates a type I acute aortic dissection with the dissection flap (white open arrow) extending into the sinuses of Valsalva (V9.1).

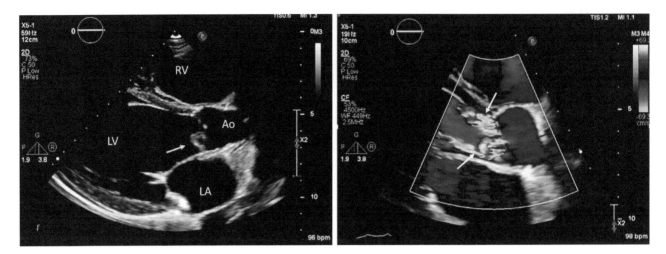

FIGURE 9.3 Severe aortic regurgitation due to infective endocarditis. Two-dimensional (left panel) and color Doppler (right panel) echocardiography display of acute severe aortic insufficiency (white arrows) due to valve destruction from a vegetation on the non-coronary cusp of the aortic valve (yellow arrow) (V9.2A, V9.2B, V9.2C). Ao: aorta; LA: left atrium; LV: left ventricle; RV: right ventricle.

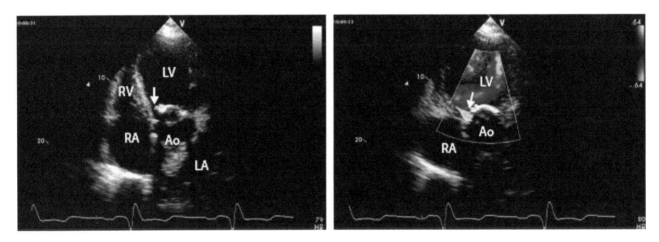

FIGURE 9.4 Severe paravalvular aortic insufficiency from bioprosthetic valve dehiscence. Transthoracic apical five-chamber view demonstrates a dehiscence (arrow) of a bioprosthetic aortic valve (left panel) (V9.3A). At the site of the dehiscence (arrow), a turbulent jet (arrow) of paravalvular aortic insufficiency can be noted on color Doppler (right panel) (V9.3B). Ao: aorta; LA: left atrium; LV: left ventricle; RA: right atrium; RV: right ventricle.

(Images and videos provided by IS.)

cardiac catheterization, or after spontaneous rupture of prior valve fenestrations.[9–12]

Prosthetic aortic valve dysfunction (see Chapter 12) can result in acute AI through either a valvular or a paravalvular mechanism. In mechanical valves, endocarditis can cause dehiscence of the prosthesis, resulting in paravalvular AI. In addition, acute thrombus formation or chronic pannus overgrowth can result in an inability of the prosthesis to close properly, leading to severe valvular AI. Acute AI can occur in bioprosthetic aortic valves due to endocarditis (Figure 9.4, (V9.3A, V9.3B) or due to valve degeneration resulting in acute leaflet tear, prolapse, or perforation. As compared to native valves, bioprosthetic aortic valves can have more rapid of a progression of structural valve deterioration, including progression to severe regurgitation, particularly amongst those known to have prior evidence of bioprosthetic valve calcification.[13]

TRANSTHORACIC ECHOCARDIOGRAPHIC EVALUATION OF SUSPECTED ACUTE AI

Echocardiography has become an indispensable tool to confirm the presence of AI, assess its severity, and provide information regarding the cause. The presence of AI can easily be ascertained from color and spectral Doppler echocardiography. Similarly, the severity of AI in the acute setting can be determined by the combination of two-dimensional and Doppler echocardiography (Table 9.1).[14] It is important to display *simultaneous electrocardiography* on the emergency

TABLE 9.1 Echocardiographic Signs in Severe Acute Aortic Insufficiency

Two-dimensional and M-mode echocardiography

Parasternal long-axis view

Flail valve leaflet (viewed prolapsing below annular plane)

Early pre-systolic closure of the mitral valve

Anterior mitral valve leaflet fluttering on M-mode

Typically normal left ventricular dimensions (LVEDD, LVESD) and function (LVEF)

Color Doppler assessment

Parasternal long-axis view

Proximal color jet width >65% of LVOT

Vena contracta >0.6 cm

Diastolic mitral regurgitation

EROA >0.3 cm² by PISA method

Parasternal short-axis view

Color jet cross-sectional area: LVOT cross-sectional area ratio of >0.6

Spectral Doppler assessment

Continuous-wave Doppler

Aortic valve

Dense regurgitant velocity envelope compared to forward velocity envelope

Pressure half-time of regurgitant envelope of <200 ms

Regurgitant volume >60 mL or regurgitant fraction >50%

Descending thoracic aorta and abdominal aorta

Holodiastolic flow reversal

Pulsed-wave and tissue Doppler

Mitral inflow restrictive filling pattern

Diastolic mitral regurgitation

Abbreviations: EROA, effective regurgitant orifice area; LVEDD, left ventricular end-diastolic dimension; LVEF, left ventricular ejection fraction; LVESD, left ventricular end-systolic dimension; LVOT, left ventricular outflow tract.

echocardiogram, as many features of acute severe AI are visible in late diastole, and the timing of these features can most easily be ascertained by electrocardiography.

The color Doppler examination of the aortic valve provides the simplest approach for the determination of the presence and severity of insufficiency.[14] The characteristics of the color flow jet in the left ventricular outflow tract (LVOT) can provide information about the *vena contracta*. The vena contracta, the narrowest width of the jet as it exits the regurgitant orifice, provides an indirect yet accurate measure of the regurgitant aortic orifice and is relatively independent of flow. For AI assessment by transthoracic echo, this is best visualized from the parasternal long-axis view. A value of >0.6 cm is indicative of severe aortic regurgitation (Figure 9.5A).[5]

In the parasternal views, the ratio of the height (long axis) or area (short axis) of the regurgitant jet to the LVOT measurements is thus used to determine severity. If the height of the jet width is greater than 65% of the LVOT or if the cross-sectional area ratio is >0.6 of the LVOT, severe insufficiency is considered to be present (Figure 9.5, A-B).[5,14,15] The proximal isovelocity surface area (PISA) method[5,16] may also be used to calculate the effective regurgitant orifice area (EROA) by the following formula:

$$EROA = \frac{Flow\ rate}{Peak\ AI\ velocity} = \frac{2\pi r^2 * aliasing\ velocity}{Peak\ AI\ velocity}$$

In this equation, *r* represents the radius of the PISA zone at the aliasing velocity (Figure 9.5, C-D). By this formula, an EROA of ≥0.3 cm² may be considered severe regurgitation.[5,14] In Figure 9.5, panel C demonstrates a PISA radius of 1.36 cm at an aliasing velocity of 30.8 cm/s in the parasternal long-axis view. Panel D demonstrates a peak velocity of the continuous-wave Doppler regurgitant jet from the apical five-chamber view of 4.0 m/s. These parameters yield an EROA of 0.89 cm², consistent with severe AI.

Two-dimensional and spectral Doppler tracings also provide other adjunctive signs that can assist in the determination of the severity of regurgitation. A very dense spectral

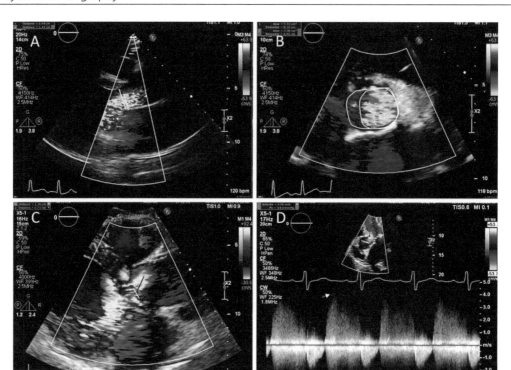

FIGURE 9.5   Quantitative transthoracic echocardiographic parameters of severe aortic insufficiency. (A) Percentage of the height of the AI regurgitant jet to the LVOT dimension >65% in the parasternal long-axis view. (B) Ratio of the cross-sectional area of the AI regurgitant jet to the LVOT cross-sectional area >0.6 in the parasternal short-axis view. (C) Vena contracta (white line) of 0.75 cm supports severe AI. (C, D) Calculation of the effective regurgitant orifice area (EROA) utilizing the proximal isovelocity surface area (PISA) (C, black line, 1.36 cm) at an aliasing velocity of −30.8 cm/s and a peak AI velocity of 4.0 m/s (arrow in D) yields an EROA of 0.89 cm², consistent with severe AI.

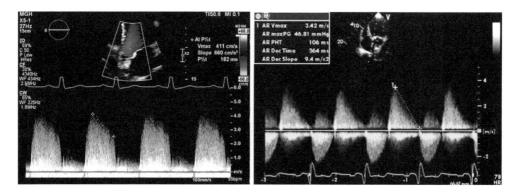

FIGURE 9.6   Pressure half-time method to evaluate AI severity. Continuous-wave Doppler analysis of the aortic regurgitant jet from the apical five-chamber view in two different patients reveals a pressure half-time of 182 ms (left panel) and 106 ms (right panel), both consistent with severe AI.

Doppler AI velocity profile and a short pressure half-time (<200 ms) usually signify hemodynamically severe acute AI (Figure 9.6).[5,14] The dense spectral signal and the short pressure half-time of the AI velocity profile on continuous-wave Doppler are not specific findings of severe AI. The pressure half-time is determined by not only the amount of regurgitation but also the compliance of the receiving chamber (left ventricle) and the peripheral aortic resistance. For example, even a mild degree of AI emptying into a stiff left ventricle can result

in a shortened pressure half-time. In addition, in instances of technically challenging transthoracic windows, a prosthetic aortic valve with acoustic shadowing, or a severely eccentric aortic regurgitant jet, color Doppler may underappreciate the severity of acute AI. Since the forward flow through the aortic valve is increased, continuous-wave Doppler may demonstrate elevated transvalvular velocities (Figure 9.7, B). If the appearance of an aortic valve is without calcified thickened leaflets or restricted opening of the native or prosthetic leaflets, then these increased transvalvular velocities are due to the effect of AI and not reflective of valvular stenosis. In this scenario, a dense continuous-wave Doppler regurgitant jet with short pressure half time (Figure 9.7, C) in context of an elevated LVOT velocity by pulsed-wave Doppler (Figure 9.7, D) may raise clinical suspicion for acute severe AI, particularly in the tachycardic patient with clinical symptoms.

Holodiastolic flow reversal in the descending thoracic aorta (obtained from the suprasternal notch window) and in the abdominal aorta (obtained from the subcostal window) will also be seen in severe insufficiency (Figure 9.8). While spectral Doppler (pulsed-wave or continuous-wave Doppler) of the descending thoracic and abdominal aorta may be difficult to interpret in the context of artifact above and below the baseline, color Doppler with persistent reversal of flow in late diastole (Figure 9.8, A and C) can provide more definitive evidence. If color flow is not seen in late diastole, it is important to drop the color scale to a Nyquist limit <40–50 cm/s, which may allow for visualization of the flow reversal. Regurgitant fractions and volumes can also be calculated to determine severity by a variety of methods, though may be less reliable or useful in emergency settings.[14,17]

Echocardiographic *assessment of the mitral valve* will also provide clues about hemodynamically significant aortic regurgitation. 2D transthoracic echocardiography may demonstrate restricted diastolic opening of the mitral valve, particularly the anterior leaflet of the mitral valve due to the aortic regurgitant jet (V9.4A, V9.4B). The transmitral pulsed-wave and tissue Doppler flow patterns may show a *restrictive pattern*, signifying early rapid equilibration of LA and LV diastolic pressures.[18] In acute AI, *early mitral valve closure* may occur as LV diastolic pressure exceeds LA pressure early in the cardiac cycle.[19,20] If this occurs, *diastolic mitral regurgitation* may be observed and may further signify acute severe insufficiency of the aortic valve.[21] The findings of early mitral valve closure, restrictive transmitral flow patterns, and diastolic mitral regurgitation may be more specific to acute AI than in a chronic, compensated severe AI. In the parasternal long-axis view, M-mode echocardiography across the mitral valve may reveal *fluttering of the anterior leaflet* during diastole due to direct contact from the aortic regurgitant jet (Figure 9.9) (V9.4B). M-mode echocardiography also can be useful to visualize early mitral valve closure prior to end-diastole (as determined by simultaneous electrocardiography).[22]

The *left ventricular size and systolic function* are important to measure, as the size of the left ventricle in acute AI is often near normal and the systolic function is normal or hyperdynamic, in comparison to chronic severe AI, in which the ventricle is markedly dilated with depressed systolic function.[23] However, ventricular dilation may be present in acute AI in those patients with previous valve or coronary disease that may have contributed to preexisting ventricular dilation.

Last, the *presence of pericardial effusion* should be noted, as a new pericardial effusion in context of acute AI may raise clinical suspicion for aortic dissection, even when a dissection flap cannot be directly observed by TTE.

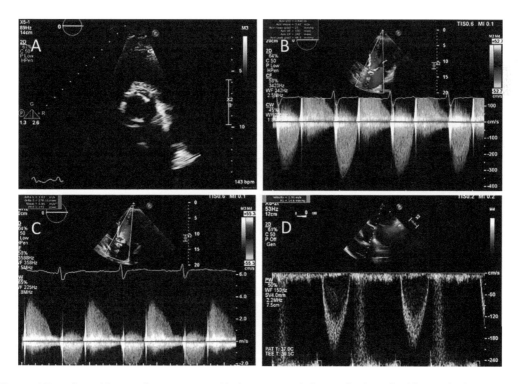

FIGURE 9.7 Spectral Doppler evidence of acute severe AI. A parasternal short-axis view of a bioprosthetic aortic valve has no evidence of thickened or immobilized leaflets (A). From the apical five-chamber view, elevated aortic valve velocity (peak velocity 3.5 m/s) and mean gradient (27 mmHg) are noted on continuous-wave Doppler analysis (B). The dense continuous-wave Doppler signal of the regurgitant jet (C) with a short pressure half time (175 ms) and an elevated velocity across the left ventricular outflow tract by pulsed-wave Doppler analysis (D, 1.9 m/s) raise suspicion for severe AI.

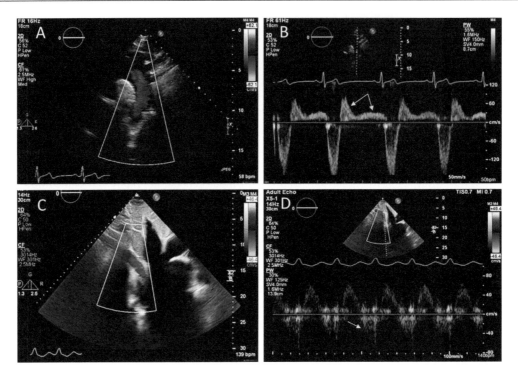

FIGURE 9.8 Holodiastolic flow reversal in the descending thoracic and abdominal aorta. Suprasternal notch view demonstrating holodiastolic flow reversal in the descending thoracic aorta by red color Doppler (A) and spectral Doppler (B, yellow arrows). Abdominal aorta visualized from the subcostal view with demonstration of holodiastolic flow reversal by blue color Doppler in diastole (C) and spectral Doppler (D, yellow arrow).

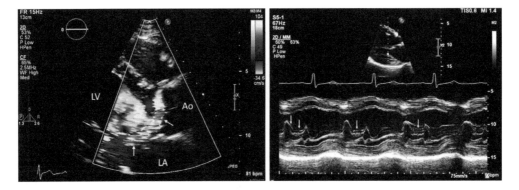

FIGURE 9.9 Anterior mitral valve fluttering due to aortic regurgitant jet. (A) Parasternal long-axis color Doppler demonstrates an eccentric regurgitant jet (yellow arrow) directed at the anterior mitral valve leaflet (white arrow). (B) M-mode echocardiogram demonstrating fluttering (yellow arrows) of the mitral valve in diastole due to effects of an aortic regurgitant jet.

UTILIZATION OF TRANSESOPHAGEAL ECHOCARDIOGRAPHY

Although the mentioned parameters can often be elucidated by transthoracic echocardiography (TTE), some clinical situations may warrant the use of transesophageal echocardiography (TEE) for the determination of the *mechanism and severity of acute AI.* For example, TEE is an important modality for the evaluation of *aortic dissection*, and it can determine the presence of dissection, type, location of entry and/or exit flow of the false lumen, and severity and mechanism of AI.[8] Possible mechanisms of acute severe AI in the context of aortic dissection, which may require TEE for definitive determination, include (1) dilation of the sinotubular junction resulting in incomplete leaflet closure due to tethering, (2) leaflet prolapse when the dissection extends into the aortic sinuses of Valsalva and disrupts normal leaflet support, and (3) prolapse of the dissection flap across normal aortic leaflet structure.[8]

Furthermore, TEE is a more sensitive modality for the diagnosis of *valvular endocarditis and its complications.* In prosthetic valve AI, TTE imaging may be limited due to shadowing from the prosthesis. In these situations, TEE is invaluable in the *assessment of prosthetic valve AI* in order to understand the mechanism and severity and confirm relative contributions of valvular or perivalvular regurgitation (V9.3A, V9.3B, V9.4D, V9.4E). Therefore, the use of TTE or TEE in the evaluation of acute AI will depend on the clinical setting, operator experience, availability, and regional practice patterns.

ECHOCARDIOGRAPHY AS A GUIDE TO MANAGEMENT

Elucidation of the *mechanism of acute AI*, especially in acute aortic dissection, is important, as this may influence *surgical approach.*[6] Whereas prompt surgery for proximal aortic dissection is well established, the approach (i.e., replacement versus repair) to the associated AI is less clear. When there is a reversible mechanism such as geometric distortion of the valve in aortic root dilation, repair with valve preservation may be feasible. In contrast, when fixed abnormalities of the valve, such as calcification or marked thickening are found by TEE, aortic valve replacement is usually recommended. Specifically, several options may exist: (1) when incomplete leaflet closure because of a dilated root is observed, valve repair may involve narrowing of the dilated aorta with a graft[24]; (2) resuspension of aortic leaflets at the commissures can be performed when leaflet prolapse is seen; (3) when intimal flap prolapse is seen to cause AI, corrective repair may involve replacement of the ascending aorta without aortic valve replacement.

In addition, if the acute aortic regurgitation is secondary to aortic dissection, perioperative TEE can provide information about *dynamic complications,* such as development of *pericardial effusion* or *rapid expansion of the aortic root.*

The *postoperative TEE* can provide important information (V14.5A, V14.5B, V14.13D, V14.13E) regarding competence of the prosthetic aortic valve, integrity of aortic graft anastomosis, pericardial fluid collections, and ventricular size and function (see Chapter 14).

If *endocarditis* is complicated by severe acute AI (V12.9A, V12.9B, V12.9C, V12.9D), in general, surgery should not be delayed when hemodynamic compromise is clinically evident.[25] Perioperative TEE can elucidate the mechanism of AI, which frequently results from valve destruction and/or leaflet perforation. A careful examination for *abscess* in the surrounding tissue is an important component of the preoperative TEE. Aortic valve replacement, with or without aortic root replacement, is the standard treatment for acute severe aortic regurgitation resulting from aortic valve endocarditis.

Last, patients with acute AI due to native valve or bioprosthetic valve degeneration (either surgical or transcatheter valves) who are of high or prohibitive surgical risk may be candidates for *transcatheter aortic valve replacement* or

valve-in-valve transcatheter aortic valve replacement.[26,27] Transthoracic and transesophageal echocardiography are crucial for diagnostic imaging and intraprocedural guidance in these patients (Chapter 22). Pre-procedural imaging should evaluate mechanism of AI, exclude abnormalities of the aortic root and ascending aorta, assess location of coronary artery ostia in relation to AV leaflet lengths, and rule out severe paravalvular regurgitation (in patients with bioprosthetic valves being evaluated for valve-in-valve procedure).

SUMMARY

Acute severe AI is a medical and surgical emergency that often complicates acute aortic syndromes, aortic valvular endocarditis, or rapid degeneration of prosthetic valves. Transthoracic and transesophageal echocardiography are definitive diagnostic tools to determine the etiology of aortic valve pathology, and there are a variety of qualitative and quantitative echocardiographic methods to diagnose severe AI, particularly in the acute and emergent setting. The information obtained by emergent echocardiographic study is invaluable in management strategies and surgical decision-making.

LIST OF VIDEOS

https://routledgetextbooks.com/textbooks/9781032157009/chapter-9.php

VIDEO 9.1 **Acute aortic insufficiency in aortic dissection:** A midesophageal view of the ascending aorta and left ventricular outflow tract from a transesophageal echocardiogram. The intimal flap of a type I aortic dissection is observed with resultant acute aortic insufficiency noted on color Doppler.

VIDEO 9.2A **Echocardiographic imaging of acute aortic insufficiency in infective endocarditis (1/3).** A transthoracic parasternal long-axis view identifies a mobile vegetation on the non-coronary cusp of the aortic valve resulting in severe aortic regurgitation (see also Videos 9.2B and 9.2C).

VIDEO 9.2B **Echocardiographic imaging of acute aortic insufficiency in infective endocarditis (2/3).** The leaflet appears to have an aneurysm and perforation (see also Videos 9.2A and 9.2C).

VIDEO 9.2C   Echocardiographic imaging of acute aortic insufficiency in infective endocarditis (3/3). Intraoperative transesophageal echocardiogram confirms infective endocarditis with leaflet aneurysm formation, leaflet perforation and valve malcoaptation leading to both regurgitation at leaflet margins and through the perforation (see also Videos 9.2A and 9.2B).

VIDEO 9.3A   Acute aortic insufficiency caused by dehiscence of aortic valve bioprosthesis (1/2): Transthoracic apical five-chamber view demonstrates a dehiscence of the aortic valve bioprosthesis. Note that the prosthesis appears unstable, with rocking movements during the cardiac cycle. At the site of the dehiscence, turbulent jet of paravalvular severe aortic insufficiency can be noted on color Doppler (see Video 9.3B). *(Video provided by IS.)*

VIDEO 9.3B   Acute aortic insufficiency caused by dehiscence of aortic valve bioprosthesis (2/2): Transthoracic apical five-chamber view demonstrates a turbulent jet of paravalvular aortic insufficiency on color Doppler, caused by dehiscence of the aortic valve bioprosthesis (see Video 9.3A). Note that the prosthesis is unstable, with rocking movements during the cardiac cycle. Pressure half-time of the regurgitant envelope was 106 ms, indicating acute severe aortic insufficiency (see Figure 9.4 in the book). *(Video provided by IS.)*

VIDEO 9.4A   Acute bioprosthetic aortic insufficiency due to structural valve degeneration (1/5). Transthoracic echocardiograms (shown here and on Videos 9.4B and 9.4C) demonstrate severe bioprosthetic aortic valve insufficiency of unknown etiology. Note the restriction of the anterior mitral valve leaflet opening in diastole. Transesophageal echocardiograms (shown on Videos 9.4D and 9.4E) diagnose the etiology of the regurgitation to be due to flail prosthetic leaflet with severe aortic insufficiency consistent with degeneration of the bioprosthetic valve.

VIDEO 9.4B   Acute bioprosthetic aortic insufficiency due to structural valve degeneration (2/5). Transthoracic echocardiograms (shown here and on Videos 9.4A and 9.4C) demonstrate severe bioprosthetic aortic valve insufficiency of unknown etiology. Note the restriction of the anterior mitral valve leaflet opening in diastole. Transesophageal echocardiograms (shown on Videos 9.4D and 9.4E) diagnose the etiology of the regurgitation to be due to flail prosthetic leaflet with severe aortic insufficiency consistent with degeneration of the bioprosthetic valve.

VIDEO 9.4C   Acute bioprosthetic aortic insufficiency due to structural valve degeneration (3/5). Transthoracic echocardiograms (shown here and on Videos 9.4A and 9.4B) demonstrate severe bioprosthetic aortic valve insufficiency of unknown etiology. Note the restriction of the anterior mitral valve leaflet opening in diastole. Transesophageal echocardiograms (shown on Videos 9.4D and 9.4E) diagnose the etiology of the regurgitation to be due to flail prosthetic leaflet with severe aortic insufficiency consistent with degeneration of the bioprosthetic valve.

VIDEO 9.4D   Acute bioprosthetic aortic insufficiency due to structural valve degeneration (4/5). Transthoracic echocardiograms (shown on Videos 9.4A, 9.4B, and 9.4C) demonstrate severe bioprosthetic aortic valve insufficiency of unknown etiology. Note the restriction of the anterior mitral valve leaflet opening in diastole.

Transesophageal echocardiograms (shown here and on Video 9.4E) diagnose the etiology of the regurgitation to be due to flail prosthetic leaflet with severe aortic insufficiency consistent with degeneration of the bioprosthetic valve.

VIDEO 9.4E   Acute bioprosthetic aortic insufficiency due to structural valve degeneration (5/5). Transthoracic echocardiograms (shown on Videos 9.4A, 9.4B, and 9.4C) demonstrate severe bioprosthetic aortic valve insufficiency of unknown etiology. Note the restriction of the anterior mitral valve leaflet opening in diastole. Transesophageal echocardiograms (shown here and on Video 9.4D) diagnose the etiology of the regurgitation to be due to flail prosthetic leaflet with severe aortic insufficiency consistent with degeneration of the bioprosthetic valve.

VIDEO 9.5A   Acute aortic insufficiency in infective endocarditis (1/2): This long-axis transesophageal view of the ascending aorta demonstrates vegetations attached to the aortic valve, prolapsing into the left ventricular outflow tract and causing poor leaflet coaptation in diastole (shown here). Acute aortic insufficiency can be noted on color Doppler; a wide vena contracta of the regurgitant jet of 12 mm indicates severe aortic insufficiency (see Video 9.5B). *(Video provided by IS.)*

VIDEO 9.5B   Acute aortic insufficiency in infective endocarditis (2/2): This long-axis transesophageal view of the ascending aorta on color Doppler demonstrates jet of acute aortic insufficiency caused by infective endocarditis of the aortic valve (see Video 9.5A). Note a wide vena contracta of the regurgitant jet of 12 mm, indicating severe aortic insufficiency. *(Video provided by IS.)*

REFERENCES

1. Rahimtoola SH. Recognition and management of acute aortic regurgitation. Heart Dis Stroke 1993;2:217–21.
2. Stout KK, Verrier ED. Acute valvular regurgitation. Circulation 2009;119:3232–41.
3. Mokadam NA, Stout KK, Verrier ED. Management of acute regurgitation in left-sided cardiac valves. Tex Heart Inst J 2011;38:9–19.
4. Carabello BA, Crawford FA Jr. Valvular heart disease. N Engl J Med 1997;337:32–41.
5. Otto CM, Nishimura RA, Bonow RO, et al. 2020 AHA/ACC guideline for the management of patients with valvular heart disease: Executive summary: A report of the American College of Cardiology/American Heart Association Joint Committee on Clinical Practice Guidelines. Circulation 2021;143(5):e35–71.
6. Morganroth J, Perloff JK, Zeldis SM, Dunkman WB. Acute severe aortic regurgitation. Pathophysiology, clinical recognition, and management. Ann Intern Med 1977;87:223–32.
7. Bonow RO, Nishimura RA. Aortic Regurgitation. In: Libby P., Bonow R.O., Mann D.L., Braunwald E. (eds). Braunwald's Heart Disease: A Textbook of Cardiovascular Medicine, 12th ed. Philadelphia: Elsevier, 2022.
8. Movsowitz HD, Levine RA, Hilgenberg AD, Isselbacher EM. Transesophageal echocardiographic description of the mechanisms of aortic regurgitation in acute type A aortic dissection: Implications for aortic valve repair. J Am Coll Cardiol 2000;36:884–90.

9. Blaszyk H, Witkiewicz AJ, Edwards WD. Acute aortic regurgitation due to spontaneous rupture of a fenestrated cusp: Report in a 65-year-old man and review of seven additional cases. Cardiovasc Pathol 1999;8:213–6.

10. Javeed N, Shaikh J, Patel M, Rezai F, Wong P. Catheter-induced acute aortic insufficiency with hemodynamic collapse during PTCA: An unreported complication. Cathet Cardiovasc Diagn 1997;42:305–7.

11. Unal M, Demirsoy E, Gogus A, Arbatli H, Hamzaoglu A, Sonmez B. Acute aortic valve regurgitation secondary to blunt chest trauma. Tex Heart Inst J 2001;28:312–4.

12. Isner JM. Acute catastrophic complications of balloon aortic valvuloplasty. J Am Coll Cardiol 1991;17:1436–44.

13. Zhang B, Salaun E, Cote N, et al. Associaton of bioprosthetic aortic valve leaflet calcification on hemodynamic and clinical outcomes. J Am Coll Cardiol 2020;76(15):1737–48.

14. Zoghbi WA, Adams D, Bonow RO, et al. Recommendations for noninvasive evaluation of native valvular regurgitation. J Am Soc Echocardiogr 2017;30(4):303–71.

15. Perry GJ, Helmcke F, Nanda NC, Byard C, Soto B. Evaluation of aortic insufficiency by Doppler color flow mapping. J Am Coll Cardiol 1987;9:952–9.

16. Thomas JD. Doppler echocardiographic assessment of valvular regurgitation. Heart 2002;88:651–7.

17. Zoghbi WA, Enriquez-Sarano M, Foster E, et al. Recommendations for evaluation of the severity of native valvular regurgitation with two-dimensional and Doppler echocardiography. J Am Soc Echocardiogr 2003;16:777–802.

18. Vilacosta I, San Roman JA, Castillo JA, et al. Retrograde atrial kick in acute aortic regurgitation. Study of mitral and pulmonary venous flow velocities by transthoracic and transesophageal echocardiography. Clin Cardiol 1997;20:35–40.

19. Botvinick EH, Schiller NB, Wickramasekaran R, Klausner SC, Gertz E. Echocardiographic demonstration of early mitral valve closure in severe aortic insufficiency. Its clinical implications. Circulation 1975;51:836–47.

20. Meyer T, Sareli P, Pocock WA, Dean H, Epstein M, Barlow J. Echocardiographic and hemodynamic correlates of diastolic closure of mitral valve and diastolic opening of aortic valve in severe aortic regurgitation. Am J Cardiol 1987;59:1144–8.

21. Downes TR, Nomeir AM, Hackshaw BT, Kellam LJ, Watts LE, Little WC. Diastolic mitral regurgitation in acute but not chronic aortic regurgitation: Implications regarding the mechanism of mitral closure. Am Heart J 1989;117:1106–12.

22. Hamirani YS, Dietl CA, Voyles W, et al. Acute aortic regurgitation. Circulation 2012;126:1121–6.

23. Mann T, McLaurin L, Grossman W, Craige E. Assessing the hemodynamic severity of acute aortic regurgitation due to infective endocarditis. N Engl J Med 1975;293:108–13.

24. David TE, Feindel CM, Bos J. Repair of the aortic valve in patients with aortic insufficiency and aortic root aneurysm. J Thorac Cardiovasc Surg 1995;109:345–51.

25. Sareli P, Klein HO, Schamroth CL, et al. Contribution of echocardiography and immediate surgery to the management of severe aortic regurgitation from active infective endocarditis. Am J Cardiol 1986;57:413–8.

26. Sawaya FJ, Deutsch MA, Seiffert M, et al. Safety and efficacy of transcather aortic valve replacement in the treatment of pure aortic regurgitation in native valves and failing surgical bioprosthesis. JACC Cardiovasc Interv 2017;10:1048–56.

27. Yoon SH, Schmidt T, Bleiziffer S, et al. Transcatheter aortic valve replacement in pure native aortic valve regurgitation. J Am Coll Cardiol 2017;70:2752–63.

Echocardiography in acute mitral regurgitation

10

Tomasz Baron and Frank A. Flachskampf

Key Points

- The presence of a clear structural abnormality of the mitral valve on echo (such as a flail leaflet with the tip of the leaflet appearing in the left atrium during systole) predicts severe mitral regurgitation, even if the color Doppler appearance is ambiguous. Conversely, the absence of any identifiable morphologic abnormality makes severe regurgitation unlikely.
- Apart from the proximal jet width (vena contracta), a well-formed, large, consistently imaged proximal acceleration zone on the ventricular side of a mitral regurgitant lesion or systolic retrograde pulmonary venous flow predicts severe regurgitation. High E-waves and increased pulmonary pressures are also regularly present.
- Definitive evaluation of regurgitation in a prosthetic mitral valve usually requires transesophageal imaging.

CLINICAL AND PATHOPHYSIOLOGIC BACKGROUND

Acute severe mitral regurgitation is a cardiovascular emergency encountered in several clinical scenarios (Table 10.1). Because of systolic regurgitation into the left atrium, there is an acute volume overload and, consequently, pressure overload of the left atrium, leading to an acute increase in pulmonary capillary pressure. This is reflected in the typical high systolic V-wave in the pulmonary wedge pressure tracing, exceeding double the value of the mean wedge pressure. The pressure increase leads to acute pulmonary edema and, propagating backward or "upstream," to acute pulmonary hypertension and right heart failure. Acute mitral regurgitation can be conceptually understood primarily as left ventricular backward failure, leading secondarily to tachycardia, hypotension,

forward failure, and cardiogenic shock. Characteristically, the left ventricle is *normal size* and left ventricular *global function is hyperkinetic*, unless there is additional left

TABLE 10.1 Etiology of Acute Mitral Regurgitation

Infective endocarditis with valvular destruction
Papillary muscle rupture after myocardial infarction
Degenerative chordal rupture, particularly in mitral valve prolapse
Mitral prosthetic dysfunction

- Bioprosthetic degeneration
- Bioprosthetic endocarditis with leaflet destruction
- Ring abscess with large paraprosthetic leak or prosthetic dehiscence
- Prosthetic thrombosis with fixed position of the occluder
- Fracture of prosthetic valve with occluder embolization

Rare causes: trauma, postoperative suture dehiscence, postvalvotomy regurgitation, and others

---

DOI: 10.1201/9781003245407-10

ventricular disease. This contrasts with chronic mitral regurgitation, which leads to progressive left ventricular dilation and systolic dysfunction.

Typical clinical signs of mitral regurgitation include a holosystolic murmur over the apex and axilla. However, in the setting of cardiogenic shock and severe pulmonary edema caused by acute mitral regurgitation, the murmur may be barely audible, and its loudness is not predictive of the severity of regurgitation. Rapidly progressive ("flash") pulmonary edema, tachycardia, and forward failure with cardiogenic shock are hallmarks of the condition. Even in the absence of a loud murmur, these signs, together with one of the aforementioned typical scenarios (see Table 10.1), are strongly suggestive of acute mitral regurgitation. The diagnostic tool of choice is echocardiography, which should be performed quickly and conclusively, proceeding to transesophageal echocardiography (TEE) if doubts remain after transthoracic imaging. The definitive therapy is surgery, consisting of repair or replacement of the regurgitant valve or prosthesis. Before surgical correction, supportive measures include diuretics, mechanical ventilation with positive end-expiratory pressure for pulmonary edema, and lowering of blood pressure to reduce afterload (with nitroprusside or another rapidly acting drug), unless the patient is already hypotensive. An excellent bridge to surgery is intra-aortic balloon counterpulsation, which decreases systolic afterload and increases diastolic systemic pressure. If feasible, it should be instituted once the diagnosis of severe acute mitral regurgitation is clear, possibly before cardiogenic shock ensues.

GOALS OF ECHOCARDIOGRAPHY IN ACUTE MITRAL REGURGITATION

Severe acute mitral regurgitation is usually not difficult to recognize, because typically both a large jet of mitral regurgitation and also morphologic evidence that the valve is grossly abnormal are present.[1-3] The emergency echo examination of the mitral valve should attempt to answer *two essential questions:*

- Is there *severe* mitral regurgitation?
- What is the *mechanism*?

If transthoracic echo is inconclusive in answering these questions with confidence, TEE should be performed without delay (V10.1A, V10.1B, V10.1C, and V10.1D). If an acute mitral prosthesis dysfunction is suspected, TEE should be used right away. The most important views are the lower transesophageal views, which allow one to scan systematically the whole prosthesis and its circumference for abnormalities.

DOPPLER ECHOCARDIOGRAPHIC FEATURES OF ACUTE SEVERE MITRAL REGURGITATION

Important Doppler features of *severe* mitral regurgitation to look for typically include the following:

- A regurgitation jet of at least moderate size on color Doppler. Eccentric jets represent more severe regurgitation than central jets of the same size. Because the size of the color Doppler jet depends directly on the pressure gradient, the jet actually decreases in size with diminishing systolic blood pressure and rising left atrial pressure, whereas the regurgitant lesion remains the same. As in chronic conditions, the jet size alone therefore may be misleading.

- Reversal or severe blunting of systolic pulmonary venous inflow. Pulmonary vein flow can be recorded by pulsed-wave Doppler in the right upper pulmonary vein from the apical, four-chamber view (V10.2) or, by TEE, in the left or right upper pulmonary veins. Reverse flow in the pulmonary vein can often already be seen on color Doppler. This is a highly specific but not sensitive sign of severe regurgitation (if it is present, severe regurgitation is almost ensured, but if it is lacking, there may still be severe regurgitation).

- A reproducible, large (over 1 cm²) proximal isovelocity surface area (PISA) on the ventricular side of the regurgitant lesion is usually seen even with the highest color Doppler aliasing velocities. For details on how to quantitatively use the proximal convergence zone, the reader is referred to systematic overviews.

- If there is a reproducible, clearly delineated jet, its minimal width at its origin (proximal jet width, vena contracta) exceeds 7 mm. In many cases, however, as in prosthetic valve dehiscence, this width is not clearly visualizable. However, it is usually obvious that the jet width is large. Only four-chamber views or long-axis views should be used for evaluation, because the jet width may be large in the two-chamber view even with moderate mitral regurgitation.

- A rare sign of very severe mitral regurgitation is a "shoulder" in the continuous-wave profile of mitral regurgitation, caused by a rapid decrease in late systolic velocities. Hence, the usually symmetric bell shape of the regurgitation profile becomes distorted and looks more triangular. This notch reflects the massive left atrial pressure increase in late systole resulting from the regurgitation and, therefore, a late systolic decrease in ventriculoatrial pressure gradient.

MORPHOLOGIC FEATURES OF ACUTE SEVERE MITRAL REGURGITATION

The whole valve and the subvalvular apparatus must be examined for one of the following disease scenarios.

Chordal rupture

Chordal rupture may occur as a degenerative complication or as a complication of infective endocarditis in mitral valve prolapse or, more rarely, in a normal valve. The uniform consequence is (partial or total) flail of the affected leaflet, with a regurgitant jet directed away from the affected leaflet (Figure 10.1) (V10.3A, V10.3B, and V10.3C). The ruptured chorda is often seen moving erratically in the left atrium during systole and in the left ventricle in diastole. The distinction between a degenerative and an endocarditic cause of a ruptured chorda, especially in the presence of a diffusely thickened valve, as in classic mitral valve prolapse, usually cannot be made with confidence on echocardiographic grounds alone, unless clear vegetations or a perforation is present. The presence or absence of general signs of infective endocarditis (fever, positive blood cultures, and serum markers of systemic inflammation, such as elevated blood sedimentation rate or C-reactive protein) is of critical importance in these cases. With TEE, the location of a prolapse or flail with the origin of the regurgitant jet can often be localized well in the transgastric, short-axis view of the left ventricle, or else through careful scanning of the whole mitral valve from a low transesophageal four-chamber view position with stepwise increments in cross-section angle, or by three-dimensional TEE with *en face* or angled *en face* views of the mitral valve from the atrial side (V13.35B). A break in the continuity of the subvalvular apparatus, as in chordal or papillary muscle rupture, is often best visualized in the transgastric, two-chamber view at approximately 90°, the transesophageal,

two-chamber view (at 60–90°), or the transesophageal long-axis view (at 120–150°) (V10.4A and V10.4B).

Papillary muscle rupture

Papillary muscle rupture occurs in approximately 1% of acute myocardial infarcts (see Chapter 3), mostly with infarctions of the posterior circulation, in the first days after infarction, although it may occur very early; it is accompanied by rapid hemodynamic deterioration (V10.5A and V10.5B). The *posteromedial* papillary muscle, which is variably perfused by the right or circumflex coronary artery,[2,3] is far more frequently affected than the anterolateral. Actual rupture of the whole papillary muscle is very rare and mostly catastrophic; what usually is designated papillary muscle rupture instead is the ischemic rupture of *one of the heads* of the posteromedial papillary muscle (V3.3 and V3.4A). It can be seen rapidly moving with the mitral leaflets, being displaced into the left atrium in systole and returning to the left ventricle in diastole. Transthoracic imaging usually is sufficient for diagnosis if there is a reasonable echo window (Figure 10.2)

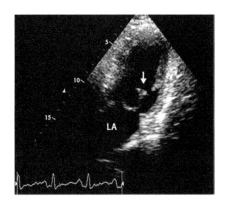

FIGURE 10.2 Transthoracic modified apical view showing detached head (arrow) of the ruptured posteromedial papillary muscle in the left ventricular cavity (V10.6). LA: left atrium.

(Image and video provided by IS.)

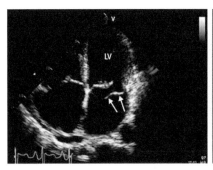
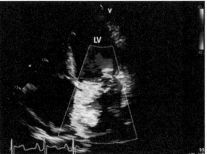

FIGURE 10.1 Transthoracic apical four-chamber view demonstrating posterior mitral leaflet flail caused by degenerative chordal rupture with completely lost coaptation between the mitral leaflets during systole (left panel) (V10.3B). Note the ruptured chord (left arrow) attached to the posterior mitral leaflet (right arrow). Color Doppler shows a large eccentric turbulent mitral regurgitation jet directed toward interatrial septum, away from the affected leaflet (right panel) (V10.3C). Severe mitral regurgitation could be predicted based on a two-dimensional study. LV: left ventricle.

(Images and videos provided by PMM.)

(V10.6). The size of the infarct-induced wall motion abnormality often is not large, leaving global ventricular function normal or near normal.

Infective endocarditis with valve destruction

Infective endocarditis can lead to *perforation of a leaflet* or to *chordal rupture* with flail of the affected leaflet (Figures 10.3 and 10.4) (V10.7A, V10.7B, V10.8A, V10.8B, and V10.8C). In mitral valve prostheses, it can lead to perforation or flail of bioprosthetic leaflets or to dehiscence of all types of prosthetic valves (see later). Usually, there are other morphologic signs of endocarditis: leaflet thickening, vegetations, pseudoaneurysms, or abscess (Figures 10.5 and 10.6) (V10.9A and V10.9B). Although severe regurgitation is generally considered a relatively late event in endocarditis, staphylococci in particular may produce severe regurgitant lesions within a few days or less.

Mitral prosthetic dysfunction

Depending on the type of prosthesis, the following possibilities for acute mitral prosthesis regurgitation exist[4]:

- *Bioprosthetic degeneration or endocarditis*. The time-dependent wear-and-tear lesions of bioprostheses may often remain silent before a large tear suddenly manifests as torrential regurgitation (V14.4A, V14.4B, V14.4C, V14.4D). The degenerative tear can lead to leaflet prolapse or flail or to perforation. In contrast, infective endocarditis affects bioprosthetic leaflets in a similar manner to native valve leaflets, leading to thickening, vegetations, or perforation. The differential diagnosis of pure degeneration and endocarditic lesions is not possible by echocardiography alone. For example, tears can lead to prolapsing leaflet segments that may mimic vegetations, and endocarditic leaflet thickening may closely resemble degenerative changes.

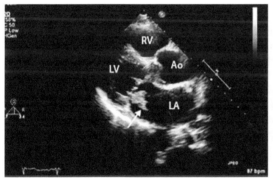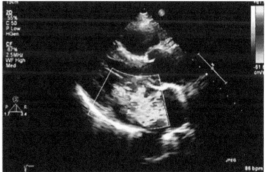

FIGURE 10.3 Transthoracic parasternal long-axis view showing large vegetation (arrow) adherent to atrial side of the posterior leaflet (left panel). Note the absence of left atrial and left ventricular dilation (V10.7A). Color Doppler shows acute severe mitral regurgitation (right panel) (V10.7B). Ao: aorta; LA: left atrium; LV: left ventricle; RV: right ventricle.

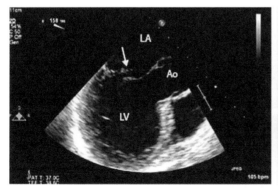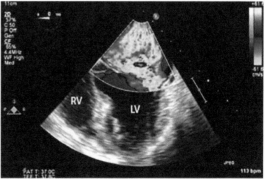

FIGURE 10.4 Transesophageal echocardiographic midesophageal long-axis view showing flail (arrow) of the posterior mitral leaflet (left panel). Note also the pronounced thickening of the tip of the anterior leaflet, which probably is also a result of endocarditis (V10.8B). Note that neither the left atrium nor the left ventricle is clearly enlarged. Transesophageal echocardiographic midesophageal four-chamber view with color Doppler showing severe eccentric mitral regurgitation corresponding to posterior leaflet flail (right panel) (V10.8C). Ao: aorta; LA: left atrium; LV: left ventricle; RV: right ventricle.

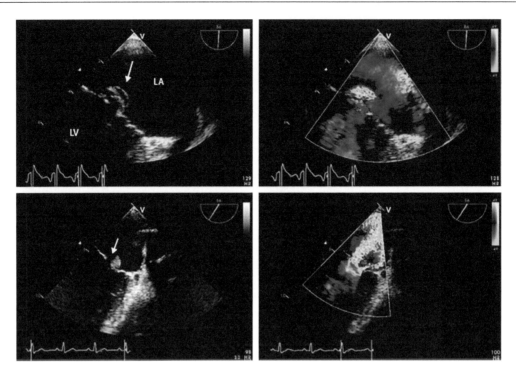

FIGURE 10.5   A 36-year-old woman with a history of recurrent urinary tract infections was referred to cardiologist because of high fever and new-onset systolic heart murmur best heard over the apex of the heart. Transesophageal echocardiographic two-chamber view showed a large vegetation and an aneurysm of A2 scallop of the mitral valve (upper left panel) (V10.9A). Color Doppler revealed mild mitral regurgitation with pooling of the blood in the aneurysm of the A2 scallop (upper right panel). Blood cultures were positive for *Enterococcus faecalis*, which was sensitive to empirically started antibiotics. However, after 9 days of antibiotic treatment, the patient developed abrupt dyspnea with intensifying of heart murmur. Transesophageal echocardiography was immediately performed again (V10.9B), revealing the rupture (arrow) of the aneurysm of the anterior mitral leaflet (left panel) with severe mitral regurgitation (lower right panel). The patient was referred to emergent cardiac surgery and underwent mitral valve replacement. Intraoperative findings confirmed the echocardiographic diagnosis (see Figure 10.6). LA: left atrium; LV: left ventricle.

(Images and videos provided by VC.)

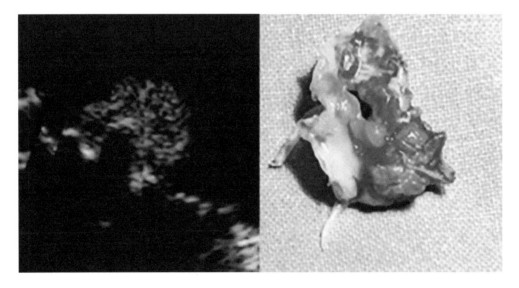

FIGURE 10.6   Zoom view of the vegetation and the aneurysm of the A2 scallop of the anterior mitral leaflet (left panel) and the anterior leaflet excised during cardiac surgery (right panel). Note the vegetations and the hole at the center of the specimen, representing the site of the rupture. For details, see Figure 10.5.

(Images provided by VC.)

- *Prosthetic ring endocarditis with prosthetic dehiscence.* Infective endocarditis of valvular prostheses preferentially leads to ring abscesses, particularly, but not exclusively, in mechanical prostheses. Ring abscesses destroy the anchoring of the prosthesis in its bed. Depending on the extensiveness of the dehiscence, regurgitation may ensue, ranging from paravalvular leakage (V12.10A, V12.10B) to dehiscence, defined as abnormal mobility ("rocking") of the whole prosthesis, to embolism of the entire prosthesis. Abnormal mobility can be best seen by careful back-and-forth review of the prosthesis motion on two-dimensional echo over a full cardiac cycle. By TEE, and particularly by three-dimensional TEE, usually the dehiscence can be directly identified as a break in continuity between the prosthetic ring and the paravalvular tissue (Figure 10.7) (V10.10E), giving rise to a large paraprosthetic regurgitant jet.
- Dehiscence may also occur without endocarditis as the result of suture insufficiency in the early postoperative period (V10.10A, V10.10B, V10.10C, V10.10D, and V10.10E).
- Mechanical (and rarely, biologic) *prosthetic thrombosis* sometimes leaves the occluder or leaflets in a fixed, half-shut position, leading to both stenosis and regurgitation (see Chapter 12). By careful apical imaging, abnormal occluder mobility can often be ascertained in tilting-disk or bileaflet prostheses in the mitral position. In case

of doubt, TEE should be performed. Unless cardiac output is already very low, continuous-wave spectral Doppler shows clearly elevated mean diastolic transprosthetic velocities yielding gradients well above 5 ± 3 mmHg, which is the normal range for mechanical prostheses in the mitral position at normal heart rates. This is at least partly a result of the additional regurgitant volume flowing through the prosthesis in diastole. In many cases, thrombus can be directly seen on the atrial side of the prosthesis by TEE, but lack of clearly visualizable thrombotic material by no means excludes thrombosis of the valve. The decisive finding of prosthetic thrombosis is *impaired leaflet mobility, not thrombus visualization* (V12.5). Pannus is very difficult to distinguish from thrombus by echo alone (V12.3), although it has been reported that pannus is more echodense than thrombus, and the diagnosis should rather be made by considering the acuity of the condition, anticoagulation status, embolic events, and so on.

- A very rare cause of acute massive prosthetic dysfunction is prosthetic strut fracture leading to embolization of the occluder. This has been seen in a series of Björk-Shiley tilting-disk valves (60–70° convexo-concave mitral prosthesis no. 29 implanted during the years 1979–1986) and exceptionally in other valves. The occluder often embolizes to the abdominal aorta. The event is mostly fatal because of overwhelming mitral regurgitation.

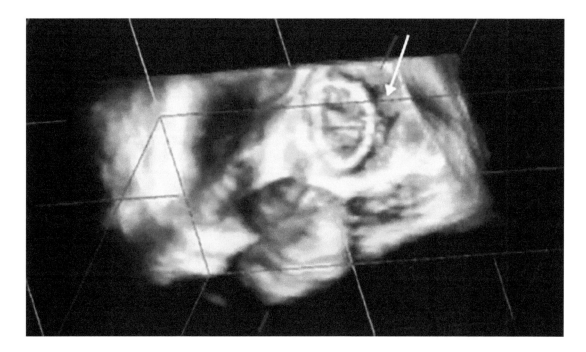

FIGURE 10.7 Three-dimensional transesophageal echocardiographic en face image (looking from the left atrial side) showing a large mitral ring dehiscence (arrow) from approximately 12–6 o'clock (V10.10E).

ECHOCARDIOGRAPHIC FEATURES OF ACUTE VERSUS CHRONIC MITRAL REGURGITATION

Importantly, the following typical features of severe *chronic* mitral regurgitation are missing in acute regurgitation:

- Regardless of the severity of regurgitation, neither the left atrium nor the left ventricle is necessarily enlarged. At least initially, sinus rhythm is mostly preserved. However, the presence of enlargement does not exclude acute regurgitation because concomitant or previous disease (as when a prosthesis is present) may have led to chamber enlargement.
- Global left ventricular dysfunction is not a typical feature of acute mitral regurgitation, and typically there is left ventricular hyperkinesis as a response to the volume load of acute regurgitation. However, left ventricular dysfunction does not exclude this condition because there may be concomitant myocardial disease.

DIFFERENTIAL DIAGNOSIS

The combination of a well-pumping left ventricle with dyspnea and/or pulmonary edema may also be present in the following:

- Hypertensive crisis
- Atrial fibrillation with rapid ventricular rate
- Cardiac tamponade
- Acute aortic regurgitation
- Constrictive pericarditis
- Acquired shunt lesion, such as postinfarction ventricular septal defect
- Noncardiac pulmonary edema (as by fluid volume overload) and others

LIST OF VIDEOS

https://routledgetextbooks.com/textbooks/9781032157009/chapter-10.php

VIDEO 10.1A   Perforation of the anterior mitral leaflet (1/4): Transthoracic apical four-chamber view showing thickening, mild to moderate calcification, and sclerosis of the mitral leaflets, particularly anterior. There is also a suspicious, not clearly visible, loss in continuity of the anterior leaflet (see also Videos 10.1B, 10.1C, and 10.1D). *(Video provided by IS.)*

VIDEO 10.1B   Perforation of the anterior mitral leaflet (2/4): Color Doppler of the mitral valve in transthoracic apical four-chamber view showing an eccentric and turbulent mitral regurgitation jet passing through most likely the perforated anterior mitral leaflet. Note that blood flow creates a large proximal acceleration zone (PISA) above the anterior mitral leaflet level as it goes from the left ventricle to the left atrium (see also Videos 10.1A, 10.1C, and 10.1D). *(Video provided by IS.)*

VIDEO 10.1C   Perforation of the anterior mitral leaflet (3/4): Transesophageal echocardiography clearly shows a perforation of the midportion of the anterior mitral leaflet (see also Videos 10.1A, 10.1B, and 10.1D). *(Video provided by IS.)*

VIDEO 10.1D   Perforation of the anterior mitral leaflet (4/4): Transesophageal echocardiography demonstrates a large and eccentric mitral regurgitation jet passing through the perforated anterior mitral leaflet (see also Videos 10.1A, 10.1B, and 10.1C). *(Video provided by IS.)*

VIDEO 10.2   Reverse flow in the pulmonary vein: Transthoracic apical four-chamber view showing severe mitral regurgitation (left panel) with reverse flow in the pulmonary vein during systole detected with pulsed-wave Doppler (right panel). *(Video provided by IS.)*

VIDEO 10.3A   Degenerative chordal rupture and flail of the posterior mitral leaflet (1/3): Transthoracic apical long-axis view demonstrating posterior mitral leaflet flail caused by chordal rupture with completely lost coaptation between the mitral leaflets during systole. Severe mitral regurgitation could be predicted based on this two-dimensional study. Note the erratically moving ruptured chord attached to the flail posterior leaflet (see also Videos 10.3B and 10.3C). *(Video provided by PMM.)*

VIDEO 10.3B   Degenerative chordal rupture and flail of the posterior mitral leaflet (2/3): Transthoracic apical four-chamber view demonstrating posterior mitral leaflet flail caused by chordal rupture with completely lost coaptation between the mitral leaflets during systole. Severe mitral regurgitation could be predicted based on this two-dimensional study. Note the erratically moving ruptured chord attached to the flail posterior leaflet (see also Videos 10.3A and 10.3C). *(Video provided by PMM.)*

VIDEO 10.3C   Degenerative chordal rupture and flail of the posterior mitral leaflet (3/3): Color Doppler of the mitral valve in transthoracic apical four-chamber view shows a large eccentric turbulent mitral regurgitation jet directed toward the interatrial septum, away from the affected leaflet. Severe mitral regurgitation could be predicted based on two-dimensional study (see also Videos 10.3A and 10.3B). *(Video provided by PMM.)*

VIDEO 10.4A   Degenerative chordal rupture and flail of the posterior mitral leaflet (1/2): Transesophageal echocardiographic four-chamber view demonstrating posterior mitral leaflet flail caused by chordal rupture with completely lost coaptation between the mitral leaflets during systole. Severe mitral regurgitation (see Video 10.4B) could be predicted based on this two-dimensional study. Note vigorously contracting left ventricle consistent with acute regurgitation.

VIDEO 10.4B   Degenerative chordal rupture and flail of the posterior mitral leaflet (2/2): Color Doppler transesophageal echocardiography of the mitral valve in apical four-chamber view shows a wide (vena contracta 12 mm) eccentric turbulent mitral regurgitation jet directed toward the interatrial septum (away from the affected posterior leaflet), with a large proximal acceleration zone (PISA), indicating severe regurgitation (could be predicted based on two-dimensional study) (see Video 10.4A).

VIDEO 10.5A   Papillary muscle rupture caused by posterior myocardial infarction (1/2): Transesophageal scanning from modified short- to long-axis view shows the tip of a papillary muscle attached to the anterior mitral leaflet, prolapsing back into the left atrium in systole. Note hyperkinetic global systolic function of the left ventricle, corresponding to a relatively small infarction and acute volume loading (see also Video 10.5B).

VIDEO 10.5B   Papillary muscle rupture caused by posterior myocardial infarction (2/2): Color Doppler transesophageal echocardiography shows severe mitral regurgitation (first part of the video) and tip of a papillary muscle attached to the anterior mitral leaflet, prolapsing back into the left atrium in systole (second part of the video, color off) (see also Video 10.5A).

VIDEO 10.6   Papillary muscle rupture caused by inferoposterior myocardial infarction: Transthoracic modified apical view showing detached head of the posteromedial papillary muscle rapidly moving with the mitral leaflets during cardiac cycle. Note the relatively preserved global ventricular function and akinesis of the papillary muscle region resulting from infarction. *(Video provided by IS.)*

VIDEO 10.7A   Mitral valve endocarditis (1/2): Transthoracic parasternal long-axis view showing large vegetation adherent to atrial side of the posterior leaflet. Note hyperkinetic left ventricle, which is not dilated (see also Video 10.7B).

VIDEO 10.7B   Mitral valve endocarditis (2/2): Color Doppler shows acute severe mitral regurgitation (see also Video 10.7A).

VIDEO 10.8A   Mitral valve endocarditis (1/3): Transthoracic echocardiographic parasternal long-axis view zoomed on mitral valve. A vegetation can be seen on the left atrial side of the mitral valve, which originates from the tip of the posterior leaflet (see also Videos 10.8B and 10.8C).

VIDEO 10.8B   Mitral valve endocarditis (2/3): Transesophageal echocardiographic midesophageal long-axis view showing flail of the posterior mitral leaflet. Note also the pronounced thickening of the tip of the anterior leaflet, which probably is also a result of endocarditis. Note that neither the left atrium nor the left ventricle is clearly enlarged and that there is hyperkinetic left ventricular contraction caused by volume loading (see also Videos 10.8A and 10.8C).

VIDEO 10.8C   Mitral valve endocarditis (3/3): Transesophageal echocardiographic midesophageal four-chamber view with color Doppler showing severe eccentric mitral regurgitation corresponding to posterior leaflet flail (see also Videos 10.8A and 10.8B).

VIDEO 10.9A   Rupture of the aneurysm of the anterior mitral leaflet caused by acute endocarditis (1/2): A 36-year-old woman with a history of recurrent urinary tract infections was referred to cardiologist because of high fever and new-onset systolic heart murmur best heard over the apex of the heart. This transesophageal echocardiographic two-chamber view showed a large vegetation and an aneurysm of A2 scallop of the mitral valve. Color Doppler revealed mild mitral regurgitation with pooling of the blood in the aneurysm of the A2 scallop (shown here). Blood cultures were positive for *Enterococcus faecalis*, which was sensitive to empirically started antibiotics. However, after 9 days of antibiotic treatment, the patient developed abrupt dyspnea with intensifying heart murmur. Transesophageal echocardiography was immediately performed again (see Video 10.9B), revealing the rupture of the aneurysm of the anterior mitral leaflet with severe mitral regurgitation. The patient was referred to emergent cardiac surgery and underwent mitral valve replacement. Intraoperative findings confirmed the echocardiographic diagnosis (see Figure 10.6 in the book). *(Video provided by VC.)*

VIDEO 10.9B   Rupture of the aneurysm of the anterior mitral leaflet caused by acute endocarditis (2/2): A 36-year-old woman with a history of recurrent urinary tract infections was referred to cardiologist because of high fever and new-onset systolic heart murmur best heard over the apex of the heart. Transesophageal echocardiographic two-chamber view showed a large vegetation and an aneurysm of A2 scallop of the mitral valve. Color Doppler revealed mild mitral regurgitation with pooling of the blood in the aneurysm of the A2 scallop (see Video 10.9A). Blood cultures were positive for *Enterococcus faecalis*, which was sensitive to empirically started antibiotics. However, after 9 days of antibiotic treatment, the patient developed abrupt dyspnea with intensifying heart murmur. Transesophageal echocardiography was immediately performed again (shown here), revealing the rupture of the aneurysm of the anterior mitral leaflet with severe mitral regurgitation. The patient was referred to emergent cardiac surgery and underwent mitral valve replacement. Intraoperative findings confirmed the echocardiographic diagnosis (see Figure 10.6 in the book). *(Figure and video provided by VC.)*

VIDEO 10.10A   Dehiscent mitral ring after mitral valve repair, with acute severe mitral regurgitation (1/5): Zoom of the mitral valve in transthoracic four-chamber view. The surgical ring is seen "floating" between the mitral leaflets, with independent motion (see also Videos 10.10B, 10.10C, 10.10D, and 10.10E).

VIDEO 10.10B   Dehiscent mitral ring after mitral valve repair, with acute severe mitral regurgitation (2/5): Transthoracic echocardiographic color Doppler shows severe mitral regurgitation caused by mitral ring dehiscence (see also Videos 10.10A, 10.10C, 10.10D, and 10.10E).

VIDEO 10.10C   Dehiscent mitral ring after mitral valve repair, with acute severe mitral regurgitation (3/5): Transesophageal echocardiography, four-chamber view. Note that the lateral aspect of the mitral ring is detached from the mitral valve (see also Videos 10.10A, 10.10B, 10.10D, and 10.10E).

VIDEO 10.10D   Dehiscent mitral ring after mitral valve repair, with acute severe mitral regurgitation (4/5): Transesophageal echocardiographic color Doppler shows severe mitral regurgitation caused by mitral ring dehiscence (see also Videos 10.10A, 10.10B, 10.10C, and 10.10E).

VIDEO 10.10E   Dehiscent mitral ring after mitral valve repair, with acute severe mitral regurgitation (5/5): Three-dimensional transesophageal echocardiographic en face image (looking from the left atrial side) showing a large mitral ring dehiscence from approximately 12–6 o'clock (see also Videos 10.10A, 10.10B, 10.10C, and 10.10D).

REFERENCES

1. Flachskampf FA, Badano L, Daniel WG, et al. Recommendations for transoesophageal echocardiography—update 2010. Eur J Echocardiogr 2010; 11:461–76.
2. Flachskampf FA, Wouters PF, Edvardsen T, et al. Recommendations for transoesophageal echocardiography: EACVI update 2014. Eur Heart J Cardiovasc Imaging 2014; 15:353–65.
3. Zoghbi WA, Adams D, Bonow RO, et al. Recommendations for noninvasive evaluation of native valvular regurgitation: a report from the American Society of Echocardiography developed in collaboration with the Society for Cardiovascular Magnetic Resonance. J Am Soc Echocardiogr 2017;30:303–71.
4. Zoghbi WA, Chambers JB, Dumesnil JG, et al. Recommendations for evaluation of prosthetic valves with echocardiography and Doppler ultrasound: a report from the American Society of Echocardiography's Guidelines and Standards Committee and the Task Force on Prosthetic Valves, developed in conjunction with the American College of Cardiology Cardiovascular Imaging Committee, Cardiac Imaging Committee of the American Heart Association, the European Association of Echocardiography, a registered branch of the European Society of Cardiology, the Japanese Society of Echocardiography and the Canadian Society of Echocardiography, endorsed by the American College of Cardiology Foundation, American Heart Association, European Association of Echocardiography, a registered branch of the European Society of Cardiology, the Japanese Society of Echocardiography, and Canadian Society of Echocardiography. J Am Soc Echocardiogr 2009; 22:975–1014.

Echocardiography in obstruction of native valves

11

Emily K. Zern and Michael H. Picard

Key Points

- Obstruction of native valves is a rare event and usually involves obstruction by tumors, thrombi, or vegetations.
- Symptoms and signs are nonspecific and can range from fatigue to sudden cardiac death.
- Echocardiography provides a rapid diagnosis of the presence of and degree of valvular obstruction utilizing a combination of two-dimensional, three-dimensional, and color and spectral Doppler echocardiography.

Acute and chronic obstruction of native cardiac valves is a rare diagnosis caused by tumors, thrombi, endocarditis, or compression of the heart by extracardiac masses. The clinical presentation depends on the location and severity of obstructed valve, chronicity of the obstruction, and comorbid medical conditions of the patient. As valvular obstruction can mimic a syndrome similar to that of valvular stenosis, patients may present with chest discomfort, decreased exercise capacity, dyspnea, syncope or presyncope, arrhythmia, or sudden death. Clinical examination may vary from a soft murmur alone to decompensated heart failure and hemodynamic compromise. This chapter will review the most common acquired causes of native valve obstructions and discuss the echocardiographic evaluation of a patient with a suspected valvular obstruction.

ECHOCARDIOGRAPHIC ASSESSMENT

Transthoracic echocardiography (TTE) is a readily available first-line imaging modality that may assist in the diagnosis of obstruction, provide clues to the underlying pathology based on location and appearance, quantify the severity of obstruction, and provide supporting data regarding the need for, urgency of, and type of intervention.

A primary role of the urgent echocardiogram is to distinguish between obstruction of the native valve and other conditions with similar clinical presentations, such as native valve stenosis or conditions that may mimic valvular obstruction (e.g., hypertrophic obstructive cardiomyopathy, subvalvular membranes, or other congenital heart disease). Assessment of the mass by TTE should include identification of the location, mobility, size, and number of masses that may be obstructing a valve. When able, the extent and origin of the mass should be defined, though this may not be possible if the mass arises from outside of standard imaging view (e.g., the systemic or pulmonary venous circulation). A pericardial effusion may accompany malignant cardiac tumors, and standard evaluation for cardiac tamponade should be performed in these instances. In addition, the use of *ultrasound-enhancing agents* (UEA) (echocardiographic contrast) can be a helpful tool for further assessment of cardiac masses. The difference in perfusion with UEA between vascular and nonvascular tumors or thrombus may provide additional diagnostic information prior to further imaging studies.

DOI: 10.1201/9781003245407-11

Spectral Doppler assessment is a crucial component of the echocardiographic evaluation of an obstructive mass. The degree of valvular obstruction (pressure gradients and peak velocity) should be quantified by continuous-wave and pulsed-wave Doppler analysis. Spectral Doppler can quantify effects of the obstruction or mass itself on the heart and surrounding structures, such as systemic or pulmonic venous obstruction or elevation of the right heart and pulmonary arterial pressures. If visualization of the valvular obstruction is limited or the origin and extent of the masses obstructing the valves cannot be well assessed with TTE, *transesophageal echocardiography* (TEE) provides important value.

CARDIAC TUMORS

Almost any type of cardiac tumor can cause some degree of obstruction of native cardiac valves and the inflow and/or outflow tracts of both ventricles. Primary cardiac tumors are rare with a reported incidence of 1,380 out of 100 million individuals, and up to 90% are benign.[1,2] In contrast, secondary tumors are 22 to 132 times more common, and by definition due to their distant spread, are considered malignant.[1] A review of 12,485 autopsies revealed an incidence of primary tumors of 0.056% and of secondary tumors of 1.23%.[3]

Primary cardiac benign tumors

Cardiac myxoma

Cardiac myxoma is the most frequent adult primary cardiac tumor, accounting for nearly 50% of primary cardiac tumors, and the most common cause of obstruction of the native valves.[4,5] The vast majority of cardiac myxomas originate as a solitary tumor in the left atrium, commonly mobile and attached by a stalk to the fossa ovalis of the interatrial septum, though these masses can occur elsewhere in the left atrial wall and mitral valve leaflets. Cardiac myxomas also can occur rarely in the other three cardiac chambers.[5,6]

Familial myxomas, such as the Carney complex, account for nearly 7% of myxomas and are more likely to be multiple and have unusual locations.[6] Although classified as benign, familial myxomas can have a dramatic natural history.

Up to 80% of patients with atrial myxoma have obstructive symptoms, typically related to the mitral valve (Figure 11.1) (V11.1, V11.2, V11.3).[7,8] Dyspnea, symptoms of heart failure, malaise, and fever are the most common presenting symptoms. Even though the mitral valve is the most common valve affected, obstruction or partial obstruction of the tricuspid valve, pulmonic valve, and right ventricular outflow tract have been described.[8–11] Focused cardiac ultrasound examination (FoCUS) can detect the tumor (V18.6), but comprehensive echocardiography accurately defines the size, location, mobility, attachment site, and hemodynamic consequences

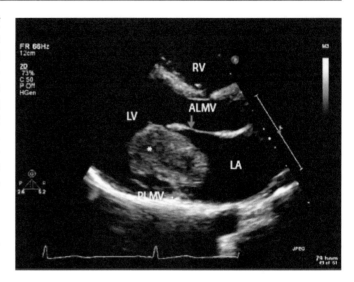

FIGURE 11.1 Transthoracic parasternal long-axis view demonstrating cardiac myxoma obstructing the mitral valve. LA: left atrium; LV: left ventricle; ALMV: anterior leaflet of mitral valve; PLMV: posterior leaflet of mitral valve; RV: right ventricle; *: myxoma.

of myxomas. When two-dimensional TTE does not show the attachment site of the tumor, two-dimensional TEE, or three-dimensional TTE or TEE echocardiography can provide additional information.[12]

Surgical resection of the obstructing tumor remains the treatment of choice. Echocardiographic follow-up after resection is necessary because a small percentage of tumors recur (approximately 10–15%).[1]

Papillary fibroelastoma

Papillary fibroelastoma is a more rare primary cardiac tumor, constituting 11.5% of all primary cardiac tumors.[2,13] They are pedunculated masses, typically found on the downstream side of valves (95% on the aortic and mitral valves) (V13.20A, V13.20B) and more commonly are found incidentally on echocardiograms performed for an alternative indication or after an embolic phenomenon.[13] Rarely, papillary fibroelastomas may present with partial valve obstruction.[14] Surgical treatment (even in asymptomatic patients) should be considered for larger papillary fibroelastomas (>1 cm), given the consequences of potential complications, such as coronary, cerebral, or systemic embolization.

Rhabdomyoma

Rhabdomyoma is the most common primary cardiac tumor in children but is extremely rare in adults. Rhabdomyomas are often associated with tuberous sclerosis, and typically they are multiple, involving the atria and ventricles and both the left and right heart.[6,15,16] They tend to be intramyocardial and, on echocardiography, are well-circumscribed with signal characteristics slightly different from the surrounding myocardium.[6]

Although histologically benign, rhabdomyomas can be functionally malignant if blood flow is obstructed, and this has been observed in some degree in up to one-quarter of infants, usually in those not associated with tuberous sclerosis.[16,17] As these tumors are most commonly located in the left ventricle and interventricular septum, the left ventricular outflow tract is the most common location of the obstruction, and obstruction of either semilunar or atrioventricular valves is rare. The number of tumors, their size, and their location in relation to intracardiac structures, as well as the severity of obstruction, are all well characterized by echocardiography. Spontaneous regression is more common in young patients under the age of 2 years. Because of partial or complete spontaneous regression of these tumors in up to 33.6% of cases, surgical treatment is typically reserved only for those with severe obstruction or life-threatening arrhythmia.[16,18]

Fibroma

Fibromas are the second most common primary ventricular tumor, more common in infants.[1,19] The tumors are usually solitary and located within either ventricular septum or ventricular free wall and can mimic hypertrophic cardiomyopathy. Index of suspicion for this tumor should be higher in patients with familial adenomatous polyposis and Gorlin syndrome (in which fibromas may be of atrial origin).[1] On echocardiography, they are well-demarcated, highly reflective, and noncontractile. Calcification of the central portion of the tumor of this tumor is one of the distinguishing features of fibroma. Even though a significant percentage of patients are asymptomatic, they may present with arrhythmias, heart failure, syncope, or sudden death.[6] The tumor may cause the obstruction of the left and right ventricular outflow tracts, but obstruction of aortic and pulmonic valves is rarer. Treatment often involves surgery due to the increased risk for arrhythmias and sudden death (and unlike rhabdomyomas, cardiac fibromas do not spontaneously regress).

Primary cardiac malignant tumors

In general, malignant cardiac tumors are extremely rare, encompassing less than 10% of all primary cardiac tumors. Treatment is usually a combination of surgery, chemotherapy, and/or radiation, and generally, survival of patients who present with these malignant tumors are poor, less than 50% at 12 months from the time of diagnosis.[20]

Sarcomas

Sarcomas represent more than two-thirds of the primary malignancies of the heart.[1,21] There are multiple subtypes including angiosarcomas, rhabdosarcomas, leiomyosarcomas, fibrosarcomas, synovial sarcomas, and undifferentiated sarcomas. Most common cardiac locations and sites of obstruction vary by subtype. *Angiosarcomas* are the most common subtype, with a predilection for the right atrium and pericardium, and after filling the right atrium, they can infiltrate into the tricuspid valve (resulting in obstruction) and the right ventricle.[1,6] Patients may present with symptoms of right heart failure due to the obstruction (Figure 11.2) (V11.4A, V11.4B, V11.4C). *Rhabdomyosarcomas* are the most common pediatric malignancy and often affect the valves, thus presenting with symptoms of obstruction.[1] *Osteosarcomas, fibrosarcomas, liposarcomas, leiomyosarcomas, and undifferentiated sarcomas* are often located in the left atrium and can grow to obstruct the mitral valve.[1,22–24]

Although surgical resection can be attempted, the long-term prognosis of these tumors is often poor, as symptoms often develop late in the disease course, and 80% of these patients have systemic metastasis at time of presentation.[22]

Metastatic cardiac tumors

Metastatic cardiac tumors (sometimes referred to as *secondary* cardiac tumors) are significantly more frequent than primary

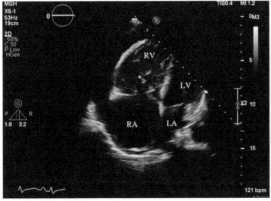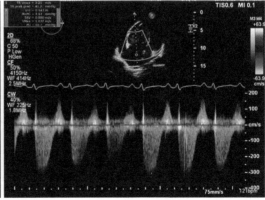

FIGURE 11.2 Large malignant sarcoma in the right ventricle. Transthoracic apical four-chamber view demonstrating large right ventricular mass compared to relatively compressed left ventricle and left atrium (left panel) (V11.4A). The right ventricular mass obstructs tricuspid valve opening during diastole (peak gradient across the tricuspid valve 11 mmHg, mean gradient 4 mmHg) (right panel) (V11.4B, V11.4C). Pathology consistent with high-grade undifferentiated pleomorphic sarcoma. LA: left atrium; LV: left ventricle; RA: right atrium; RV: right ventricle; *: sarcoma.

cardiac tumors. Metastases spread to the heart via direct extension and hematogenous, lymphatic, and transvenous routes. Carcinomas of the lung (Figure 11.3) (V11.5), breast, and esophagus; renal cell carcinoma; malignant melanoma (Figure 11.4); and lymphoma and leukemia are among the most frequent to metastasize to the heart.[25] Some studies suggest that the right side is more frequently involved, whereas other studies suggest equal involvement of the right- and left-sided chambers.[26-29] Direct metastatic obstruction of the valves is a rare phenomenon though has been reported (Figures 11.3 and 11.4).[1,25] Given the wide variety of scenarios and rarity of the phenomenon, the treatment modality should be individualized. Prognosis of patients with metastatic heart involvement remains poor.

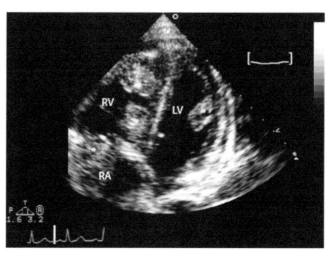

FIGURE 11.4   Off-axis apical four-chamber view demonstrating metastatic melanoma obstructing tricuspid valve. LA: left atrium; RA: right atrium; RV: right ventricle; *: metastasis.

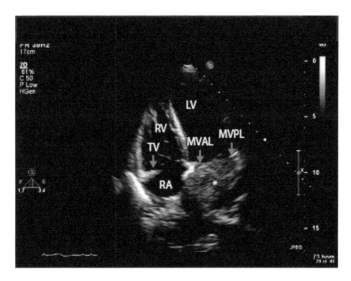

FIGURE 11.3   Four-chamber view showing metastatic undifferentiated epithelial lung carcinoma obstructing the mitral valve. LA: left atrium; LV: left ventricle; MVAL: mitral valve, anterior leaflet; MVPL: mitral valve, posterior leaflet; RA: right atrium; RV: right ventricle; TV: tricuspid valve; *: carcinoma.

THROMBI

Intracardiac thrombi can rarely cause native valve obstruction (Figure 11.5) (V11.6A, V11.6B). Intracardiac thrombus formation may be associated with multiple conditions including atrial fibrillation, myocardial heart disease (e.g., myocardial infarctions, apical aneurysms, dilated cardiomyopathies, Chagas disease), infiltrative or endocardial heart disease (eosinophilic myocarditis, endomyocardial fibrosis, cardiac amyloidosis), valvular heart disease (e.g., mitral stenosis, tricuspid stenosis), hypercoagulable states, endocarditis, and foreign bodies within the cardiac chambers.[30,31] Native aortic valve thrombosis is an extremely rare

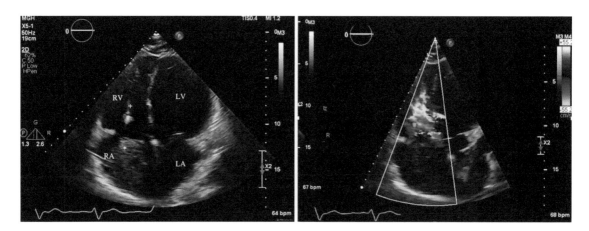

FIGURE 11.5   Large right atrial thrombus in a patient with dilated cardiomyopathy, defibrillator lead, and antiphospholipid antibody syndrome. Right atrial thrombus (left panel) (V11.6A) resulted in partial obstruction of superior vena cava flow and mimicked tricuspid valve stenosis with visible flow acceleration across the tricuspid valve (right panel) (V11.6B). LA: left atrium; LV, left ventricle; RA: right atrium; RV: right ventricle; *: thrombus; +: defibrillator lead.

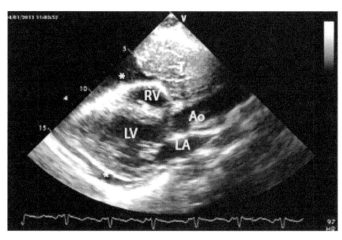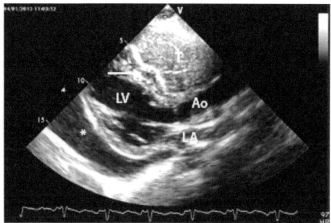

FIGURE 11.6 Extracardiac tumor compression with symptoms mimicking cardiac tamponade and hemodynamic compromise from native valve obstruction. Transthoracic parasternal long-axis view showing a large circular pericardial effusion (*) with a large tumor mass (T) with irregular edges (left panel). Tumor compresses the right ventricle (V11.7B) resulting in almost complete obliteration of the right ventricular cavity (arrow) in diastole (right panel). Right atrial collapse and swinging heart, consistent with cardiac tamponade, can also be visualized in V11.7A. The hemodynamic compromise was likely due to both obstruction by the tumor and the effects of reduced filling of the right heart due to tamponade. Histopathologic diagnosis of the tumor was lymphoma. Ao: aorta; LA: left atrium; LV: left ventricle; RV: right ventricle.

(Images and videos provided by ES.)

phenomenon, more commonly presenting with myocardial infarction rather than valvular obstruction, and approximately 30% of patients had a hypercoagulable state.[32] Right heart thrombi can also be present as a result of embolization or direct extension from the vena cavae. Multiple case reports describe thrombi obstructing mitral, aortic, and tricuspid valves; typically, these are large, free-floating thrombi. Echocardiography helps to promptly evaluate location and cause of obstruction as well as significance of hemodynamic compromise.

ENDOCARDITIS

Valvular destruction and regurgitation (see Chapters 9 and 10) are well-recognized complications of endocarditis. Obstructive valvular vegetations are rarer but must be considered in the differential diagnosis of patients with bacteremia and hemodynamic compromise. *Large bulky vegetations in the setting of fungal endocarditis* are the most common infectious lesions to obstruct native valves. Evidence of valvular obstruction by infective endocarditis has been demonstrated to be an independent risk factor for in-hospital mortality, and thus presence of valvular stenosis related to vegetation should be noted on echocardiographic exam.[32] Surgical intervention is typically indicated in cases of obstruction with severe hemodynamic compromise. Native aortic valve obstruction by *non-bacterial thrombotic endocarditis* and

Löffler endocarditis has been reported, with valvular stenosis improving after treatment with immunosuppression in the latter case.[33,34]

MIMICKERS OF VALVULAR OBSTRUCTION

Multiple conditions may mimic the symptoms and hemodynamic compromise of native valve obstruction. Compression of cardiac chambers by extracardiac masses (Figure 11.6) (V11.7A, V11.7B), pericardial effusion with tamponade, and large aortic aneurysms compressing the pulmonary artery are some of these causes.

SUMMARY

Native valve obstruction is a rare phenomenon, though it can be caused by primary or metastatic cardiac tumors, intracardiac thrombi, infective or nonbacterial endocarditis, or external compression. Presenting symptoms may vary from that of valvular stenosis of the affected valve to acute hemodynamic deterioration. Echocardiography provides a rapid evaluation of patients with native valve obstruction to provide insight into etiology and determine degree of obstruction to guide medical or surgical decision-making.

LIST OF VIDEOS

https://routledgetextbooks.com/textbooks/9781032157009/chapter-11.php

VIDEO 11.1   A 45-year-old woman with right-sided heart failure and liver failure: Transthoracic parasternal long-axis view showing a left atrial mass that obstructed the mitral valve. The patient underwent successful surgical removal of an atrial myxoma.

VIDEO 11.2   A 51-year-old woman with multiple strokes: Transesophageal four-chamber view showing a left atrial mass prolapsing into the left ventricle and causing partial obstruction of the mitral valve. The left atrial mass was attached to the lower portion of the interatrial septum and the base of anterior mitral leaflet. The patient underwent successful surgical removal of an atrial myxoma.

VIDEO 11.3   A 55-year-old man with right shoulder discomfort associated with right hand tingling: During the work-up for possible thoracic outlet obstruction, a mass was noted in the left atrium on computed tomography images. Transesophageal four-chamber view showing very large mass attached to the atrial septum and filling the left atrium. The patient underwent successful surgical removal of an atrial myxoma.

VIDEO 11.4A   Large malignant sarcoma in the right ventricle obstructs tricuspid valve opening during diastole (1/3). Transthoracic off-axis apical four-chamber (right ventricular focus, shown here) and right ventricular inflow (see Video 11.4B) views demonstrate relative tricuspid valve obstruction with flow acceleration (see Video 11.4C) due to incomplete opening of the valve leaflets in diastole (see Figure 11.2, for Doppler gradients). Pathology consistent with high-grade undifferentiated pleomorphic sarcoma.

VIDEO 11.4B   Large malignant sarcoma in the right ventricle obstructs tricuspid valve opening during diastole (2/3). Transthoracic right ventricular inflow (shown here) and off-axis apical four-chamber (right ventricular focus, see Video 11.4A) views demonstrate relative tricuspid valve obstruction with flow acceleration (see Video 11.4C) due to incomplete opening of the valve leaflets in diastole (see Figure 11.2, for Doppler gradients). Pathology consistent with high-grade undifferentiated pleomorphic sarcoma.

VIDEO 11.4C   Large malignant sarcoma in the right ventricle obstructs tricuspid valve opening during diastole (3/3). Note relative tricuspid valve obstruction with flow acceleration demonstrated by color Doppler, due to incomplete opening of the valve leaflets in diastole (see Figure 11.2, for Doppler gradients). See also Videos 11.4A and 11.4B. Pathology consistent with high-grade undifferentiated pleomorphic sarcoma.

VIDEO 11.5   Spreading of lung cancer into left atrium with obstruction of the mitral valve. Transthoracic echocardiography in a patient with lung cancer, presenting with severe dyspnea and cough, revealed a large mass, spreading through pulmonary vein into the left atrium, causing obstruction of the mitral valve in diastole. *(Video provided by SA.)*

VIDEO 11.6A   Large right atrial thrombus causing partial obstruction to flow across the tricuspid valve (1/2). This intracardiac thrombus formed in a patient with dilated cardiomyopathy, defibrillator lead, and antiphospholipid antibody syndrome (see also Video 11.5B).

VIDEO 11.6B   Large right atrial thrombus causing partial obstruction to flow across the tricuspid valve (2/2). Right atrial thrombus (see also Video 11.5A) formed in a patient with dilated cardiomyopathy, defibrillator lead, and antiphospholipid antibody syndrome, resulted in partial obstruction of superior vena cava flow and mimicked tricuspid valve stenosis with visible flow acceleration across the tricuspid valve (shown here).

VIDEO 11.7A   Extracardiac tumor compression with cardiac tamponade symptoms and hemodynamic compromise of native valve obstruction (1/2): Modified transthoracic apical four-chamber view showing large pericardial effusion, "swinging heart," and right atrial collapse—all consistent with cardiac tamponade. Transthoracic parasternal long-axis view (see Video 11.6B) showing a large circular pericardial effusion with swinging heart and a large tumor mass with irregular edges compressing the right ventricular outflow tract and resulting in almost complete obliteration of the right ventricular cavity in diastole. Histopathologic diagnosis of the tumor was lymphoma. *(Video provided by ES.)*

VIDEO 11.7B   Extracardiac tumor compression with cardiac tamponade mimicking symptoms and hemodynamic compromise of native valve obstruction (2/2): Transthoracic parasternal long-axis view showing a large circular pericardial effusion with "swinging heart" and a large tumor mass with irregular edges compressing the right ventricle and resulting in almost complete obliteration of the right ventricular cavity in diastole. Modified transthoracic apical four-chamber view (see Video 11.6A) showing large pericardial effusion, swinging heart, and right atrial collapse—all consistent with cardiac tamponade. Histopathologic diagnosis of the tumor was lymphoma. *(Video provided by ES.)*

REFERENCES

1. Tyebally S, Chen D, Bhattacharyya S, et al. Cardiac tumors. JACC Cardio Oncol 2020; 2(2): 293–311.
2. Habertheuer A, Laufer G, Wiedemann D, et al. Primary cardiac tumors on the verge of oblivion: a European experience over 15 years. J Cardiothorac Surg 2015; 10: 56.
3. Lam KY, Dickens P, Chan AC. Tumors of the heart. A 20-year experience with a review of 12,485 consecutive autopsies. Arch Pathol Lab Med 1993; 117(10): 1027–1031.
4. Elbardissi AW, Dearani JA, Daly RC, et al. Survival after resection of primary cardiac tumors: a 48-year experience. Circulation 2008; 118(14 Suppl): S7–S15.

5. Keeling IM, Oberwalder P, Anelli-Monti M, et al. Cardiac myxomas: 24 years of experience in 49 patients. Eur J Cardiothorac Surg 2002; 22(6): 971–977.

6. Bruce CJ. Cardiac tumours: diagnosis and management. Heart 2011; 97: 151–160.

7. Pinede L, Duhaut P, Loire R. Clinical presentation of left atrial cardiac myxoma. A series of 112 consecutive cases. Medicine (Baltimore) 2001; 80(3): 159–172.

8. Reynen K. Cardiac myxomas. N Engl J Med 1995; 333(24): 1610–1617.

9. Xiao ZH, Hu J, Zhu D, Shi YK, Zhang EY. Tricuspid valve obstruction and right heart failure due to a giant right atrial myxoma arising from the superior vena cava. J Cardiothorac Surg 2013; 8: 200.

10. Özeren M, Düzgü CM, Bugra O, Toker M, Yücel E. Myxoma originating from right ventricular apex obstructing ventricular inflow. Gazi Med J 2002; 13: 199–202.

11. Riera JM, Vila IC, Serrano JM, et al. Right ventricular myxoma. A rare case of pulmonary stenosis. Rev Esp Cardiol 1996; 49: 153–154.

12. Reddy VK, Faulkner M, Bandarupalli N, et al. Incremental value of live/real time three-dimensional transthoracic echocardiography in the assessment of right ventricular masses. Echocardiography 2009; 26(5): 598–609.

13. Gowda RM, Khan IA, Nair CK, Mehta NJ, Vasavada BC, Sacchi TJ. Cardiac papillary fibroelastoma: a comprehensive analysis of 725 cases. Am Heart J 2003; 146: 404–410.

14. Thomas MR, Jayakrishnan AG, Desai J, Monaghan MJ, Jewitt DE. Transesophageal echocardiography in the detection and surgical management of a papillary fibroelastoma of the mitral valve causing partial mitral valve obstruction. J Am Soc Echocardiogr 1993; 6: 83–86.

15. Begnetti M, Gow RM, Haney I, Mawson J, Williams WG, Freedom RM. Pediatric primary benign cardiac tumors: a 15-year review. Am Heart J 1997; 134(6): 107–114.

16. Verhaaren H, Vanakker O, De Wold D, Suys B, François K, Matthys D. Left ventricular outflow obstruction in rhabdomyoma of infancy: meta-analysis of the literature. J Pediatr 2003; 143: 258–263.

17. Black MD, Kadletz M, Smallhorn JF, Freedom RM. Cardiac rhabdomyomas and obstructive left heart disease: histologically but not functionally benign. Ann Thorac Surg 1998; 65: 1388–1390.

18. Bosi G, Lintermans JP, Pellegrino PA, Svaluto-Moreolo G, Vliers A. The natural history of cardiac rhabdomyoma with and without tuberous sclerosis. Acta Paediatr 1996; 85(8): 928–931.

19. Elbardissi AW, Dearani JA, Daly RC, et al. Survival after resection of primary cardiac tumors: a 48-year experience. Circulation 2008; 118(14 Suppl): S7–S15.

20. Sultan I, Bianco V, Habertheuer A, et al. Long-term outcomes of primary cardiac malignancies: multi-institutional results from the National Cancer Database. J Am Coll Cardiol 2020; 75(18): 2338–2347.

21. Burke A. Primary malignant cardiac tumors. Semin Diagn Pathol 2008; 25: 39–46.

22. Shanmugam G. Primary cardiac sarcoma. Eur J Cardiothorac Surg 2006; 29(6): 925–932.

23. Araoz PA, Eklund HE, Welch TJ, Breen JF. CT and MR imaging of primary cardiac malignancies. Radiographics 1999; 19(6): 1421–1434.

24. Silverman NA. Primary cardiac tumors. Ann Surg 1980; 191(2): 127–138.

25. Reynen K, Köckeritz U, Strasses RH. Metastases to the heart. Ann Oncol 2004; 15(3): 375–381.

26. Prichard RW. Tumors of the heart; review of the subject and report of 150 cases. AMA Arch Pathol 1951; 51(1): 98–128.

27. DeLoach JF, Haynes JW. Secondary tumors of heart and pericardium. Review of the subject and report of one hundred thirty seven cases. AMA Arch Int Med 1953; 91(2): 224–249.

28. Goudie RB. Secondary tumours of the heart and pericardium. Br Heart J 1955; 17(2): 183–188.

29. Scott RA, Garvin CF. Tumors of the heart and pericardium. Am Heart J 1939; 17: 431–436.

30. Waller BF, Grider L, Rohr TM, McLaughlin T, Taliercio CP, Fetters J. Intracardiac thrombi: frequency, location, etiology, and complications: a morphologic review—Part I. Clin Cardiol 1995; 18(8): 477–479.

31. Waller BF, Rohr TM, McLaughlin T, Grider L, Taliercio CP, Fetters J. Intracardiac thrombi: frequency, location, etiology, and complications: a morphologic review—Part II. Clin Cardiol 1995; 18(8): 530–534.

32. Alajaji W, Hornick J, Malek E, Klein AL. The characteristics and outcomes of native aortic valve thrombosis: a systematic review. J Am Coll Cardiol 2021; 78(8): 811–824.

33. Alaiti MA, Hoit BD. Nonbacterial thrombotic endocarditis. Echocardiography 2015; 32(6): 1051–1052.

34. Yamamoto M, Seo Y, Ishizu T, Aonuma K. Reversible aortic valve stenosis with Löffler endocarditis. Eur Heart J. 2018; 39(24): 2332.

Emergency echocardiography in patients with prosthetic valves

12

Mauro Pepi and Frank A. Flachskampf

Key Points

- Suspected malfunction or endocarditis of a prosthetic valve should prompt transthoracic and/or transesophageal examination.
- Obstruction and regurgitation may coexist, as when the occluder is thrombotically immobilized.
- If there is suspicion of obstruction in a mechanical valve, the occluder opening should be closely scrutinized, including examination by cinefluoroscopy, and the thrombus should be sought.
- Sudden new regurgitation can be a result of structural deterioration, endocarditis, or thrombosis.

Prosthetic-valve-related emergencies may be caused by *prosthetic valve obstruction* of varying degrees and acuities, *prosthetic valve regurgitation* of varying degrees and acuities, *infective endocarditis, embolism,* or a *combination* of these.

PROSTHETIC VALVE THROMBOSIS

Prosthetic valve (PV) thrombosis remains a constant source of postoperative morbidity and mortality. Despite recent advances in diagnostic methods, obstructive and nonobstructive PV thrombosis continues to be a challenge.[1–5]

Thrombosis occurs both in mechanical and biological prostheses,[6] leading especially in the former to predominant stenosis with or without some regurgitation depending on the dynamics of the prosthetic leaflet(s). In biological prostheses, subclinical thrombosis (i.e., occurrence of valve related thrombi without clinical symptoms) is more frequent than previously thought and may occur with minimal or no elevation in transvalvular gradients but nevertheless may lead to embolic complications and the development of pannus and hence, over time, to obstruction.[6,7]

The onset of symptoms may be very variable, gradual, or sudden. In fact, symptoms and clinical findings depend on how rapidly the prosthetic obstruction develops and on the severity of obstruction. Symptoms include dyspnea, generalized weakness, or, in cases of rapid progression of obstruction, pulmonary edema, or shock and cerebral as well as coronary or peripheral embolization.

DOI: 10.1201/9781003245407-12

The incidence of PV thrombosis is twice as high in the mitral than aortic position, and it is even higher in the tricuspid position, independently of the prosthesis type. Echocardiography should focus on determining movement of the occluder(s), and Doppler gradients across the valve. Moreover, mechanisms determining obstruction (thrombus, pannus, or both) may be identified in addition to the hemodynamic consequences of obstruction (left ventricular function, right ventricular function, and pulmonary systolic pressure).[1]

In the presence of clinical suspicion of PV thrombosis, transthoracic echocardiography should be immediately performed, and transesophageal echocardiography (TEE) and other diagnostic tests (including cinefluoroscopy) are generally recommended after this first-step approach. However, in patients with cardiogenic shock and in ventilated patients, TEE should be immediately performed.

Doppler gradients

PV obstruction may be suspected if the Doppler-derived *gradients are clearly higher* than those given for a normal prosthetic model of the same outer diameter and with comparable transprosthetic flow conditions. Therefore, tables with normal values of different prosthetic models may be very useful in comparing gradients in individual cases, but because of high variability in gradients, particularly in the aortic position, it is more important to evaluate and *compare* (when available) gradients obtained in acute conditions with previous Doppler gradients from the same patient. Gradient drop indicates successful thrombolysis in cases of PV thrombosis (Figure 12.1). It is therefore very important to perform Doppler echocardiographic follow-up early postoperatively to facilitate detection of changes in Doppler gradients. Although an *increased mean gradient* is the hallmark of PV thrombosis, approximately up to 20% of patients with mitral PV thrombosis (excluding those with nonobstructive thrombosis) have a normal Doppler gradient at rest.[2,3] This occurs mainly or exclusively in patients with bileaflet prostheses in the mitral position; therefore, *inspection of disk motion* by transthoracic echocardiography (V12.1A, V12.1C), TEE (V12.2) or cinefluoroscopy (V12.1B, V12.1D) is mandatory. In patients with aortic prostheses, the opposite situation may occur: as a result of the well-known pressure-recovery phenomenon (overestimation of Doppler gradient when compared with invasive true pressure drop caused by distal pressure recovery), very high gradients may be observed, particularly with small models even in normally functioning prostheses.[4,5] Furthermore, direct observation of disk motion in mechanical aortic prostheses is difficult even with TEE and is often inconclusive.

New parameters have been proposed to differentiate aortic valve prosthetic obstruction (AVPO) from prosthetic high-functional gradient or PV mismatch. In particular, these include delayed peak systolic velocity, leading to longer acceleration time (AT) and higher AT-to-ejection time (ET) ratios (AT/ET). AT (>95 ms) and AT/ET (>0.32) have the best accuracy (range 87–94%) in identifying AVPO.[8,9] Moreover, significant

intraprosthetic aortic regurgitation is usually associated with aortic thrombosis or pannus and is uncommon in PV mismatch.

Transthoracic Doppler evaluation must be performed using both flow-dependent parameters (e.g., V_{max}, EOA) as well as flow-independent parameters (e.g., AT, ET, AT/ET). Together they provide a measure of PV function independent of cardiac output variation. The combined use of flow dependent and flow independent parameters allows a better discrimination between normal PV, prosthesis-patient-mismatch phenomenon, and PV obstruction.[10,11]

The continuity equation can be used to estimate mitral and aortic valve areas, and pressure half-time may be used to evaluate tricuspid and mitral PV function. The pressure half-time depends also on PV type; although it may not give an accurate valve area, it is useful in tracking changes for an individual patient (for example, comparison with early normal postoperative values presumably reflecting normal PV function). The continuity equation is particularly useful when transvalvular flow is decreased, as in patients with left ventricular dysfunction.

For assessment of all these data in acute conditions, it is very important to evaluate from the parasternal window the *basic linear measurements*, including the left ventricular outflow tract (to be inserted into the continuity equation), and to measure gradients of the mitral and aortic prostheses in the four- and five-chamber apical views. From these views, abnormal flow jets (very thin and turbulent inflow jet[s] for the obstructed mitral valve and/or abnormal regurgitant jets for the mitral and aortic prostheses) should be searched for.

All these data may be also easily obtained by the TEE, and in this regard, transthoracic parameters may facilitate a focused and goal-oriented TEE study to visualize prosthetic jets to confirm or complete the diagnosis. For regurgitation, the transthoracic approach is very useful to evaluate the severity of the regurgitant lesion for aortic prostheses, and TEE may further improve recognition of the site of the regurgitant jet (intraprosthetic or paraprosthetic). The site and severity of mitral valve prosthetic jets are easily assessed by TEE studies (see also the following section on PV regurgitation).

Disk motion and excursion

A reduced or absent leaflet motion associated with an increased pressure gradient is the hallmark of PV thrombosis. *Cinefluoroscopy* is better suited than echocardiography to evaluate precisely the actual valve opening and closing angles (V12.1B, V12.1D). However, thanks to recent advances in transducers and ultrasound units, transthoracic echocardiography (V12.1A, V12.1C), and TEE (V12.2) now allow visualization of disk motion in a large number of cases. Typically, in multiple cross-sectional views (from the parasternal and apical views, *including off-axis views*), persistent restriction of prosthetic disk opening may be observed with M-mode and two-dimensional (2D) and three-dimensional (3D) echo. Altered mobility may involve one or both disks in bileaflet models (with different levels of alteration—from stuck leaflet to mild alteration of disk excursion) or the single occluder in a

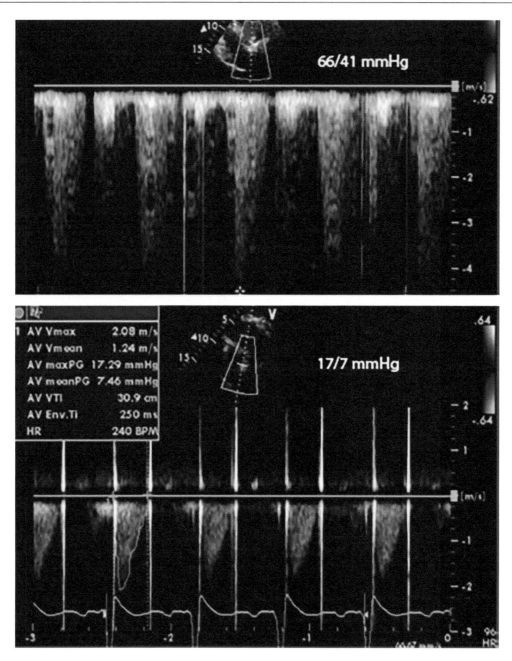

FIGURE 12.1   An 83-year-old woman with a mechanical aortic valve prosthesis was admitted to the coronary care unit with suddenly developed cardiogenic shock. Prosthetic valve clicks were not audible, and international normalized ratio was 3.59. Transthoracic echocardiography (TTE) revealed immobile prosthetic aortic disks (V12.1A) with systolic pressure gradients over the valve of 66/41 mmHg (upper panel) and a moderate central aortic regurgitation jet. On cinefluoroscopy, prosthetic disks looked stuck in a "middle" position (V12.1B). At this point, thrombolysis was administered. After 3 hours, valve clicks were audible. On control TTE, normal disk motion (V12.1C) and drop of systolic gradient over the valve to 17/7 mmHg was registered. The next morning, the patient was stable and extubated. The only adverse event that occurred was minor hematuria. On control fluoroscopy (V12.1D), regular opening of the artificial valve disks was registered.

(Image and videos provided by BI.)

single-disk (or ball) prosthesis. Even with recent transthoracic improvements in quality, TEE is significantly more accurate in detecting occluder motion, particularly in the mitral position (V12.2). Disk motion should be evaluated carefully throughout the studies, because it is not uncommon to observe cases with *intermittent* restriction of prosthetic disk opening. In these cases, M-mode, 2D, 3D, and Doppler may detect varying degrees and delays in the opening of the disk and associated intermittent increase of transprosthetic gradients.

In patients with symptoms of suspected PV dysfunction, the *integration of TTE and cinefluoroscopy* (V12.1A, V12.1B) appears to be a feasible and valuable strategy to assess PV function. This approach plays a pivotal role in diagnosis of relevant PV dysfunction and selection of patients who need further assessment with TEE or cardiac computed tomography (CT).[12]

Prosthetic valve thrombus and pannus

TEE (2D and 3D) is a sensitive and accurate tool for diagnosing PV thrombosis or pannus (Figure 12.2) (V12.3, V12.4), including the characteristics and mechanisms producing *obstruction* (Figure 12.3) (V12.5). Moreover, in cases with *embolism* (see Chapter 13) without clinical and echocardiographic signs of obstruction, TEE, or less frequently TTE, allow detection of nonobstructive thrombosis (V13.37).

Thrombus is defined as a distinct mass of abnormal echoes attached to the prosthesis and clearly seen throughout the cardiac study. The site, size, mobility, and signal characteristics of the mass should be annotated. Through multiple views and multiplane angle rotation, the extension and size of the thrombus may be evaluated and the area of the mass calculated. The ultrasound density of the mass may be classified as *soft or dense*. These echocardiographic parameters, in association with clinical data, may allow distinction between the *pannus and thrombus*.[13] This is essential to determine the underlying cause of PV dysfunction and to indicate optimal management of PV obstruction (surgery versus thrombolysis). Duration of symptoms, anticoagulation status, and ultrasound intensity of the mass obstructing mechanical prosthesis can, in fact, help to distinguish these two entities, even though recognition of the pannus is still difficult. Patients with thrombus have shorter time intervals from valve insertion to malfunction, shorter duration of symptoms, and lower rate of anticoagulation. Pannus formation is more common in the aortic position. On echocardiography, thrombi are in general larger than the pannus and appear as a soft mass, whereas the pannus is more echodense (increased reflectivity). A recent meta-analysis showed that in acquired PV obstruction caused by thrombosis, mass detection by TEE and leaflet restriction detected by cinefluoroscopy were observed in the majority of cases (96% and 100%, respectively).[14] In contrast, in acquired PV obstruction free of thrombosis (pannus), leaflet restriction detected by cinefluoroscopy was absent in some cases (17%), and mass detection by TEE was absent in the majority of cases (66%). In case of mass detection by TEE, predictors for obstructive thrombus masses (compared with pannus) were leaflet restriction, soft echo density, and increased mass length. In situations of inconclusive echocardiography computed tomography may correctly detect pannus or thrombus based on the morphologic aspects and localization.

Moreover, TEE may also reveal other complications such as the coexistence of left atrial and/or left atrial appendage thrombi, which may be associated particularly with severe mitral prosthetic obstruction.

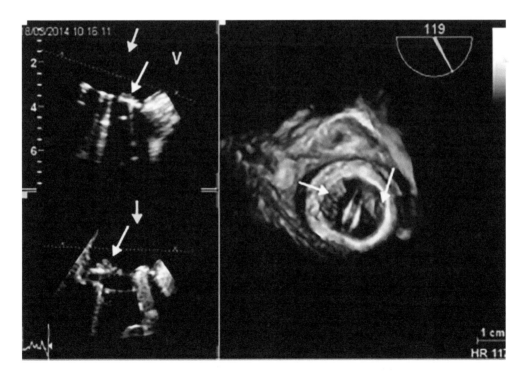

FIGURE 12.2 Biplane two-dimensional transesophageal echocardiography (TEE) showing a bileaflet mechanical mitral valve prosthesis with normal motion of both disks (V12.3). Note the presence of the mass (thrombus or pannus) on the atrial side of the prosthesis (white arrows, upper and lower left panels) that does not appear to affect the valve function (V12.3). Two masses (larger at the left side and smaller at the right side of the prosthesis) can be better appreciated with 3D TEE (white arrows, right panel) (V12.3).

(Image and video provided by BAP.)

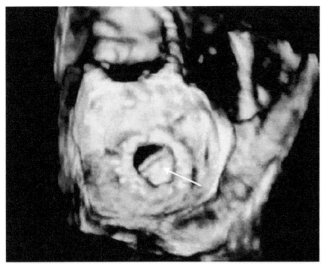

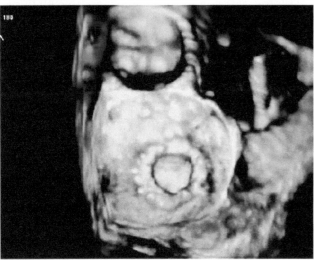

FIGURE 12.3 Images of the mechanical bileaflet mitral valve prosthesis from the atrial side (surgical view) obtained via 3D TEE, with the aorta positioned in the upper part of the view and the tricuspid valve positioned on the right (a catheter has been inserted into the right cavities), showing complete blockage of one of the two disks. Note the absence of motion of one of the disks (arrow) during cardiac cycle (diastole, upper panel; systole, lower panel) (V12.5).

Management of prosthetic valve thrombosis

Surgical intervention has been the traditional way to treat PV thrombosis. More recently, thrombolysis has been reported to be an effective alternative treatment option.[15–17] Successful thrombolysis has been demonstrated in a recent large trial in 83.2% of cases.[18] Success of thrombolysis was associated with a shorter time interval after surgery, but not with New York Heart Association functional class, position of the thrombosed valve, bileaflet versus monoleaflet valve design, mobility of the thrombus, suboptimal international normalized ratio on admission, or previous aspirin use.

Echocardiographic data (including Doppler data, disk mobility, and thrombus or pannus) are extremely useful in choosing the best therapeutic intervention (V13.3, V13.4). *Thrombus size* is an independent predictor of outcome when thrombolysis is attempted.[18,19] Patients with a small thrombus (area of the thrombus of <0.8 cm^2) have essentially no or minimal complications with thrombolysis. Patients with functional classes III and IV benefit even more by *quantification of thrombus burden*. In this subgroup with high surgical mortality, a small thrombus detected by TEE identifies patients with low complication and low death rates who may benefit from thrombolysis as a first-line therapy. On the other hand, patients in functional classes III and IV with larger thrombi (>0.8 cm^2) need assessment of total surgical risk but are, in general, candidates for valve surgery. Furthermore, *disk motion* may predict the efficacy of thrombolytic treatment.[20] In mitral valve thrombosis (bileaflet prostheses), hypomobile leaflets always recover regardless of symptom duration and extent of disk motion reduction, whereas completely blocked leaflets, particularly in late PV thrombosis, do not respond to thrombolysis. Therefore, echocardiography (and cinefluoroscopy) may predict the results of thrombolysis by accurately defining the amount of restriction in disk motion. In bileaflet prostheses with one leaflet blocked and the other hypomobile (without contraindication because of a very large thrombus), thrombolysis may be used to restore normal movement to the hypomobile leaflet, to improve the patient's clinical and hemodynamic condition before surgery.

These observations clearly indicate the *importance of a complete* TTE and TEE evaluation. The key for diagnosis and making decision for medical versus surgical treatment is not only the presence of an increased gradient but also accurate evaluation of thrombus size, leaflet motion, and coexistence of atrial thrombi. Both cinefluoroscopy (V12.1B) and cardiac CT (V12.6) are excellent alternatives for the assessment of leaflet motion.

PROSTHETIC VALVE REGURGITATION

All mechanical prostheses and practically all bioprostheses show minor regurgitation already when functioning normally. In mechanical prostheses, there is a closure backflow by the closing motion of the occluder (disk or leaflets), and an additional leakage flow after closure because of small leaks between the occluder and the ring or struts incorporated by design to ensure mobility and continuous flushing to prevent microthrombi. These small leaks may be picked up on spectral and color Doppler and show regurgitant jet patterns typical of valve types,[21] but they usually can be easily distinguished from major regurgitation. In bioprostheses, there is also minimal regurgitation similar to native "physiologic" regurgitation. The following mechanisms are involved when severe and often acute regurgitation occurs in a valve prosthesis:

- *Structural damage.* The prototype of this mechanism is embolism of the occluder after strut fracture, leading to absence of any valve mechanism. For instance, this event occurred in some early Björk-Shiley valves, but it occurs rarely in other mechanical valves. In bioprostheses, tears or ruptures in degenerated leaflets may also lead to sudden development of severe regurgitation.

- *Ring dehiscence and large paravalvular leaks.* Suture insufficiency may lead to abnormal motion of the entire prosthesis ("rocking") (V9.3A, V9.3B, V12.7A, V12.7B, V12.14A, V12.14B), which itself is mechanically intact but produces regurgitation by a large gap between the periannular tissue and the prosthesis ring. There is a continuum from paravalvular leak to dehiscence, although the latter is usually restricted to valves that move abnormally in toto. Infective endocarditis (see later) of the prosthetic ring may lead to paravalvular leaks or dehiscence (V12.8A, V12.8B, V12.8C, V12.8D, V12.8E).
- *Fixation of the occluder* in a semiopen or semiclosed position by thrombosis, pannus, or other reasons, such as large vegetations. In these cases, there is often also an obstruction, but regurgitation may be clinically more evident.
- *Infective endocarditis* (see the following section) can directly destroy bioprosthetic leaflets, leading to prolapse, flail, defects, or rupture of entire bioprosthetic leaflets.

The typical echocardiographic signs of prosthetic regurgitation are summarized in Table 12.1. The clinical consequences of acute severe prosthetic regurgitation correspond to those of acute regurgitation of the respective native valve, with prominent backward failure and pulmonary congestion or edema for aortic and mitral prostheses and possible additional forward failure or full-fledged cardiogenic shock. In extremely severe regurgitation, typical murmurs such as the systolic murmur of mitral regurgitation may be absent or inaudible as a result of the massively reduced cardiac output.

The severity of regurgitation can be assessed by the same criteria used to define the severity of native valvular regurgitation. Thanks to the technological improvement of the 3D TEE, an increasingly realistic imaging of the leaflets of mechanical and biological prostheses has been provided in recent years. One of the advantages of this rapidly evolving technique is that it allows visualization from both the atrial and ventricular perspective (Figure 12.4). Three-dimensional TEE also allows obtaining a panoramic view of the suture ring, leaflets, and discs and may also show the exact number, site, size, and shape (circular, linear, crescent or irregular) of the PV leaflets. One of these imaging tools, the *transillumination*, makes it possible to change the lighting conditions and therefore to improve contrast, to change shadows and to add more depth perception. Moreover, the addition of color Doppler allows visualization of the flow trajectory, while *transparency* peels away layers to see the jet origin (Figure 12.5).

TABLE 12.1   Echocardiographic Signs of Mitral and Aortic Prosthetic Valve Regurgitation

Echocardiographic signs of mitral prosthetic regurgitation
- Structural damage to the prosthesis, such as torn bioprosthetic leaflet, leaflet defect, or loss or immobilization of occluder in mechanical valves. The cause is degenerative, material failure (mechanical prostheses), or infective endocarditis.
- Paravalvular interruption of continuity at the level of the sewing ring. If a relatively small section of the ring circumference has lost its anchoring in the tissue, a paravalvular leak is present, with varying severity of regurgitation. If the section is big enough to produce rocking of the whole prosthesis, typically >40% of the circumference, this is termed *dehiscence*, and severe regurgitation is always present.
- Forward flow is increased, with increased transmitral flow velocities, mimicking prosthetic obstruction. The prosthesis-specific pressure half-time, however, is not markedly changed. Note that regurgitation and true obstruction may coexist, as in prosthetic thrombosis.
- Proximal jet width is related to regurgitation severity as in native mitral regurgitation. A cutoff of 6–7 mm is usually chosen to separate severe, "surgical" regurgitation from lesser degrees.
- The presence of a reproducible, large (>1 cm²) proximal isovelocity surface area (PISA) indicates the presence of substantial regurgitation.
- Reversal of systolic pulmonary venous inflow (high specificity and modest sensitivity).
- In very severe regurgitation, there may be a "shoulder" in the continuous-wave signal of mitral regurgitation, indicating a steep rise in left atrial pressure in late systole.

Echocardiographic signs of aortic prosthetic regurgitation
- Structural damage to the prosthesis, such as torn bioprosthetic leaflet, leaflet defect, or loss or immobilization of occluder in mechanical valves. The cause is degenerative, material failure (mechanical prostheses) or infective endocarditis.
- Paravalvular interruption of continuity at the level of the sewing ring, with consecutive paravalvular leak or dehiscence.
- Premature mitral valve closure (no A-wave) and shortened mitral E-wave deceleration.
- Forward flow is increased, with increased transaortic flow velocities, mimicking prosthetic obstruction. Note that regurgitation and true obstruction may coexist, as in prosthetic thrombosis.
- Proximal jet width is related to regurgitation severity, as in native aortic regurgitation, but usually is very difficult to gauge owing to shadowing and jet artifacts.
- The presence of a reproducible, large (>1 cm²) PISA on the aortic side indicates the presence of substantial regurgitation.
- Shortened pressure half-time (<250 ms) of the continuous-wave Doppler signal of aortic regurgitation indicates severe regurgitation.
- Holodiastolic flow reversal in the ascending and particularly the descending aorta is a clear sign of severe aortic regurgitation (high specificity and moderate sensitivity).

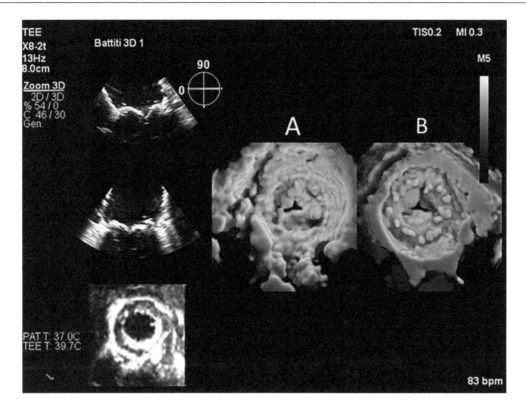

FIGURE 12.4   3D TEE of a biological mitral valve prosthesis in a patient with severe mitral stenosis and regurgitation. Simultaneous views from the left ventricle (A) and left atrium (B, surgical view) showing degeneration of the leaflets, resulted in severe stenosis (note very small valve orifice).

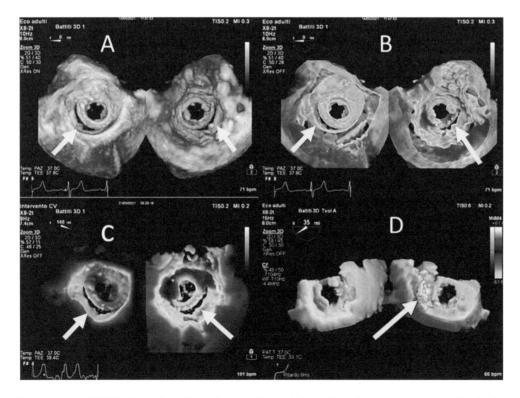

FIGURE 12.5   Simultaneous 3D TEE views from the left ventricle and from the left atrium (surgical view) of a biological mitral valve prosthesis with a paravalvular leak. (A) *Standard 3D visualization* with an abnormal paravalvular space (arrows). (B) Same views in *transparency* mode. (C) Same views in *transillumination* mode. (D) Same views with added color flow which confirms the leakage (arrow).

Immediate echocardiography is mandatory. In most cases, the yield of TEE is markedly higher than TTE, and the clinical urgency makes a definitive diagnosis imperative. The techniques and methods to judge prosthetic regurgitation are not fundamentally different from the assessment of native valves (see also Chapters 9 and 10).[21] However, artifacts and shadowing from valve prostheses and the fact that these patients very frequently have pathologically altered cardiac morphology make assessment considerably more difficult. It should be remembered that shadowing from a mitral prosthesis will often obscure mitral prosthetic regurgitation when viewed from an apical TTE window. The presence of a large proximal convergence zone on the ventricular and therefore unobstructed side of the prosthesis may indicate paravalvular leakage. Use of parasternal and subcostal windows therefore is mandatory, and TEE is recommended. Contrary to its superiority for mitral regurgitation, assessment of aortic regurgitation (e.g., after transcatheter aortic valve implantation—TAVI) with TEE may be very difficult; among other reasons, this is because of difficult alignment of the continuous-wave cursor with the direction of regurgitant flow, although often additional information is obtained (e.g., vegetation due to infective endocarditis and abscess).

PROSTHETIC VALVE INFECTIVE ENDOCARDITIS

PV endocarditis has an incidence of approximately 1% during the first year and less than 0.5% per patient and year thereafter. Due to difficulties in PV imaging, detection of vegetations and other signs of endocarditis is more challenging than in native valves. *The suspicion of PV endocarditis should therefore always prompt TEE.* Furthermore, the presence of a fever or systemic inflammatory signs in a patient with heart valve prostheses should always raise the suspicion of prosthetic endocarditis. Rapid diagnosis is particularly critical if staphylococcal bacteremia is found. TEE allows thorough assessment, particularly of the atrial side of mitral prostheses (V13.36A, V13.36B), and also better evaluation of aortic prostheses. It has been convincingly shown that the diagnostic accuracy of TEE for the detection of small vegetations, particularly abscesses, is markedly higher than that of transthoracic echo.[22] Typical signs of infective prosthetic endocarditis include the following:

- *Vegetations.* These are mobile, irregular masses attached to prosthetic structures, most often on the low-pressure side (atrial side in mitral prostheses; ventricular side on aortic prostheses) (V13.18A, V13.18B). Their maximal linear dimension correlates roughly with complications, particularly risk of embolism, and outcomes. Very large vegetations may cause obstruction, although this is rare (V14.4A, V14.4B, V14.4C). The echodensity

correlates roughly with acuity of the disease; fresh vegetations have the echodensity of myocardium or less, and old vegetations are often calcified (V12.12).
- *Abscesses.* These are perivalvular cavities (Figure 12.6) (V12.9A, V12.9B, V12.9C, V12.9D) or localized perivalvular tissue thickening. Their presence and extent are greatly underestimated by transthoracic echo and often even by TEE. Ring abscesses are typical of mechanical prostheses. The cavities may or may not have access to heart chambers or the ascending aorta and may create pseudoaneurysm (V12.13A, V12.13B, V12.13C, V12.13D) or fistulas between heart chambers.
- *Defects (holes) in bioprosthetic leaflets creating regurgitation.*
- *Paraprosthetic leaks and prosthetic dehiscence* (V12.10A, V12.10B) (Figure 12.7) (V12.11). This is discussed in the section on prosthetic valve regurgitation.
- *Pericardial effusion.* Small effusions often signal bacterial tissue invasion.

Because prosthetic endocarditis practically mandates *urgent surgical* valve replacement due to its poor responsiveness to antibiotic treatment, it is very important to furnish to the surgeon complete information about the extent of endocarditis and the presence of complications. All valves have to be systematically evaluated for the signs of endocarditis.

On the other hand, *negative TEE is a strong argument against the presence of infective endocarditis, but it does not completely rule out the disease.* There may be vegetations too small to be visualized, acoustic shadowing, or artifacts from the prosthesis. However, negative repeat TEE after a few days (5–7 days) has a very high negative predictive value to rule out endocarditis.

TAVI AND THE ROLE OF EMERGENCY ECHOCARDIOGRAPHY

TAVI has evolved into standard therapy for elderly and/or high-risk patients with severe aortic valve stenosis who require valve replacement. Moreover, recently TAVI has been also indicated in patients with intermediate or even low risk. Nonetheless, the procedure still bears specific risks for complications that may critically influence the outcome. In this regard, echocardiography (both TTE and TEE) is extremely useful in rapid recognition of several complications (see also Chapter 22). Besides vascular complications, cardiac tamponade, aortic root rupture and coronary obstruction may occur during intraprocedural or periprocedural periods. All these complications may be immediately recognized by TEE (if the patient is monitored in general anesthesia); otherwise, TEE should be performed quickly.[23]

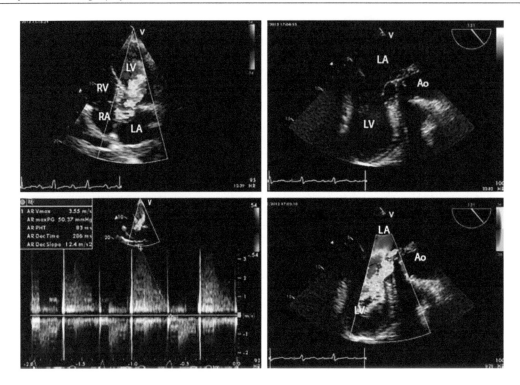

FIGURE 12.6 A 59-year-old man underwent aortic valve replacement (St. Jude no. 21) 9 months before presentation. At admission, he complained of fatigue and dyspnea; he was febrile (38.5°C), with basal rales and systolic and diastolic heart murmur. Color Doppler in the transthoracic apical five-chamber view revealed torrential aortic regurgitation jet (upper left panel) (V12.9A) with a pressure half-time of the regurgitation signal of 83 ms (lower left panel), consistent with severe acute aortic regurgitation. Emergent transesophageal echocardiography showed perivalvular pseudoaneurysm formation (*) and prosthetic valve dehiscence (V12.9B, V12.9C, V12.9D). The patient underwent urgent cardiac surgery but died after several days in sepsis and with multiorgan failure. Ao: aorta; LA: left atrium; LV: left ventricle; RA: right atrium; RV: right ventricle.

(Image and videos provided by PMM.)

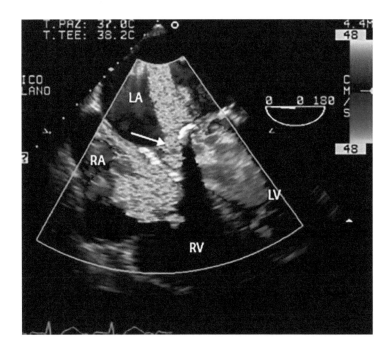

FIGURE 12.7 Paraprosthetic mitral regurgitation. (V12.11). Transesophageal echocardiography shows severe mitral regurgitation in a patient with mechanical mitral valve prosthesis, with the origin of the jet (arrow) outside of the prosthetic annulus, indicating a prosthetic valve dehiscence. There is also associated severe tricuspid regurgitation.

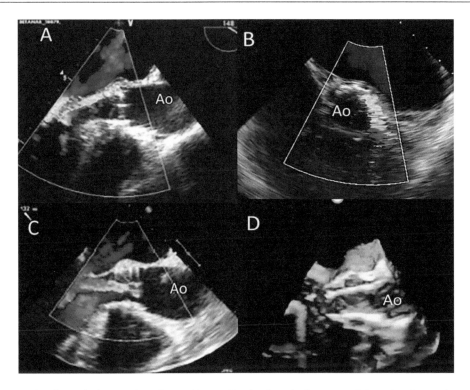

FIGURE 12.8   Intraprocedural TEE during TAVI performed immediately after deployment of the valve. Regurgitant jet due to paraprosthetic leak in the long-axis (A) and short-axis (B) views. (C) Transprosthetic regurgitation. (D) Incomplete expansion of the device (3D TEE).

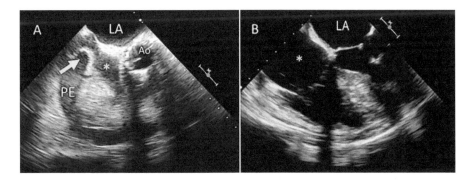

FIGURE 12.9   Cardiac tamponade due to right ventricular perforation during TAVI. (A) TEE showing pericardial effusion (PE) with right atrial collapse (arrow). (B) Immediate pericardiocentesis resulted in complete disappearance of pericardial effusion with normal right atrial cavity on control TEE. Ao: aorta; LA: left atrium; *: right atrial cavity.

Cardiac tamponade may occur due to perforation of the RV (Figure 12.9), of the LV or related to annular rupture. Echo-guided pericardiocentesis should be immediately performed or if unfeasible or the complication involved the aortic annulus or the aortic wall (aortic dissection) surgery may be indicated.

Moreover, paraprosthetic aortic regurgitation (AR) after TAVI has been identified as an important prognostic determinant. AR can be classified into transvalvular and paravalvular forms (Figure 12.8) (V14.9A, V14.9B), and TTE or TEE may differentiate type and severity of the lesion (see Chapter 22 for more details).[23]

LIST OF VIDEOS

VIDEO 12.1A   Thrombosis of mechanical aortic valve prosthesis (1/4): An 83-year-old woman with a mechanical aortic valve prosthesis admitted to the coronary care unit with suddenly developed cardiogenic shock. Prosthetic valve clicks were not audible, and international normalized ratio was 3.59. Transthoracic echocardiography (TTE) revealed immobile aortic prosthetic disks with systolic pressure gradients over the valve of 66/41 mmHg (see Figure 12.1 in the book) and a moderate central aortic regurgitation jet. On cinefluoroscopy (see Video 12.1B), prosthetic disks looked stuck in a "middle" position. At this point thrombolysis was administered. After 3 hours, valve clicks were audible. On control TTE, normal disk motion (see Video 12.1C) and systolic gradient over drop over the valve to 17/7 mmHg was registered (see Figure 12.1 in the book). The next morning, the patient was stable and extubated. The only adverse event that occurred was minor hematuria. On control fluoroscopy (see Video 12.1D), regular opening of the artificial valve disks was registered. *(Video provided by BI.)*

VIDEO 12.1B   Thrombosis of mechanical aortic valve prosthesis (2/4): Cinefluoroscopy in a patient with suspected prosthetic valve obstruction and suddenly developed cardiogenic shock demonstrates valve disks stuck in a "middle" position (see also Videos 12.1A, 12.1C, and 12.1D), indicating valve obstruction, presumably by thrombus. *(Video provided by BI.)*

VIDEO 12.1C   Thrombosis of mechanical aortic valve prosthesis (3/4): On control transthoracic echocardiography, 3 hours after successful thrombolysis in a patient with obstruction of the aortic prosthesis and suddenly developed cardiogenic shock (see Videos 12.1A, 12.1B, and 12.1D), normal disk motion with no significant systolic gradient over the valve (17/7 mmHg) was registered (see Figure 12.1 in the book). *(Video provided by BI.)*

VIDEO 12.1D   Thrombosis of mechanical aortic valve prosthesis (4/4): On control cinefluoroscopy, 3 hours after successful thrombolysis in a patient with obstruction of the aortic valve prosthesis and suddenly developed cardiogenic shock (see Videos 12.1A, 12.1B, and 12.1C), normal movements of the prosthetic aortic valve disks were registered. *(Video provided by BI.)*

VIDEO 12.2   Prosthetic mitral valve dysfunction from pannus causing obstruction: Transesophageal echocardiography reveals the alteration of both mitral valve disks. Specifically, one leaflet (left side in this view) is stuck, whereas the other shows incomplete diastolic opening. Despite the absence of thrombus inside the prosthesis, the echodense image on the left ventricular side of the prosthesis suggest the presence of pannus that limits disk motion, causing severe prosthetic obstruction.

VIDEO 12.3   Thrombosis of prosthetic mitral valve: Biplane two-dimensional transesophageal echocardiography (TEE) shows a bileaflet mitral prosthesis with normal motion of both disks (upper and lower left panels). Note the presence of the mass (thrombus or pannus) on the atrial side of the prosthesis that does not appear to affect the valve function. Two masses (larger at the left side and smaller at the right side of the prosthesis) can be better appreciated by three-dimensional TEE (right panel). *(Video provided by BAP.)*

VIDEO   12.4   Prosthetic aortic valve thrombosis: Transesophageal echocardiography long-axis view (at 133°) showing the presence of a large mobile thrombus attached to the ventricular side of the prosthesis, protruding into the left ventricular outflow tract.

VIDEO   12.5   Prosthetic mitral valve dysfunction: Three-dimensional transesophageal echocardiography showing complete blockage of one of the two disks of a mechanical bileaflet mitral valve prosthesis. The mitral valve prosthesis is imaged in a surgical view (from left atrial side) with the aorta positioned in the upper part of the view, and the tricuspid valve (a catheter has been inserted into the right heart cavities) positioned on the right.

VIDEO   12.6   Cardiac computed tomography (CT) of the bileaflet mitral valve prosthesis: Cardiac CT shows normal disk motion of the bileaflet mitral valve prosthesis. *(Video provided by RV.)*

VIDEO 12.7A   Dehiscence of aortic valve bioprosthesis (1/2): Zoom transesophageal echocardiographic view showing "rocking" movements of the aortic valve bioprosthesis from ring dehiscence causing severe acute aortic regurgitation (see also Videos 12.7B, 9.3A, and 9.3B).

VIDEO 12.7B   Dehiscence of aortic valve bioprosthesis (2/2): Transesophageal echocardiographic long-axis view showing severe aortic regurgitation by color Doppler caused by ring dehiscence of the aortic valve bioprosthesis (see also Videos 12.7A, 9.3A and 9.3B).

VIDEO 12.8A   Paravalvular leak of a bileaflet mechanical aortic valve prosthesis (1/5): A 63-year-old woman with mechanical aortic valve prosthesis (St. Jude no. 19) was admitted to the coronary care unit with pulmonary edema and irregular tachycardia (130 bpm, atrial fibrillation). Transthoracic echocardiography revealed left ventricle of normal size (end-diastolic diameter, 49 mm; end-systolic diameter, 39 mm) and global systolic function, with restrictive transmitral flow pattern (E/A 2.7, DT 135 ms). The motion of prosthetic valve leaflets looked normal, but color Doppler showed significant turbulent jet of aortic regurgitation that appeared to be paravalvular (shown here). Pressure half-time of the regurgitant signal was 230 ms. Transesophageal echocardiography in a modified short-axis view of the base of the heart revealed the presence of an unusual echo-free space at the posterior part of the prosthetic ring (see Video 12.8B), where turbulent flow can be noted (see Video 12.8C). The gap between the periannular tissue and the prosthesis ring is seen also in the modified four-chamber view (see Video 12.8D), with significant paravalvular aortic regurgitation (see Video 12.8E). The patient was managed conservatively.

VIDEO 12.8B   Paravalvular leak of a bileaflet mechanical aortic valve prosthesis (2/5): Transesophageal echocardiography in a modified short-axis view of the base of the heart in a patient with bileaflet mechanical aortic valve prosthesis showing the presence of an unusual echo-free space at the posterior prosthetic ring, where the origin of a turbulent jet was noted on color Doppler (see Video 12.8C), indicating paravalvular leak (see also Videos 12.8A, 12.8D, and 12.8E).

VIDEO 12.8C   Paravalvular leak of a bileaflet mechanical aortic valve prosthesis (3/5): Transesophageal echocardiography in a modified short-axis view of the base of the heart in a patient with a bileaflet mechanical aortic valve prosthesis showing a turbulent jet by color Doppler at the site of the unusual echo-free space at the posterior prosthetic ring (see Video 12.8B), indicating paravalvular leak (see also Videos 12.8A, 12.8D, and 12.8 E).

VIDEO 12.8D   Paravalvular leak of a bileaflet mechanical aortic valve prosthesis (4/5): Modified four-chamber transesophageal echocardiographic view in a patient with a bileaflet mechanical aortic valve prosthesis showing the gap between the periannular tissue and the prosthesis ring where the origin of a turbulent jet was noted on color Doppler (see Video 12.8C), indicating paravalvular leak (see also Videos 12.8A, 12.8B, and 12.8E).

VIDEO 12.8E   Paravalvular leak of a bileaflet mechanical aortic valve prosthesis (5/5): Modified four-chamber transesophageal echocardiographic view in a patient with a bileaflet mechanical aortic valve prosthesis showing a turbulent jet of significant paravalvular aortic regurgitation by color Doppler (see also Videos 12.8A, 12.8B, 12.8C, and 12.8D).

VIDEO 12.9A   Perivalvular pseudoaneurysm of the prosthetic aortic valve (1/4): A 59-year-old man underwent aortic valve replacement (St. Jude no. 21) 9 months before presentation. At admission, he complained of fatigue and dyspnea; he was febrile (38.5°C), with basal rales and systolic and diastolic heart murmur. Color Doppler in the transthoracic apical five-chamber view revealed torrential aortic regurgitation with a pressure half-time of 83 ms (see Figure 12.4 in the book), consistent with severe acute aortic regurgitation. The cause of aortic regurgitation could not be detected by transthoracic echocardiography. However, emergent transesophageal echocardiography showed perivalvular pseudoaneurysm formation and prosthetic valve dehiscence (see Videos 12.9B, 12.9C, and 12.9D). The patient underwent urgent cardiac surgery but died after several days in sepsis and with multiorgan failure. *(Video provided by PMM.)*

VIDEO 12.9B   Perivalvular pseudoaneurysm of the prosthetic aortic valve (2/4): This transesophageal long-axis view reveals a pulsatile perivalvular echo-free space that communicates with the lumen, indicating pseudoaneurysm formation (see zoom view Video 12.9C). Severe aortic regurgitation due to prosthetic aortic valve dehiscence was seen on color Doppler (see Videos 12.9A and 12.9D). The patient underwent urgent cardiac surgery but died after several days in sepsis and with multiorgan failure. *(Video provided by PMM.)*

VIDEO 12.9C   Perivalvular pseudoaneurysm of the prosthetic aortic valve (3/4): Zoom view of the perivalvular pseudoaneurysm of the prosthetic aortic valve (see also Videos 12.9A, 12.9B, and 12.9D). *(Video provided by PMM.)*

VIDEO 12.9D   Perivalvular pseudoaneurysm of the prosthetic aortic valve (4/4): Color Doppler in a transesophageal long-axis view revealed severe aortic regurgitation caused by perivalvular pseudoaneurysm formation and prosthetic aortic valve dehiscence (see Videos 12.9A, 12.9B, and 12.9C). The patient underwent urgent cardiac surgery but died after several days in sepsis and with multiorgan failure. *(Video provided by PMM.)*

VIDEO 12.10A   Paravalvular leak in a suspected prosthetic valve endocarditis (1/2): Transthoracic echocardiographic apical long-axis view in a patient with congestive heart failure and suspected

prosthetic valve endocarditis showing the gap between the periannular tissue and the mitral prosthesis ring, with paravalvular mitral regurgitation (see Video 12.10B). *(Video provided by IS.)*

VIDEO 12.10B   Paravalvular leak in a suspected prosthetic valve endocarditis (2/2): Transthoracic echocardiographic apical long-axis view in a patient with congestive heart failure and suspected prosthetic valve endocarditis showing the jet of paravalvular mitral regurgitation through the gap between the periannular tissue and the mitral prosthesis ring (see Video 12.10A). *(Video provided by IS.)*

VIDEO 12.11   Paraprosthetic mitral regurgitation: Transesophageal echocardiography showing a severe mitral regurgitation in a patient with mechanical mitral valve prosthesis, with the origin of the jet outside of the prosthetic annulus, indicating a prosthetic valve dehiscence. Note also associated severe tricuspid regurgitation.

VIDEO 12.12   Multiple transesophageal echocardiographic views of a mobile mass attached to mitral valve prosthesis: Different transesophageal echocardiographic views allow excellent visualization of the mitral valve from the atrial aspect without interference by acoustic shadow from the prosthetic material. These transesophageal echocardiographic views show mobile masses attached to the prosthetic mitral valve consistent with thrombi or vegetations with high embolic potential. Eccentric jet of mitral regurgitation can be seen by color Doppler (left lower panel).

VIDEO 12.13A   Infective endocarditis of the aortic valve prosthesis complicated by abscess and perivalvular pseudoaneurysm formation (1/4). TEE showing drained periannular abscess of the mechanical aortic valve prosthesis drained into the left ventricular outflow tract resulted in perivalvular pseudoaneurysm formation (see Videos 12.13B, 12.13C, and 1213 D). *(Video provided by ISr and MS.)*

VIDEO 12.13B   Infective endocarditis of the aortic valve prosthesis complicated by abscess and perivalvular pseudoaneurysm formation (2/4). TEE with color Doppler showing pathologic turbulence inside perivalvular pseudoaneurysm cavity (see Videos 12.13A, 12.13C, and 12.13D). *(Video provided by ISr and MS.)*

VIDEO 12.13C   Infective endocarditis of the aortic valve prosthesis complicated by abscess and perivalvular pseudoaneurysm formation (3/4). TEE in short axis showing drained periannular abscess of the mechanical aortic valve prosthesis drained into the left ventricular outflow tract resulted in perivalvular pseudoaneurysm formation (see Video 12.13A, 12.13B and 12.13D). *(Video provided by ISr and MS.)*

VIDEO 12.13D   Infective endocarditis of the aortic valve prosthesis complicated by abscess and perivalvular pseudoaneurysm formation (4/4). TEE in short axis with color Doppler showing pathologic turbulence inside perivalvular pseudoaneurysm cavity (see Video 12.13A, 12.13B and 12.13C). *(Video provided by ISr and MS.)*

VIDEO 12.14A   Acute aortic insufficiency caused by dehiscence of an aortic valve bioprosthesis (1/2): Transthoracic apical five-chamber view demonstrates a dehiscence of the aortic valve bioprosthesis. Note that the prosthesis appears unstable, with rocking movements during the cardiac cycle. At the site of the dehiscence, turbulent jet of paravalvular severe aortic insufficiency can be noted on color Doppler (see Video 12.14B). *(Video provided by IS.)*

VIDEO 12.14B　Acute aortic insufficiency caused by dehiscence of an aortic valve bioprosthesis (2/2): Transthoracic apical five-chamber view demonstrates a turbulent jet of paravalvular aortic insufficiency on color Doppler, caused by dehiscence of the aortic valve bioprosthesis (see Video 12.14A). Note that the prosthesis is unstable, with rocking movements during the cardiac cycle. Pressure half-time of the regurgitant envelope was 106 ms, indicating acute severe aortic insufficiency. *(Video provided by IS.)*

REFERENCES

1. Zoghbi WA, Chambers JB, Dumesnil JG, et al. Recommendations for evaluation of prosthetic valves with echocardiography and Doppler ultrasound: a report from the American Society of Echocardiography's Guidelines and Standards Committee and the Task Force on Prosthetic Valves, developed in conjunction with the American College of Cardiology Cardiovascular Imaging Committee, Cardiac Imaging Committee of the American Heart Association, the European Association of Echocardiography, a registered branch of the European Society of Cardiology, the Japanese Society of Echocardiography and the Canadian Society of Echocardiography, endorsed by the American College of Cardiology Foundation, American Heart Association, European Association of Echocardiography, a registered branch of the European Society of Cardiology, the Japanese Society of Echocardiography, and Canadian Society of Echocardiography. J Am Soc Echocardiogr 2009; 22:975–1014.
2. Montorsi P, De Bernardi F, Muratori M, Cavoretto D, Pepi M. Role of cine-fluoroscopy, transthoracic and transesophageal echocardiography in patients with suspected prosthetic heart valve thrombosis. Am J Cardiol 2000; 85:58–64.
3. Montorsi P, Cavoretto D, Parolari A, Muratori M, Alimento M, Pepi M. Diagnosing prosthetic mitral valve thrombosis and the effect of the type of prostheses. Am J Cardiol 2002; 90:73–6.
4. Baumgartner H, Khan S, DeRobertis M, Czer L, Maurer G. Discrepancies between Doppler and catheter gradients in aortic prosthetic valves in vitro: a manifestation of localized gradients and pressure recovery. Circulation 1990; 82:1467–75.
5. Baumgartner H, Schima H, Tulzer G, Kuhn P. Effect of stenosis geometry on the Doppler-catheter gradient relation in vitro: a manifestation of pressure recovery. J Am Coll Cardiol 1993; 21:1018–25.
6. Makkar RR, Fontana G, Jilaihawi H, et al. Possible subclinical leaflet thrombosis in bioprosthetic aortic valves. N Engl J Med 2015; 373(21):2015–24.
7. Egbe AC, Pislaru SV, Pellikka PA, et al. Bioprosthetic valve thrombosis versus structural failure: clinical and echocardiographic predictors. J Am Coll Cardiol 2015; 66:2285–94.
8. Muratori M, Montorsi P, Maffessanti F, et al. Dysfunction of bileaflet aortic prosthesis: accuracy of transthoracic echocardiography versus fluoroscopy. JACC Cardiovasc Imaging 2013; 6:62–71.
9. Ben Zekry S, Saad RM, Ozkan M, et al. Flow acceleration time and ratio of acceleration time to ejection time for prosthetic aortic valve function. JACC Cardiovasc Imaging 2011; 4·1161–70.
10. Muratori M, Fusini L, Mancini ME, et al. The role of multimodality imaging in left-sided prosthetic valve dysfunction. J Cardiovasc Dev Dis 2022; 9:12.
11. Lancellotti P, Pibarot P, Chambers J, et al. Recommendations for the imaging assessment of prosthetic heart valves: a report from the European Association of Cardiovascular Imaging endorsed by the Chinese Society of Echocardiography, the Inter-American Society of Echocardiography, and the Brazilian Department of Cardiovascular Imaging. Eur Heart J Cardiovasc Imaging 2016; 17(6):589–90.
12. Muratori M, Fusini L, Ali SG, et al. Detection of mechanical prosthetic valve dysfunction. Am J Cardiol 2021; 150:101–9.
13. Barbetseas J, Nagueh SF, Pitsavos C, et al. Differentiating thrombus from pannus formation in obstructed mechanical prosthetic valves: an evaluation of clinical, transthoracic and transesophageal echocardiographic parameters. J Am Coll Cardiol 1998; 32:1410–7.
14. Tanis W, Habets J, van den Brink RB, Symersky P, Budde RP, Chamuleau SA. Differentiation of thrombus from pannus as the cause of acquired mechanical prosthetic heart valve obstruction by non-invasive imaging: a review of the literature. Eur Heart J Cardiovasc Imaging 2014; 15(2):119–29.
15. Lengyel M, Fuster V, Keltai M, et al. Guidelines for management of left-sided prosthetic valves thrombosis: a role for thrombolytic therapy. J Am Coll Cardiol 1997; 30:1521–6.
16. Lengyel M, Vandor L. The role of thrombolysis in management of left-side prosthetic valve thrombosis: a study of 85 cases diagnosed by transesophageal echocardiography. J Heart Valve Dis 2001; 10:636–49.
17. Shapira Y, Herz I, Vaturi M, et al. Thrombolysis is an effective and safe therapy in stuck bileaflet mitral valves in the absence of high-risk thrombi. J Am Coll Cardiol 2000; 35:1874–80.
18. Özkan M, Gündüz S, Biteker M, et al. Comparison of different TEE-guided thrombolytic regimens for prosthetic valve thrombosis. The TROIA Trial. JACC Cardiovasc Imaging 2013; 6:206–16.
19. Tong A, Roudaut R, Ozkan M, et al. Transesophageal echocardiography improves risk assessment of thrombolysis of prosthetic valve thrombosis: results of the international PRO-TEE registry. J Am Coll Cardiol 2004; 43:77–84.
20. Montorsi P, Cavoretto D, Alimento M, Muratori M, Pepi M. Prosthetic mitral valve thrombosis: can fluoroscopy predict the efficacy of thrombolytic treatment? Circulation 2003; 108(Suppl II):79–84.
21. Flachskampf FA, Guerrero JL, O'Shea JP, Weyman AE, Thomas JD. Patterns of normal transvalvular regurgitation in mechanical valve prostheses. J Am Coll Cardiol 1991; 18:1493–8.
22. Daniel WG, Mügge A, Martin RP, et al. Improvement in the diagnosis of abscesses associated with endocarditis by transesophageal echocardiography. N Engl J Med 1990; 324:795–800.
23. Möllmann H, Kim W-K, Kempfert J, Walther T, Hamm C. Complications of transcatheter aortic valve implantation (TAVI): how to avoid and treat them. Heart 2015; 101:900–8.

Echocardiography in detecting cardiac sources of embolism

13

Maria João Andrade and Justiaan Swanevelder

Key Points

- Standard comprehensive transthoracic echocardiography (TTE) and transesophageal echocardiography (TEE) with or without contrast should be performed in all patients with stroke or transient ischemic attack of presumed embolic cause.
- Cardiac thrombi, vegetations, tumors, and complex atheromas should be searched for in the left atrium, left atrial appendage, left ventricle, and aorta in patients with embolic strokes and transient ischemic attacks.
- Advances in ultrasound investigation capabilities (contrast, real-time 3D, strain) further improve the etiological work-up and evaluation of the putative sources of emboli in patients with embolic stroke.

Stroke is one of the leading causes of death and disability in developed countries. Investigation of the source of embolic stroke is crucial to prevent further insults and to provide therapeutic guidance. The EACVI recommendations on cardiovascular imaging for the detection of embolic sources, endorsed by the Canadian Society of Echocardiography were recently updated.[1]

Approximately 15–30% of ischemic strokes are cardioembolic and can be suspected on clinical and neuroimaging grounds (i.e., abrupt onset of neurological symptoms with lack of preceding transitory ischemic attack in patients with atrial fibrillation, striking stroke severity in the elderly, a typical territorial distribution of infarcts with multiplicity in space and age, or other signs of systemic thromboembolism). In a vast majority of cases, including patients with atrial fibrillation, native valve diseases or valvular prosthesis, or post–myocardial infarction or patients with cardiomyopathies, the source of emboli are cardiac thrombi. Less frequently systemic embolism may result from secondary embolization of a cardiac tumor, the migration of infected valvular vegetations in patients with infective endocarditis or embolization of an atherosclerotic plaque from the aorta.

The list of cardiac conditions/diseases that may be associated with a risk for cardioembolism is shown in Table 13.1. Of note, the actual echocardiographic finding of a potential cardiac source of embolism does not always imply that the stroke is cardioembolic, since patients frequently suffer from both atherosclerotic cerebrovascular disease and heart disease and sometimes more than one potential source of embolism is present. Although, echocardiographic detection of a potential embolic source (e.g., thrombus, vegetations of infective endocarditis, cardiac tumors) may be helpful in planning patient management in certain clinical scenarios,[1] the presence of conditions, such as atrial septal aneurysm, patent foramen ovale, complex aortic atheroma, or spontaneous echo contrast, does not necessarily imply definitive therapeutic strategies since available data are controversial in guiding the optimal approach.

DOI: 10.1201/9781003245407-13

161

TABLE 13.1   Conditions and Diseases Associated with High, Low, or Uncertain Risk for Cardioembolism

HIGH RISK	LOW OR UNCERTAIN RISK
Atrial fibrillation or flutter	Mitral valve prolapse
Myocardial infarction *(recent or with LV aneurysm)*	Mitral annulus calcifications
Cardiomyopathies (all)	Calcified aortic stenosis
Infective endocarditis	Patent foramen ovale (PFO)
Rheumatic mitral stenosis	Atrial septal aneurysm (w/o PFO)
Prosthetic valves (mechanical)	Spontaneous echo contrast ("smoke sign")
Cardiac masses (except calcifications): *thrombi, tumors, infective or marantic vegetations*	Valvular strands/Lamb's excrescences
Complex aortic atherosclerotic plaques (atheromas)	Atrial septal pouch

Transthoracic echocardiography (TTE) is the initial imaging modality of choice for evaluation of the cardiac sources of embolus. If no identified source is found on TTE, contrast transesophageal echocardiography (TEE) should be done promptly (ideally within 48 hours) according to the clinical context. The superiority of TEE appears dependent on the patient's age and could be useful to identify small size or questionable abnormalities beyond the resolution of TTE. TEE is particularly useful to identify the presence of left atrial (LA) and left atrial appendage (LAA) thrombogenic status, represented by the presence of thrombi, spontaneous echo contrast, LAA sludge or dysfunction. A meta-analysis of 27 studies aimed to assess the values of TEE for cryptogenic stroke revealed the detection of findings that prompted the introduction of anticoagulant therapy in up to one-third of patients.[2]

Cardiac computed tomography (CT) and magnetic resonance imaging (MRI) may be considered in addition of TTE and TEE for the detection of a cardiac source of embolism in specific situations or as valuable alternatives, such as before procedures of ablation of atrial arrhythmias and percutaneous LAA closure. Although CT has the limitation of radiation exposure, both tests are less invasive than TEE with a comparable diagnostic accuracy for detecting LAA thrombosis.[3,4] CMR is more sensitive than TTE for the detection of intraventricular thrombi after myocardial infarction (MI).[5]

MAJOR CARDIAC SOURCES OF EMBOLISM

Left atrial thrombi

The left atrium and particularly LAA (an embryonic remnant of the primordial LA) are the most common sites for intracardiac thrombus formation in patients presenting with embolic stroke (V13.29A, V13.29B). They are mostly seen in patients with atrial fibrillation (AF) and mitral stenosis. AF is the most frequently dysrhythmia for which risk stratification of thromboembolic events is based on clinical risk scores, mainly $CHADS_2$ or CHA_2DS_2-VASc.[6] While TTE is recommended in all patients with AF to identify possible underlying cardiac disease, TEE is mandatory for the diagnosis and exclusion of LA and LAA thrombus.

Spontaneous echocardiographic contrast (SEC) defined as dynamic "smoke-like" slowly swirling echo densities (V13.1) are often associated with thrombus.[7] TTE and TEE may contribute further to predict the risk of ischemic stroke through evaluation of LA and LAA function (by LA global longitudinal strain and emptying LAA velocities <20 cm/seg on pulsed-wave Doppler) but also LV ejection fraction <35% and complex aortic plaques.[8]

Rheumatic valve disease is still common in developing countries. Systemic embolization, mostly cerebral, occurs in 10–20% of patients with mitral stenosis. Age, AF, LA enlargement, and the presence of SEC are all related with the risk for embolization.[9] Oral anticoagulation therapy with vitamin K antagonists is mandatory when AF complicates mitral stenosis.[10]

Especially, chamber dilation combined with AF promotes LA thrombus formation. LA dilation occurs in many disorders, such as rheumatic mitral valve disease (V13.1), valvular and nonvalvular AF, and cardiomyopathies. Embolic risk has been stratified with $CHADS_2$ or CHA_2DS_2-VASc score, and the LA should be fully examined in patients with high scores.[10,11] Although TTE visualizes the LA cavity well, usually it is not satisfactory in detecting LA thrombus, especially when they are in the LAA (V13.2) or when an artificial mitral prosthesis is in place (V13.3, V13.4).

The *shape* of the LAA varies, and sometimes the appendage has multiple lobes. A study examining 500 normal autopsy hearts demonstrated that the most frequent occurrence was a two-lobe left atrial appendage (54%), although a three- or four-lobe appendage was also common (26%).[12] In order not to miss smaller thrombi in the left atrial appendage, its whole structure should be visualized from all angles by multiplane TEE (Figure 13.1) (V13.27A, V13.27B). Observation from multiple planes also helps to differentiate actual thrombus from pectinate muscles (Figure 13.2) or echocardiographic artifact. Biase et al., using CT or MRI, classified the *left atrial*

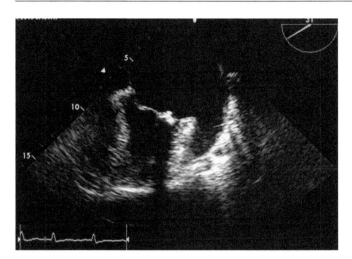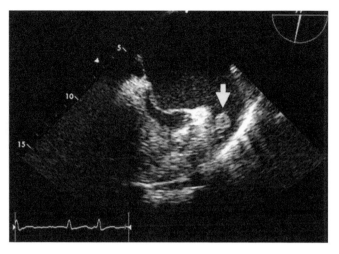

FIGURE 13.1   Multiple TEE views are needed to depict the whole image of left atrial appendage in search for thrombus. TEE view at 31 degrees shows LAA free of thrombus (left panel) (V13.27A), while at 77 degrees thrombus can be detected in the LAA (right panel) (V13.27B).

(Images and videos provided by PMM.)

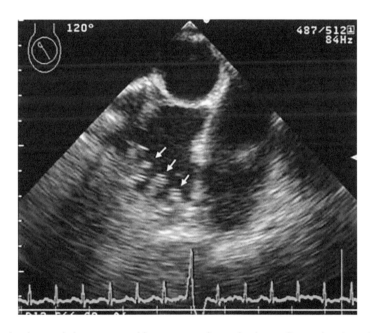

FIGURE 13.2   Pectinate muscles (arrows) demonstrated by transesophageal echocardiography viewed at 120°.

appendage morphology in patients with drug-refractory atrial fibrillation into four categories: cactus, chicken wing, windsock, and cauliflower. They found that the chicken wing morphology was less likely to cause an embolic event even after controlling for comorbidities and CHADS$_2$ score. Compared with chicken wing morphology, cactus was 4 times, windsock 4.5 times, and cauliflower 8 times more likely to cause a stroke or transient ischemic attack.[13]

The presence of LAA dysfunction supports a diagnosis of thrombus, whereas normal function suggests the alternative. Many studies have shown an association between LAA dysfunction and stroke. LAA function has been assessed with several methods, including appendage flow velocities, appendage wall velocity, and left atrial and atrial appendage myocardial strain. In patients without cardiac abnormalities, the mean *emptying flow velocity* of the LAA (V13.28), measured by pulsed-wave Doppler echocardiography, is 50–60 cm/s, and the mean filling velocity is 40–50 cm/s.[14] Appendage thrombi are more prevalent in patients with low flow velocities of ≤20 cm/s (Figure 13.3) than in those with higher velocities.[15] LAA *wall velocity* is measured by tissue Doppler echocardiography. The velocity is significantly lower in patients with AF having thrombus in the LAA than in those without.[16] In a study where LAA *strain and strain*

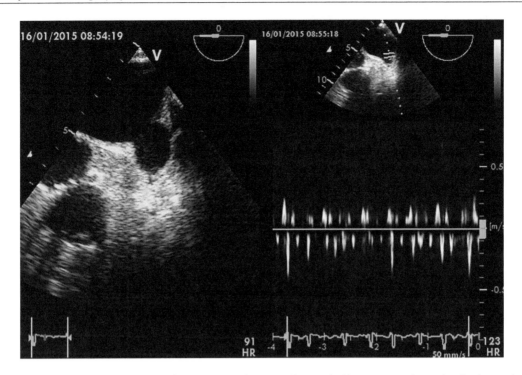

FIGURE 13.3   Low left atrial appendage (LAA) flow velocities (<20 cm/s) recorded by transesophageal pulsed Doppler echocardiography, indicating high risk of thrombus formation.

(Images provided by PMM.)

rate with tissue Doppler echocardiography were investigated, they correlated well with LAA appendage velocity and were significantly lower in patients with LAA thrombus than those without.[17] Left atrial strain determined by speckle tracking echocardiography, also correlated well with LAA flow velocity and morphology assessed by TEE and predicted the presence of LAA thrombus even in patients with sinus rhythm.[18,19]

Another important marker of LAA dysfunction is the presence of *spontaneous echocardiographic contrast ("smoke sign")*, displayed as a swirling intracavitary motion of sluggish blood flow (V13.1, V13.31). Spontaneous contrast is caused by rouleaux formation of red blood cells and implies blood stasis. Of note, its presence may be sensitive but is not a specific sign of thrombus formation. The term *LAA sludge* is used for intracavitary echodensity, continuously seen throughout the cardiac cycle, with gelatinous appearance, giving the impression of impending precipitation, but without a discrete organized thrombus. It has been shown that spontaneous echocardiographic contrast was seen in 75% of patients with LAA emptying velocity of less than 20 cm/s. Moreover, prevalence of neurologic events was much higher in patients with spontaneous echocardiographic contrast (20.5%) than in those without (5.7%).[15]

Although the LAA is the most common site of the thrombus formation, it can also present in the left atrial body (V13.5). Left atrial body thrombi are rarely found in the path of the pulmonary venous or mitral regurgitation flow which wash them out. Exceptionally rarely, floating ball thrombus can be found in the left atrial cavity, usually requiring urgent surgery (V13.6).

Differential diagnosis between LA thrombus and tumor might be challenging (V13.30A, V13.30B, V13.30C).

In the presence of *prosthetic valve thrombosis*, especially in the mitral position, thrombi are often difficult to identify by TTE. TTE can demonstrate an elevated transprosthetic gradient suggesting prosthetic valve obstruction or regurgitation, but the cause of the prosthetic dysfunction is often undefined. In such cases, TEE is essential to improve visualization of the prosthesis from the atrial side, without the interposition of acoustic shadows (V13.3, V13.4). Differential diagnosis between prosthetic valve thrombus versus vegetations might be difficult (V13.37).

Left ventricular thrombi

After a myocardial infarction (MI) or in the setting of dilated cardiomyopathy, stagnant blood flow may occur in the left ventricle leading to thrombus formation (V13.7, V13.8, V13.11, V18.17B).

Myocardial infarctions affect the anterior wall, or the apex of the left ventricle have a higher rate of left ventricular thrombus (LVT) formation, which generally arises within 10 days following the infarction. (Figure 13.4) (V13.32).

The risk of ischemic stroke in patients presenting with an anterior MI and an LVT is 12% in the month following the MI and seems to be higher if the thrombus is pedunculated and mobile (V13.9).[20] In the absence of AF and heart failure, the

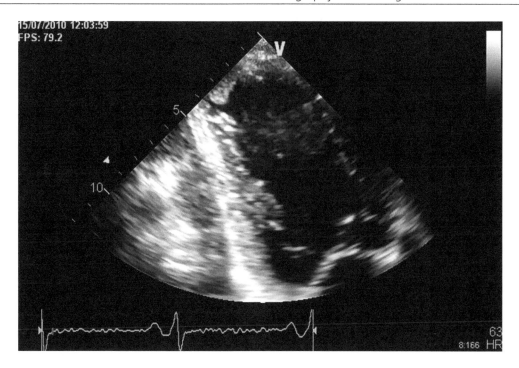

FIGURE 13.4 Left ventricular apical thrombus in a patient with recent anterior myocardial infarction. Note the spontaneous echocardiographic contrast ("smoke sign") in the LV cavity, indicating stagnant blood flow (V13.32).

risk of systemic embolism decreases markedly in the subsequent months.

Irrespective of their cause, all dilated cardiomyopathies can be complicated by an LVT, whose incidence ranges from 11% to 44%[21] (V13.11). The risk of embolic events is related to the degree of LV dysfunction SD and to the presence of AF.

TTE performance for LVT detection depends on the clinical indication of the echocardiogram and the sensitivity of TTE increases when a contrast agent is used (V13.10).[22] CMR has higher sensitivity for identification of LVT and should be used when TTE is of suboptimal quality or when the TTE is negative in the setting of significant clinical suspicion.[23] Repeated TTE is indicated to monitor resolution of LVT after 4–6 weeks of anticoagulation.

TEE has a little additional benefit to offer in detection of left ventricular thrombus, mainly because of the distance from the transducer to the thrombus and the limited ventricular views of the transesophageal approach. Apical thrombus can easily be overlooked because in routine midesophageal TEE views the left ventricle is often foreshortened and the apex not well visualized. However, when TTE is of poor image quality, the deep transgastric TEE view may have value to visualize the left ventricular apex.

Aortic arch atheromatous plaques

Thrombus from any atherosclerotic plaque surface or plaque material itself detached from the aortic wall may cause systemic embolization.[24] Less frequently, embolic material can originate from calcified aortic valve or mitral annuli (Figure 13.5) (V13.12). Plaques in the aortic arch may cause stroke and the search for complex aortic atheromas by TTE, and especially by TEE, should routinely be done as a part of a diagnostic work-up of patients with ischemic stroke and peripheral embolization. Suprasternal TTE may be helpful for the preliminary screening of atherosclerotic plaques in the aortic arch and indicate the need for a more detailed TEE search (V13.13A, V13.13B, and V13.13C). Patients with stroke may also have more than one potential source of embolism detectable by echocardiography (V13.34A, V13.34B). Mobility, size, and morphology of a plaque are important predictors of embolization. Protruding or pedunculated aortic atheromas or mobile lesions and atherosclerotic plaques of 4 mm or greater are at a higher risk of embolization.[25] In such cases, it seems prudent to avoid invasive catheter-based procedures or to modify the approach (radial instead of femoral) according to plaque localization (Figure 13.6) (V13.14A, V13.14B). Three-dimensional TEE may provide better appreciation of the size, shape, and mobility of aortic atheromas (V13.15).

Vegetations

In infective endocarditis (IE), embolic events related to the migration of infected vegetations are a frequent and life-threatening complication, occurring in 20–50% of patients.[26] Echocardiography (TTE and TEE) is the first-line imaging modality for the diagnosis allowing to identify vegetations (V13.16, V13.17) and other characteristic of lesions (Figure 13.7) (V13.33A, V13.33B, V13.33C).

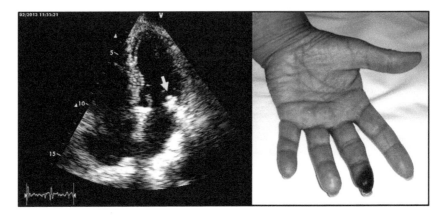

FIGURE 13.5 Transthoracic apical four-chamber view showing a small mobile mass (thrombus or atheroma) attached to the calcified posterior mitral annulus, with high embolic potential (left panel) (see also V13.12). This chronic hemodialysis patient presented with left-hand peripheral embolism (right panel) and no clinical or laboratory signs of systemic infection.

(Images and videos provided by IS.)

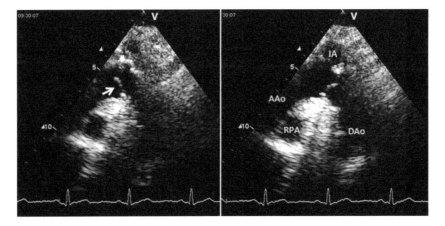

FIGURE 13.6 Transthoracic echocardiographic suprasternal views reveal highly mobile aortic arch atheroma (arrow) just opposite from the origin of innominate artery (IA) and left carotid artery. Note the strikingly different position of the mobile atheroma in the aortic lumen in different frames (left panel versus right panel), indicating high mobility. This patient with chest pain was scheduled coronary angiography. However, based on echocardiographic findings, he was considered at high risk of cerebral or peripheral embolism and was switched to CT coronary angiography (V13.14A, V13.14B). AAo: ascending aorta; DAo: descending aorta; RPA: right pulmonary artery.

(Images and video provided by VC.)

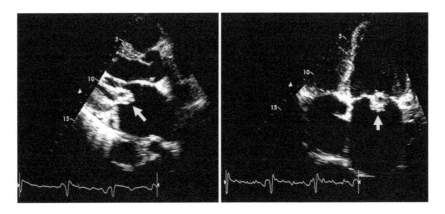

FIGURE 13.7 Large vegetation on the posterior mitral leaflet is shown (arrows) in parasternal long-axis (left panel) and apical four-chamber (right panel) transthoracic echocardiographic views (V13.33A, V13.33B, V13.33C).

(Images and videos provided by IS.)

Nowadays, the sensitivity for the diagnosis of vegetations in native and prosthetic valves is 70% and 50%, respectively, for TTE and 96% and 92%, respectively, for TEE.[27] Specificity has been reported to be around 90% for both TTE and TEE. Identification of vegetations may be difficult in the presence of pre-existing valvular lesions, prosthetic valves (V13.36A, V13.36B), small vegetations (V13.37), and IE-affecting intra-cardiac devices. TEE significantly improves the sensitivity to detect a vegetation especially in patients with valve prosthesis (V13.18A, V13.18B) Therefore, virtually all patients clinically suspected of IE should undergo TEE.[26,28] It has been shown that three-dimensional TEE provides enhanced appreciation of the full length, the shape and precise attachment of vegetation in comparison with two-dimensional examination (Figure 13.8) (V13.35A, V13.35B).[29]

Several factors have been associated with an increased risk of embolism in patients with IE. Among them, the size and mobility (V13.38A, V13.38B) of the vegetations are the most potent independent predictors of a new embolic event, especially in *Staphylococcus aureus* infection.[30] Based on the study of 847 patients with an 8.5% six-month incidence of new embolism, a simple "embolic risk calculator" was proposed to estimate the embolic risk in patients with IE on admission to the hospital.[31]

Because the risk of embolism is particularly high during the first days after the initiation of antibiotic therapy, the benefit of surgery will be greatest during the first week of antibiotic therapy, when the embolic rate is highest.[26,32]

Sterile vegetations composed of fibrin-platelet thrombi are common in patients with advanced cancer (*marantic endocarditis*) and systemic lupus erythematosus (*Libman-Sacks endocarditis*). These vegetations, although less destructive and rarely causing valvular dysfunction, are prone to systemic embolization.[33]

Lambl's excrescences are only weakly correlated with stroke risk. Their discovery during work-up for a cryptogenic stroke should not discourage the search for another possible cause. It has no effect on patient management.[1]

Of note, isolated and uncomplicated mitral valve prolapse should not be considered as a potential cardiac source of embolism.[1]

Cardiac tumors

Primary cardiac tumors are rare, the diversity of their clinical presentation depending on histology, size, and location. Until they obstruct heart chambers or valves or cause embolization, arrhythmias, or cardiac tamponade, cardiac tumors may remain asymptomatic or manifest by constitutional symptoms.[34] Echocardiography is the first-line imaging modality for diagnosis of cardiac tumors, TEE being often necessary for morphological details.

Eighty percent of all primary heart tumors are benign and *myxoma* is the most common primary benign cardiac tumor (70%). Myxoma is typically located in the left atrium, with a narrow fibrovascular stalk to the fossa ovalis region of the interatrial septum (Figure 13.9) (V13.19A and V13.19B). As opposed to thrombi, their echogenicity is usually not homogeneous (V13.39A, V13.39B, V13.39C), with echolucent and calcification areas. In general, the mobility, friability, and tendency for thrombus formation relate to propensity for embolization. It has been shown that the incidence of embolism is significantly higher in the *polypoid type* (soft and irregular shape and independent mobility, 58%) than in the *round type* (solid and round shape, immobile, 0%).[35,36] Due to the high

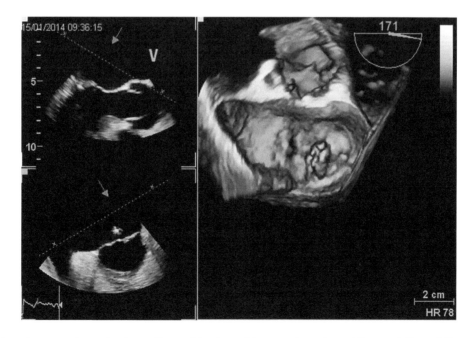

FIGURE 13.8   Biplane transesophageal echocardiographic view of large, extremely mobile vegetation of the posterior mitral valve leaflet with high embolic potential (left panel) with three-dimensional reconstruction (right panel) (V13.35A, V13.35B).

(Image and videos provided by BAP.)

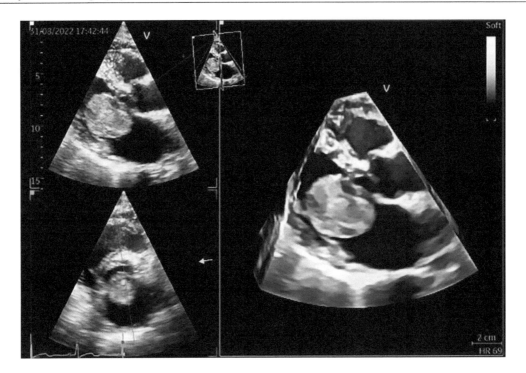

FIGURE 13.9 Three-dimensional transthoracic parasternal view showing a large nonhomogeneous mass in the left atrium, attached to the interatrial septum. During diastole, the tumor moves into the left ventricle through the mitral valve, causing valvular obstruction (V13.19A, V13.19B).

embolic potential (risk of systemic embolization in up to 75% of patients), surgical resection is indicated.[37]

Papillary fibroelastoma is the second most frequent primary benign tumor, representing 10% of cardiac tumors found in autopsy series. These tumors are usually small (1–2 cm) with a preferential location in the aortic valve, followed by the mitral valve (V13.20A and V13.20B). On gross inspection, such tumors have a characteristic frondlike appearance, resembling a sea anemone. Although papillary fibroelastoma occurs in all age groups, it is most seen in elderly patients supporting the hypothesis that papillary fibroelastoma may represent a degenerative process. Regardless of their size, they are very mobile tumors with a high embolic potential, manifesting as transient ischemic or cerebrovascular accidents, myocardial infarction, or syncope. Surgery is usually indicated in cases of location in the left heart.[38]

ATRIAL SEPTAL ANOMALIES AND PARADOXICAL EMBOLISM

Atrial septal aneurysm (ASA)

Atrial septal aneurysm (ASA) is defined as a >10 mm excursion into the RA or LA from the plane of the atrial septum, or a combined total excursion of 15 mm.[39] The incidence of ASA in the general population is around 2% as estimated by TTE,

rising to 4.6% in TEE studies and to 7.2% in patients undergoing TEE after an ischemic stroke.[40,41] The link between ASA and PFO is well established, with approximately 60% of patients presenting with ASA plus PFO.[42] (V13.21, V13.23). The mechanisms proposed to explain the link between ASA and systemic embolism include a thrombus in the ASA, a paradoxical embolism from a venous thrombus through a PFO or coexisting paroxysmal AF.[43]

Patent foramen ovale (PFO)

PFO is a flap-like opening between the septum primum and septum secundum at the fossa ovalis. The reported prevalence of PFO in the general population is 25%, increasing to over 50% in patients with cryptogenic stroke.[43,44] Due to the gradient between the LA and right atrium, the PFO is usually closed, and no shunting is seen. Under certain hemodynamic conditions, such as elevated right atrial (RA) pressure and with provocative maneuvers to increase RA pressure, such as cough and the Valsalva maneuver, a right-to-left shunt can be seen. Due to its wide availability, non-invasiveness, and reasonable sensitivity, TTE is the primary method to investigate the presence of right-to-left shunting through a PFO. To differentiate intracardiac shunting from transpulmonary passage of bubbles, PFO is proven only if agitated saline contrast is observed crossing the atrial septum or appear in the LA within three cardiac cycles after complete opacification of the RA (V13.22).[45,46] If contrast TTE is negative in patients with cryptogenic stroke or TIA, TEE can demonstrate right-to-left shunt flow across a PFO with very high accuracy (sensitivity of 89%, specificity of 91%), either with color Doppler (V13.40A, V13.40B) or contrast echocardiography (V13.23).[47] Of note, even better sensitivity and specificity of TTE (89% and 70%) versus TEE (35% and 56%) have been recently reported, if both applied with agitated saline contrast and the Valsalva maneuver.[48] Although sometimes difficult to perform in patients with recent stroke, the Valsalva maneuver with contrast agent should be performed during both TTE and TEE examination. Elevated LA pressure reduces the rate of PFO detection.[49] PFO size, shunt severity, presence of ASA, and atrial septal hypermobility can be linked to a causal role of PFO in stroke.[50]

Recent studies have shown that among adults after cryptogenic stroke, closure of a PFO with an ASA or large interatrial shunt was associated with a lower rate of recurrent ischemic strokes than medical therapy alone during extended follow-up.[51–53]

Left atrial septal pouch (LASP)

LASP is defined as a recess opening into the LA due to incomplete fusion of the cranial segment of the overlap between the septum primum and septum secundum, in the absence of an interatrial shunt at rest or with Valsalva maneuver release. LASP is identified by TEE and although it has been speculated about a causal relationship with ischemic stroke, results from retrospective studies were not conclusive.[54]

Paradoxical embolism

Deep vein thrombosis is very important as a cause of pulmonary thromboembolism with potential paradoxical systemic embolism. Paradoxical embolism occurs when there is embolic transit from the systemic venous circulation to the systemic arterial circulation through a right-to-left shunt, such as a PFO or atrial septal defect. In the setting of systemic embolism, the documentation of a thrombus straddling the PFO confirms a paradoxical embolism (V13.24, V13.41, V13.42). The optimal choice of treatment remains challenging.[55] Rarely, the source of paradoxical embolism may be mobile masses (vegetation or thrombus) attached to catheters or pacemaker leads (V13.25 and V13.26).

LIST OF VIDEOS

VIDEO 13.1   Spontaneous echo contrast: Transthoracic echocardiography in parasternal long-axis view from a patient with severe rheumatic valvular disease affecting both the mitral and the aortic valves. Note the abundant spontaneous echocardiographic contrast inside the left atrium indicating blood stasis.

VIDEO 13.2   Thrombus in the left atrial appendage. Transesophageal echocardiography. At 90 degrees, a thrombus is shown in the left atrial appendage of a patient with dilated left atrium and atrial fibrillation.

VIDEO 13.3   Mechanical mitral prosthesis thrombosis. TEE focused view of a bi-leaflet mechanical mitral prosthesis where one of the disks is still, blocked by a thrombus. Because it did not resolve with appropriate anticoagulation, an operation was needed that confirmed prosthetic thrombosis.

VIDEO 13.4   Biological mitral prosthesis thrombosis. TEE focused view of a biological prosthesis in mitral position showing thickening of the cusps, one of which completely fixed. A mass suggestive of thrombus may be seen in the ventricular side of the prosthesis. The patient presented with heart failure and improved after anticoagulation therapy.

VIDEO 13.5   Left atrium body thrombus. TEE shows a large thrombus in the body of the left atrium in a patient with cardiomyopathy and atrial fibrillation after a cerebral embolic event. Note the spontaneous echo contrast ("smoke sign").

VIDEO 13.6   Free-floating ball thrombus. TEE shows free-floating ball thrombus in the left atrium in a patient with prosthetic mitral valve with extremely high embolic potential. In cases like this, urgent surgery is usually required. Note also spontaneous echo contrast ("smoke sign").

VIDEO 13.7   Left ventricular thrombus and spontaneous echo contrast after myocardial infarction. TTE shows an apical left ventricular aneurysm with thrombus and spontaneous echo contrast ("smoke sign") in the left ventricular cavity, in a patient after a recent large myocardial infarction.

VIDEO 13.8   Apical left ventricular thrombus. TTE shows a protruding mass consistent with thrombus in the dyskinetic apex of the left ventricle after recent myocardial infarction.

VIDEO 13.9   Highly mobile left ventricular thrombus: Transthoracic echocardiography shows a round, highly mobile mass consistent with thrombus in the akinetic apex of a left ventricle after myocardial infarction.

VIDEO 13.10   Contrast echocardiography: left ventricular apical thrombus: In this patient with dilated cardiomyopathy and very poor global LV function transthoracic echocardiography with injecting contrast (lower left and right panels), apical LV thrombus was detected. Note the better delineation of LV endocardial borders with contrast and defect in the LV apex indicating thrombus.

VIDEO 13.11   Left ventricular thrombus in dilated cardiomyopathy: In this patient with dilated cardiomyopathy and very poor global left ventricular (LV) function, an apical LV thrombus can be seen on transthoracic echocardiography (upper left and lower panels). Note that thrombus can be better visualized using nonstandard, angled views of the apex (right lower panel).

VIDEO 13.12   Masses attached to the calcified posterior mitral annulus in a patient with left-hand peripheral embolism: In a patient with left-hand peripheral embolism (shown in Figure 13.6 in the book), transthoracic echocardiography four-chamber view shows small mobile mass (thrombus or atheroma) attached to the calcified posterior mitral annulus, with high embolic potential. *(Video provided by IS.)*

VIDEO 13.13A   Transesophageal echocardiography in a patient with transient ischemic attack (TIA) (1/3): In this patient with TIA, complex atheroma in the aortic arch was detected on suprasternal transthoracic echocardiography view (shown here). Transesophageal echocardiographic study showed extremely mobile plaque in the aortic arch not seen with transthoracic echocardiography (see Video 13.13B), as well as complex aortic atheromas in descending aorta (see Video 13.13C). *(Video provided by VC.)*

VIDEO 13.13B   Transesophageal echocardiography in a patient with transient ischemic attack (TIA) (2/3): In this patient with TIA, complex atheroma in the aortic arch was detected on suprasternal transthoracic echocardiographic view (see Video 13.13A). Transesophageal echocardiographic study shows extremely mobile plaque in the aortic arch not seen with transthoracic echocardiography (shown here), as well as complex aortic atheromas in descending aorta (see Video 13.13C). *(Video provided by VC.)*

VIDEO 13.13C   Transesophageal echocardiography in a patient with transient ischemic attack (TIA) (3/3): In this patient with TIA, complex atheroma in the aortic arch was detected on suprasternal transthoracic echocardiographic view (see Video 13.13A). Transesophageal echocardiographic study shows extremely mobile plaque in the aortic arch not seen with transthoracic echocardiography (see Video 13.13B), as well as complex aortic atheromas in descending aorta (shown here). *(Video provided by VC.)*

VIDEO 13.14A   Highly mobile aortic atheroma (1/2): This transthoracic echocardiographic suprasternal view reveals highly mobile aortic arch atheroma (shown here) just opposite to the origin of the innominate artery and left carotid artery (see also Video 13.14B) in a patient with chest pain scheduled for coronary angiography. The patient was considered at high risk of cerebral or peripheral embolism and therefore directed to CT coronary angiography. *(Video provided by VC.)*

VIDEO 13.14B   Highly mobile aortic atheroma (2/2): Transthoracic echocardiographic suprasternal zoom view reveals highly mobile aortic arch atheroma (see also Video 13.14A) just opposite to the origin of the innominate artery and left carotid artery (shown here) in a patient with chest pain scheduled for coronary angiography. The patient was considered at high risk of cerebral or peripheral embolism and therefore directed to CT coronary angiography. *(Video provided by VC.)*

VIDEO 13.15   Mobile aortic atheroma by three-dimensional transesophageal echocardiography. Three-dimensional transesophageal echocardiographic imaging of mobile aortic atheroma allows excellent assessment of its size, shape, and mobility.

VIDEO 13.16   Mitral valve vegetation. TTE apical two-chamber view from a patient admitted with pulmonary edema, cardiogenic shock, and multiple embolic infarctions on CT scan. A very large and mobile vegetation is seen in the atrial face of the mitral valve. Blood cultures were positive for methicillin-sensitive *Staphylococcus aureus*. The patient underwent emergent mitral valve replacement.

VIDEO 13.17   Aortic valve vegetations. TTE parasternal long-axis view in a patient with infective endocarditis. Aortic valve vegetations can be appreciated, with severe valve destruction causing torrential regurgitation. Urgent aortic valve replacement was needed for worsening heart failure.

VIDEO 13.18A   Mechanical mitral prosthesis with vegetation. Biplane TEE demonstrates an extremely mobile vegetation attached to the atrial side of the mechanical prosthetic mitral annulus with high embolic potential (see also Video 13.18B).

VIDEO 13.18B   Mechanical mitral prosthesis with vegetation. 3D-TEE view of the same patient as in Video 13.18A, showing the mobile vegetation attached to the mechanical prosthesis.

VIDEO 13.19A   Left atrial myxoma (1/2). Three-dimensional transthoracic parasternal view showing a large nonhomogeneous mass in the left atrium, attached to the interatrial septum. During diastole, the tumor moves to the left ventricle through the mitral valve causing valvular obstruction (see also Video 13.19B).

VIDEO 13.19B   Left atrial myxoma (2/2). Three-plane apical view showing the same tumor as in Video 13.19A.

VIDEO 13.20A   Papillary fibroelastoma (1/2). Biplane transesophageal views of a small and very mobile papillary fibroelastoma attached to the arterial side of the aortic valve (see also Video 13.20B).

VIDEO 13.20B   Papillary fibroelastoma (2/2). Three-dimensional view of the same tumor as in Video 13.20A. Location and mobility increase embolic potential.

VIDEO 13.21   Atrial septal aneurysm and PFO: An atrial septal aneurysm is shown in different transthoracic echocardiographic views. Note the small amount of left-to-right flow across the patent foramen ovale (PFO) demonstrated with color Doppler (left lower video). The presence of the atrial septal aneurysm in addition to PFO has been associated with a marked increase in recurrent unexplained neurologic events. *(Video provided by PMM.)*

VIDEO 13.22   PFO demonstrated with contrast (TTE with contrast). Transthoracic apical four-chamber view in a young patient after a suspected cardioembolic stroke. Note the presence of atrial septal aneurysm. After intravenous agitated saline infusion, contrast is observed in the left atrium immediately after complete opacification of the right atrium, confirming the presence of a PFO.

VIDEO 13.23   Atrial septal aneurysm and PFO (TEE with contrast). Transesophageal views focused on the interatrial septum. Note the presence of exuberant atrial septal aneurysm. After intravenous agitated saline infusion and with Valsalva maneuver to increase right atrial pressure, contrast is observed in the left atrium, confirming the presence of a PFO.

VIDEO 13.24   Thrombus crossing through PFO. In a patient with recent stroke, biplane TEE shows a very long and mobile thrombus crossing from the right to the left atrium through a PFO.

VIDEO 13.25   Pacemaker wire mass: This transthoracic echocardiographic four-chamber view shows mobile masses (thrombi or vegetations) attached to the pacemaker wire in the right heart. In case of increased right atrial pressure and patent foramen ovale, paradoxical embolism may occur. *(Video provided by MMP.)*

VIDEO 13.26   Hickman catheter mass: Note a mobile mass (possibly vegetation) in the right atrium attached to the Hickman catheter placed in the superior vena cava in a febrile patient.

VIDEO 13.27A   Imaging of the left atrial appendage (LAA) (1/2): Multiple transesophageal echocardiographic views are needed to depict the whole image of the left atrial appendage in search for thrombus. Transesophageal echocardiographic view at 31° shows LAA free of thrombus, whereas at 77° (see Video 13.27B) thrombus can be detected in the LAA. *(Video provided by PMM.)*

VIDEO 13.27B   Imaging of the left atrial appendage (LAA) (2/2): Multiple transesophageal echocardiographic views are needed to depict the whole image of the left atrial appendage in search for thrombus. Transesophageal echocardiography at 77° shows thrombus in the LAA, whereas at 31° (see Video 13.27A) the LAA appears free of thrombus. *(Video provided by PMM.)*

VIDEO 13.28   Low flow velocities in the left atrial appendage: Transesophageal echocardiographic views at different angles of the left atrial appendage show spontaneous echo contrast and thrombus. Note the low emptying flow velocities (<20 cm/s) recorded by pulsed-wave Doppler (right lower panel). *(Video provided by PMM.)*

VIDEO 13.29A   Left atrial appendage thrombus with subsequent right femoral artery embolism (1/2): Transesophageal echocardiographic midesophageal two-chamber long-axis view. Visualization of the left ventricle and left atrial appendage with left upper pulmonary vein (left panels). Note a large mass at the entrance of the left atrial appendage. Three-dimensional transesophageal echocardiographic en face view from the left atrial perspective (right panel) showing the thrombus appearing from the left atrial appendage (at 2 o'clock) in a patient with constrictive pericarditis (see also Video 13.29B). A few days later, the patient had right femoral artery embolism. *(Video provided by VP.)*

VIDEO 13.29B   Magnetic resonance imaging (MRI) in a patient with right femoral artery embolism (2/2): MRI four-chamber view showing thickened and calcified pericardium in a patient with constrictive pericarditis and right femoral artery embolism (see also Video 13.29A). *(Video provided by VP.)*

VIDEO 13.30A   Transesophageal echocardiography (TEE) of the left atrium in a patient with VVI pacemaker, atrial fibrillation, and recent stroke (1/3): On cardiac computed tomography, two masses were seen in the left atrium and the patient was referred for TEE. On TEE images, masses both in the left atrial appendage and in the body of the left atrium can be seen. The presence of the mass in the appendage may indicate that the more likely diagnosis is thrombus as opposed to cardiac tumors (myxomas). In this case, the mass significantly reduced in size (see Videos 13.30B and 13.30C) after 3 weeks of anticoagulation, indicating a thrombotic origin. *(Video provided by BP.)*

VIDEO 13.30B   Transesophageal echocardiography (TEE) of the left atrium in a patient with VVI pacemaker, atrial fibrillation, and recent stroke (2/3): On cardiac computed tomography, two masses were seen in the left atrium and the patient was referred for TEE. On TEE images, masses both in the left atrial appendage and in the body of the left atrium can be seen (see Video 13.30A). The presence of the mass in the appendage may indicate that the more likely diagnosis is thrombus as opposed to cardiac tumors (myxomas). In this case, the mass significantly reduced in size (shown here; see also Video 13.30C) after 3 weeks of anticoagulation, indicating a thrombotic origin. *(Video provided by BP.)*

VIDEO 13.30C   Transesophageal echocardiography (TEE) of the left atrium in a patient with VVI pacemaker, atrial fibrillation, and recent stroke (3/3): On cardiac computed tomography, two masses were seen in the left atrium and the patient was referred for TEE. On TEE images, masses both in the left atrial appendage and in the body of the left atrium can be seen (see Video 13.30A). The presence of the mass in the appendage may indicate that the more likely diagnosis is thrombus as opposed to cardiac tumors (myxomas). In this case, the mass significantly reduced in size (shown here; see also Video 13.30B) after 3 weeks of anticoagulation, indicating a thrombotic origin. *(Video provided by BP.)*

VIDEO 13.31   Free-floating ball thrombus: Transesophageal echocardiography shows free-floating ball thrombus in the left atrium in a patient with prosthetic mitral valve with extremely high embolic potential. In cases like this, urgent surgery is usually required. Note also spontaneous echo contrast ("smoke sign").

VIDEO 13.32   Apical left ventricular thrombus: Transthoracic echocardiography shows a protruding mass consistent with thrombus in the dyskinetic apex of the left ventricle after recent myocardial infarction. Note the poor global left ventricular function with spontaneous echo contrast ("smoke sign").

VIDEO 13.33A   Large vegetation on the posterior mitral leaflet (1/3): It can be seen in transthoracic echocardiographic parasternal long-axis (shown here), short-axis (see Video 13.33B), and four-chamber (see Video 13.33C) views. *(Video provided by IS.)*

VIDEO 13.33B   Large vegetation on the posterior mitral leaflet (2/3): It can be seen in transthoracic echocardiographic short-axis (shown here), parasternal long-axis (see Video 13.33A), and four-chamber (see Video 13.33C) views. *(Video provided by IS.)*

VIDEO 13.33C   Large vegetation on the posterior mitral leaflet (3/3): It can be seen in transthoracic echocardiographic four-chamber (shown here), parasternal long-axis (see Video 13.33A), and short-axis (see Video 13.33B) views. *(Video provided by IS.)*

VIDEO 13.34A   A patient with embolic stroke with possible multiple sources of emboli (1/2): In this patient with embolic stroke and aortic valve sclerosis, in addition to a mobile mass attached to calcified posterior mitral annulus (atheroma or thrombus) seen in transthoracic four-chamber view (shown here), thick atheroma was detected in the aortic arch with mobile parts from suprasternal transthoracic echocardiographic view (see Video 13.34B). *(Video provided by IS.)*

VIDEO 13.34B   A patient with embolic stroke with possible multiple sources of emboli (2/2): In this patient with embolic stroke and aortic valve sclerosis, in addition to a mobile mass attached to calcified posterior mitral annulus (atheroma or thrombus) seen in transthoracic four-chamber view (see Video 13.34A), thick atheroma was detected in the aortic arch with mobile parts from suprasternal transthoracic echocardiographic view (shown here). *(Video provided by IS.)*

VIDEO 13.35A   Posterior mitral leaflet vegetation (1/2): Transesophageal echocardiography (TEE) shows a large, mobile posterior mitral leaflet vegetation. Although the length of this posterior mitral leaflet vegetation can be measured by two-dimensional TEE, the full length, shape, and precise attachment are easier to appreciate with three-dimensional TEE (see Video 13.35B). *(Video provided by BAP.)*

VIDEO 13.35B   Posterior mitral leaflet vegetation (2/2): Although the length of this posterior mitral leaflet vegetation can be also measured by two-dimensional transesophageal echocardiography (TEE) (see Video 13.35A), the full length, shape, and precise attachment are easier to appreciate with three-dimensional TEE (shown here, right panel). *(Video provided by BAP.)*

VIDEO 13.36A   Prosthetic mitral valve vegetation (1/2): This biplane transesophageal echocardiographic view demonstrates a large, extremely mobile vegetation of the prosthetic mitral valve with high embolic potential (see also Video 13.36B). *(Video provided by BAP.)*

VIDEO 13.36B   Prosthetic mitral valve vegetation (2/2): This three-dimensional transesophageal echocardiographic view demonstrates a large, mobile vegetation of the prosthetic mitral valve with high embolic potential (see also Video 13.36A). *(Video provided by BAP.)*

VIDEO 13.37   Prosthetic mitral valve mass: Transthoracic echocardiography shows small mobile mass (vegetation vs. thrombus) attached to prosthetic mitral valve in a patient with fever and signs of embolic episodes on cerebral computed tomography. Note the very poor left ventricular function.

VIDEO 13.38A   Focused cardiac ultrasound (FoCUS) examination with a handheld imaging device in a 35-year-old man on a chronic hemodialysis program 6 days after stroke (1/2): The patient was transferred to the cardiology department because of dyspnea and a new murmur. A large vegetation on the aortic valve was immediately noted (presumably the source of embolic stroke), with significant acute aortic insufficiency causing acute heart failure (see Video 13.38B). *(Video provided by IS.)*

VIDEO 13.38B   Focused cardiac ultrasound (FoCUS) examination with a handheld imaging device in a 35-year-old man on a chronic hemodialysis program 6 days after stroke (2/2): The patient was transferred to the cardiology department because of dyspnea and a new murmur. A large vegetation on the aortic valve was immediately noted (presumably the source of embolic stroke) (see Video 13.38A), with significant acute aortic insufficiency causing acute heart failure (shown here). *(Video provided by IS.)*

VIDEO 13.39A   Left atrial myxoma (1/3): Multiple transthoracic echocardiographic views showing a large nonhomogeneous mass in the left atrium, attached to the interatrial septum (see also Videos 13.39B and 13.39C). *(Video provided by BAP.)*

VIDEO 13.39B   Left atrial myxoma (2/3): Multiple transesophageal echocardiographic views showing a large nonhomogeneous mass in the left atrium, attached to the interatrial septum (see also Videos 13.39A and 13.39C). *(Video provided by BAP.)*

VIDEO 13.39C   Left atrial myxoma (3/3): Three-dimensional transesophageal echocardiographic atrial view of a large left atrial myxoma (right panel) (see also Videos 13.39A and 13.39B). *(Video provided by BAP.)*

VIDEO 13.40A   Patent foramen ovale (1/2): This transesophageal echocardiographic view of the interatrial septum shows left-to-right flow through the patent foramen ovale (see also Video 13.40B).

VIDEO 13.40B   Patent foramen ovale (2/2): This zoom transesophageal echocardiographic view of the interatrial septum shows left-to-right flow through the patent foramen ovale (see also Video 13.40A).

VIDEO 13.41   Thrombus lodged in the patent foramen ovale: In a patient with recent stroke, transthoracic echocardiographic four-chamber view shows mobile mass in the right atrium representing thrombus lodged in the patent foramen ovale. *(Video provided by BP.)*

VIDEO 13.42   Thrombus stuck in the PFO. TEE shows a large and mobile thrombus stuck in the PFO. *(Video provided by MPo.)*

REFERENCES

1. Cohen A, Donal E, Delgado V, et al. EACVI recommendations on cardiovascular imaging for the detection of embolic sources: endorsed by the Canadian Society of Echocardiography. Eur Heart J Cardiovasc Imaging 2021;22(6):e24–e57.

2. McGrath ER, Paikin JS, Motlagh B, et al. Transesophageal echocardiography in patients with cryptogenic ischemic stroke: a systematic review. Am Heart J 2014;168:706–12.
3. Zou H, Zhang Y, Tong J, Liu Z. Multidetector computed tomography for detecting left atrial/left atrial appendage thrombus: a meta-analysis. Intern Med J 2015;45:1044–53.
4. Chen J, Zhang H, Zhu D, et al. Cardiac MRI for detecting left atrial/left atrial appendage thrombus in patients with atrial fibrillation: meta-analysis and systematic review. Herz 2019;44:390–7.
5. Roifman I, Connelly KA, Wright GA, Wijeysundera HC. Echocardiography vs cardiac magnetic resonance imaging for the diagnosis of left ventricular thrombus: a systematic review. Can J Cardiol 2015;31:785–91.
6. Lip GYH, Nieuwlaat R, Pisters R, et al. Refining clinical risk stratification for predicting stroke and thromboembolism in atrial fibrillation using a novel risk factor-based approach: the euro heart survey on atrial fibrillation. Chest 2010;137:263–72.
7. Soulat-Dufour L, Lang S, Etienney A, et al. Correlation between left atrial spontaneous echocardiographic contrast and 5-year stroke/death in patients with non-valvular atrial fibrillation. Arch Cardiovasc Dis 2020;113:525–33.
8. Leung M, van Rosendael PJ, Abou R, et al. Left atrial function to identify patients with atrial fibrillation at high risk of stroke: new insights from a large registry. Eur Heart J 2018;39:1416–25.
9. Negi PC, Sondhi S, Rana V, et al. Prevalence, risk determinants and consequences of atrial fibrillation in rheumatic heart disease: 6 years hospital based-Himachal Pradesh- Rheumatic Fever/Rheumatic Heart Disease (HP-RF/RHD) Registry. Indian Heart J 2018;70:S68–S73.
10. Iung B, Leenhardt A, Extramiana F. Management of atrial fibrillation in patients with rheumatic mitral stenosis. Heart 2018;104:1062–8.
11. Camm AJ, Kirchhof P, Lip GYH, et al. Guidelines for the management of atrial fibrillation. Eur Heart J 2010;31:2369–429.
12. Veinot JP, Harrity PJ, Gentile F, et al. Anatomy of the normal left atrial appendage. A quantitative study of age-related changes in 500 autopsy hearts: implications for echocardiographic examination. Circulation 1997;96:3112–5.
13. Biase LD, Santangeli P, Anselmino M, et al. Does the left atrial appendage morphology correlate with the risk of stroke in patients with atrial fibrillation? Results from a multicenter study. J Am Coll Cardiol 2012;60:531–8.
14. Agmon Y, Khandheria BK, Gentile F, Seward JB. Echocardiographic assessment of the left atrial appendage. J Am Coll Cardiol 1999;34:1867–77.
15. Leung DY, Black IW, Cranney GB, et al. Prognostic implications of left atrial spontaneous echo contrast in nonvalvular atrial fibrillation. J Am Coll Cardiol 1994;24:755–62.
16. Tamura H, Watanabe T, Hirono O, et al. Low wall velocity of left atrial appendage measured by trans-thoracic echocardiography predicts thrombus formation caused by atrial appendage dysfunction. J Am Soc Echocardiogr 2010;23:545–52.
17. Sevimli S, Gundogdu F, Arslan S, et al. Strain and strain rate imaging in evaluating left atrial appendage function by transesophageal echocardiography. Echocardiography 2007;24:823–9.
18. Leong DP, Penhall A, Perry R, et al. Speckle-tracking strain of the left atrium: a transoesophageal echocardiographic validation study. Eur Heart J Cardiovasc Imaging 2013;14:898–905.
19. Karabay CY, Zehir R, Güler A, et al. Left atrial deformation parameters predict left atrial appendage function and thrombus in patients in sinus rhythm with suspected cardioembolic stroke: a speckle tracking and transesophageal echocardiography study. Echocardiography 2013;30:572–81.
20. Vaitkus PT, Barnathan ES. Embolic potential, prevention and management of mural thrombus complicating anterior myocardial infarction: a meta-analysis. J Am Coll Cardiol 1993;22:1004–9.
21. Donal E, Delgado V, Bucciarelli-Ducci C, et al. 2016–18 EACVI Scientific Documents Committee. Multimodality imaging in the diagnosis, risk stratification, and management of patients with dilated cardiomyopathies: an expert consensus document from the European Association of Cardiovascular Imaging. Eur Heart J Cardiovasc Imaging 2019;20:1075–93.
22. Wada H, Yasu T, Sakakura K, et al. Contrast echocardiography for the diagnosis of left ventricular thrombus in anterior myocardial infarction. Heart Vessels 2014;29:308–12.
23. Weinsaft JW, Kim HW, Crowley AL, et al. LV thrombus detection by routine echocardiography: insights into performance characteristics using delayed enhancement CMR. JACC Cardiovasc Imaging 2011;4:702–12.
24. Saric M, Kronzon I. Aortic atherosclerosis and embolic events. Curr Cardiol Rep 2012;14:342–9.
25. Di Tullio MR, Sacco RL, Savoia MT, Sciacca RR, Homma S. Aortic atheroma morphology and the risk of ischemic stroke in a multiethnic population. Am Heart J 2000;139 (2 Pt 1):329–36.
26. Delgado V, Ajmone Marsan N, de Waha S, Bonaros N, Brida M, Burri H, et al.; ESC Scientific Document Group. 2023 ESC Guidelines for the management of endocarditis. Eur Heart J 2023;44(39):3948–42.
27. Habib G, Badano L, Tribouilloy C, et al. Recommendations for the practice of echocardiography in infective endocarditis. Eur J Echocardiogr 2010;11:202–19.
28. Bruun NE, Habib G, Thuny F, Sogaard P. Cardiac imaging in infectious endocarditis. Eur Heart J 2014;35:624–32.
29. Berdejo J, Shibayama K, Harada K, et al. Evaluation of vegetation size and its relationship with embolism in infective endocarditis: a real-time 3-dimensional transesophageal echocardiography study. Circ Cardiovasc Imaging 2014;7(1):149–54.
30. Di Salvo G, Habib G, Pergola V, et al. Echocardiography predicts embolic events in infective endocarditis. J Am Coll Cardiol 200;37:1069–76.
31. Hubert S, Thuny F, Resseguier N, et al. Prediction of symptomatic embolism in infective endocarditis: construction and validation of a risk calculator in a multicenter cohort. J Am Coll Cardiol 2013;62(15):1384–92.
32. Kang DH, Kim YJ, Kim SH, et al. Early surgery versus conventional treatment for infective endocarditis. N Engl J Med 2012;366(26):2466–73.
33. Liu J, Frishman WH. Nonbacterial thrombotic endocarditis: pathogenesis, diagnosis, and management. Cardiol Rev 2016;24:244–7.
34. Poterucha TJ, Kochav J, O'Connor DS, et al. Cardiac tumors: clinical presentation, diagnosis, and management. Curr Treat Options in Oncol 2019;20:66.
35. Colin GC, Gerber BL, Amzulescu M, et al. Cardiac myxoma: a contemporary multimodality imaging review. Int J Cardiovasc Imaging 2018;34:1789–808.
36. Ha JW, Kang WC, Chung N, et al. Echocardiographic and morphologic characteristics of left atrial myxoma and their relation to systemic embolism. Am J Cardiol 1999;83:1579–82.
37. Obrenovic-Kircanski B, Mikic A, Parapid B, et al. A 30-year-single-center experience in atrial myxomas: from presentation to treatment and prognosis. Thorac Cardiovasc Surg 2013;61:530–6.

38. Cianciulli TF, Soumoulou JB, Lax JA, et al. Papillary fibroelastoma: clinical and echocardiographic features and initial approach in 54 cases. Echocardiography 2016;33:1811–7.

39. Mügge A, Daniel WG, Angermann C, et al. Atrial septal aneurysm in adult patients. A multicenter study using transthoracic and transcsophageal echocardiography. Circulation 1995;91:2785–92.

40. Agmon Y, Khandheria BK, Meissner I, et al. Frequency of atrial septal aneurysms in patients with cerebral ischemic events. Circulation 1999;99:1942–4.

41. McGrath ER, Paikin JS, Motlagh B, et al. Transesophageal echocardiography in patients with cryptogenic ischemic stroke: a systematic review. Am Heart J 2014;168:706–12.

42. Berthet K, Lavergne T, Cohen A, et al. Significant association of atrial vulnerability with atrial septal abnormalities in young patients with ischemic stroke of unknown cause. Stroke 2000;31:398–403.

43. Homma S, Sacco RL. Patent foramen ovale and stroke. Circulation 2005;112:1063–72.

44. Overell JR, Bone I, Lees KR. Interatrial septal abnormalities and stroke: a meta-analysis of case-control studies. Neurology 2000;55:1172–9.

45. Pinto FJ. When and how to diagnose patent foramen ovale. Heart 2005;91:438–40.

46. Di Tullio MR. Patent foramen ovale: echocardiographic detection and clinical relevance in stroke. J Am Soc Echocardiogr 2010;23:144–55.

47. Mojadidi MK, Bogush N, Caceres JD, et al. Diagnostic accuracy of transesophageal echocardiogram for the detection of patent foramen ovale: a meta-analysis. Echocardiography 2014;31:752–8.

48. Takaya Y, Nakayama R, Akagi T, et al. Importance of saline contrast transthoracic echocardiography for evaluating large right-to-left shunt in patent foramen ovale associated with cryptogenic stroke. Int J Cardiovasc Imaging 2022;38:515–20.

49. Siostrzonek P, Lang W, Zangeneh M, et al. Significance of left-sided heart disease for the detection of patent foramen ovale by transesophageal contrast echocardiography. J Am Coll Cardiol 1992;19:1192–6.

50. Pristipino C, Sievert H, D'Ascenzo F, et al. European position paper on the management of patients with patent foramen ovale. General approach and left circulation thromboembolism. Eur Heart J 2019;40:3182–95.

51. Mas J-L, Derumeaux G, Guillon B, et al. Patent foramen ovale closure or anticoagulation vs. antiplatelets after stroke. N Engl J Med 2017;377:1011–21.

52. Saver JL, Carroll JD, Thaler DE, et al. Long-term outcomes of patent foramen ovale closure or medical therapy after stroke. N Engl J Med 2017;377:1022–32.

53. Søndergaard L, Kasner SE, Rhodes JF, et al. Patent foramen ovale closure or antiplatelet therapy for cryptogenic stroke. N Engl J Med 2017;377:1033–42.

54. Hołda MK, Krawczyk-O_zo´g A, Koziej M, et al. Left-sided atrial septal pouch is a risk factor for cryptogenic stroke. J Am Soc Echocardiogr 2018;31:771–6.

55. Fauveau E, Cohen A, Bonnet N, Gacem K, Lardoux H. Surgical or medical treatment for thrombus straddling the patent foramen ovale: impending paradoxical embolism? Report of four clinical cases and literature review. Arch Cardiovasc Dis 2008;101:637–44.

Emergency intraoperative and postoperative echocardiography

14

Patrick Collier, Zoran B. Popovic, and Brian P. Griffin

Key Points

- Emergent intraoperative echocardiography (IOE) may be requested for evaluation of an emergency case when there was not sufficient time for adequate preoperative assessment or when an emergent situation arises during an elective surgical procedure.
- Emergent IOE should be performed with a goal-orientated individual approach.
- Intraoperative hemodynamic changes may have a profound effect on valvular lesions, especially the severity of mitral regurgitation. If necessary, the hemodynamic situation should be manipulated to determine the true or potential severity of a valvular lesion.
- Both transthoracic and transesophageal echocardiography can be used for intraoperative or postoperative assessment of cardiac function, unexplained and sudden hemodynamic deterioration, suspicion of pericardial tamponade, cardiac ischemia, assessment of perioperatively placed ventricular assist devices, and a range of other scenarios.

Echocardiography has been used in the operating room since the early 1980s. A number of features make it the preferred intraoperative imaging modality. It is portable, fast, and compact; does not involve radiation; and provides hemodynamic and anatomical data. Intraoperative echocardiography (IOE) is used primarily within the cardiothoracic operating room but can also be a valuable tool when unexpected situations arise during noncardiac surgery. In emergent operative cases, IOE provides vital diagnostic information for the surgeon to help guide surgical intervention. In addition, it provides rapid anatomical and physiologic information in the event of a sudden change in hemodynamic status either before or after surgical intervention.

INTRAOPERATIVE ECHOCARDIOGRAPHY IMAGING APPROACHES

There are three approaches to emergent IOE.

Transesophageal approach

Transesophageal echocardiography (TEE) is the most widely used IOE technique. The probe is typically inserted

DOI: 10.1201/9781003245407-14

after induction of anesthesia and tracheal intubation, remaining in place for the duration of surgery. TEE imaging is performed without interference with the surgical field. Pre-pump intraoperative TEE findings correlate well with surgical observations, significant discrepancies being reported in ~ 2.5% of cases.[1] Still, it is important to be aware of the following *potential pitfalls* when performing intraoperative TEE:

1. It can be difficult to pass the TEE probe if the operation is in progress.
2. Inadequate imaging may result from abnormal anatomy wherein a hiatal hernia prevents adequate apposition between the probe and the esophagus or when prosthetic structures cause shadowing of cardiac structures.
3. Interference by electrocautery or electric saws makes interpretation of all Doppler signals impossible and results in minor distortion of two-dimensional (2D) images.
4. No useful imaging is possible while the heart is at a standstill during cardiopulmonary bypass (CPB).

Epicardial approach

Epicardial IOE refers to imaging using a high-frequency (3.0–7.0 MHz) transducer placed directly on the heart. The probe is placed in a sterile sleeve, and an acoustic interface is made with acoustic gel and a wet epicardial surface. An acoustic stand-off, such as a sterile saline bag, is necessary when imaging structures are near the probe, such as the anterior wall of the ascending aorta. Epicardial imaging is superior to TEE for evaluating the ascending aorta for atheroma or focal dissection and for assessing the interventricular septum and determining gradients across the left ventricular outflow tract (LVOT). In most circumstances, epicardial imaging is performed only if TEE is not feasible or if TEE imaging is suboptimal.[2] The *disadvantages* of epicardial imaging are as follows:

1. It interferes with cardiac surgery.
2. There is only limited time available for imaging.
3. Imaging of structures close to the transducer may be difficult to assess.
4. Imaging may alter hemodynamic parameters if force is applied when the probe is placed on the heart.

However, in emergent situations, the benefit of obtaining vital anatomical and hemodynamic information usually offsets such relative disadvantages.

Transthoracic approach

Transthoracic imaging can be used either before induction of anesthesia or after chest closure when the TEE probe has been removed, typically when rapid assessment is requested to evaluate an acute hemodynamics. However, imaging quality is usually impaired given prone position and limited acoustic windows due to shielding by chest drains and dressing.

REQUIREMENTS FOR INTRAOPERATIVE ECHOCARDIOGRAPHY

Equipment

Ideally, an ultrasound machine interfaced with all necessary transducers and software dedicated solely to IOE should be available at all times in the operating room. Sterile sleeves and acoustic gel should be available for epicardial imaging.

Personnel

By definition, emergent IOE is used to make critical decisions in the operating room; thus, an especially proficient and experienced operator is necessary. Persons performing emergent IOE not only require experience in TEE imaging but should also be familiar with transthoracic and epicardial imaging and with the potential surgical approaches. Skilled operators are typically cardiac anesthesiologists or cardiologists who have received training as outlined in the guideline documents of the respective professional societies.

Approach

Emergent IOE should be performed with a *goal-orientated approach*. First, the question necessitating IOE must be addressed by the modality best suited to answer it. For example, if there is concern about an intraoperative aortic dissection, epicardial imaging may be best, especially if there is difficulty in optimally visualizing the ascending aorta by TEE. The initial portion of the study should focus on thorough imaging of the aorta in multiple planes, and then a complete yet expedient echocardiographic examination should follow. Investigation of all important structures is vital to ensure that no critical information is omitted. We advocate the *routine use of contrast* (agitated saline mixed with blood) in the right heart to ascertain the presence or absence of intracardiac shunting (most commonly a patent foramen ovale [PFO]) for all. Once the study is completed, a record of the examination should be made. After cessation of CPB, the same examination technique as used preoperatively should be performed.

IOE has the following aspects that *differ* from a study in the echocardiographic laboratory:

1. Echocardiography is performed simultaneously with the operation; room lighting and/or space for the machine and echocardiographer may be suboptimal.

2. Radiofrequency interference from other devices, especially those for diathermy, may hinder acquisition.
3. Patient's hemodynamics can change quickly in the operating room.

It is prudent to share information *only* once it has been verified from as many imaging planes as possible. This principle is especially pertinent to emergent IOE because major surgical management decisions are based on the data revealed by it.

INDICATIONS FOR EMERGENCY INTRAOPERATIVE ECHOCARDIOGRAPHY

A request for emergent IOE may be for diagnostics in a case in which there was not sufficient time for adequate preoperative assessment or when an emergent situation arises during an elective surgical procedure (Table 14.1). Such a request may occur at any of the following *four stages* during cardiac operations (the approach and likely findings at each of these stages are discussed later):

1. *Induction of anesthesia* and positioning of vascular access and diagnostic catheters
2. *Pre-pump*—from the time of induction until the patient is put on CPB
3. *Post-pump*—at the end of the main procedure after the patient is weaned from CPB
4. *Before transfer* to the intensive care unit (ICU)—interval from immediate weaning from CPB to leaving the operating room and returning to the ICU

In addition to its diagnostic role, IOE can be used to monitor response to therapeutic maneuvers (e.g., "de-airing" of the left side of the heart after CPB),[3] and pharmacologic interventions in the setting of left ventricular (LV) dysfunction.

As different operative procedures give rise to specific concerns, we review them individually later in the text. A good example of the overall variability of clinical scenarios when emergent IOE is needed is given in a series of consecutive patients requiring emergent intraoperative TEE. The most common reasons were hemodynamic instability, preoperative evaluation, chest trauma, and unexplained intraoperative hypoxemia. New findings were disclosed in 80% patients, with an alteration of the planned surgical procedure in 23%.[4] Evaluation of hemodynamic instability is a category 1 indication for IOE in the task force report of American Society of Echocardiography and Society of Cardiovascular Anesthesiologists.[5]

TABLE 14.1 Indications for Emergency Intraoperative Echocardiography

Emergency surgery with insufficient time for adequate preoperative assessment
1. Cardiac surgery
   Acute myocardial ischemia requiring emergent revascularization
   Ischemic complications (ventricular septal defect, cardiac rupture, papillary muscle rupture)
   Acute valvular failure (endocarditis, prosthetic malfunction)
   Pericardial disease (tamponade)
2. Surgery of great vessels
   Acute aortic dissection
   Aortic aneurysm rupture
3. Noncardiac surgery
   Hemodynamic instability
   New electrocardiographic changes
   Unexpected operative findings involving the heart or great vessels

Elective cardiac surgery requiring emergent intraoperative imaging
1. At induction
   Hemodynamic collapse
   New electrocardiographic changes
   Unexplained hemodynamics
2. Pre-pump
   Unexpected surgical findings
   Calcification at the cannulation site
   Hemodynamic compromise
   Positioning of diagnostic catheters
3. Post-pump
   Difficulty in weaning
   Unexpected arrhythmia
   New electrocardiographic changes
   Hemodynamic compromise
   Positioning of diagnostic or therapeutic aids
4. Before return to intensive care unit
   Hemodynamic compromise

Induction of anesthesia

Problems at induction of anesthesia are rare in experienced cardiothoracic surgical centers. Nevertheless, as the complexity of cardiac surgical procedures and severity of comorbid conditions increases, the potential for hemodynamic compromise at this stage of the procedure remains. Typical problems include drug reactions, myocardial ischemia, arrhythmia, and hypotension. Less common problems include a catastrophe during vascular catheter placement or the development/worsening of pericardial tamponade. In the critical care setting, TEE has been shown to provide hemodynamic information independent of and in addition to that provided by a pulmonary artery catheter.[6] Many patients undergoing cardiac surgery have tenuous hemodynamics and/or severe coronary artery disease. The hemodynamic effects of anesthetic drugs can result in hemodynamic instability and/or collapse. In addition, physiologic stresses at induction increase the risk of myocardial ischemia. Continuous electrocardiographic monitoring has limitations for the detection of myocardial ischemia, especially in patients with known coronary artery disease and abnormal resting electrocardiogram (ECG). As wall motion abnormalities develop before ECG changes in the setting of early ischemia, identification of RWMA is more sensitive for the detection of ischemia than are ECG changes alone.[7] At this phase of the operation, the TEE probe is typically not in place, and a rapidly performed transthoracic echocardiogram may help by identifying changes in global LV systolic function and/or new LV RWMA.

Pre-pump

After induction of anesthesia and mechanical ventilation, rapid deployment of the TEE probe is usually feasible. It is at this stage of surgery that emergency diagnostic imaging is most used. In the true emergent cardiac case, IOE may represent the sole means of preoperative assessment. While the study should focus initially on the acute problem, it is vital to perform a rapid, comprehensive examination of all valves, chambers, and the aorta. In addition, an agitated saline bolus injection for the detection of right-to-left shunting is performed to detect a potential PFO, which, if significant, is usually closed because there is a non-negligible risk of hypoxemia resulting from right-to-left shunting in the postoperative period.

Studies have shown that IOE alters surgical management in 9–19% of cases, and it becomes critical in emergent cases without comprehensive preoperative assessment.[4,8] In other cases requiring emergent surgery in which presurgical echocardiography was performed, IOE is used to confirm findings, ensure that no changes have occurred, and confirm that there are no other additional findings.

ACUTE MYOCARDIAL ISCHEMIA AND MECHANICAL COMPLICATIONS RELATED TO MYOCARDIAL ISCHEMIA

Emergent coronary revascularization is one of the most important indications for pre-pump emergent IOE. Most commonly, patients are transfers from the cardiac catheterization laboratory, after a percutaneous coronary intervention (PCI) complication has caused acute ischemia not amenable to percutaneous salvage. Occasionally, a patient with acute myocardial infarction (AMI) with failed primary PCI will present. As with all IOE studies, a rapid and comprehensive examination should be performed to identify coexisting problems. This is especially important in these patients because they typically have not had an opportunity for a comprehensive preoperative examination.

Acute mechanical complications after AMI include ventricular septal rupture (VSR), acute papillary muscle rupture, and rupture of the LV free wall (see also Chapter 3). Typically, the patient is hemodynamically unstable and often has had limited and incomplete preoperative evaluation.

Ventricular septal rupture

In the thrombolytic era, VSR has become less common (0.2% incidence, compared with 1–3% historically) but occurs earlier (median of 1 day after infarction, compared with 3–5 days historically).[9] VSR occurs only where there is transmural myocardial infarction. (Figure 14.1) (V14.1A, V14.1B, V14.1C, V14.1D). Age, female gender, history of hypertension, and lack

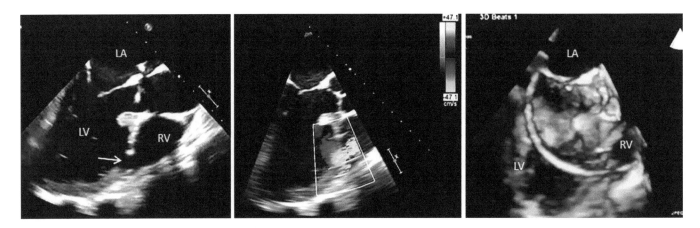

FIGURE 14.1   Ventricular septal rupture. Transesophageal echocardiographic two-dimensional image (left panel) shows large ventricular septal rupture (arrow) caused by extensive acute transmural hemorrhagic myocardial infarction of the anteroseptal wall (7–10 days in evolution) (V14.1A). Color Doppler revealed turbulent flow with left-to-right shunt (middle panel, V14.1B). During attempted three-dimensional TEE-guided percutaneous repair of the ventricular septal defect (right panel, V14.1C), the patient developed acute hypotension and a new large pericardial effusion (V14.1D). Resuscitation attempts for cardiac tamponade were unsuccessful. Hemopericardium and extension of the ventricular septal rupture to LV perforation were diagnosed at subsequent autopsy. LA: left atrium; LV: left ventricle; RV: right ventricle.

of prior history of myocardial ischemia increase the risk of VSR. Patients typically present with acute pulmonary edema, RV failure, and a new murmur. Currently, the most favored approach is surgery albeit exact timing (early vs. emergent) is controversial. While the diagnosis has usually been made before arrival in the operating room, diagnostic insight is often limited, and IOE is necessary to locate and define the extent of the defect. A color Doppler of the entire interventricular septum is mandatory to localize the defect because these defects may be difficult to appreciate by 2D imaging alone. A VSR associated with an anterior infarct occurs in the region of the apical septum and is best visualized with either the transgastric short-axis apical or a midesophageal four-chamber view while those associated with inferior infarcts involve the posteroinferior basal septum and can be seen in either the LV transgastric short-axis view or the four-chamber midesophageal view.

VSR defects are classified as simple or complex. *Simple defects* are those that have a direct course across the septum with one discrete color flow jet and are more frequent with anterior infarcts. *Complex defects* tend to be associated with a large area of myocardial necrosis, with multiple serpiginous defects traversing the septum (more common with inferoposterior infarcts). If they involve the basal septum, they may be associated with mitral and/or tricuspid dysfunction.[9] The width of the color jet correlates with the size of the defect at surgery.[9] TEE also provides additional information, including assessing LV and RV function and estimating right ventricular systolic pressure (RVSP). It is important to exclude other mechanical complications of the infarct, including free-wall and/or papillary muscle rupture.

Patients with inferoposterior defects have a higher mortality, as these infarcts are often associated with RV infarction, are more complex, and more challenging to repair.[9]

Acute ischemic mitral regurgitation

Acute MR accompanying AMI has varying etiology. *Papillary muscle necrosis with partial or complete rupture* results in severe MR (Figure 14.2) (V14.2A, V14.2B, V14.2C, V14.2D, V14.2E) and is associated with a poor prognosis unless there is urgent surgical intervention. Patients present with acute pulmonary edema, hypotension, and respiratory failure. Often the murmur is relatively soft. The patients are usually taken to the operating room emergently, and intraoperative TEE is performed during surgical preparation. Papillary muscle rupture most commonly occurs in the setting of a limited inferior wall myocardial infarction. The posteromedial papillary muscle is particularly vulnerable to ischemia because it is supplied by a single coronary artery, the posterior descending. The anterolateral papillary muscle is less vulnerable because of dual supply by left anterior descending and left circumflex arteries. Echocardiographically, LV appears small and hyperdynamic, with the area of inferior wall infarction often difficult to spot. Typically, the head of the papillary muscle is seen prolapsing into the left atrium in association with torrential MR. As each papillary muscle provides chordae to both leaflets, rupture of

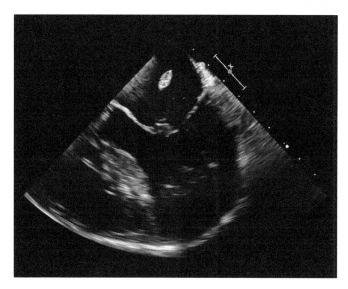

FIGURE 14.2 Papillary muscle rupture. Transesophageal echocardiographic two-dimensional image shows a bulky mobile echodensity consistent with a head of ruptured papillary muscle after delayed presentation of inferior wall myocardial infarction (V14.2A, V14.2B), associated with acute severe mitral regurgitation (V14.2C). The patient underwent successful mitral valve replacement (V14.2D) with persistence of a large inferior regional wall motion abnormality postoperatively (V14.2E).

the posteromedial papillary muscle results in prolapse or flail of both leaflets (posterior aspects). The flail head of the papillary muscle is not always appreciated and may remain tethered or entangled within the chordae. In this situation, the presence of severe MR with a hyperdynamic left ventricle and a short-axis view demonstrating a "missing" posteromedial papillary muscle is diagnostic. In less severe cases, if only one head of the papillary muscle is torn, detailed assessment of the subvalvular mitral apparatus from multiple views to confirm the underlying cause is needed. Because the area of infarction is often small, the long-term prognosis is relatively good if surgery is successful.

Acute papillary muscle dysfunction caused by infarction or ischemia in the LV territory adjacent to the insertion of the papillary muscle can also result in MR. In the setting of a large infarct (most commonly anterior), LV dilation can result in a *disruption of the normal* subvalvular *geometry*, with apical displacement of the papillary muscles, resulting in tethering of the subvalvular apparatus and causing MR. The latter two causes of MR are less likely to present emergently with acute MR.

Left ventricular free-wall rupture

Acute rupture of the LV free wall occurs in ~3% of transmural infarcts and is rapidly fatal; it is one of the primary causes of sudden death after infarction (Figure 14.3) (V14.3A, V14.3B, V14.3C, V14.3D, V14.3E, V14.3F). In some cases, an "incomplete" rupture occurs, providing a window for emergent surgical intervention. This most commonly occurs in the setting of a posterolateral wall infarct, associated with left circumflex or left anterior descending artery occlusion. A nonfatal rupture typically occurs at the junction of the infarcted and normal myocardium, creating a narrow indirect channel through the myocardium to the epicardium, with pericardial containment and creation of a pseudoaneurysm. Typical symptoms are recurrent chest pain, hypotension, emesis, restlessness, and bradycardia. Echocardiography typically demonstrates some degree of pericardial effusion with or without the appearance of intrapericardial thrombus. This appearance in the setting of an AMI is highly specific for cardiac rupture.[10] Direct visualization of the communication is not always possible, although there may be the appearance of a channel by 2D echo with some limited flow by color Doppler. Echocardiographic features suggestive of tamponade are often noted.

ACUTE VALVE DISEASE

Acute mitral regurgitation

In the absence of ischemia, acute MR may occur as a result of disruption at any level of the valve or subvalvular apparatus (Table 14.2). *Chordal rupture with flail leaflet* and severe MR can occur spontaneously in severe myxomatous disease, chest trauma, or, occasionally, without any apparent cause. Intraoperative echocardiographic assessment of MR has several

TABLE 14.2   Causes of Acute Valvular Regurgitation

Acute mitral regurgitation
Mitral annulus
    Endocarditis with abscess
Mitral leaflet
    Endocarditis—perforation or vegetation preventing complete leaflet closure
    Invasive procedures—percutaneous balloon mitral valvotomy
Chordae tendineae
    Myxomatous mitral valve disease
    Blunt trauma or direct trauma
    Endocarditis
    Spontaneous rupture
Papillary muscle
    Papillary muscle rupture
    Acute papillary muscle dysfunction secondary to ischemia/infarction
    Trauma

Acute aortic regurgitation
Leaflet abnormalities
    Traumatic rupture
    Acute endocarditis
    Acute prosthetic valve dysfunction
    Post—aortic balloon valvuloplasty
Aortic root or ascending aorta abnormalities
    Acute aortic dissection
Perivalvular leak or dehiscence of prosthetic valves

goals, including assessment of MR severity, determination of its mechanism, evaluation of associated features, and determination of the potential for repair. It is vital to recognize that MR is a

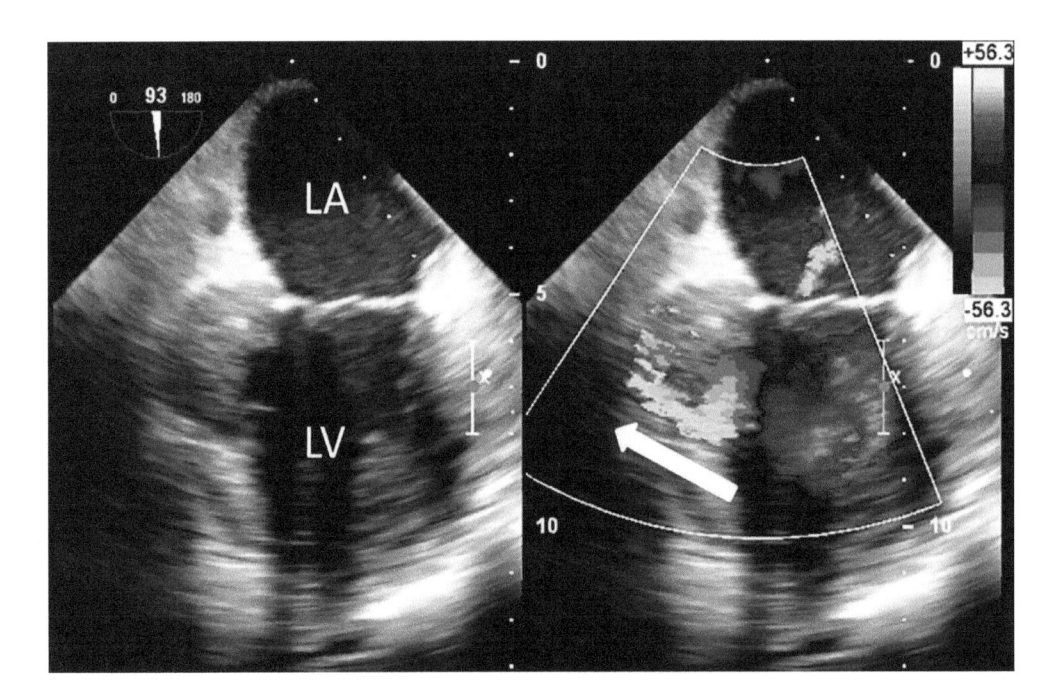

FIGURE 14.3   Complicated LV free-wall rupture. After a delayed-presentation inferior wall myocardial infarction, inferior LV free-wall rupture was detected. The arrow highlights the direction of the abnormal flow in color compare mode (two-dimensional, left panel; color Doppler, right panel; V14.3A and V14.3B). However, preoperative transesophageal echocardiography in the operating room identified a new complication—namely, intramural dissection of the right ventricular free wall (V14.3C and V14.3D), with flow communication to the right ventricle (V14.3E and V14.3F)—at which point a plan to attempt surgical repair was abandoned. LA: left atrium; LV: left ventricle.

dynamic condition, the severity of which can vary. Intraoperative decrease in afterload and systolic blood pressure can artificially reduce MR severity and may require phenylephrine afterload challenge.[11] Valve repair is most likely in patients with myxomatous degeneration and is less likely in a patient with valve calcification, extensive fibrosis, leaflet destruction caused by endocarditis, or anterior leaflet pathology (see also Chapter 10).

Acute aortic regurgitation

Causes of acute aortic regurgitation (AR) are best divided into leaflet and aortic abnormalities (Table 14.2). Acute AR imposes a sudden increase in stroke volume that the LV is required to produce, with the LV end-diastolic pressure increasing acutely, causing dyspnea and pulmonary edema. Most commonly, acute AR results from an *aortic dissection*. The role of IOE in the setting of acute AR is to define the anatomy of the aortic valve and ascending aorta, determine the cause and the severity of AR, assess LV function, and exclude other abnormalities. In the presence of relatively normal leaflets, as with an acute aortic dissection, successful repair of the valve is possible (see also Chapter 9).

Endocarditis

Valve surgery is indicated urgently in patients with endocarditis and severe valvular dysfunction with any of the following: congestive heart failure, presence of an abscess or fistula, large vegetations (>10 mm) that are either increasing or not

changing in size, recurrent embolic events, and resistant infection (Figure 14.4) (V14.4A, V14.4B, V14.4C, V14.4D). In the setting of hemodynamic instability and known endocarditis, many patients may have had only limited opportunity to have an updated echocardiographic study to define the anatomy and extent of infection before arriving in the operating room. IOE can define the extent of infection, location and size of any abscess, and the involvement of or spread to other valves or chambers. Infection can spread from one valve to another, most commonly in the setting of a regurgitant jet of AR hitting the anterior mitral valve leaflet and setting up a satellite focus of infection. The spread can also occur from extension of infection through the fibrous skeleton of the heart. The process may progress to abscess, pseudoaneurysm, or fistula formation. Echocardiographically, an abscess appears as an echolucent cavity in the perivalvular region, with limited intracavitary flow by color Doppler. The wall of an abscess can break down, resulting in communication with contiguous chambers, with fistula formation from either the LVOT to the right ventricle or right atrium (Gerbode defect) or from the aorta to the left atrium or right ventricle. Perivalvular infection of a mitral valve can occasionally cause mitral annular abscess or spread of infection to the aortic valve.

Acute prosthetic valve failure

Patients with prosthetic valves may present with either primary or secondary valve failure (see also Chapter 12). Primary *mechanical valve failure* is rare, although strut failure resulting in disk embolization may occur, especially with single

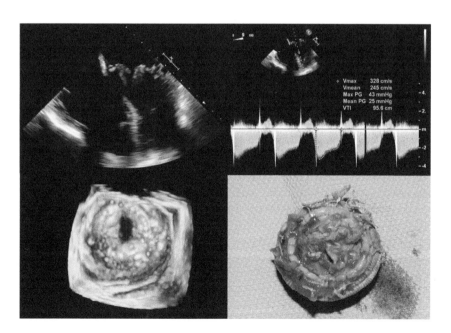

FIGURE 14.4 Prosthetic mitral valve endocarditis and severe acute mitral stenosis. Gross thickening and mobile echodensities (upper left panel, two-dimensional transesophageal echocardiography [TEE]; lower left panel, three-dimensional TEE (V14.4A and V14.4C) on a bioprosthetic mitral valve from endocarditis caused by methicillin-sensitive *Staphylococcus aureus*, which resulted in near-obstructive acute severe mitral stenosis with high transvalvular gradients (upper right panel) (V14.4B and V14.4C). This was treated successfully with redo mitral valve replacement (V14.4D) and antibiotic therapy. Surgically removed diseased bioprosthesis (lower right panel).

tilting-disk valves. This is usually immediately catastrophic. In the unusual case wherein the patient gets to the operating room, absence of the valve occluder and overwhelming regurgitation at the prosthetic valve are encountered. *Bioprosthetic valve degeneration* may lead to a sudden acute flail cusp requiring urgent reintervention. This is readily recognized with emergency TEE. *Acute thrombosis of a mechanical valve* can result in acute valvular dysfunction. Emergent surgery carries significant mortality but is usually recommended in younger patients with left-sided prostheses and fewer comorbidities because of the embolic risk attendant on thrombolysis. These patients may present emergently to surgery with minimal investigation because of extreme hemodynamic failure. TEE is sensitive and accurate in the diagnosis of prosthetic valve thrombosis,[12] typically demonstrating a mass with associated obstruction of the valve occluder(s) and typically high gradients across the valve.

Mechanical and bioprosthetic valves are at a similar risk of *endocarditis*, with an annual rate of ~0.5%.[13] Compared with native valve, prosthetic valve endocarditis is more likely to be complicated by abscess and perivalvular destruction, leading to the risk of valve dehiscence. Endocarditis on a bioprosthetic valve, as with a native valve, can result in *leaflet destruction and regurgitation*. Severe perivalvular regurgitation in prosthetic valve endocarditis carries a grave prognosis, and emergent surgery is often indicated. In addition to assessment of the infected valve, a comprehensive examination is warranted to exclude other valve involvement and to document LV function.

PERICARDIAL DISEASE

Patients with cardiac tamponade and hemodynamic instability (see also Chapter 8) can present to the operating room if percutaneous drainage is not feasible or failed. In the operating room, echocardiography is used to confirm tamponade and define the location and extent of fluid. In patients *after cardiac surgery, a loculated effusion*, even if small, can result in hemodynamic compromise. Demonstration of respiratory variation of mitral and tricuspid pulsed-wave Doppler may be difficult in the operating room. RV diastolic collapse is the most specific echocardiographic sign of cardiac tamponade, with RA collapse occasionally helpful but less specific. With elevated right-sided pressures seen with pulmonary hypertension, RV collapse will not occur until higher values of intrapericardial pressure are reached. In addition, it is important to look for atypical echocardiographic features such as left atrial (LA) collapse and/or localized echodense masses suggestive of pericardial thrombus.

AORTIC DISSECTION

Acute aortic dissection (see also Chapter 6) is a common reason for emergent IOE. Any dissection involving the ascending aorta requires emergent surgery, as conservative treatment has ~1% per hour mortality within the first 48 hours. While there are a number of classifications to describe the locations of the dissection flap, it is preferable to describe the anatomical location of the flap and, most important, whether it involves the ascending aorta (Stanford type A or DeBakey type I or II—65% of acute dissections), or whether it arises in the descending aorta (Stanford type B, DeBakey type III), for which initial medical therapy is the usual strategy (see Figure 6.1). The diagnosis of acute ascending dissection is typically made preoperatively via TEE, or computed tomography (CT). However, patients with suspected acute aortic dissection and acute hypotension may arrive in the operating room with minimal preoperative evaluation. Acute hypotension in the setting of a dissection is most likely a result of aortic wall rupture or cardiac tamponade. Intraoperative TEE and, if necessary, epicardial imaging permit complete imaging of the ascending aorta, aortic valve, and left ventricle. In addition to defining the location of the origin of the intimal flap in the ascending aorta and the extent of spread of the dissection in the aortic arch, great vessels, and descending aorta, IOE can probe for complications. Acute AR can occur because of proximal extension of the dissection flap (resulting in disruption of leaflet suspension), annular dilation in patients with aortic dilation, or prolapse of the intimal flap through aortic valve interfering with cusp coaptation.

A detailed examination of the aortic valve to *assess its involvement and suitability for valve repair* is necessary. A prolapsing, "normal"-appearing leaflet resulting from involvement by the dissection of the cusp base can usually be repaired (resuspended) with a high likelihood of success.[14] Both coronary ostia should be searched for, as involvement of one or both coronary arteries by acute dissection occurs in 10–20% of cases. Adequate visualization of the coronary ostia is not always possible, with success rates of 88% for the left main stem and 50% for the right coronary artery.[15] In addition, assessment of other pathologies is necessary especially in syndromic patients.

CALCIFICATION AT THE CANNULATION SITE

Calcifications of the ascending aorta may make placement of the bypass cannula difficult and increase the risk of embolism (see Chapter 13). Furthermore, cross-clamping of a calcified aorta may lead to catastrophic embolization. Intraoperative aortic palpation and TEE are inaccurate methods for detecting atheroma in the ascending aorta. *Epicardial imaging* provides a detailed and accurate assessment of the relevant portion of the aorta. Based on the echocardiographic appearance, the approach to cannula insertion and/or cross-clamping may be modified.

HEMODYNAMIC COMPROMISE

Pre-pump

Acute hemodynamic compromise in the pre-pump period has precipitants similar to those at induction of anesthesia. Acute myocardial ischemia with new RWMA is the most common cause in both emergent and nonemergent cases. IOE can provide qualitative assessment of depleted intravascular volume by visualization of a small, hypercontractile, "empty" LV cavity. The progression of an aortic dissection causing acute AR or rupture can precipitate hemodynamic collapse. Similarly, progression of the emergent lesion requiring intervention (e.g., enlarging VSR, progression from a partial to a complete papillary muscle rupture, valvular dehiscence) can precipitate acute emergencies. When opening the chest in patients with prior coronary artery bypass grafting, there is a risk of damage to previously grafted arteries, especially internal mammary grafts, which often lie close to the sternum. This may lead to acute arterial hemorrhage and ischemia, culminating in rapid hemodynamic compromise. Emergency echocardiography may help determine the volume status and onset of RWMA in this situation. Patients with large ascending aortic aneurysms adherent to the sternum are also at risk of iatrogenic rupture with sternotomy.

Hemodynamic instability post-pump

Post-pump IOE is typically performed after the aortic cross-clamp has been removed and CPB has been weaned, but before removal of the arterial and venous CPB cannulae and before administration of protamine, so that if a major problem is found, CPB can be rapidly reinstituted. Post-pump IOE has the following four aims to

1. confirm the *success* of the surgical procedure (such as competency of valve repair),
2. evaluate for *intracardiac air*,
3. document satisfactory *LV and RV function*,
4. evaluate for any potential *complications*.

Emergently, IOE can be requested for unexplained difficulty in weaning off CPB, or sudden acute hemodynamic deterioration (either unexplained hypotension or refractory malignant arrhythmia) after a transient period of hemodynamic stability after coming off pump.

A variety of factors can cause hemodynamic instability during weaning off CPB, with echocardiography useful as diagnostic and a monitoring tool.[16]

Early after cessation of CPB, there may be *global LV systolic dysfunction* owing to residual effects of hyperkalemic cardioplegia or to widespread myocardial ischemia.

A *new RWMA post-pump* is usually a result of *embolization of intracardiac air* but can be a residual effect of the *cardioplegia*. Air can embolize down either coronary artery, but because of its superior position in the supine patient, the right coronary artery is most commonly affected. IOE is sensitive for the detection of intracardiac air, which is most commonly located at the LV apex, with a characteristic "firefly" appearance, or is seen entering the left atrium from the pulmonary veins.[3] If very severe, the entire LV cavity may be filled with a snowstorm-like effect. Typically, this improves with time but may require maintaining CPB support longer until the air has cleared and LV function improves. The surgeon will typically try to vent the air with needle puncture of the LV chamber and vent with the aortic CPB cannula until the air has dissipated.

Isolated left anterior descending and/or left circumflex territory ischemia caused by air is unusual and gives rise to the concern that there is a problem with the vessel or bypass graft, external compression of the vessel, compromise of the left coronary artery ostium, or embolization of particulate material from within the heart. The persistence of an inferior RWMA after the air has been removed and the inferior wall has had time to recover from air embolization gives rise to these same concerns. With RWMA immediately after coronary artery bypass, the implicated coronary artery or graft may require intervention, as *post-pump RWMA* are associated with adverse events in one-third of cases.[17]

In *unexplained hemodynamic instability* postoperatively, the *ascending aorta* should be screened for evidence of acute injury such as intramural hematoma (Figure 14.5) (V14.5A, V14.5B) or dissection, which may complicate removal of the aortic CPB cannula. Attention also needs to be paid to the right ventricle because *post-pump RV dysfunction* may result from residual or inadequate cardioplegia, or any cause of right coronary artery obstruction or interruption. IOE can also be used to *assess intracardiac volume*, and an empty hypercontractile left ventricle in a hypotensive patient should suggest volume replacement as the initial resuscitative measure. Other potential causes of acute hemodynamic instability and specific complications that can occur after certain cardiac procedures are outlined in Table 14.3. A rapid assessment of all valves to document any *new significant regurgitation* is necessary. In the setting of unexplained hypoxemia, significant *shunting* can occur across a PFO, especially if right heart pressures are elevated, and this should always be looked for.

Hemodynamic instability after mitral valve repair

Hemodynamics post mitral valve repair is influenced by multiple pathologies.

A *decrease in LV systolic function after correction of MR* is not unusual, especially in those with severe MR and pre-pump subnormal LV function. This is a result of unmasking of pre-pump contractile dysfunction concealed by the reduced afterload associated with severe MR.

LVOT obstruction caused by systolic anterior motion (SAM) of the mitral valve happens in 3–9% of valve repairs

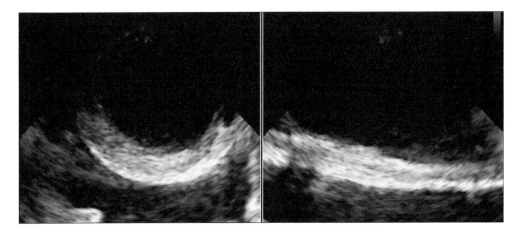

FIGURE 14.5 Acute perioperative aortic intramural hematoma. During post-pump intraoperative transesophageal echocardiography, gross thickening of the aortic wall was identified, representing acute perioperative intramural hematoma in the proximal descending aorta (V14.5A and V14.5B).

TABLE 14.3 Potential Post-Pump Findings in a Patient with Hemodynamic Instability

Any cardiac surgical procedure
  New regional wall motion abnormality
  Major change in global LV function
  Intracardiac air
  Acute valvular regurgitation
  Acute aortic dissection
  PFO with significant right-to-left shunt
  Cardiac tamponade (after closure of the chest)
Coronary artery bypass grafting (CABG)
  Dissection at graft insertion
Mitral valve repair
  Acute repair failure or annuloplasty ring dehiscence
  LVOT obstruction caused by SAM
  Acute left circumflex occlusion caused by a suture
  Significant residual atrial septal defect
  Mitral stenosis
Valve replacement
  Mitral
  Aortic
  Acute valve dehiscence
  Mechanical strut occlusion or failure to open
  Intracardiac fistula
  LV pseudoaneurysm or rupture
  Left atrial dissection
  Strut obstruction of LVOT
  Coronary ostial obstruction
Surgical myectomy
  Ventricular septal defect
  Residual LVOT obstruction
Residual mitral regurgitation

Abbreviations: LV, left ventricular; LVOT, left ventricular outflow tract; PFO, patent foramen ovale; SAM, systolic anterior motion.

(Figure 14.6) (V14.6A, V14.6B, V14.6C, V14.6D, V14.6E, V14.6F, and V14.6G).[18] High gradients across the LVOT can occur and result in severe hypotension, secondary MR, and inability to wean the patient from CPB. It is a dynamic condition, and its severity can be exacerbated by inotropes and/or volume depletion. It is caused by anterior displacement of the mitral coaptation line and is associated with myxomatous valve disease (especially large leaflets and bileaflet prolapse), small hyperdynamic left ventricle, and the use of a stiff annuloplasty ring.[18] While SAM is easily visualized by TEE, the gradient produced by SAM may be difficult to measure, with the best alignment usually being from a deep transgastric view. Occasionally, epicardial imaging is necessary. Initial treatment involves withdrawal of inotropes, volume repletion, and the use of beta-blockers. If the condition persists, a sliding annuloplasty (reducing the height of the posterior leaflet) or valve replacement may be necessary.

Occasionally, *suture dehiscence after repair* results in MR. If it occurs at the site of leaflet resection in the posterior leaflet, it can simulate a *posterior leaflet perforation*. Rarely, the *annuloplasty ring can dehisce*, and this is shown by increased mobility of the ring with MR originating outside the ring.

The *left circumflex artery* runs in the atrioventricular groove near the lateral aspect of the mitral annulus, and there is a small risk of ensnaring it when suturing the ring.

Finally, in limited incision mitral valve surgery, the mitral valve is typically approached through the interatrial septum, and inadequate closure may infrequently result in *significant shunting.*

Hemodynamic instability after valve replacement

Historically, it was common to have residual LV systolic dysfunction after mitral valve replacement before the importance of preserving the subvalvular apparatus was appreciated. In a current era, early hemodynamic instability from prosthetic valve dysfunction is unusual. This can involve *primary valve dysfunction*, when one or both of the disks in a mechanical valve or the leaflets in a bioprosthetic valve fail to open. This

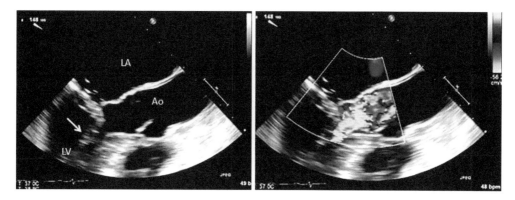

FIGURE 14.6 Postoperative systolic anterior motion (SAM) of the mitral valve. After initial mitral valve repair, hemodynamic compromise was noted resulting in difficulty weaning off cardiopulmonary bypass. SAM of the mitral valve leaflets was identified (arrow) by intraoperative transesophageal echocardiography (left panel, V14.6A) with flow acceleration in the LVOT (right panel, V14.6B). An aggressive sliding annuloplasty was then performed, which resolved the SAM (V14.6C and V14.6D) but resulted in moderate mitral regurgitation (V14.6D and V14.6E). A final decision was made to replace the valve with a low-profile bioprosthetic valve (V14.6F and V14.6G). Ao: aorta; LA: left atrium; LV: left ventricle.

usually resolves spontaneously with increasing filling pressures. Occasionally, if suture material or residual valve apparatus is *interfering* with valve function, MR may result, and a second pump-run may be required to correct this.

Acute valve dehiscence is extremely rare but can be seen with severe endocarditis with extensive perivalvular tissue destruction.

A rare complication of mitral valve replacement is *LV rupture or pseudoaneurysm* often presenting as acute hemodynamic collapse post-pump. This complications is more likely in patients with extensive annular calcification or after repeated mitral valve surgery. A pseudoaneurysm appears as a small saccular cavity communicating with the LV along the posterior aspect of the mitral valve annulus, and it requires redo surgery. *LA wall dissection* is a related complication with similar predisposing factors, reflected by echocardiography in the appearance of a cavity within the left atrium with a linear echodensity consistent with a dissection flap. Rarely, after mitral bioprosthetic insertion in a patient with a small left ventricle, *LV outflow obstruction resulting from the struts of the bioprosthesis* is seen.

Hemodynamic impairment after myectomy

After myectomy, hemodynamic impairment may result from an inadequate resection of muscle with *residual LV outflow obstruction and SAM*. This usually requires further removal of muscle or, if this is impossible, mitral valve intervention or even replacement with a low-profile valve. If the resection of muscle is too large, *ventricular septal defect* with left-to-right shunting may result. This may be difficult to detect without using multiple views and may require epicardial imaging for detection.

Visualization of septal perforator transection is normal after myectomy; it consists of a low-velocity flow from the septum into the left ventricle and should not be mistaken for ventricular septal defect.

Hemodynamic instability before leaving the operating room

Hemodynamic instability after the chest is closed and the patient is being prepared for transfer to the ICU is *typically caused by factors similar to those immediately post-pump*. At this stage, the TEE probe has been removed. An initial approach may be to try to identify problem with transthoracic imaging; however, this is often difficult in patients after surgery, with impediments, such as chest drains and bandages impeding the conventional imaging windows. If necessary, the TEE probe may need to be reinserted. *Intracardiac air* is unlikely to be the culprit, unless significant residual air was seen on final post-pump imaging.

Chest closure can change the anatomical orientation of the heart and, more importantly, of bypass grafts, and there is a risk of *graft kinking or compression*. A likelier cause of acute hemodynamic compromise is *cardiac tamponade*. This may be heralded by increased drainage through the chest tubes. A *localized collection at a critical point* (such as behind the left atrium) (Figure 14.7) (V14.7A, V14.7B, and V14.7C, V14.8A, V14.8B, and V14.8C) or the rapid collection of a relatively small volume of fluid can cause disproportionate hemodynamic compromise.

Placement of supporting devices

Emergent IOE may be requested to assist with the placement of intravascular catheters and cardiac assist devices. In the operating room, IOE can sometimes be of assistance in visualizing the location of a *pulmonary artery catheter* that cannot be easily passed into the correct position in the pulmonary artery and can demonstrate coiling in the right atrium or ventricle. TEE is often used to confirm the correct location of the distal tip of the balloon of an *intra-aortic balloon pump*, which is just distal to the origin of the left subclavian artery.

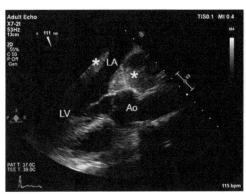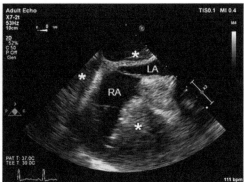

FIGURE 14.7   Post-cardiac surgery hematoma. A large post-cardiac surgery hematoma (*) around the left and right atria, aortic root, and right pulmonary artery (V14.7C), compressing the left (left panel, V14.7A) and both left and right atria (right panel, V14.7B). Ao: aorta; LA: left atrium; LV: left ventricle; RA, right atrium.

Ventricular assist devices

Before implantation of a left ventricular assist device (LVAD), IOE should recognize potential issues.[19] *Severe RV dysfunction* gives rise to concerns that the right ventricle will be unable to maintain sufficient forward cardiac output and filling of the left heart. The LVAD pump inflow cannula is typically placed in the LV apex, with the pump outflow cannula returning blood to the ascending aorta (see Figure 15.2). Evaluation of the *LV apex for thrombus* and the *ascending aorta for atheroma* is important. In addition, the *presence and severity of AR* are important. If AR is significant, corrective aortic valve surgery will be required. Finally, if a *PFO* is identified, it should be closed because when the pump is implanted and LA pressure falls, blood can be shunted from right to left.

Immediately after implantation of an LVAD, IOE should show the *aortic valve either not opening or opening infrequently as it is effectively bypassed*. Flows into the inflow and from the outflow *cannula* should be documented, with flows being less than 2 m/s for both. Increased flow velocity at the inflow cannula may be caused by *angulation and partial obstruction of the cannula*, which may require repositioning if this is affecting pump flow. Finally, the post-pump IOE should evaluate *RV function*, and exclude evidence of *PFO and aortic dissection*.

TRANSESOPHAGEAL ECHOCARDIOGRAPHY-GUIDED INTERVENTIONS IN THE HYBRID OPERATING ROOM

By definition, a hybrid operating room allows for easy conversion of percutaneous procedures to open-heart surgery if necessary. Intraoperative TEE commonly plays a key role in guidance of the percutaneous procedures (see Chapter 22)

and early identification of complications should they arise— for example, with *transcatheter aortic valve replacement* (V14.9A, V14.9B, V14.10A, V14.10B), *percutaneous mitral valve repair using E-clip, pacemaker lead extraction*, and *paravalvular leak closure* (Figure 14.8) (V14.11A, V14.11B, V14.11C, V14.11D).

INTRAOPERATIVE ECHOCARDIOGRAPHY DURING NONCARDIAC SURGERY

Emergency echocardiography is occasionally requested during noncardiac surgery. In elective noncardiac surgery cases, patients have already had a diagnostic work-up to exclude underlying cardiac problems, especially if there is a suggestion from the past history that the patient's cardiovascular status may be of concern. However, unexpected situations do arise.

The noncardiac procedures where echocardiography is likely to be required usually are vascular procedures, especially those involving aorta, thoracic procedures involving lung carcinoma, surgery to remove suspected renal carcinoma, and major gastrointestinal operations.

IOE is usually requested in the setting of *hemodynamic instability* (V14.12A and V14.12B), which, for nonthoracic surgery, is typically a result of *myocardial ischemia precipitated by acute changes in intravascular volume and/or blood pressure*. During major vascular surgery, reduction in preload from reduction in venous return and increase in afterload from aortic cross-clamping may lead to afterload mismatch, with severe reduction in ventricular function. This is especially the case with suprarenal aortic surgery. These findings may be exacerbated by acidosis from tissue underperfusion. Distinguishing this from severe ischemia may be difficult, but the *global rather than regional* ventricular dysfunction is helpful in differentiation. Improvement in function usually occurs in response to removal of the aortic cross-clamp.

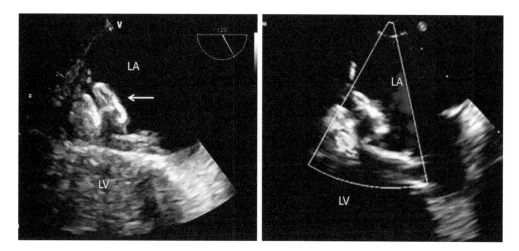

FIGURE 14.8 Percutaneous paravalvular prosthetic mitral valve leak closure. Severe paravalvular mitral regurgitation (V14.11A) was identified in a patient with advanced heart failure and severe hemolysis causing pigment nephropathy. After being deemed too high-risk for open reoperation, the patient was brought to a hybrid operating room for TEE-guided percutaneous paravalvular mitral valve leak closure. A 12 mm Amplatzer vascular plug was deployed without interference of prosthetic mitral valve disk motion (V14.11B), and the device (arrow) appeared well seated (V14.11C). Interval follow-up TEE showed sustained diminution of the paravalvular leak (right panel, V14.11D). LA: left atrium; LV: left ventricle.

Occasionally during abdominal or thoracic surgery, extension of a disease process from these cavities into the mediastinum and cardiac chambers or great vessels requires elective or emergency IOE. Conditions in which this may be required include lung tumors invading the heart directly or via the pulmonary veins or renal tumors propagating along the inferior vena cava.

INFLUENCE ON PATIENT MANAGEMENT

IOE has a demonstrated impact on patient management. In a series of >3,000 predominantly elective cardiac surgical patients, a *new information* was found on pre-pump intraoperative TEE in 14% of patients, primarily due to identification of a PFO.[20] In post-pump studies, new information was found after surgery in 6% of patients, which resulted in additional procedure or hemodynamic management in 4%.[20] In a series of 66 patients who underwent emergent IOE, TEE showed new information in 80% of cases, with alteration to the planned procedure in 23%.[4]

POSTOPERATIVE COMPLICATIONS AND THEIR DETECTION

Postoperative TEE is indicated for assessment of cardiac function particularly in the setting of non-diagnostic transthoracic echocardiogram (limited endocardial definition is not infrequent in this setting and can relate to many factors, such as chest wall tenderness, bandages, and inability to adjust position). Other indications include unexplained, sudden hemodynamic deterioration, suspicion of pericardial tamponade, cardiac ischemia, assessment of perioperatively placed ventricular assist devices and a range of other scenarios.[21] Reflecting these higher risk indications for postoperative TEE, it has, not surprisingly, been demonstrated that the need to perform postoperative TEE comes with significantly worse outcomes than those without the need to do so.[21] The diagnostic yield of postoperative TEE in intensive care patients ranges from 36 to 58%, with therapeutic impact in 19–33% and surgical impact in 7–17%.[21]

Some of the examples of the use of echocardiography in the postoperative period are the following: detection of postoperative biventricular dysfunction (V14.13A) mediastinal hematoma (V14.13B), postoperative tamponade (V14.13C), iatrogenic postoperative aortic dissection (V14.13D, V14.13E), postoperative systolic anterior motion of the mitral valve with dynamic LVOT obstruction (V14.13F, V14.13G), and postoperative assessment of ventricular assist device (V14.13H).

CONCLUSIONS AND RECOMMENDATIONS

Emergent IOE is a powerful diagnostic tool that has wide applicability to various operating room environments. The challenge to the operator is to quickly use the best available modality that has the highest likelihood of answering the anatomical or hemodynamic questions that arise during surgery. As new technological developments continue to change and improve both the surgical and echocardiographic specialties, the operator will need to strive to ensure similar adaptive changes; this will require practicality, frugality, and creativity in use of emergent IOE. Emergency IOE will probably have an increasingly important role in the operating room in the future. As the complexity of cardiac and noncardiac surgery increases and as operative patients continue to become older and sicker, there will be a greater role for the rapid, accurate anatomical and hemodynamic data that echocardiography provides.

LIST OF VIDEOS

https://routledgetextbooks.com/textbooks/9781032157009/chapter-14.php

VIDEO 14.1A   Complicated ventricular septal rupture (1/4): Extensive acute transmural hemorrhagic myocardial infarction of the anteroseptal wall (7–10 days in evolution) complicated by a large ventricular septal rupture, as seen with two-dimensional (shown here) and color Doppler (see Video 14.1B) (see also Videos 14.1C, and 14.1D).

VIDEO 14.1B   Complicated ventricular septal rupture (2/4): Extensive acute transmural hemorrhagic myocardial infarction of the anteroseptal wall (7–10 days in evolution) complicated by a large ventricular septal rupture, as seen with color Doppler (see also Videos 14.1A,

VIDEO 14.1C   Complicated ventricular septal rupture (3/4): During attempted three-dimensional TEE-guided percutaneous repair of the ventricular septal defect (shown here), the patient developed acute hypotension and a new large pericardial effusion (see Video 14.1D). Resuscitation attempts for cardiac tamponade were unsuccessful. Hemopericardium and extension of the ventricular septal rupture to LV perforation were diagnosed at subsequent autopsy (see also Videos 14.1A and 14.1B).

VIDEO 14.1D   Complicated ventricular septal rupture (4/4): During attempted three-dimensional TEE-guided percutaneous repair of the ventricular septal defect (see Video 14.1C), the patient developed acute hypotension and a new large pericardial effusion (shown here). Resuscitation attempts for cardiac tamponade were unsuccessful. Hemopericardium and extension of the ventricular septal rupture to LV perforation were diagnosed at subsequent autopsy (see also Videos 14.1A and 14.1B).

VIDEO 14.2A   Posteromedial papillary muscle rupture (1/5): After a delayed-presentation inferior wall myocardial infarction, a bulky mobile echodensity can be seen traversing the mitral valve by two-dimensional (shown here) and three-dimensional transesophageal echocardiography (see Video 14.2B) associated with acute severe mitral regurgitation (see Video 14.2C). The patient underwent successful mitral valve replacement (see Video 14.2D) with persistence of a large inferior regional wall motion abnormality postoperatively (see Video 14.2E).

VIDEO 14.2B   Posteromedial papillary muscle rupture (2/5): After a delayed-presentation inferior wall myocardial infarction, a bulky mobile echodensity can be seen traversing the mitral valve by two-dimensional (see Video 14.2A) and three-dimensional transesophageal echocardiography (shown here) associated with acute severe mitral regurgitation (see Video 14.2C). The patient underwent successful mitral valve replacement (see Video 14.2D) with persistence of a large inferior regional wall motion abnormality postoperatively (see Video 14.2E).

VIDEO 14.2C   Posteromedial papillary muscle rupture (3/5): Acute severe mitral regurgitation after a delayed-presentation inferior wall myocardial infarction (shown here). A bulky mobile echodensity can be seen traversing the mitral valve by two-dimensional (see Video 14.2A) and three-dimensional transesophageal echocardiography (see Video 14.2B). The patient underwent successful mitral valve replacement (see Video 14.2D) with persistence of a large inferior regional wall motion abnormality postoperatively (see Video 14.2E).

VIDEO 14.2D   Posteromedial papillary muscle rupture (4/5): The patient underwent successful mitral valve replacement (shown here) after posteromedial papillary muscle rupture (see Videos 14.2A, 14.2B, and 14.2C) with persistence of a large inferior regional wall motion abnormality postoperatively (see Video 14.2E).

VIDEO 14.2E   Posteromedial papillary muscle rupture (5/5): Persistence of large inferior regional wall motion abnormality (shown here) after successful mitral valve replacement (see Video 14.2D) as a result of posteromedial papillary muscle rupture (see Videos 14.2A, 14.2B, and 14.2C).

VIDEO 14.3A   Complicated LV free-wall rupture (1/6): After a delayed-presentation inferior wall myocardial infarction, inferior LV free-wall rupture was detected by two-dimensional transesophageal echocardiography (TEE; shown here) and color Doppler (see Video 14.3B). However, preoperative TEE in the operating room identified a further new complication—namely, intramural dissection of the right ventricular free wall (see Videos 14.3C and 14.3D) with flow communication to the right ventricle (see Videos 14.3E and 14.3F)—at which point a plan to attempt surgical repair was abandoned.

VIDEO 14.3B   Complicated LV free-wall rupture (2/6): After a delayed-presentation inferior wall myocardial infarction, inferior LV free-wall rupture was detected by two-dimensional transesophageal echocardiography (TEE; see Video 14.3A) with abnormal flow by color Doppler (shown here). However, preoperative TEE in the operating room identified a further new complication—namely, intramural dissection of the right ventricular free wall (see Videos 14.3C and 14.3D) with flow communication to the right ventricle (see Videos 14.3E and 14.3F)—at which point a plan to attempt surgical repair was abandoned.

VIDEO 14.3C   Complicated LV free-wall rupture (3/6): After a delayed-presentation inferior wall myocardial infarction, inferior LV free-wall rupture was detected by two-dimensional transesophageal echocardiography (TEE; see Video 14.3A) with abnormal flow by color Doppler (see Video 14.3B). However, preoperative TEE in the operating room identified a further new complication—namely, intramural dissection of the right ventricular free wall (shown here; see also Video 14.3D) with flow communication to the right ventricle (see Videos 14.3E and 14.3F)—at which point a plan to attempt surgical repair was abandoned.

VIDEO 14.3D   Complicated LV free-wall rupture (4/6): After a delayed-presentation inferior wall myocardial infarction, inferior LV free-wall rupture was detected by two-dimensional transesophageal echocardiography (TEE; see Video 14.3A) with abnormal flow by color Doppler (see Video 14.3B). However, preoperative TEE in the operating room identified a further new complication—namely, intramural dissection of the right ventricular free wall (shown here; see also Video 14.3C) with flow communication to the right ventricle (see Videos 14.3E and 14.3F)—at which point a plan to attempt surgical repair was abandoned.

VIDEO 14.3E   Complicated LV free-wall rupture (5/6): After a delayed-presentation inferior wall myocardial infarction, inferior LV free-wall rupture was detected by two-dimensional transesophageal echocardiography (TEE; see Video 14.3A) with abnormal flow by color Doppler (see Video 14.3B). However, preoperative TEE in the operating room identified a further new complication—namely, intramural dissection of the right ventricular free wall (see Videos 14.3C and 14.3D) with flow communication to the right ventricle (shown here; see also Video 14.3F)—at which point a plan to attempt surgical repair was abandoned.

VIDEO 14.3F   Complicated LV free-wall rupture (6/6): After a delayed-presentation inferior wall myocardial infarction, inferior LV free-wall rupture was detected by two-dimensional transesophageal echocardiography (TEE; see Video 14.3A) with abnormal flow by color Doppler (see Video 14.3B). However, preoperative TEE in the operating room identified a further new complication—namely, intramural dissection of the right ventricular free wall (see Videos 14.3C and 14.3D) with flow communication to the right ventricle (shown here; see also Video 14.3E)—at which point a plan to attempt surgical repair was abandoned.

VIDEO 14.4A   Prosthetic mitral valve endocarditis and severe acute mitral stenosis (1/4): Gross thickening and mobile echodensities (shown here) on a bioprosthetic mitral valve resulting from endocarditis from methicillin-sensitive *Staphylococcus aureus*, which caused near-obstructive acute severe mitral stenosis (see Videos 14.4B and 14.4C). This was treated successfully with redo mitral valve replacement (see Video 14.4D) and antibiotic therapy.

VIDEO 14.4B   Prosthetic mitral valve endocarditis and severe acute mitral stenosis (2/4): Gross thickening and mobile echodensities (see Video 14.4A) on a bioprosthetic mitral valve resulting from endocarditis from methicillin-sensitive *Staphylococcus aureus*, which caused near-obstructive acute severe mitral stenosis (shown here; see also Video 14.4C). This was treated successfully with redo mitral valve replacement (see Video 14.4D) and antibiotic therapy.

VIDEO 14.4C   Prosthetic mitral valve endocarditis and severe acute mitral stenosis (3/4): Three-dimensional transesophageal echocardiography shows gross thickening and mobile echodensities on a bioprosthetic mitral valve resulting from endocarditis caused by methicillin-sensitive *Staphylococcus aureus*, which caused near-obstructive acute severe mitral stenosis (see also Videos 14.4A and 14.4B). This was treated successfully with redo mitral valve replacement (see Video 14.4D) and antibiotic therapy.

VIDEO 14.4D   Prosthetic mitral valve endocarditis and severe acute mitral stenosis (4/4): Successful redo mitral valve replacement for bioprosthetic mitral endocarditis caused by methicillin-sensitive *Staphylococcus aureus* resulting in near-obstructive acute severe mitral stenosis (see also Videos 14.4A, 14.4B and 14.4C).

VIDEO 14.5A   Acute perioperative aortic intramural hematoma (1/2): During post-pump intraoperative transesophageal echocardiography, gross thickening of the aortic wall was identified, representing acute perioperative intramural hematoma in the proximal descending aorta (shown here) and the aortic arch (see Video 14.5B).

VIDEO 14.5B   Acute perioperative aortic intramural hematoma (2/2): During post-pump intraoperative transesophageal echocardiography, gross thickening of the aortic wall was identified, representing acute perioperative intramural hematoma in the aortic arch (shown here) and the proximal descending aorta (see Video 14.5A).

VIDEO 14.6A   Postoperative systolic anterior motion (SAM) of the mitral valve (1/7): After initial mitral valve repair, hemodynamic compromise resulting in difficulty weaning off cardiopulmonary bypass was noted. SAM of the mitral valve leaflets was identified by intraoperative transesophageal echocardiography (shown here) with flow acceleration in the LVOT (see Video 14.6B). An aggressive sliding annuloplasty was then performed, which resolved the SAM and LV outflow obstruction (see Videos 14.6C and 14.6D) but resulted in moderate mitral regurgitation (see Videos 14.6D and 14.6E). A final decision was made to replace the valve with a low-profile bioprosthetic valve (see Videos 14.6F and 14.6G).

VIDEO 14.6B   Postoperative systolic anterior motion (SAM) of the mitral valve (2/7): After initial mitral valve repair, hemodynamic compromise resulting in difficulty weaning off cardiopulmonary bypass was noted. SAM of the mitral valve leaflets was identified by intraoperative transesophageal echocardiography (see Video 14.6A) with flow acceleration in the LVOT (shown here). An aggressive sliding annuloplasty was then performed, which resolved the SAM and LV outflow obstruction (see Videos 14.6C and 14.6D) but resulted in moderate mitral regurgitation (see Videos 14.6D and 14.6E). A final decision was made to replace the valve with a low-profile bioprosthetic valve (see Videos 14.6F and 14.6G).

VIDEO 14.6C   Postoperative systolic anterior motion (SAM) of the mitral valve (3/7): After initial mitral valve repair, hemodynamic compromise resulting in difficulty weaning off cardiopulmonary bypass was noted. SAM of the mitral valve leaflets was identified by intraoperative transesophageal echocardiography (see Video 14.6A) with flow acceleration in the LVOT (see Video 14.6B). An aggressive sliding annuloplasty was then performed, which resolved the SAM and LV outflow obstruction (shown here and in Video 14.6D) but resulted in moderate mitral regurgitation (see Videos 14.6D and 14.6E). A final decision was made to replace the valve with a low-profile bioprosthetic valve (see Videos 14.6F and 14.6G).

VIDEO 14.6D   Postoperative systolic anterior motion (SAM) of the mitral valve (4/7): After initial mitral valve repair, hemodynamic compromise resulting in difficulty weaning off cardiopulmonary bypass was noted. SAM of the mitral valve leaflets was identified by intraoperative transesophageal echocardiography (see Video 14.6A) with flow acceleration in the LVOT (see Video 14.6B). An aggressive sliding annuloplasty was then performed, which resolved the SAM and LV outflow obstruction (shown here and in Video 14.6C) but resulted in moderate mitral regurgitation (shown here and in Video 14.6E). A final decision was made to replace the valve with a low-profile bioprosthetic valve (see Videos 14.6F and 14.6G).

VIDEO 14.6E   Postoperative systolic anterior motion (SAM) of the mitral valve (5/7): After initial mitral valve repair, hemodynamic compromise resulting in difficulty weaning off cardiopulmonary bypass was noted. SAM of the mitral valve leaflets was identified by intraoperative transesophageal echocardiography (see Video 14.6A) with flow acceleration in the LVOT (see Video 14.6B). An aggressive sliding annuloplasty was then performed, which resolved the SAM and LV outflow obstruction (see Videos 14.6C and 14.6D) but resulted in moderate mitral regurgitation (shown here and in Video 14.6D). A final decision was made to replace the valve with a low-profile bioprosthetic valve (see Videos 14.6F and 14.6G).

VIDEO 14.6F   Postoperative systolic anterior motion (SAM) of the mitral valve (6/7): After initial mitral valve repair, hemodynamic compromise resulting in difficulty weaning off cardiopulmonary bypass was noted. SAM of the mitral valve leaflets was identified by intraoperative transesophageal echocardiography (see Video 14.6A) with flow acceleration in the LVOT (see Video 14.6B). An aggressive sliding annuloplasty was then performed, which resolved the SAM and LV outflow obstruction (see Videos 14.6C and 14.6D) but resulted in moderate mitral regurgitation (see Videos 14.6D and 14.6E). A final decision was made to replace the valve with a low-profile bioprosthetic valve (shown here and in Video 14.6G).

VIDEO 14.6G   Postoperative systolic anterior motion (SAM) of the mitral valve (7/7): After initial mitral valve repair, hemodynamic compromise resulting in difficulty weaning off cardiopulmonary bypass was noted. SAM of the mitral valve leaflets was identified by intraoperative transesophageal echocardiography (see Video 14.6A) with flow acceleration in the LVOT (see Video 14.6B). An aggressive sliding annuloplasty was then performed, which resolved the SAM and LV outflow obstruction (see Videos 14.6C and 14.6D) but resulted in moderate mitral regurgitation (see Videos 14.6D and 14.6E). A final decision was made to replace the valve with a low-profile bioprosthetic valve (shown here and in Video 14.6F).

VIDEO 14.7A   Post-cardiac surgery hematoma (1/3): Transesophageal echocardiographic long-axis view showing a large post-cardiac surgery hematoma around the left and right atria, aortic root, and right pulmonary artery, compressing the left atrium (shown here, at 2 o'clock) (see also Videos 14.7B and 14.7C).

VIDEO 14.7B   Post-cardiac surgery hematoma (2/3): Transesophageal echocardiographic view of both atria showing a large

post-cardiac surgery hematoma around the left and right atria, aortic root, and right pulmonary artery, compressing both the left and right atria (shown here) (see also Videos 14.7A and 14.7C).

VIDEO 14.7C   Post-cardiac surgery hematoma (3/3): Transesophageal echocardiographic short-axis view at the level of aortic valve showing a large post-cardiac surgery hematoma around the aortic root and right pulmonary artery (see also Videos 14.7A and 14.7B).

VIDEO 14.8A   Post-cardiac surgery hematoma behind left atrium (1/3): Transthoracic echocardiographic two-chamber view showing a large hematoma compressing the left atrium in an asymptomatic patient 4 days after cardiac surgery. The patient was treated conservatively (see also Videos 14.8B and 14.8C). *(Video provided by GA.)*

VIDEO 14.8B   Post-cardiac surgery hematoma behind left atrium (2/3): Transthoracic echocardiographic four-chamber view showing a large hematoma compressing the left atrium in an asymptomatic patient 4 days after cardiac surgery. The patient was treated conservatively (see also Videos 14.8A and 14.8C). *(Video provided by GA.)*

VIDEO 14.8C   Post-cardiac surgery hematoma behind left atrium (3/3): Transesophageal echocardiographic four-chamber midesophageal view showing a large hematoma compressing the left atrium in an asymptomatic patient 3 weeks after cardiac surgery (see also Videos 14.8A and 14.8B). The patient was treated conservatively. *(Video provided by GA.)*

VIDEO 14.9A   Transcatheter aortic valve replacement (TAVR) complication (1/2): After TAVR, distortion of prosthetic valve leaflet coaptation was noted on transesophageal echocardiography, with severe acute aortic regurgitation and acute hemodynamic decompensation (see also Video 14.9B). *(Video provided by GA.)*

VIDEO 14.9B   Transcatheter aortic valve replacement (TAVR) complication (2/2): After TAVR, distortion of prosthetic valve leaflet coaptation was noted on transesophageal echocardiography, with severe acute aortic regurgitation and acute hemodynamic decompensation (see Video 14.9A). Immediate implantation of the second prosthetic valve resulted in an excellent result (shown here). *(Video provided by GA.)*

VIDEO 14.10A   Transcatheter aortic valve replacement (TAVR) complication (1/2): Transesophageal echocardiography showing free-floating aortic valve prosthesis in the LV cavity after failure of positioning of the valve during TAVR. The patient underwent emergency surgical aortic valve replacement with an excellent outcome (see Video 14.10B). *(Video provided by GA.)*

VIDEO 14.10B   Transcatheter aortic valve replacement (TAVR) complication (2/2): After failure of positioning of the prosthetic aortic valve during TAVR (see Video 14.10A), the patient underwent emergency surgical aortic valve replacement with an excellent outcome (shown here). *(Video provided by GA.)*

VIDEO 14.11A   Percutaneous paravalvular mitral valve leak closure (1/4): Severe paravalvular mitral regurgitation was identified in a patient with advanced heart failure and severe hemolysis causing pigment nephropathy (shown here). After being deemed too high-risk for open reoperation, the patient was brought to a hybrid operating room for TEE-guided percutaneous paravalvular mitral valve leak closure. A 12 mm Amplatzer vascular plug was deployed without interference of prosthetic mitral valve disk motion (see Video 14.11B), and the device appeared well seated (see Video 14.11C). Interval follow-up TEE showed sustained diminution of the paravalvular leak (see Video 14.11D).

VIDEO 14.11B   Percutaneous paravalvular mitral valve leak closure (2/4): Severe paravalvular mitral regurgitation (see Video 14.11A) was identified in a patient with advanced heart failure and severe hemolysis causing pigment nephropathy. After being deemed too high-risk for open reoperation, the patient was brought to a hybrid operating room for TEE-guided percutaneous paravalvular mitral valve leak closure. A 12 mm Amplatzer vascular plug was deployed without interference of prosthetic mitral valve disk motion (shown here), and the device appeared well seated (see Video 14.11C). Interval follow-up TEE showed sustained diminution of the paravalvular leak (see Video 14.11D).

VIDEO 14.11C   Percutaneous paravalvular mitral valve leak closure (3/4): Severe paravalvular mitral regurgitation (see Video 14.11A) was identified in a patient with advanced heart failure and severe hemolysis causing pigment nephropathy. After being deemed too high-risk for open reoperation, the patient was brought to a hybrid operating room for TEE-guided percutaneous paravalvular mitral valve leak closure. A 12 mm Amplatzer vascular plug was deployed without interference of prosthetic mitral valve disk motion (see Video 14.11B), and the device appeared well seated (shown here). Interval follow-up TEE showed sustained diminution of the paravalvular leak (see Video 14.11D).

VIDEO 14.11D   Percutaneous paravalvular mitral valve leak closure (4/4): Severe paravalvular mitral regurgitation (see Video 14.11A) was identified in a patient with advanced heart failure and severe hemolysis causing pigment nephropathy. After being deemed too high-risk for open reoperation, the patient was brought to a hybrid operating room for TEE-guided percutaneous paravalvular mitral valve leak closure. A 12 mm Amplatzer vascular plug was deployed without interference of prosthetic mitral valve disk motion (see Video 14.11B), and the device appeared well seated (see Video 14.11C). Interval follow-up TEE showed sustained diminution of the paravalvular leak (shown here).

VIDEO 14.12A   Hemodynamic instability during noncardiac surgery (1/2): A patient with hypertrophic cardiomyopathy undergoing noncardiac surgery became hypotensive. Transesophageal echocardiographic transgastric long-axis view showed systolic anterior motion (SAM) with turbulence in the LVOT and small LV cavity, indicating hypovolemia (see also Video 14.12B). *(Video provided by JS.)*

VIDEO 14.12B   Hemodynamic instability during noncardiac surgery (2/2): A patient with hypertrophic cardiomyopathy undergoing noncardiac surgery became hypotensive. Transesophageal echocardiographic transgastric short-axis view showed obliteration of the LV cavity in systole, indicating severe hypovolemia (see also Video 14.12A). *(Video provided by JS.)*

VIDEO 14.13A   Postoperative biventricular dysfunction. TEE showing dilated right ventricle with poor systolic function. Left ventricle is unloaded with the Impella device.

VIDEO 14.13B   Postoperative mediastinal hematoma. TEE revealed a large mass compressing right atrium, consistent with mediastinal hematoma.

VIDEO 14.13C   Postoperative pericardial tamponade. On biplane imaging, fluid is seen adjacent to the right atrium (left panel), with invagination of right atrial wall into the right atrial cavity, simulating the appearance of right atrial mass (right panel).

VIDEO 14.13D   Postoperative new aortic dissection. TEE revealed intimal flap in the aortic lumen indicating occurrence of iatrogenic aortic dissection, which can be seen both in transverse (left panel) and longitudinal view (right panel) of the aorta. Note the spontaneous echo contrast in the false (bigger) aortic lumen.

VIDEO 14.13E   Postoperative new aortic dissection (with color Doppler). TEE with color Doppler in the patient presented on Video 14.13D showing intra-aortic flow in a true and false lumen.

VIDEO 14.13F   Postoperative systolic anterior motion of the mitral valve. TEE revealed systolic anterior motion of the mitral valve in the postoperative period causing dynamic obstruction of the LVOT. Hypovolemia might be considered.

VIDEO 14.13G   Postoperative systolic anterior motion of the mitral valve (with color Doppler). TEE with color Doppler revealed turbulent flow in the LVOT due to dynamic obstruction caused by systolic anterior motion of the mitral valve. Note also consecutive mild mitral regurgitation. Hypovolemia might be considered.

VIDEO 14.13H   Postoperative ventricular assist device assessment. Impella device is seen appropriately placed across the aortic valve with the outlet placed just above the aortic valve, and inlet approximately 3.5 cm below the valve.

REFERENCES

1. Chaliki HP, Click RL, Abel MD. Comparison of intraoperative transesophageal echocardiographic examinations with the operative findings: prospective review of 1918 cases. J Am Soc Echocardiogr 1999; 12:237–40.
2. Stewart WJ, Currie PJ, Salcedo EE, et al. Intraoperative Doppler color flow mapping for decision-making in valve repair for mitral regurgitation. Technique and results in 100 patients. Circulation 1990; 81:556–66.
3. Duff HJ, Buda AJ, Kramer R, Strauss HD, David TE, Berman ND. Detection of entrapped intracardiac air with intraoperative echocardiography. Am J Cardiol 1980; 46:255–60.
4. Brandt RR, Oh JK, Abel MD, Click RL, Orszulak TA, Seward JB. Role of emergency intraoperative transesophageal echocardiography. J Am Soc Echocardiogr 1998; 11:972–7.
5. Cahalan MK, Stewart W, Pearlman A, et al. American Society of Echocardiography and Society of Cardiovascular Anesthesiologists task force guidelines for training in perioperative echocardiography. J Am Soc Echocardiogr 2002; 15:647–52.

6. Poelaert JI, Trouerbach J, De Buyzere M, Everaert J, Colardyn FA. Evaluation of transesophageal echocardiography as a diagnostic and therapeutic aid in a critical care setting. Chest 1995; 107:774–9.

7. Battler A, Froelicher VF, Gallagher KP, Kemper WS, Ross J. Dissociation between regional myocardial dysfunction and ECG changes during ischemia in the conscious dog. Circulation 1980; 62:735–44.

8. Sheikh KH, Bengtson JR, Rankin JS, de Bruijn NP, Kisslo J. Intraoperative transesophageal Doppler color flow imaging used to guide patient selection and operative treatment of ischemic mitral regurgitation. Circulation 1991; 84:594–604.

9. Crenshaw BS, Granger CB, Birnbaum Y, et al. Risk factors, angiographic patterns, and outcomes in patients with ventricular septal defect complicating acute myocardial infarction. GUSTO-I (Global Utilization of Streptokinase and TPA for Occluded Coronary Arteries) Trial Investigators. Circulation 2000; 101:27–32.

10. López-Sendón J, González A, López de Sá E, et al. Diagnosis of subacute ventricular wall rupture after acute myocardial infarction: sensitivity and specificity of clinical, hemodynamic and echocardiographic criteria. J Am Coll Cardiol 1992; 19:1145–53.

11. Grewal KS, Malkowski MJ, Piracha AR, et al. Effect of general anesthesia on the severity of mitral regurgitation by transesophageal echocardiography. Am J Cardiol 2000; 85:199–203.

12. Dzavik V, Cohen G, Chan KL. Role of transesophageal echocardiography in the diagnosis and management of prosthetic valve thrombosis. J Am Coll Cardiol 1991; 18:1829–33.

13. Hammermeister KE, Henderson WG, Burchfiel CM, et al. Comparison of outcome after valve replacement with a bioprosthesis versus a mechanical prosthesis: initial 5 year results of a randomized trial. J Am Coll Cardiol 1987; 10:719–32.

14. Movsowitz HD, Levine RA, Hilgenberg AD, Isselbacher EM. Transesophageal echocardiographic description of the mechanisms of aortic regurgitation in acute type A aortic dissection: implications for aortic valve repair. J Am Coll Cardiol 2000; 36:884–90.

15. Ballal RS, Nanda NC, Gatewood R et al. Usefulness of transesophageal echocardiography in assessment of aortic dissection. Circulation 1991; 84:1903–14.

16. Reichert CL, Visser CA, Koolen JJ, et al. Transesophageal echocardiography in hypotensive patients after cardiac operations. Comparison with hemodynamic parameters. J Thorac Cardiovasc Surg 1991; 104:321–6.

17. Leung JM, O'Kelly B, Browner WS, Tubau J, Hollenberg M, Mangano DT. Prognostic importance of postbypass regional wall-motion abnormalities in patients undergoing coronary artery bypass graft surgery. SPI Research Group. Anesthesiology 1989; 71:16–25.

18. Lee KS, Stewart WJ, Lever HM, Underwood PL, Cosgrove DM. Mechanism of outflow tract obstruction causing failed mitral valve repair. Anterior displacement of leaflet coaptation. Circulation 1993; 88:II24–9.

19. Scalia GM, McCarthy PM, Savage RM, Smedira NG, Thomas JD. Clinical utility of echocardiography in the management of implantable ventricular assist devices. J Am Soc Echocardiogr 2000; 13:754–63.

20. Click RL, Abel MD, Schaff HV. Intraoperative transesophageal echocardiography: 5-year prospective review of impact on surgical management. Mayo Clin Proc 2000; 75:241–7.

21. Schmidlin D, Schuepbach R, Bernard E, Ecknauer E, Jenni R, Schmid ER. Indications and impact of postoperative transesophageal echocardiography in cardiac surgical patients. Crit Care Med 2001; 29(11):2143–8.

Echocardiography in mechanical circulatory support

15

David G. Platts and Gregory M. Scalia

Key Points

- Echocardiography is essential in identification of candidates for mechanical circulatory support (MCS) and provides key information for the management of critically ill patients with implanted assist devices.
- Echocardiography is used for preoperative assessment, guidance during MCS device insertion, detection of complications, and guidance during weaning and explantation of the device.
- Complications detectable by echocardiography, often associated with hemodynamic instability, include thrombosis, device malfunction, cannula displacement or malalignment, pulmonary embolism, aortic dissection, cardiac tamponade, and hypovolemia.
- The nonphysiologic nature of the circulation in patients with MCS requires unique understanding and interrogation.

Patients with severe acute or chronic cardiorespiratory failure are increasingly being treated with short- and long-term forms of mechanical circulatory support (MCS).[1–3] Internal and external mechanical pumps and blood oxygenators have sustained life while transplant donor organs are obtained or the heart/lungs of the patient recover. Destination therapy is increasingly being utilized in patients, where organ recovery is not expected and transplantation is contra-indicated, with the implantation of durable long term MCS devices is the definitive from of treatment.[4] Despite the benefits of MCS, these patients can be complex to manage, and they have complications that can result in significant morbidity and mortality, including bleeding, thrombosis, and infection.

Throughout the journey of MCS for a patient, echocardiography is fundamental in their management.[5,6] The nonphysiologic nature of the circulation in these patients and anatomy of these devices requires a unique understanding of their structure and function and how to assess the MCS, patient, and MCS-patient interface, as outlined in this chapter. The most recent Appropriate Use Criteria for Echocardiography[7] has the highest score of 9 (highly appropriate) for echocardiography in aspects of managing a patient with MCS. Institutions that perform MCS require an echocardiography service that is readily available, plus experienced in the evaluation of these critically unwell patients. Additionally, close collaboration and communication between critical care, cardiology, echocardiologists, pulmonology, and cardiothoracic surgery is required to optimize the outcomes of these complex patients.

DOI: 10.1201/9781003245407-15

VENTRICULAR ASSIST DEVICES

Ventricular assist devices (VAD) are a specialized form of mechanical cardiac support used to manage selected patients with severe refractory heart failure.[8,9] This area has evolved significantly over the past two decades. Optimal patient selection/timing, choice of device and peri and postoperative management are key to favorable patient outcomes. Echocardiography provides the clinician with a safe, accurate, well-tolerated technique that can be performed at the bedside, which is fundamental to the management of patients supported with a VAD.[10–12] Both transthoracic (TTE) and transesophageal echocardiography (TEE) are utilized in MCS assessment, depending upon the indication, image quality, and clinical situation of the patient. Advanced echocardiographic imaging modes, such as contrast enhanced TTE, three-dimensional (3D) echocardiography, and strain/myocardial mechanics, also have an important role in selected patients pre and post MCS insertion.

MCS devices can be grouped or classified based on their duration, location, flow characteristics, or generation.[8,13] The commonest form of circulatory support worldwide is counterpulsation using an intra-aortic balloon pump (IABP). This chapter focuses on the advanced forms of MCS—durable ventricular assist devices (VAD) (Figure 15.1), extra corporeal membrane oxygenation (ECMO), and percutaneous micro-axial flow pumps (such as the Impella). The vast majority of MCS devices now are continuous flow ventricular assist devices[14] which are smaller, more durable, better tolerated and result in improved outcomes than the earlier pulsatile devices.[15,16] Recent advances in pump

design and recognition of the benefits of pulsatility, have resulted in pumps now having an intrinsic "pulse," such as the Abbott HeartMate 3, which has pulsatility built into its continuous flow at an equivalent rate of 30 beats per minute. The commonest VAD type is a left-sided VAD (LVAD), but a right-sided VAD (RVAD) or a total artificial heart (TAH) may also be implanted.

There are several key indications for VAD insertion. They may be inserted as a bridge to transplant, bridge to decision, bridge to candidacy, bridge to recovery, and destination therapy.[17] The relative frequency of these indications has also changed recently, with destination therapy now being the commonest indication for VAD insertion in the USA.[14]

Preoperative echocardiographic assessment

Ventricular structure and function

Echocardiography is fundamental in the quantification of left ventricular (LV) structure and function prior to the insertion of an LVAD. The LV ejection fraction and stroke volume are usually severely reduced in patients being considered for LVAD insertion. Assessment of LV morphology is important prior to LVAD insertion. Due to the cannulation of the LV apex, it is important to understand the apical morphology and to ensure there is no thrombus present. TTE is the imaging modality of choice to assess the LV apex with contrast enhanced imaging being used to help to assess for thrombus.[18,19] Excessive trabeculation may also be detected and require surgical excision at the time of LVAD implant to ensure it does not interact with the inflow cannula/blood flow.

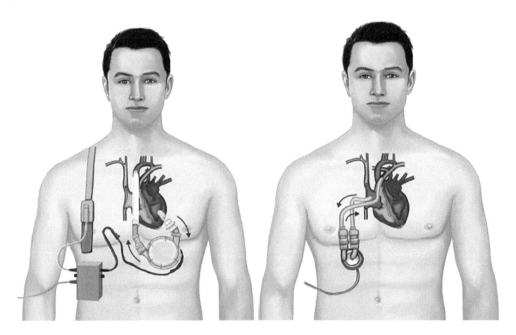

FIGURE 15.1 Schematic illustration of ventricular assist devices. Left ventricular assist device (LVAD) (left panel): blood from the left ventricle enters the LVAD, which pumps it further to the ascending aorta. The pump is connected via flexible cable to an externally worn controller and battery packs that provide power to both pump and controller. Right ventricular assist device (RVAD) (right panel): blood from the right atrium enters the RVAD, which pumps it further to the pulmonary artery.

(Artwork provided by SUP.)

Right heart failure in the early post-LVAD stage is a strong adverse prognostic marker.[20,21] Prior to LVAD insertion, the right heart is carefully evaluated. An LVAD can improve right ventricular (RV) function (primarily by improving hemodynamics and reducing pulmonary vascular resistance) or it may worsen RV function (due to increased venous return and preload). Numerous multifaceted scoring systems have also been developed to help quantify the risk of RV failure.[22–25] Parameters that have been used to help predict RV function following LVAD insertion include right heart dimensions, degree of tricuspid regurgitation, RV-LV end-diastolic dimension ratio, RV fractional area change, and reduced right heart myocardial mechanics using myocardial mechanics/strain.[26–28] Recently, a EUROMACS right-sided heart failure risk score has been evaluated and validated utilizing a combination of clinical, hematologic, hemodynamic, and RV echocardiographic parameters to help predict right-sided heart failure after implantation of a continuous flow LVAD.[29] Patients with severe fixed pulmonary hypertension are not candidates for LVAD insertion or heart transplantation but may be a candidate for heart-lung transplantation. Sometimes an LVAD may be inserted to reduce reversible elevated trans-pulmonary gradients to convert a patient from non-candidacy to candidacy for heart transplantation ("bridge to candidacy").

Intracardiac shunts

Prior to insertion of a VAD, it is important to evaluate for an intracardiac shunt, which may cause right to left shunting (and hence hypoxia/cyanosis) along with increasing the risk of paradoxical embolization. If detected, these cardiac shunts can be repaired at the time of LVAD insertion. Shunts at the atrial level are due to either an atrial septal defect or patent foramen ovale (V13.40A, V13.40B), may not become evident until the LVAD operates. If an LVAD is being inserted following left heart failure following an acute myocardial infarction, it is important to carefully evaluate the interventricular septum to exclude a post infarct ventricular septal defect (see Chapter 3).

Assessment of the ascending aorta

Careful evaluation of the ascending aorta is important prior to LVAD insertion. The outflow graft of the LVAD device is connected via an end to side anastomosis onto the ascending aorta (Figure 15.1). If the ascending aorta is significantly dilated (>45 mm) when an LVAD is inserted, this would need to be replaced with a Dacron graft. Aortic dissection flaps need to be excluded and significant atherosclerotic disease needs to be identified and avoided (V13.14A, V13.14B). TEE usually provides images of sufficient quality to assess for ascending aortic atheroma (V13.15).[30] High-frequency (15 MHz) linear transducers can also be used to perform direct epiaortic echocardiography to visualize the ascending aorta to help position the LVAD outflow cannula anastomosis site. Preoperative CT aortography may also be useful in assessing for aortic anatomy and disease.

Assessment of cardiac valves

Preoperative evaluation of the cardiac valves is important prior to LVAD insertion. Dysfunction of any of the cardiac valves may potentially adversely affect LVAD function. Additionally, the presence of a mechanical valve replacement complicates the situation due to the increased risk of valve thrombosis from potentially slower intracardiac blood flow. A mechanical valve replacement is removed at the time of surgery and replaced with a tissue valve.

Assessment of any aortic regurgitation (AR) is particularly important prior to an LVAD implantation. AR of moderate or greater severity requires correction at the time of LVAD implantation otherwise there be significant recirculation from ventricle to pump to aorta and back to ventricle. This is especially relevant with the longer duration of LVAD implantation and destination therapy. The aortic valve can be replaced with a tissue aortic valve or in some cases it has been oversewn, though this is now rare. AR may also occur subsequent to LVAD insertion[31] as the valve is often in the permanently closed state with a continuous high aorta to left ventricular pressure gradient[32,33] (Figure 15.2). There are multiple hemodynamic and histopathologic factors that can result in AR post LVAD.[34]

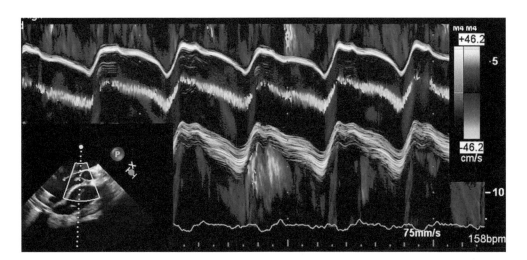

FIGURE 15.2   Color M-mode image of mild, continuous aortic regurgitation in a patient with a HeartWare LVAD.

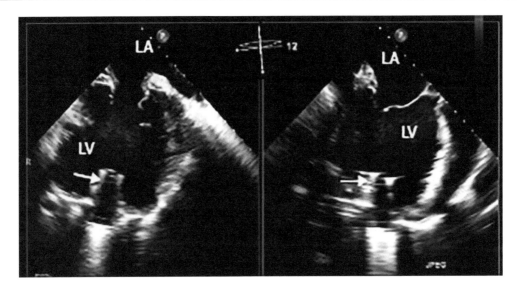

FIGURE 15.3   Biplane TEE showing a HeartWare LVAD inflow cannula (arrows) positioned in the LV. Note that the LV inflow cannula is free of surrounding structures and is orientated toward the mitral inflow (V15.1). LA: left atrium; LV: left ventricle.

Post-VAD AR can result in reduced effectiveness of the MCS support and elevated LV filling pressures. Traditional AR quantification methods using echocardiography may be difficult to apply. Newer parameters such as diastolic flow acceleration and the systolic to diastolic velocity ratio of the outflow cannula may improve assessment of AR post LVAD.[35] Management of post-VAD AR can be complex and includes medical therapy, VAD settings alteration, surgical aortic valve replacement, TAVI or ultimately transplantation.

Patients being assessed for VAD implantation often have varying degrees of tricuspid regurgitation. The decision to intervene in tricuspid regurgitation is a difficult one. Post-LVAD insertion, at higher pump speeds, venous return to the right heart is significantly increased. Pulmonary vascular resistance (PVR) can be calculated using echocardiography. Documentation of a reduction in the PVR following LVAD insertion (a reduction in the right ventricular afterload) is an important prognostic maker and sequential evaluation of this should be performed after LVAD insertion.[36]

If there is significant mitral stenosis, this may reduce LVAD filling. Consequently, at the time of LVAD implantation, a tissue mitral valve replacement or commissurotomy may be required. However, mitral stenosis is a rare finding prior to LVAD insertion.[37]

Mitral regurgitation is very common in heart failure and in the potential LVAD patient population.[38] However, with adequate LV decompression following LVAD insertion, the degree of mitral regurgitation usually decreases[33,39] and surgical intervention is very rarely required.

Guidance during VAD insertion

Echocardiography plays a fundamental role during intraoperative evaluation of VAD insertion. Important components to this evaluation are cannula positioning, assessment of cannula

flow, determining adequate cardiac chamber decompression, assessment of RV function, and excluding air with the circuit or cardiac chambers. All VADs have an inflow cannula and an outflow cannula (usually via a Gore-Tex graft as an end to side anastomosis to the aorta) (Figure 15.1). Intraoperative TEE is used to *ensure satisfactory positioning of the inflow cannula*, allowing for unobstructed flow into the cannula (Figure 15.3) (V15.1). The cannula should not be in direct contact with ventricular walls or mitral valvular or subvalvular apparatus. Real-time 3D TEE can provide rapid, multi-planar spatial assessment/orientation of the access cannula (V15.2).

Flow from the VAD travels via the outflow cannula made from reinforced synthetic material that is anastomosed to the ascending aorta (for an LVAD) (V15.3) or the pulmonary artery (for an RVAD). *Complications associated with the outflow cannula* are rare but may include extrinsic compression or incorrect surgical positioning or attachment to the great vessels, causing kinking and hence obstruction to outflow. Very rarely there may be thrombus formation within the outflow graft.

Following VAD insertion, it is important that TEE is used to determine that the circuit and cardiac chambers have been *de-aired*. There are numerous surgical and device site locations that can allow entry of air into the circulation. Any residual air may result in systemic embolization. As the right coronary artery (RCA) is a more anterior structure, air preferentially embolizes down this vessel, potentially resulting in LV and/or RV dysfunction and significant arrhythmias. RCA air may also cause transient but significant RV dysfunction, which can then compromise LVAD filling and result in low flows and LV suction. In this situation, the patient may need to be rested back on cardiopulmonary bypass, the heart de-aired and the LVAD then recommenced.

Once the VAD has been inserted and support commenced, it is important to use color and spectral Doppler imaging to *evaluate cannula flows*. In the HeartWare continuous flow LVAD, Doppler analysis of the inflow is unhelpful due to the presence of significant color artifact. Other continuous flow

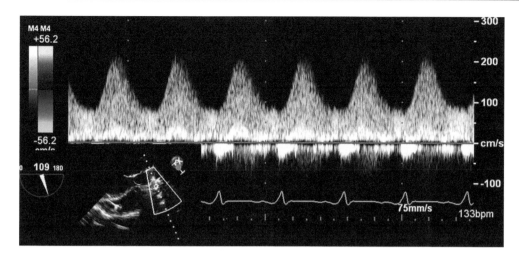

FIGURE 15.4   Spectral Doppler image of a HeartWare LVAD outflow into the ascending aorta. Note the continuous but biphasic pattern consistent with a degree of native pulsatility/contractility in addition to the continuous flow provided by the LVAD.

LVADs (such as the axial flow HeartMate II) typically have a continuous but phasic inflow pattern with a normal velocity being less than 2 m/s.[40,41] It is important to carefully assess the outflow signal. This is usually evaluated using pulsed-wave Doppler interrogation with the sample volume placed 1 cm proximal to the aortic anastomosis (Figure 15.4) (V15.3). The morphology and velocity of the trace depends upon the preload, afterload, cannula diameter, and contribution of native cardiac function. With increasing levels of native cardiac function, the spectral Doppler outflow waveform becomes more pulsatile. The usual outflow velocity for a continuous flow HeartWare device is 1.4 m/s, with a range of 1.0–1.9 m/s.[42,43]

Once inserted, echocardiography is very useful in *determining the optimal pump speed*. This can be done by adjusting the pump settings to optimize hemodynamics while watching the degree of LV unloading. This is a dynamic process and involves interaction between the implanting surgeon, echocardiologist, anesthetist, and perfusionist. Echocardiographic parameters evaluated include the LV dimensions, degree of mitral regurgitation, interventricular septal motion, right heart size and function, and amount of aortic valve opening or pulsatility.[44] *Insufficient pump speeds* will result in a non-decompressed LV, rightward bowing of the interventricular septum and ongoing severe mitral regurgitation, if already present. *Excessive pump speeds* will result in a "sucked down" LV and increased leftward shift of the interventricular septum. This may also cause excessive venous return to the right heart, resulting in right heart dilatation and impairment.

It is also important to recognize that that *loading conditions can vary* significantly within the same patient in the early stages of LVAD insertion. This includes a significant difference between the sternum/chest being open versus closed. Other acute hemodynamic variables occur between being in theatre, ventilated in ICU, non-ventilated on inotropes, and finally as an ambulatory outpatient. As such, at each stage there is often the need to optimize the LVAD setting depending upon their physiologic state.[45]

Detection of complications

Echocardiography is usually the first investigation used to assess for VAD dysfunction/complications. Complications may be classified as either VAD specific complications, patient related issues and complications secondary to the pump-patient interface. Common complications include thrombus, bleeding, device malfunction, cannula displacement or malalignment and infection. Other potential causes for hemodynamic instability in VAD patients include pulmonary embolus, a hypertensive crisis, aortic dissection, and hypovolemia. TEE is often required to assess for *tamponade or localized pericardial collections* (V15.4, V15.5A, V15.5B). Diffuse sternal and mediastinal bleeding may cause an anterior collection, which may cause significant cardiac or VAD component compression. A silicone membrane is often placed over the heart-LVAD complex to protect it during the repeat sternotomy for transplantation or explantation of the LVAD. This will appear and a bright, echodense linear structure. An anterior mediastinal hematoma (causing cardiac compression) may occur either posterior or anterior to this membrane.

Thrombus formation is a serious complication that may occur in patients supported on a VAD. There may be thrombus formation around or within the VAD inflow cannula or within the device itself.[46] If sufficiently large, thrombus may impede VAD function, up to the level of complete VAD failure. VAD thrombosis can result in hemolysis due to the increased turbulent flow. It may also be a source of cardioembolism.

Pump thrombosis can result in serious morbidity or mortality. Treatment options include thrombolysis (local or systemic), pump exchange, or urgent cardiac transplantation listing. It can be a difficult diagnosis to make, especially as it is not possible to directly visualize intradevice thrombus. There are multiple clinical, biochemical, VAD metrics (such as power and derived flow), and indirect echocardiographic features that help in the diagnosis of VAD thrombosis. Indirect echocardiographic features include a dilated LV, rightward shift of the interventricular septum, regular aortic opening, and an increase in the degree of mitral regurgitation. There may also be visualized spontaneous echo contrast or left heart thrombus, either associated with or separate to the VAD cannula. One focus is on performing "ramp studies," where LV size and function, along with aortic valve opening, are quantified during incremental increased in VAD speeds, to help determine the presence of pump thrombosis.[47] Very rarely, air may enter the VAD circuit and result in significant air embolism.[48] The Abbott HeartMate 3 LVAD is a fully magnetically levitated centrifugal pump which is a commonly inserted form of MCS.[49] The rotor remains in a stable position with a range of speeds. It is intrapericardial and has a cardiac output up to 10 L/min and provides an asynchronous pulse of 30 BPM. It has a relatively larger blood flow pathway. These device characteristics have the aim of reducing pump thrombosis and providing some of the physiologic benefits of a degree of circulatory pulsatility.[50–52]

VAD patients are at an increased risk of *infection*, both locally and systemically. Sites of infection include on and around the cannula, mediastinum, drive line or native cardiac valves or other implantable cardiac devices. TEE is usually required to assess for VAD associated infection. VAD driveline infection is a common and serious issue, with associated increased complications and may be controlled but not eradicated until the VAD is removed.

Ascending aortic dissection can occur after LVAD insertion but is rare. It can be due to the relatively high velocity jet from the VAD return cannula into the ascending aorta, with resultant high shear forces, or secondary to the actual anastomosis site. It is very rare for there to be complications from the aortic anastomosis site but occasionally there may be mild stenosis. Despite the Gore-Tex graft used being circular, the final anastomosis morphology is often more elliptical (Figure 15.5).

Pump failure is a rare but life-threatening condition. There are several causes for pump failure including controller malfunction, an interruption of the power supply and intrinsic problems with the actual pump, including severe pump thrombosis. As there is a connection from the aorta to the LV via the LVAD circuit that does not have a valve system, pump failure may be evident by diastolic retrograde or regurgitant flow from the aorta through the pump, into the LV.

Cardiac tamponade may occur, especially in the earlier postoperative stage due to the acuity of the anticoagulation and recent surgical status and any associated coagulopathy. This may present as hemodynamic compromise with low flow alarms, suction alarms, low mean arterial pressures and loss of pulsatility. Echocardiography is the investigation of choice to assess for tamponade in MCS patients. It may be challenging to diagnose as the usual spectral Doppler parameters can be unreliable in this clinical situation, device artifacts may limit hemodynamic assessment and small focal collections may be significant. The key is to evaluate for a collection that may compromise LVAD filling, and this may in the left or right atrium or RV. *Diffuse mediastinal bleeding* can also be an issue and present with tamponade. Tamponade in MCS requires prompt diagnosis with echocardiography and urgent surgical decompression (V15.4, V15.5A, V15.5B).

VAD optimization, weaning, and explantation

Following insertion of a VAD, the settings may need to be optimized. It is not a "set and forget" scenario. Demands on the patient and the VAD vary and this may require optimization of VAD settings.[53] Every patient should have an *individualized optimization strategy and sequential reassessment* of the profile. This is done to unload the LV, optimize systemic circulatory support and decrease pulmonary congestion. There are numerous complementary techniques in the optimization of an LVAD. These include several echocardiographic parameters but, also importantly, numerous hemodynamic variables obtained via right heart catheterization.[54–56]

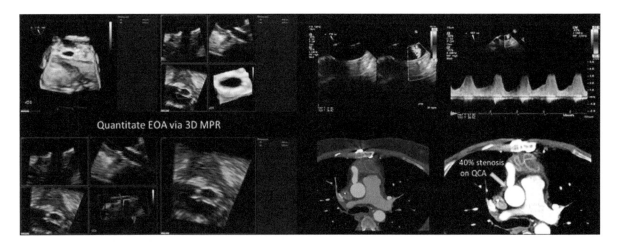

FIGURE 15.5 Examples of 2D and 3D TEE images of a HeartWare LVAD outflow graft/anastomosis to the ascending aorta. Note the capacity of echocardiography to evaluate both anatomy/morphology of the anastomosis as well as the velocity/waveform of the LVAD outflow.

Following VAD implantation, the patient may proceed to transplant or if there is sufficient myocardial recovery, the VAD may be explanted, although this is rare. However, it is unusual for there to be sufficient recovery for LVAD explanation to occur.[57] Determination of myocardial recovery is a complex and dynamic field, and a constellation of clinical, biochemical, hematological, hemodynamic, and echocardiographic variables are analyzed to help assess recovery.[58] However, there is a relative paucity of data to guide clinicians as to the optimal method of assessing recovery. As the LV is in an unloaded state, it is difficult to accurately quantify recovery without monitoring response while *performing an incremental reduction* in VAD support. There are several protocols used to assess for recovery, but these can vary between units and there is currently no standardized approach for VAD weaning.[59] Echocardiographic parameters that can be utilized in assessing myocardial recovery include LV ejection fraction, stroke volume, ventricular dimensions, LV pulsatility/aortic valve opening, and right heart size and function evaluation. Dobutamine stress echocardiography has also been used to help determine myocardial recovery.[60,61]

support for days to weeks and even months.[64] ECMO may be instituted in multiple settings: the critical care unit, cardiac catheter suite, or emergency department, the operating room and even rarely at the site of arrest in the community. ECMO was first utilized in the 1970s and is now a rapidly evolving technique with regular improvements in devices and management as well as alterations in appropriate patient selection.[65]

Echocardiography plays a fundamental role throughout the care of a patient supported on ECMO.[66] It provides information that helps in patient selection, guides insertion and placement of cannula, assesses progress, detects complications and helps in evaluating cardiac recovery and the weaning of ECMO support.[67] The use of ECMO in critically unwell patients is likely to increase. As such, echocardiography staff who work within units that have an ECMO program will need to develop a *specific set of skills* to image these unique patients. This particularly applies to understanding the technique, recognizing the appearance of various cannula on echocardiography and be cognizant of specific complication of ECMO.

EXTRACORPOREAL MEMBRANE OXYGENATION (ECMO)

Extracorporeal membrane oxygenation (ECMO) is a modified form of cardiopulmonary bypass used to provide cardiac and/or respiratory support in selected patients that have not responded to maximal medical support.[62,63] While typically used in the short term, it can provide cardiopulmonary

Modes of ECMO

There are broadly two types of ECMO, venovenous (VV ECMO) and venoarterial (VA ECMO) (Figure 15.6).[68] Patients with respiratory failure (but with intact cardiac function) can be supported with VV ECMO alone. De-oxygenated blood is drained from the venous system into the ECMO circuit, where gas exchange occurs and it is then returned oxygenated to the venous system, usually close to the right atrium. Patients with cardiac (with or without respiratory failure) are

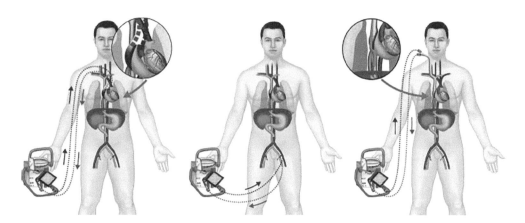

FIGURE 15.6 Modes of ECMO. Left panel: in central VA ECMO, deoxygenated (blue) blood is drained from the right atrium, and after oxygenation and carbon dioxide removal, it is returned (pink) to the arterial circulation via a pressured cannula placed centrally in the ascending aorta. Middle panel: in peripheral VA ECMO, deoxygenated (blue) blood is drained from the venous system via a large (e.g., femoral) vein, and after oxygenation, it is returned to the arterial circulation via a pressured cannula placed peripherally in a large (e.g., femoral) artery. Right panel: in VV ECMO, using a single dual-chamber venous cannulation strategy, deoxygenated (blue) blood is drained from the venous system (superior and inferior vena cava) into the ECMO circuit, where gas exchange occurs, and is then returned oxygenated (pink) to the venous system through an outflow exit orifice into the right atrium. This type of ECMO does not provide hemodynamic support.

(Artwork provided by SUP.)

supported with VA ECMO. In this form of ECMO, deoxygenated blood is drained from the right atrium, either by direct surgical cannulation or via a cannula placed in a major vein with the tip sitting in the right atrium. Oxygenation and carbon dioxide removal occur within the oxygenator and then it is returned to the arterial circulation, via a pressured cannula placed centrally in the ascending aorta or peripherally in a large artery.

There are *five main components* to an ECMO circuit: (1) an access cannula to drain blood from the venous system, (2) a rotary blood pump and controlling unit, (3) an oxygenator for gas exchange, (4) a blood temperature control unit and (5) a return cannula to return the blood back to the venous or arterial system.

There are *multiple cannulation options* available with ECMO, but they can be broadly classified into central and peripheral cannulation. Central cannulation occurs at the time of cardiac surgery and involves cannulation under direct vision into a large vessel, such as the pulmonary artery or ascending aorta. Peripheral cannulation involves insertion of the cannula into a peripheral vessel, such as the femoral artery or femoral vein and is typically performed using a percutaneous technique. However, peripheral cannulation may occur with surgical placement of the cannula into the vessel or via a Gore-Tex side or "chimney" graft.

Echocardiography prior to ECMO commencement

In critically unwell patients, echocardiography can help evaluate for clinical conditions that may account for the patient's instability, such as cardiac tamponade or ventricular failure. Conditions that can impact on the insertion of arterial cannula can also be identified by echocardiography, such as severe aortic dissection and significant atherosclerotic disease in the aorta. Anatomic issues that may complicate or preclude right-sided cannula placement can also be detected by echocardiography, including tricuspid valve stenosis, significant intracardiac shunts, prominent Chiari network, and the presence of an implantable cardiac devices (e.g., pacemaker, cardioverter-defibrillator). In severe respiratory conditions requiring VV ECMO support, echocardiography also helps by assessing the LV and thereby determining if VA ECMO rather than VV ECMO is needed.

Echocardiography during ECMO cannulation and initiation

Cannulation and initiation of ECMO are frequently guided using echocardiography, providing real-time feedback on cannula positioning and impact on ventricular function. Due to limited spatial resolution and depth penetration, TTE may be insufficient, and a TEE may be required. For peripheral VV ECMO using a femoral vein approach, the ideal location

for the access (inflow) cannula tip is in the proximal inferior vena cava. For the return (outflow) cannula, the ideal position is in the mid-right atrium and clear of any right heart structures. Echocardiographic guidance for placement of VV ECMO cannula can help reduce the occurrence of recirculation where the access cannula is more proximally than the return cannula (or they are too close together) resulting in oxygenated blood being drawn back into the ECMO circuit (Figure 15.7) (V15.6).

During peripheral ECMO cannulation, guidewires are visualized by TEE in the inferior vena cava and within the descending thoracic aorta. The presence of an intraluminal aortic wire is key because these patients are often critically unwell, and the implanting physician may not have pulsatile/ oxygenated blood to confirm arterial puncture. Additionally, prior to the insertion of large bore cannula, it is imperative that the intraluminal location of the guidewire is confirmed. Biplane imaging and 3D imaging can also help in identifying wires as the shadow artifacts of a wire can result in some confusion. Appropriate identification and location of a venous guidewire is also important. The wire should not be in the right ventricle, down a hepatic vein or across the interatrial septum, all places where a guide wire could easily end up, resulting in potential cardiac damage from the wire or misplacement of the venous cannula (Figure 15.8) (V15.7). Placement of dual lumen cannula requires careful guidance using imaging.[69,70] Cannula displacement or misplacement can have significant adverse effects including ineffective delivery of ECMO support, recirculation, and cardiac or vascular trauma.

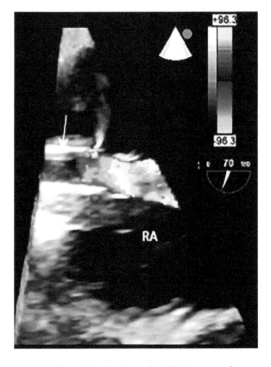

FIGURE 15.7 2D and color Doppler TEE image of an appropriately positioned VV ECMO outflow/return cannula (arrow) in the right atrium (RA). Note the main outflow color jet at the tip and multiple side hole jets (V15.6).

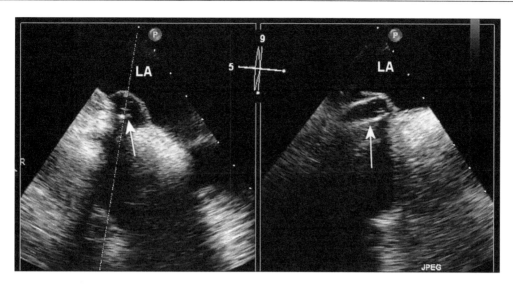

FIGURE 15.8   Biplane TEE of venoarterial ECMO access cannula (arrows) inserted too far into the right atrium and onto the interatrial septum (V15.7). This may both potentially compromise ECMO outflow as well as increase the risk of cardiac trauma. LA: left atrium.

Echocardiography and monitoring of response to ECMO

When ECMO is initiated, there are various changes in hemodynamics and loading, with a reduction in LV preload but an increase in LV afterload when VA ECMO is commenced. During VV ECMO, the pulmonary circulation receives blood with increased oxygen content with no significant change to the RV preload and no adverse effect in hemodynamics in the normal left heart. VV ECMO increases the mixed venous oxygen saturation. It is often difficult in assessing the RV systolic pressure when on VV ECMO as the return cannula flow into the right atrium can prevent reliable assessment of a tricuspid regurgitant jet. Sepsis may result in severe RV dysfunction, compounded by increased pulmonary vascular resistance in response to hypoxia.

Patients supported with ECMO are critically unwell, and there may be factors that contraindicate or significantly increase the risk of TEE. Such factors would include a coagulopathy, thrombocytopenia, and mucosal oedema. Complicating this picture is the relatively high incidence of non-diagnostic TTE studies (approximately 25%) in the critical care complex.[18,71] In this situation, contrast enhanced TTE may salvage a nondiagnostic study and convert it to a diagnostic study when assessing for cardiac chamber size/function/morphology.[72–75] Contrast-enhanced TTE by improving the blood-myocardial interface is particularly useful in determining ventricular structure, function, morphology, and detection of ventricular thrombus.

Echocardiography and detection of ECMO complications

While ECMO can be a life-saving form of therapy, there may be significant associated complications. Echocardiography (especially TEE) is usually the initial investigation of ECMO complications, such as cardiac tamponade, cannula displacement or thrombosis.[76] During ECMO, the heart is in a partially bypassed state and as such evaluation of the significance of *pericardial collections and tamponade* can be challenging. Conventional Doppler parameters are not helpful in diagnosing tamponade. The key is to assess for cardiac chamber compression that may actually hinder ECMO/cannula filling and flow. Tamponade is a relatively common problem during ECMO with an incidence of 6.5% in VA ECMO and 3.1% in VV ECMO.[77] Clinical clues to the presence of tamponade include low ECMO flows, circuit "kicking" (shuddering of the ECMO circuit tubes as a result of the transmission of the compressive forces back down the tubing and column of blood), hypotension, and tachycardia.

Cannula complications are relatively common ECMO with an incidence of 4.7% in cardiac ECMO and 8.4% in respiratory ECMO.[77] Common complications include displacement, obstruction, and thrombosis. *Cannula displacement* has the potential dual consequence of reducing effective delivery of ECMO support and increasing the possibility of cardiac/vascular trauma (V15.8).

Thrombus associated with ECMO support is another serious complication and may occur in numerous locations including within the cannula, the atria, ventricles, valvular apparatus and within the aortic root. Systemic embolization and pulmonary embolization, compromise of ECMO flow and limitation of normal intracardiac flow may result. The non-vented severely impaired LV has increased afterload (in VA ECMO). Reduced LV ejection and aortic valve opening may result in stasis with thrombosis within the aortic root and/or LV, along with severe pulmonary oedema (Figure 15.9) (V15.9, V15.10). Therapeutic options to manage this situation include inotropes, altered ECMO settings, TEE-guided percutaneous balloon atrial septostomy,[78,79] IABP, percutaneous unloading with an Impella or surgical venting.

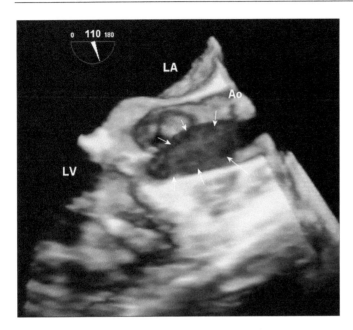

FIGURE 15.9　3D TEE image of an aortic root thrombus (arrows) in a patient on peripheral VA ECMO with an unvented non-pulsatile left ventricle (V15.10). Ao: aorta; LA: left atrium; LV: left ventricle.

A *venous cast* of the cannula may remain within the cardiac structures when the patient is decannulated from ECMO. This cast may embolize to lungs at decannulation. During surgical removal of venous cannula, the inferior vena cava should be assessed with TEE to exclude the presence of a residual venous cast. If this is missed, it may result in pulmonary embolization. If detected, however, it can be easily removed during surgery.

Echocardiography during patient recovery and weaning of support

Echocardiography plays an important role in final aspect of VA ECMO support, and that is the assessment of myocardial recovery and ability to wean from support. Echocardiography does not play a major role in the assessment of weaning from VV ECMO, other than in the evaluation of right heart structure and function. Assessment of gas exchange is the key metric in VV ECMO weaning. Following a period of VA ECMO support, returning or increasing arterial pulsatility may be a marker of cardiac recovery.

There is currently no standardized approach to weaning a patient from VA ECMO. Broadly speaking, the VA ECMO flows are slowly decreased, during which numerous hemodynamic and echocardiographic variables are assessed to help determine myocardial recovery.[80] One approach is to decrease the VA ECMO flows in 0.5 L/min increments while assessing clinical, hemodynamic, and echocardiographic parameters.[81] Due to the increased risk of circuit thrombosis at low flow rates, ECMO flows are not usually reduced below 1.0 L/min. An alternative approach is to decrease ECMO flows to 66% of

baseline for 10–15 minutes, then to 33% and/or a minimum of 1.0–1.5 L/min for another 10–15 minutes. At each stage, the LV ejection fraction, LVOT velocity time integral, transmitral Doppler E- and A-wave velocities and lateral mitral annular tissue Doppler velocities are measured.[82] If at any stage the mean arterial blood pressure falls below 60 mmHg, the support is increased back to 100% and the wean is terminated.

Myocardial recovery after weaning from VA ECMO may be suggested by the presence of the following parameters during minimal ECMO support: LV ejection fraction >20–25%, LVOT velocity time integral >10 cm, a lateral annular S′ velocity >6 cm/s, absence of LV dilatation, and no cardiac tamponade.[83,84] There has been a recent focus on echocardiographic assessment of myocardial mechanics, using velocity vector imaging, to determine ability to wean from VA ECMO.[85]

PERCUTANEOUS AXIAL FLOW PUMPS (IMPELLA®)

There are several options available for short term MCS.[86] The commonest device utilized worldwide is the *intra-aortic balloon pump* (IABP). This works on the principle of synchronized counter-pulsation and augments coronary perfusion and reduces LV afterload.

An alternative device is a catheter mounted microaxial pump, called an Impella (Figure 15.10).[87] This is an intravascular, transvalvular axial flow pump that can remain *in situ* for days to weeks. Depending upon the size, they can provide either partial or full cardiac support with the option of biventricular support as well. These devices are inserted retrogradely across the aortic valve and work by removing blood from the LV cavity and delivering it into the proximal ascending aorta (V14.13H).[88] They work in series with the ventricle and utilize the Archimedes screw principle for flow. Blood

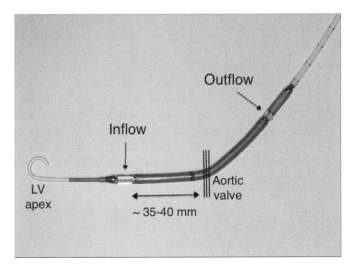

FIGURE 15.10　Impella CP device. Note the pigtail, inflow component, and outflow component. LV: left ventricular.

flow is generated by a variable speed impeller. This is graded as a "P level" of support. For the Impella CP, P0 is a stopped motor, P1 has an RPM of 23,000 RPM and can generate flow up to 1.7 L/min, while P8 has a motor speed of 44,000 RPM, which can generate flows up to 3.3 L/min. Other Impellas, such as the 5 and 5.5, provide full cardiac support with flows of ≥5 L/min. They have multiple hemodynamic benefits, including unloading the LV, increasing coronary perfusion pressure, and increasing mean arterial pressure.[89] There are numerous sizes to support the LV,[90] and there is also a right heart support device called the Impella RP (V15.14), which is inserted via access from the common femoral vein.[91,92]

The Impella is a short-term MCS option and accurate assessment of cardiac structure and function and Impella positioning is critical. The two common indications for Impella insertion are to support a high-risk percutaneous coronary intervention[93] and to manage cardiogenic shock.[94] Consequently, echocardiography is utilized frequently when managing a patient supported with an Impella (Table 15.1). Echocardiography is fundamental in multiple aspects of Impella patient care: (1) patient selection, (2) identification of contraindications, (3) guiding insertion, (4) device positioning and detection of complications, and (5) evaluation of recovery and weaning. Bedside echocardiography should be available on a 24-hour basis if a unit engages in Impella support.[95]

Prior to insertion of an Impella, there are a number of conditions detectable by echocardiography that contraindicate the insertion of the Impella. These include aortic dissection, mechanical aortic valve prosthesis, severe mitral stenosis, ventricular thrombus, and more-than-mild aortic regurgitation. During insertion, the Impella can be guided by fluoroscopy and echocardiography. The optimal views for guiding insertion are usually the parasternal long-axis view for TTE and the LV long axis for TEE. The Impella inflow should be approximately 35–40 mm below the aortic valve and the Impella outflow clearly above the aortic valve (usually around 20 mm). The Impella should ideally be as coaxial as possible to the long axis of the LV-aorta direction. The pigtail should also be free of any surrounding structures, such as the mitral subvalvular apparatus and LV walls. The inflow should also be free of contact with the mitral valve apparatus. The outflow should be within the aortic lumen rather than against the aortic wall.

Commoner indications for echocardiography are to assess Impella position (Figure 15.11) (V15.11, V15.12, V15.13, V15.14), low flow alarms, suction alarms, and hemolysis. A *suction alarm* may be due to inadequate LV filling, tamponade, incorrect Impella position, right heart failure, or support/P-levels too high. This can result in reduced Impella flows/hemodynamic support and hemolysis. Echocardiography is a key in the assessment of suction alarms as it can assess volume status, Impella position, and right heart function and check for tamponade.

Hemolysis may be a complication of Impella support, especially as the impeller may be rotating at over 40,000 RPM during high level support. This can result in shear forces acting on the red blood cell membrane, causing destruction and hemolysis. Monitoring for hemolysis occurs both clinically (such as dark urine) and biochemically (such as elevated hemolysis markers, LDH, and plasma-free hemoglobin). However, echocardiography also helps in hemolysis assessment by evaluating correct Impella positioning and checking for any associated thrombosis. If the inflow or outflow components of the Impella are against a cardiac structure (such as the mitral valve apparatus or directly onto the aortic wall), this can cause hemolysis. If the patient supported with an Impella ever had cardiopulmonary resuscitation or defibrillation, an echocardiogram should always be done post event to ensure appropriate device positioning.

Due to acute and dynamic nature of patients supported by an Impella, frequent assessment of ventricular function or ventricular recovery is often required. There is no formal standardized way on how to wean an Impella, and the protocols vary between institutions. However, they are based on the principle of a step-wise reduction in Impella support while monitoring the patient clinically, hemodynamics, and ventricular function on echocardiography. The technique of weaning an Impella depends upon the indication. During high-risk PCI when the support is brief, the wean tends to be more rapid. The P-level of support may be decreased by 2 levels every 10 minutes and if the patient remains stable at P2 for 10 minutes, the device may be removed. In cardiogenic shock or heart failure indications, the weaning occurs slower and there may be incremental reduction of support over hours, such as by decreasing the P-level by 2 steps each 2 hours and if the patient remains stable at P2 for 2 hours, the device may then be removed.

TABLE 15.1   Echocardiography during Impella Support

Pre-insertion of Impella
- Indications
- Contraindications

Post-insertion of Impella
- Confirmation of fluoroscopic location
- After moving the patient
- Suspected Impella migration
- Controller alarm (incorrect Impella position!)
- Hemolysis
- Assessment of ventricular function recovery
- Guidance during weaning

LIST OF VIDEOS

https://routledgetextbooks.com/textbooks/9781032157009/chapter-15.php

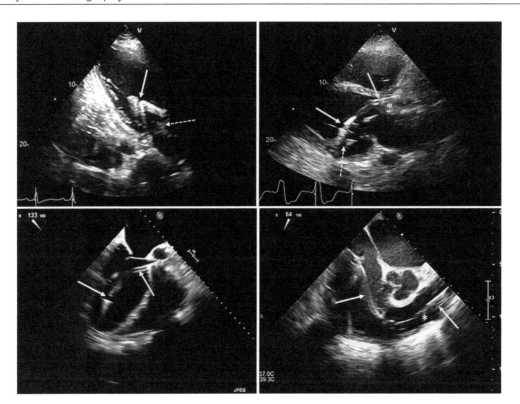

FIGURE 15.11 Upper left panel: appropriate position of Impella CP in a parasternal long-axis TTE view; note good pigtail position and Impella inflow (arrow) at an appropriate distance below the aortic valve (dotted arrow) and free of surrounding cardiac structures (V15.11). Upper right panel: parasternal long-axis TTE view with incorrect Impella position and orientation; note the Impella is too deep within the LV (white arrow: Impella inflow; yellow arrow: Impella outflow; *: aortic valve; dotted arrow: pigtail), the orientation is not coaxial with the long axis of the LV and the Impella tip/pigtail is pushing against the basal inferolateral LV wall (V15.12)—this can result in both ineffective hemodynamic support and increased risk of cardiac trauma. Lower left panel: LV long-axis TEE view showing Impella inserted too deep into the left ventricle (V15.13); note the inflow (white arrow) and outflow components (yellow arrow) of the Impella are both within the LV cavity—this would result in no effective hemodynamic support as all the unloaded LV blood is returned within the LV. Lower right panel: parasternal short-axis TEE view of an Impella RP (V15.14); note the Impella RP outflow (yellow arrow) positioned above the pulmonary valve (*), in the main pulmonary artery; white arrow indicates shaft of Impella RP, while Impella RP inflow is not visualized in this image as it is located within the very proximal inferior vena cava.

VIDEO 15.1 Biplane transesophageal echocardiography (TEE) of HeartWare inflow cannula in the left ventricular apex: Biplane TEE of HeartWare inflow cannula positioned in the left ventricular apex.

VIDEO 15.2 Real-time three-dimensional transesophageal echocardiography of HeartWare LVAD inflow cannula in the left ventricular apex: Precise position of the HeartWare LVAD inflow cannula can be appreciated by real-time three-dimensional transesophageal echocardiography. Note the central location and appropriate orientation of the inflow cannula.

VIDEO 15.3 Assessment of HeartWare LVAD outflow: Transesophageal echocardiography color Doppler assessment of Heart-Ware LVAD outflow into the ascending aorta.

VIDEO 15.4 Cardiac tamponade in a patient with a HeartWare LVAD: Note compression of the left ventricle, compromising LVAD filling.

VIDEO 15.5A Suddenly developed cardiogenic shock in a patient with left ventricular assist device (LVAD) (1/2):

A 66-year-old male patient with LVAD implanted because of terminal heart failure suddenly developed cardiogenic shock on the 18th day after LVAD implantation. Transesophageal echocardiography was performed, and modified four-chamber view (at 0°) showed a large pericardial hematoma compressing predominantly the right atrium, but also the tricuspid valve and right ventricle. A slight shifting of the interventricular septum toward the left ventricular cavity, which is small and appears "underfilled," could be noted. The inflow cannula of the LVAD is normally positioned in the left ventricular apex. In attempting to obtain midesophageal two-chamber view, at 90° (see Video 15.5B), nothing but a large pericardial hematoma could be imaged (measuring approximately 8 cm in diameter). The hematoma was evacuated during urgent surgical revision and the patient fully recovered. *(Video provided by MC.)*

VIDEO 15.5B Suddenly developed cardiogenic shock in a patient with left ventricular assist device (LVAD) (2/2): A 66-year-old male patient with LVAD implanted because of terminal heart failure suddenly developed cardiogenic shock on the 18th day after LVAD implantation. Transesophageal echocardiography was performed, and modified four-chamber view (at 0°) showed a large pericardial hematoma compressing predominantly the right atrium, but also the tricuspid valve and right ventricle (see Video 15.5A). A slight shifting of the interventricular septum toward the LV cavity, which is small and appears "underfilled," could be noted. The inflow cannula of the LVAD is normally positioned in the LV apex. In attempting to obtain midesophageal two-chamber view, at 90° (shown here) nothing but a large pericardial hematoma could be imaged (measuring approximately 8 cm in diameter). The hematoma was evacuated during urgent surgical revision and the patient fully recovered. *(Video provided by MC.)*

VIDEO 15.6   Venovenous extracorporeal membrane oxygenation (VV ECMO) outflow cannula in the right atrium: 2D and color Doppler TEE showing appropriately positioned VV-ECMO outflow/return cannula in the right atrium. Note the main outflow color jet at the tip of the cannula and multiple side hole jets.

VIDEO 15.7   Biplane transesophageal echocardiography of venoarterial extracorporeal membrane oxygenation (VA ECMO) access cannula: Note that VA access cannula has been inserted too far into the right atrium and onto the interatrial septum.

VIDEO 15.8   Cardiac tamponade after institution of peripheral venoarterial extracorporeal membrane oxygenation (VA ECMO) system: A 49-year-old male with a recent anterior myocardial infarction was presented with cardiorespiratory arrest. During cardiopulmonary resuscitation, a peripheral VA ECMO system was instituted. However, a full ECMO flow of 4.8 L was maintained only for a very short period of time, followed by the recurrence of cardiogenic shock and increase in central venous pressure. Clinically, cardiac tamponade was suspected. Transthoracic apical four-chamber view showing obliterated cavities of both right atrium and ventricle and a pericardial effusion or hematoma compressing the right heart cavities. Global left ventricular systolic function is severely impaired, with akinesia of the anterior septum, apex, and distal part of the lateral wall, with spontaneous echo contract in the left ventricular cavity. The patient was urgently taken to the operating room, where a rupture of the right ventricular free wall by the venous ECMO cannula was found and repaired. *(Video provided by MC.)*

VIDEO 15.9   Unvented left ventricle in a patient on peripheral venoarterial extracorporeal membrane oxygenation (VA ECMO): Note the absence of contractility of the left ventricle, apical thrombus, and absence of aortic valve opening.

VIDEO 15.10   Aortic root thrombus in a patient on peripheral venoarterial extracorporeal membrane oxygenation (VA ECMO): Real-time 3D transesophageal echocardiography of an aortic root thrombus in a patient on VA ECMO with an unvented left ventricle. Note also the absence of aortic valve opening.

VIDEO 15.11   Appropriate Impella position. In an apical long-axis TTE view note good pigtail position and Impella inflow at an appropriate distance below the aortic valve and free of surrounding cardiac structures.

VIDEO 15.12   Incorrect Impella position and orientation. In a parasternal long-axis TTE view note the Impella is too deep within

the LV, the orientation is not coaxial with the long axis of the LV and the Impella tip/pigtail is pushing against the basal inferolateral LV wall. This can result in both ineffective hemodynamic support and increased risk of cardiac trauma.

VIDEO 15.13   Impella too deep into the left ventricle. In an LV long-axis TEE view, note the inflow and outflow components of the Impella are both within the LV cavity. This would result in no effective hemodynamic support as all the unloaded left ventricular blood is returned within the left ventricle.

VIDEO 15.14   Parasternal short-axis TEE view of an Impella RP. Note the Impella RP outflow positioned above the pulmonary valve, in the main pulmonary artery. The Impella RP inflow is not visualized in this image as it is located within the very proximal inferior vena cava.

REFERENCES

1. Patel CB, Cowger JA, Zuckermann A. A contemporary review of mechanical circulatory support. J Heart Lung Transplant. 2014;33(7):667–74.
2. Schramm R, Morshuis M, Schoenbrodt M, Boergermann J, Hakim-Meibodi K, Hata M, et al. Current perspectives on mechanical circulatory support. Eur J Cardiothorac Surg. 2019;55(Supplement_1):i31–7.
3. Fried J, Sayer G, Naka Y, Uriel N. State of the art review: evolution and ongoing challenges of left ventricular assist device therapy. Struct Heart. 2018;2(4):262–73.
4. Nesta M, Cammertoni F, Bruno P, Massetti M. Implantable ventricular assistance systems (VAD) as a bridge to transplant or as 'destination therapy'. Eur Heart J Supp. 2021;23(Supplement_E):E99–E102.
5. Stainback RF, Estep JD, Agler DA, Birks EJ, Bremer M, Hung J, et al. Echocardiography in the management of patients with left ventricular assist devices: recommendations from the American Society of Echocardiography. J Am Soc Echocardiogr. 2015;28(8):853–909.
6. Cohen DG, Thomas JD, Freed BH, Rich JD, Sauer AJ. Echocardiography and continuous-flow left ventricular assist devices: evidence and limitations. JACC Heart Fail. 2015;3(7):554–64.
7. Douglas PS, Garcia MJ, Haines DE, Lai WW, Manning WJ, Patel AR, et al. ACCF/ASE/AHA/ASNC/HFSA/HRS/SCAI/SCCM/SCCT/SCMR 2011 appropriate use criteria for echocardiography. A report of the American College of Cardiology Foundation Appropriate Use Criteria Task Force, American Society of Echocardiography, American Heart Association, American Society of Nuclear Cardiology, Heart Failure Society of America, Heart Rhythm Society, Society for Cardiovascular Angiography and Interventions, Society of Critical Care Medicine, Society of Cardiovascular Computed Tomography, Society for Cardiovascular Magnetic Resonance American College of Chest Physicians. J Am Soc Echocardiogr. 2011;24(3):229–67.
8. Mitter N, Sheinberg R. Update on ventricular assist devices. [Miscellaneous Article]. Curr Opin Anaesthesiol. 2010;23(1):57–66.
9. Birks EJ. Left ventricular assist devices. Heart. 2010;96 (1):63–71.

10. Ammar KA, Umland MM, Kramer C, Sulemanjee N, Jan MF, Khandheria BK, et al. The ABCs of left ventricular assist device echocardiography: a systematic approach. Eur Heart J Cardiovasc Imaging. 2012;13(11):885–99.

11. Estep JD, Stainback RF, Little SH, Torre G, Zoghbi WA. The role of echocardiography and other imaging modalities in patients with left ventricular assist devices. JACC Cardiovasc imaging. 2010;3(10):1049–64.

12. Rasalingam R, Johnson SN, Bilhorn KR, Huang PH, Makan M, Moazami N, et al. Transthoracic echocardiographic assessment of continuous-flow left ventricular assist devices. J Am Soc Echocardiogr. 2011;24(2):135–48.

13. Lahpor JR. State of the art: implantable ventricular assist devices. Curr Opin Organ Transplant. 2009;14(5):554–9.

14. Kirklin JK, Naftel DC, Pagani FD, Kormos RL, Stevenson LW, Blume ED, et al. Sixth INTERMACS annual report: a 10,000-patient database. J Heart Lung Transplant. 2014;33(6):555–64.

15. Slaughter MS, Rogers JG, Milano CA, Russell SD, Conte JV, Feldman D, et al. Advanced heart failure treated with continuous-flow left ventricular assist device. N Eng J Med. 2009;361(23):2241–51.

16. Fang JC. Rise of the machines—left ventricular assist devices as permanent therapy for advanced heart failure. N Eng J Med. 2009;361(23):2282–5.

17. Slaughter MS, Pagani FD, Rogers JG, Miller LW, Sun B, Russell SD, et al. Clinical management of continuous-flow left ventricular assist devices in advanced heart failure. J Heart Lung Transplant. 2010;29(4 Suppl):S1–39.

18. Mulvagh SL, Rakowski H, Vannan MA, Abdelmoneim SS, Becher H, Bierig SM, et al. American Society of Echocardiography consensus statement on the clinical applications of ultrasonic contrast agents in echocardiography. J Am Soc Echocardiogr. 2008;21(11):1179–201.

19. Senior R, Becher H, Monaghan M, Agati L, Zamorano J, Vanoverschelde JL, et al. Contrast echocardiography: evidence-based recommendations by European Association of Echocardiography. Eur J Echocardiogr. 2009;10(2):194–212.

20. Dang NC, Topkara VK, Mercando M, Kay J, Kruger KH, Aboodi MS, et al. Right heart failure after left ventricular assist device implantation in patients with chronic congestive heart failure. J Heart Lung Transplant. 2006;25(1):1–6.

21. Fukamachi K, McCarthy PM, Smedira NG, Vargo RL, Starling RC, Young JB. Preoperative risk factors for right ventricular failure after implantable left ventricular assist device insertion. Ann Thorac Surg. 1999;68(6):2181–4.

22. Wang Y, Simon MA, Bonde P, Harris BU, Teuteberg JJ, Kormos RL, et al. Decision tree for adjuvant right ventricular support in patients receiving a left ventricular assist device. J Heart Lung Transplant. 2012;31(2):140–9.

23. Wang Y, Simon M, Bonde P, Harris BU, Teuteberg JJ, Kormos RL, et al. Prognosis of right ventricular failure in patients with left ventricular assist device based on decision tree with SMOTE. IEEE Trans Inf Technol Biomed. 2012;16(3):383–90.

24. Kormos RL, Teuteberg JJ, Pagani FD, Russell SD, John R, Miller LW, et al. Right ventricular failure in patients with the HeartMate II continuous-flow left ventricular assist device: incidence, risk factors, and effect on outcomes. J Thorac Cardiovasc Surg. 2010;139(5):1316–24.

25. Frankfurter C, Molinero M, Vishram-Nielsen JKK, Foroutan F, Mak S, Rao V, et al. Predicting the risk of right ventricular failure in patients undergoing left ventricular assist device implantation. Circulation Heart Fail. 2020;13(10):e006994.

26. Grant AD, Smedira NG, Starling RC, Marwick TH. Independent and incremental role of quantitative right ventricular evaluation for the prediction of right ventricular failure after left ventricular assist device implantation. J Am Coll Cardiol. 2012;60(6):521–8.

27. Kato TS, Jiang J, Schulze PC, Jorde U, Uriel N, Kitada S, et al. Serial echocardiography using tissue Doppler and speckle tracking imaging to monitor right ventricular failure before and after left ventricular assist device surgery. JACC Heart Fail. 2013;1(3):216–22.

28. Cohen DG, Thomas JD, Freed BH, Rich JD, Sauer AJ. Echocardiography and continuous-flow left ventricular assist devices. JACC Heart Fail. 2015;3(7):554–64.

29. Soliman OII, Akin S, Muslem R, Boersma E, Manintveld OC, Krabatsch T, et al. Derivation and validation of a novel right-sided heart failure model after implantation of continuous flow left ventricular assist devices: the EUROMACS (European Registry for Patients with Mechanical Circulatory Support) right-sided heart failure risk score. Circulation. 2018;137(9):891–906.

30. Shanewise JS, Cheung AT, Aronson S, Stewart WJ, Weiss RL, Mark JB, et al. ASE/SCA guidelines for performing a comprehensive intraoperative multiplane transesophageal echocardiography examination: recommendations of the American Society of Echocardiography Council for Intraoperative Echocardiography and the Society of Cardiovascular Anesthesiologists Task Force for Certification in Perioperative Transesophageal Echocardiography. J Am Soc Echocardiogr. 1999;12(10):884–900.

31. Bryant AS, Holman WL, Nanda NC, Vengala S, Blood MS, Pamboukian SV, et al. Native aortic valve insufficiency in patients with left ventricular assist devices. Ann Thorac Surg. 2006;81(2):e6–8.

32. Toda K, Fujita T, Domae K, Shimahara Y, Kobayashi J, Nakatani T. Late aortic insufficiency related to poor prognosis during left ventricular assist device support. Ann Thorac Surg. 2011;92(3):929–34.

33. Holman WL, Bourge RC, Fan P, Kirklin JK, Pacifico AD, Nanda NC. Influence of left ventricular assist on valvular regurgitation. Circulation. 1993;88(5 Pt 2):II309–18.

34. Fang JC, Wever-Pinzon O. Dealing with unintended consequences: continuous-flow LVADs and aortic insufficiency*. JACC Cardiovasc Imaging. 2016;9(6):652–4.

35. Grinstein J, Kruse E, Sayer G, Fedson S, Kim GH, Jorde UP, et al. Accurate quantification methods for aortic insufficiency severity in patients with LVAD. JACC Cardiovasc Imaging. 2016;9(6):641–51.

36. Lam KM, Ennis S, O'Driscoll G, Solis JM, Macgillivray T, Picard MH. Observations from non-invasive measures of right heart hemodynamics in left ventricular assist device patients. J Am Soc Echocardiogr. 2009 Sep;22(9):1055–62.

37. Chumnanvej S, Wood MJ, MacGillivray TE, Melo MFV. Perioperative echocardiographic examination for ventricular assist device implantation. Anesth Analg. 2007;105(3):583–601.

38. Koelling TM, Aaronson KD, Cody RJ, Bach DS, Armstrong WF. Prognostic significance of mitral regurgitation and tricuspid regurgitation in patients with left ventricular systolic dysfunction. Am Heart J. 2002;144(3):524–9.

39. Scalia GM, McCarthy PM, Savage RM, Smedira NG, Thomas JD. Clinical utility of echocardiography in the management of implantable ventricular assist devices. J Am Soc Echocardiogr. 2000;13(8):754–63.

40. Catena E, Milazzo F, Montorsi E, Bruschi G, Cannata A, Russo C, et al. Left Ventricular support by axial flow pump: the echocardiographic approach to device malfunction. J Am Soc Echocardiogr. 2005;18(12):1422.e7–.e13.

41. Stainback RF, Croitoru M, Hernandez A, Myers TJ, Wadia Y, Frazier OH. Echocardiographic evaluation of the Jarvik 2000 axial-flow LVAD. Texas Heart Inst J. 2005;32(3):263–70.

42. McDiarmid A, Gordon B, Wrightson N, Robinson-Smith N, Pillay T, Parry G, et al. Hemodynamic, echocardiographic, and exercise-related effects of the HeartWare left ventricular assist device in advanced heart failure. Congest Heart Fail. 2013;19(1):11–5.

43. Shah NR, Cevik C, Hernandez A, Gregoric ID, Frazier OH, Stainback RF. Transthoracic echocardiography of the HeartWare left ventricular assist device. J Cardiac Fail. 2012;18(9):745–8.

44. Estep JD, Chang SM, Bhimaraj A, Torre-Amione G, Zoghbi WA, Nagueh SF. Imaging for ventricular function and myocardial recovery on nonpulsatile ventricular assist devices. Circulation. 2012;125(18):2265–77.

45. Longobardo L, Kramer C, Carerj S, Zito C, Jain R, Suma V, et al. Role of echocardiography in the evaluation of left ventricular assist devices: the importance of emerging technologies. Curr Cardiol Rep. 2016;18(7):62.

46. Kaufmann F, Hörmandinger C, Knosalla C, Falk V, Potapov E. Thrombus formation at the inflow cannula of continuous-flow left ventricular assist devices—a systematic analysis. Artif Organs. 2022;46(8):1573–84.

47. Uriel N, Morrison KA, Garan AR, Kato TS, Yuzefpolskaya M, Latif F, et al. Development of a novel echocardiography ramp test for speed optimization and diagnosis of device thrombosis in continuous-flow left ventricular assist devices: the Columbia ramp study. J Am Coll Cardiol. 2012;60(18):1764–75.

48. Platts D, Burstow D, Hamilton Craig C, Wright G, Thomson B. Systemic air embolization originating from a pleural air leak via a left ventricular assist device cannula anastomosis site. J Am Soc Echocardiogr. 2010;23(3):341 e1–2.

49. Chatterjee A, Feldmann C, Hanke JS, Ricklefs M, Shrestha M, Dogan G, et al. The momentum of HeartMate 3: a novel active magnetically levitated centrifugal left ventricular assist device (LVAD). J Thorac Dis. 2018;10(Suppl 15):S1790–s3.

50. Cheng A, Williamitis CA, Slaughter MS. Comparison of continuous-flow and pulsatile-flow left ventricular assist devices: is there an advantage to pulsatility? Ann Cardiothorac Surg. 2014;3(6):573–81.

51. Purohit SN, Cornwell WK, Pal JD, Lindenfeld J, Ambardekar AV. Living without a pulse. Circ Heart Fail. 2018;11(6):e004670.

52. Schramm R, Zittermann A, Morshuis M, Schoenbrodt M, von Roessing E, von Dossow V, et al. Comparing short-term outcome after implantation of the HeartWare® HVAD® and the Abbott® HeartMate 3®. ESC Heart Fail. 2020;7(3):908–14.

53. Stapor M, Pilat A, Gackowski A, Misiuda A, Gorkiewicz-Kot I, Kaleta M, et al. Echo-guided left ventricular assist device speed optimisation for exercise maximisation. Heart. 2022;108(13):1055–62.

54. Imamura T, Jeevanandam V, Kim G, Raikhelkar J, Sarswat N, Kalantari S, et al. Optimal hemodynamics during left ventricular assist device support are associated with reduced readmission rates. Circ Heart Fail. 2019;12(2):e005094.

55. Couperus LE, Delgado V, Khidir MJH, Vester MPM, Palmen M, Fiocco M, et al. Pump speed optimization in stable patients with a left ventricular assist device. Asaio J. 2017;63(3):266–72.

56. Lilliu M, Onorati F, Luciani GB, Faggian G. Effects of echo-optimization of left ventricular assist devices on functional capacity, a randomized controlled trial. ESC Heart Fail. 2021;8(4):2846–55.

57. Birks EJ, Tansley PD, Hardy J, George RS, Bowles CT, Burke M, et al. Left ventricular assist device and drug therapy for the reversal of heart failure. N Eng J Med. 2006;355(18):1873–84.

58. Monteagudo Vela M, Rial Bastón V, Panoulas V, Riesgo Gil F, Simon A. A detailed explantation assessment protocol for patients with left ventricular assist devices with myocardial recovery. Interact Cardiovasc Thorac Surg. 2021;32(2):298–305.

59. Chaggar PS, Williams SG, Yonan N, Fildes J, Venkateswaran R, Shaw SM. Myocardial recovery with mechanical circulatory support. Eur J Heart Fail. 2016;18(10):1220–7.

60. Khan T, Delgado RM, Radovancevic B, Torre-Amione G, Abrams J, Miller K, et al. Dobutamine stress echocardiography predicts myocardial improvement in patients supported by left ventricular assist devices (LVADs): hemodynamic and histologic evidence of improvement before LVAD explantation. J Heart Lung Transplant. 2003;22(2):137–46.

61. Maybaum S, Mancini D, Xydas S, Starling RC, Aaronson K, Pagani FD, et al. Cardiac improvement during mechanical circulatory support: a prospective multicenter study of the LVAD Working Group. Circulation. 2007;115(19):2497–505.

62. Beckmann A, Benk C, Beyersdorf F, Haimerl G, Merkle F, Mestres C, et al. Position article for the use of extracorporeal life support in adult patients. Eur J Cardiothorac Surg. 2011;40(3):676–80.

63. Park PK, Napolitano LM, Bartlett RH. Extracorporeal membrane oxygenation in adult acute respiratory distress syndrome. Crit Care Clin. 2011;27(3):627–46.

64. Makdisi G, Wang I-W. Extra corporeal membrane oxygenation (ECMO) review of a lifesaving technology. J Thorac Dis. 2015;7(7):E166–E76.

65. MacLaren G, Combes A, Bartlett RH. Contemporary extracorporeal membrane oxygenation for adult respiratory failure: life support in the new era. Intensive Care Med. 2012;38(2):210–20.

66. Bailleul C, Aissaoui N. Role of echocardiography in the management of veno-arterial extra-corporeal membrane oxygenation patients. J Emerg Crit Care Med. 2019;3.

67. Platts DG, Sedgwick JF, Burstow DJ, Mullany DV, Fraser JF. The role of echocardiography in the management of patients supported by extracorporeal membrane oxygenation. J Am Soc Echocardiogr. 2012;25(2):131–41.

68. Fraser JF, Shekar K, Diab S, Dunster K, Foley SR, McDonald CI, et al. ECMO—the clinician's view. ISBT Sci Ser. 2012;7(1):82–8.

69. Javidfar J, Brodie D, Wang D. Use of bicavaldual-lumen-catheter for adult venovenous extracorporeal membrane oxygenation. Ann Thorac Surg. 2011;91:1763–8.

70. Javidfar J, Wang D, Zwischenberger JB, Costa J, Mongero L, Sonett J, et al. Insertion of bicaval dual lumen extracorporeal membrane oxygenation catheter with image guidance. Asaio J. 2011;57(3):203–5.

71. Reilly JP, Tunick PA, Timmermans RJ, Stein B, Rosenzweig BP, Kronzon I. Contrast echocardiography clarifies uninterpretable wall motion in intensive care unit patients. J Am Coll Cardiol. 2000;35(2):485–90.

72. Makaryus AN, Zubrow ME, Gillam LD, Michelakis N, Phillips L, Ahmed S, et al. Contrast echocardiography improves the diagnostic yield of transthoracic studies performed in

the intensive care setting by novice sonographers. J Am Soc Echocardiogr. 2005;18(5):475–80.

73. Costa JM, Tsutsui JM, Nozawa E, Morhy SS, Andrade JL, Ramires JF, et al. Contrast echocardiography can save nondiagnostic exams in mechanically ventilated patients. Echocardiography. 2005;22(5):389–94.

74. Yong Y, Wu D, Fernandes V, Kopelen HA, Shimoni S, Nagueh SF, Callahan JD, Bruns DE, Shaw LJ, Quinones MA, Zoghbi WA. Diagnostic accuracy and cost-effectiveness of contrast echocardiography on evaluation of cardiac function in technically very difficult patients in the intensive care unit. Am J Cardiol. 2002 Mar 15;89(6):711–8.

75. Platts D, Fraser JF, Mullany D, Burstow D. Left ventricular endocardial definition enhancement using perflutren microsphere contrast echocardiography during peripheral venoarterial extracorporeal membranous oxygenation. Echocardiography. 2010;27(9):E112–E4.

76. Sedgwick JF, Burstow DJ, Platts DG. The role of echocardiography in the management of patients supported by extracorporeal membranous oxygenation (ECMO). Int J Cardiol. 2010;147(Supplement 1):S16.

77. ELSO. Ann Arbor, MI 2011. Available from: www.elso.med.umich.edu/.

78. Koenig PR, Ralston MA, Kimball TR, Meyer RA, Daniels SR, Schwartz DC. Balloon atrial septostomy for left ventricular decompression in patients receiving extracorporeal membrane oxygenation for myocardial failure. J Pediatr. 1993;122(6):S95-S9.

79. O'Connor TA, Downing GJ, Ewing LL, Gowdamarajan R. Echocardiographically guided balloon atrial septostomy during extracorporeal membrane oxygenation (ECMO). Pediatr Cardiol. 1993;14(3):167–8.

80. Randhawa VK, Al-Fares A, Tong MZY, Soltesz EG, Hernandez-Montfort J, Taimeh Z, et al. A Pragmatic approach to weaning temporary mechanical circulatory support: a state-of-the-art review. JACC Heart Fail. 2021;9(9):664–73.

81. Cavarocchi NC, Pitcher HT, Yang Q, Karbowski P, Miessau J, Hastings HM, et al. Weaning of extracorporeal membrane oxygenation using continuous hemodynamic transesophageal echocardiography. J Thorac Cardiovasc Surg. 2013;146(6):1474–9.

82. Aissaoui N, Luyt CE, Leprince P, Trouillet JL, Leger P, Pavie A, et al. Predictors of successful extracorporeal membrane oxygenation (ECMO) weaning after assistance for refractory cardiogenic shock. Intensive Care Med. 2011;37(11):1738–45.

83. Aissaoui N, Luyt CE, Leprince P, Trouillet JL, Léger P, Pavie A, et al. Predictors of successful extracorporeal membrane oxygenation (ECMO) weaning after assistance for refractory cardiogenic shock. Intensive Care Med. 2011;37(11):1738–45.

84. Kim D, Jang WJ, Park TK, Cho YH, Choi J-O, Jeon E-S, et al. Echocardiographic predictors of successful extracorporeal membrane oxygenation weaning after refractory cardiogenic shock. J Am Soc Echocardiogr. 2021;34(4):414–22.e4.

85. Aissaoui N, Guerot E, Combes A, Delouche A, Chastre J, Leprince P, et al. Two-dimensional strain rate and Doppler tissue myocardial velocities: analysis by echocardiography of hemodynamic and functional changes of the failed left ventricle during different degrees of extracorporeal life support. J Am Soc Echocardiogr. 2012;25(6):632–40.

86. Rihal CS, Naidu SS, Givertz MM, Szeto WY, Burke JA, Kapur NK, et al. 2015 SCAI/ACC/HFSA/STS clinical expert consensus statement on the use of percutaneous mechanical circulatory support devices in cardiovascular care: endorsed by the American Heart Assocation, the Cardiological Society of India, and Sociedad Latino Americana de Cardiologia Intervencion; Affirmation of Value by the Canadian Association of Interventional Cardiology-Association Canadienne de Cardiologie d'intervention*. J Am Coll Cardiol. 2015;65(19):e7–e26.

87. Zein R, Patel C, Mercado-Alamo A, Schreiber T, Kaki A. A Review of the impella devices. Interv Cardiol. 2022;17:e05.

88. Glazier JJ, Kaki A. The impella device: historical background, clinical applications and future directions. Int J Angiol. 2019;28(2):118–23.

89. Nakamura M, Imamura T, Ueno H, Kinugawa K. Current indication and practical management of percutaneous left ventricular assist device support therapy in Japan. J Cardiol. 2020;75(3):228–32.

90. Burzotta F, Trani C, Doshi SN, Townend J, van Geuns RJ, Hunziker P, et al. Impella ventricular support in clinical practice: collaborative viewpoint from a European expert user group. Int J Cardiol. 2015;201:684–91.

91. Anderson M, Morris DL, Tang D, Batsides G, Kirtane A, Hanson I, et al. Outcomes of patients with right ventricular failure requiring short-term hemodynamic support with the Impella RP device. J Heart Lung Transplant. 2018;37(12):1448–58.

92. Kapur NK, Esposito ML, Bader Y, Morine KJ, Kiernan MS, Pham DT, et al. Mechanical circulatory support devices for acute right ventricular failure. Circulation. 2017;136(3):314–26.

93. Atkinson TM, Ohman EM, O'Neill WW, Rab T, Cigarroa JE. A practical approach to mechanical circulatory support in patients undergoing percutaneous coronary intervention: an interventional perspective. JACC Cardiovasc Interv. 2016;9(9):871–83.

94. Basra SS, Loyalka P, Kar B. Current status of percutaneous ventricular assist devices for cardiogenic shock. Curr Opin Cardiol. 2011;26(6):548–54.

95. Burzotta F, Trani C, Doshi SN, Townend J, van Geuns RJ, Hunziker P, et al. Impella ventricular support in clinical practice: collaborative viewpoint from a European expert user group. Int J Cardiol. 2015;201:684–91.

Echocardiography in chest trauma

16

Agatha Y. Kwon and Gregory M. Scalia

Key Points

- Echocardiography, especially transesophageal echocardiography, is a key component of diagnostic investigations after blunt or penetrating chest trauma.
- Knowing the possible mechanisms of injuries to the heart and great vessels is crucial in interpretation of echocardiographic findings.
- Echocardiographic signs are often nonspecific and may include regional (noncoronary) distribution patterns of right and/or left ventricular dysfunction, increased myocardial wall echogenicity and thickness, signs of myocardial rupture in various locations, (with or without cardiac tamponade or pseudoaneurysm formation), acute valve regurgitation, and signs of acute aortic syndrome.
- This is an area of echocardiography that should be undertaken by the most experienced operators available.

Chest trauma, whether blunt or penetrating, potentially may involve damage to the heart and great vessels with consequences that may range from simple hematoma formation to major organ disruption, hemodynamic collapse, and death. Approximately 25% of traumatic deaths are caused by cardiovascular injuries and constitutes the second most common cause of death after central nervous system injuries in polytrauma patients.[1]

Trauma to the heart and great vessels is broadly classified into two categories based on the mechanisms of injury: blunt and penetrating (Table 16.1). Blunt cardiac injuries are more common and are a consequence of impact on the chest, with or without bony injury. Penetrating cardiac injuries are a consequence of direct intrusion into the heart or great vessels by foreign objects. Iatrogenic injuries from medical procedures can also cause such injuries. Less common causes of cardiac injury include electrocution and radiation.

In general, patients with significant chest trauma will be transferred from emergency room to intensive care units for stabilization, monitoring, and diagnostic investigations. Point-of-care ultrasound (POCUS) is an established diagnostic bedside tool with portable or handheld ultrasound devices (HUDs), which are now ubiquitous in the emergency and critical care settings. Emergency ultrasound examination of the heart, often in form of focused cardiac ultrasound (FoCUS) imaging (see Chapter 19), has been repeatedly shown to confer a survival advantage in chest trauma patients by allowing rapid triage toward emergent and subsequent definitive interventions.[2,3] As with ultrasound examination in cardiac arrest (see Chapter 5), the operator should urgently assess for the "big four"—tamponade, severe left ventricular dysfunction (global/regional), severe hypovolemia, and severe right ventricular dysfunction.[2] In patients with refractory shock without a clear cause, a comprehensive transthoracic echocardiogram (TTE) should

DOI: 10.1201/9781003245407-16

TABLE 16.1 Cardiac Trauma Classification

Blunt cardiac trauma
  Myocardial contusion
  Cardiac rupture
  Valve injury
  Coronary injury or dissection

Great vessel trauma
  Aortic transection
  Pseudoaneurysm
  Dissection

Penetrating cardiac trauma
  High-velocity missiles versus stabbing injuries
  Organ and vessel perforation, rupture, and fistula formation
  Valve injury
  Cardiac tamponade

Iatrogenic injuries
  Pacemaker wire
  Catheter-based interventions
  Intra-aortic balloon pump
  Cardiopulmonary resuscitation

be considered with the goal of identifying changes that may require immediate intervention. Adequate views of the heart may not be attainable via TTE in patients with severe injuries, open chest wounds and/or chest tubes that may preclude transducer placement, and transesophageal echocardiography (TEE) may be the preferred or the only option.

ANATOMICAL AND MECHANICAL CONSIDERATIONS

Heart and surface relationships

The heart is located within the middle mediastinum and protected by the bony structures of the sternum and the third and fourth ribs (Figure 16.1). The heart is bordered anteriorly by

the right ventricle, laterally by the left ventricle, superiorly by the great vessels of the aorta and pulmonary artery, and inferiorly by the veins of the vena cava. The anterior, retrosternal position of the right ventricle makes it most vulnerable to cardiac trauma.[1] The cardiac chambers are supported and protected by the fibrous pericardial layer that extends superiorly to cover the proximal portion (3–5 cm) of the ascending aorta and pulmonary artery. There remains only a small portion of the left atrium that is not protected by the pericardial layer at the origin of the four pulmonary veins.

BLUNT CARDIAC TRAUMA

Blunt cardiac trauma (BCT) is second only to central nervous system injuries as the most frequent cause of death after impact trauma. In the non-military setting, the commonest cause of BCT is motor vehicle accidents, which accounts for over 80% of all causes of BCT.[4] *Low-velocity injuries* are seen after direct impact in contact sports, falls, horse kicks and blasts. *High-velocity injuries* occur in motor vehicle accidents, with head-on impact from steering wheel, air bag, or seat belt. Falls from great height (>3–4.5 m), including attempted suicide, can also result in high-velocity BCT.

Forces involved in blunt cardiac trauma

Rapid deceleration causes cardiac injury by *direct compression* of the heart between the sternum and the vertebral column and, due to *rapid increases in thoracic pressure* from abdominal and lower-limb compression, causing a "hydraulic ram effect"—*sudden, rapid deceleration* of the chest with the heart continuing to move forward or outward while veins that flow to the atria are fixed to the pericardial cavity and remain in place, causing shearing stresses at certain anatomic sites that lead to tear or rupture.[5]

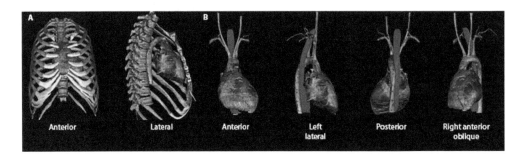

FIGURE 16.1 (A) Anatomic relationships with the ribs and costal cartilages (anterior view) and the sternum (lateral view). (B) Anatomic relationship of the esophagus (pink) with the heart and aorta. The distal ascending aorta is clearly in the far field from the transesophageal probe, whereas the distal arch is a very near-field structure.

(Images created with the Virtual Human Dissector, Touch of Life Technologies, Colorado USA.)

MYOCARDIAL CONTUSION

Myocardial contusion is an infrequent but serious complication seen in the setting of severe BCT, often accompanied by significant extracardiac injuries. It involves patchy and irregular myocyte damage, usually with epicardial hemorrhage, intramural hematoma, and bruising.[6] Because of its anterior location beneath the sternum, the *right ventricle* is the most vulnerable to this form of injury. The anteroapical portion of the left ventricle is also vulnerable, particularly from left lateral impact. Arrhythmias are a common complication, usually occurring within first 24–48 hours and are thought to result from varying combinations of increased catecholamine levels, direct damage to the conduction system, and/or hypoxic and edematous myocardial changes. Focal myocardial edema can compromise the regional myocardial microvasculature, further escalating regional myocardial dysfunction and perfusion defects. Traumatic ventricular septal defect can occur as a result of necrosis of contused myocardium, most commonly occurring in the muscular interventricular septum near the apex. Sudden cardiac death caused by ventricular arrhythmias may occur with low-energy impact to the chest wall if it coincides with a narrow window during cardiac repolarization.[7]

Echocardiographic findings

Myocardial contusion may manifest as *right or left ventricular dysfunction* and may be seen, often in a regional (noncoronary distribution), with or without *pericardial effusion* (V16.1A, V16.1B, V16.1C, V16.2A, and V16.2B).[8] The contused area may have increased echogenicity and increased thickness, and there may be associated chamber dilatation, particularly right ventricular outflow tract in right ventricular trauma. Color

Doppler echocardiography should be used to exclude the presence of ventricular septal defect (VSD). In the follow-up of patients with known myocardial contusion, it is important to rule out development of ventricular aneurysms or pseudoaneurysms, or formation of intracardiac thrombus.[9]

CARDIAC RUPTURE

Blunt cardiac rupture is defined as a full-thickness laceration of the myocardial wall. It is rare, occurring in less than 0.5% of all BCT, and is usually an autopsy finding with most victims exsanguinating before arriving in the emergency department. Rupture of the right atrium and right atrial appendage is more common due to their thin walls and anterior location.[10] Disruption of the venous-atrial junctions can also occur from deceleration force, and in rare cases, traumatic ventricular and atrial septal rupture can occur (Figure 16.2). Generally, pericardial tears lead to intrapericardial bleeding and effusion with patients suffering cardiac tamponade with massive hemodynamic collapse.

Echocardiographic findings

Point-of-care ultrasound examination of the heart may demonstrate tamponade. In some cases, the rupture may be contained by a pseudoaneurysm membrane with a blood-filled cavity in communication with the heart, usually with to-and-fro flow and thrombus within the false aneurysm. This finding should prompt the treating team to consider urgent cardiac surgery because such pseudoaneurysms are highly unstable. Complete rupture with tamponade can occur abruptly with drastic consequences.

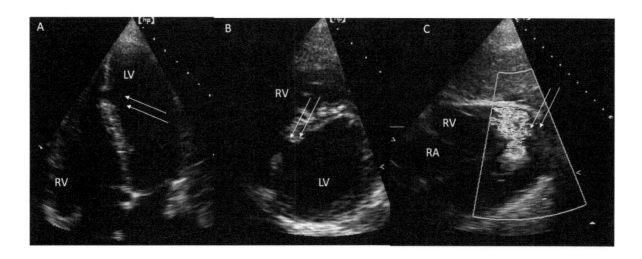

FIGURE 16.2 Traumatic apical ventricular septal defect (arrows) following blunt chest impact in a motor vehicle accident. (A) Apical four-chamber view. (B) Parasternal short-axis view. (C) Subcostal view of turbulent jet across ventricular septal defect with color Doppler (arrows). LV: left ventricle; RV: right ventricle.

VALVE INJURY

Due to higher transmural pressures on the left-sided structures, trauma to aortic and mitral valves is at greater risk for injury than the right-sided valves, with *acute regurgitation* being the commonest consequence.

Aortic valve trauma usually manifests as tears along the coaptation surface of the cusps near to the commissures resulting in tear or avulsion of a single coronary cusp from the aortic annulus, most commonly the non-coronary cusp, followed by the right-coronary cusp, and lastly, the left-coronary cusp.[11] Acute and catastrophic aortic regurgitation is the most common consequence. However, some patients develop post-traumatic aortic regurgitation which progresses slowly. Since aortic valve rupture resulting from chest trauma is often complicated with various aortic injuries, careful examination of the aorta is essential.

Mitral valve trauma most commonly involves papillary muscle rupture, which may be partial (involving one or more apical heads) or complete, chordal rupture, or more rarely laceration or perforation of the mitral valve leaflets themselves.[12,13] Traumatic papillary muscle rupture usually causes acute, severe mitral regurgitation. The timing of rupture may be immediate, secondary to compression of a full ventricle, or late, with papillary muscle contusion followed by inflammation and necrosis. When papillary muscle rupture is complete, and especially when it involves the anterolateral papillary muscle, the clinical picture is almost always hyper-acute with clinically important hemodynamic collapse, often necessitating emergency cardiac surgery.

Tricuspid valve trauma usually involves chordal rupture, anterior papillary muscle rupture, and less commonly a leaflet tear or avulsion, primarily anterior leaflet (Figure 16.3) (V16.3A, V16.3B, V16.3C).[11] Due to the compliant nature of the right ventricle, tricuspid regurgitation is often well tolerated hemodynamically, and surgical intervention may be delayed (V16.4A, V16.4B). Consequently, tricuspid valve trauma may go unnoticed until it becoming clinically apparent up to decades later after the trauma event. The pulmonary valve is seldom involved.

CORONARY INJURY OR DISSECTION

Traumatic coronary artery injury has been reported rarely but is arguably underreported due to diagnostic challenges in the setting of polytrauma and concurrent chest wall injuries. The underlying pathology thought to lead to traumatic coronary artery dissection is different from the mechanisms of spontaneous coronary artery dissection. BCT with rapid deceleration and shearing force applied to the coronary arteries causes tearing of the vascular intima, with consequent intraluminal thrombosis and obstruction, vascular rupture, embolism to the contrary arteries, and coronary spasm at the site of the injury. The resultant clinical course manifests as an acute coronary syndrome, with potential malignant ventricular arrhythmias, and even sudden cardiac death.[14] BCT may also cause myocardial infarction by rupturing pre-existing atherosclerotic coronary plaques.[15] The left anterior descending artery (LAD) is more commonly affected than the right coronary and circumflex arteries due to its proximity to the chest wall.[16] Vigorous cardiopulmonary resuscitation is also often associated with bony injury to the sternum and/or ribs. Myocardial contusion or traumatic laceration of pericardial or cardiac structures may ensue (Figure 16.4) (V16.12).

Echocardiography may offer important clues to these possibilities by identifying *regional wall motion* abnormalities of the left ventricle with or without right ventricular dysfunction.[17] Such findings may guide the treating team toward invasive coronary angiography as a matter of urgency.

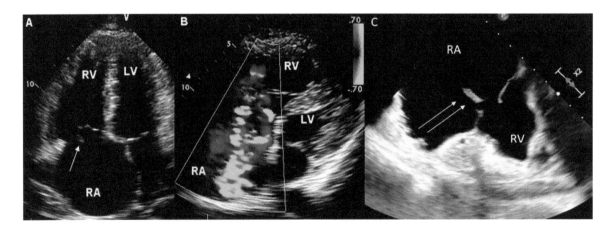

FIGURE 16.3 (A) Blunt anterior chest trauma causing rupture and flail of the anterior tricuspid valve leaflet (arrow) (V16.3A). (B) Severe tricuspid regurgitation with hugely dilated volume-overloaded right heart chambers (V16.3B). (C) TEE images of ruptured chords with a muscle fragment (arrows) (V16.3C). LA: left atrium; LV: left ventricle; RA: right atrium; RV: right ventricle.

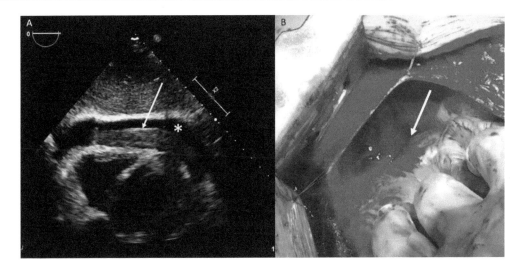

FIGURE 16.4 A 44-year-old female received cardiopulmonary resuscitation (CPR) by paramedics following a syncopal episode. She suffered a fall 3 days prior, injuring her left ribs. CT chest demonstrated left fractured ribs with a large flail segment, a hemothorax, and a pericardial effusion. Following initial pericardiocentesis of 300 mL of frank blood, subcostal echocardiographic view (V16.12) revealed a persistent large pericardial effusion (*) and a large pericardial hematoma (arrow) (A). Urgent median sternotomy revealed two punctures in the lateral pericardium and a lacerated bleeding left circumflex coronary artery (arrow), presumed secondary to rib fractures (B). The circumflex vessel was oversewn, the pericardial hematoma was evacuated, and two liters of blood was removed from the left pleural cavity.

GREAT VESSEL TRAUMA

Traumatic injury to great vessels is a common cause of sudden cardiac death after BCT. In particular, the *thoracic aorta* is most commonly injured by either narrow impact (e.g., a horse kick) or wide impact (e.g., acceleration/deceleration injury) blunt trauma. The most common causes of deceleration injuries are motor vehicle accidents and falls from a great height (>3–4.5 meters).[18] Acceleration injuries caused by pedestrians and cyclists impacting with motor vehicles are less common but well recognized.[19] Explosions may cause aortic injury by acceleration or deceleration.[20] These sudden and dramatic changes in velocity result in differential movement between adjacent thoracic structures, causing shearing-type injuries. Complete, full-thickness aortic injury typically results in immediate exsanguination. For the small subgroup of survivors, they almost invariably have an incomplete aortic injury with intact adventitia or periadvential tissues,[21] and salvage is frequently possible if aortic rupture is identified and treated early.

Anatomy and injury mechanisms

Blunt aortic trauma can occur along the entire length of the aorta, from the aortic root to the iliac bifurcation; however, the isthmus segment of the proximal descending aorta, just distal to the left subclavian artery and proximal to the third intercostal artery, is the most common aortic site of injury.

There are multiple anatomic and mechanistic reasons to account for the aortic isthmus injury. The aortic isthmus is a transition zone from the unfixed, mobile aortic arch to the fixed descending aorta, where the arch is "held down" by its attachment to the left pulmonary artery via the ligamentum arteriosum. In rapid horizontal deceleration trauma, commonly seen in motor vehicle accidents, the isthmus is predisposed to go in opposite vectors, causing torsion and traction forces, and can lead to a tear in the intima. It is also thought that weaker tensile strength exists in the tissue of the aortic isthmus, making it intrinsically more vulnerable to injury.[22] During a sudden deceleration, the aortic rupture can occur due to direct compression of the vessel from the anterior chest's fixed osseous structures (manubrium, first rib, and/or medial clavicles) and the posterior thoracic spine (the "osseous pinch" effect).[23] Simultaneous occlusion of the aorta and acute intravascular hypertension (the "water hammer" effect) is also thought to result in tears at the isthmus.[24] In rapid vertical deceleration, injuries tend to cause tears at the base of the innominate artery.

Other less common sites of aortic injury include the ascending, the distal descending, and the infrarenal abdominal aorta, however, transection of the aorta at these levels is thought to require massive degree of shearing force, usually fatal at the scene of the impact.

Echocardiographic findings

Because of the potentially lethal and legal consequences of a missed diagnosis, any diagnostic method that is used must be extremely sensitive in detecting injuries to the thoracic aorta and its branches. Moreover, because a false-positive test could lead to an unnecessary thoracotomy in an already-ill patient, the avoidance of false positive results is equally important. Thus, the diagnostic studies together must either confirm or exclude the diagnosis of aortic disruption with an exceptional degree of certainty. There must be *zero tolerance for inaccuracy.*[25]

Deceleration injuries to the aorta can result in a variety of pathological configurations. *Complete rupture or transection* of the aorta (V16.5A, V16.5B) with free intrathoracic bleeding results in rapid demise in 80–90% of cases.[26] Cases of great vessel rupture that reach a hospital and undergo imaging tend to have so-called *contained* rupture (V16.6A, V16.6B), where the bleeding has been walled off by a pseudomembrane. This configuration, like ventricular pseudoaneurysm, has inherent instability and can rupture many years after the original injury (Figure 16.5).[27]

TEE in the hands of experienced operators is an effective means of imaging the aortic arch and descending aorta, and highly sensitive and specific for the detection of aortic injury, with reported sensitivity and specificity of up to 97%.[28,29] At echocardiography, contained rupture of the aorta is best visualized from the high transesophageal views (Figure 16.5). Discontinuity or transection of the aortic arch from the descending aorta can be seen, with torn and mobile ends of the mural flap often visible within the aortic lumen. There is usually perivascular hematoma, with or without to-and-fro flow of liquid blood into a pseudoaneurysm space. In some cases, there can be obstruction to flow across the transection ("pseudocoarctation") with abnormal continuous Doppler flow pattern in proximal descending thoracic aorta and luminal narrowing on echocardiography.[30]

Blunt aortic trauma may also cause intimal tearing, similar to spontaneous dissection or intramural hematoma (Figure 16.6).[31,32] This configuration tends to have more inherent stability with a more benign course. Echocardiographic

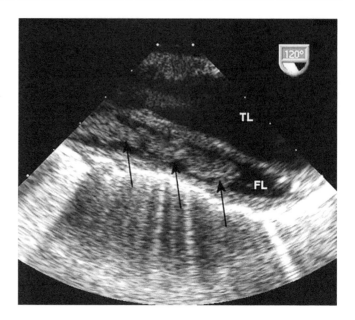

FIGURE 16.6   Traumatic aortic dissection following motor vehicle accident in young adult. Note the formed thrombus (arrows) floating in the false lumen. There was normal flow in the true lumen. FL: false lumen; TL: true lumen.

appearances are similar to those seen in spontaneous dissection (see Chapter 6).

It is extremely important to be aware that the *blind spot* in distal ascending aorta for TEE caused by the trachea and the right main bronchus can be a source of false-negative examinations for aortic trauma. *If the suspicion of aortic trauma is high, particularly if there is mediastinal hematoma, a second imaging modality such as aortography or contrast spiral computed tomographic scanning is indicated.*[33]

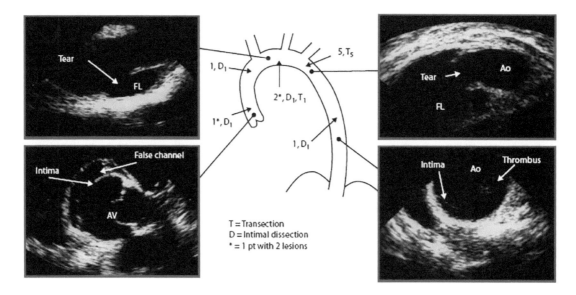

FIGURE 16.5   Clinical experience in a major cardiac trauma referral center with aortic trauma. Aortic transection and dissection are most common in the distal arch, but may be seen in the ascending aorta, mid arch, and descending aorta. Ao: aorta; AV: aortic valve; FL: false lumen.

PENETRATING CARDIAC TRAUMA

Penetrating cardiac trauma (PCT) occurs when the integrity of the heart is violated with laceration of cardiovascular structures in the trajectory of the offending object, most commonly a knife or bullet.

Typical entry sites

Penetrating injuries are especially concerning for PCT when they occur within the area known as the cardiac box (Ziedler area), an anatomic area defined superiorly by the clavicles, laterally by the midclavicular lines and inferiorly by xiphoid process.[34] However, the heart is approachable from any other thoracic site, even through the abdomen, and a cardiac injury should be suspected whenever a thoracic penetrating injury is present. Injuries to the ventral surface of the chest are most common, with consequent damage to the right ventricle.

Types of offending objects

Most PCT patients are young men presenting with stabbing or gunshot wounds. The offending object plays an important role in patient survival. Stabbing PCT with a knife is the most common form of all penetrating injuries and are considered low-velocity PCT, along with other sharp offending objects, such as screwdrivers, ice picks, nail guns, axes, and machetes. In addition to these external objects, injury can also be caused by rib displacement or the compression of sternal fragments into cardiac structures in proximity. Low-velocity PCT via stabbing wounds are not always immediately fatal and tend to only produce limited injury with damage to tissues with which they come direct contact with. Shallow knife wounds may only lacerate the pericardium and not penetrate cardiac chambers. Deeper penetrating injuries, however, will not only enter the pericardium and the cardiac chambers and may also lacerate the interventricular septum and perforate valve tissue. The hemodynamic consequence of a knife injury will therefore depend on the degree of valvular regurgitation, the size of the ventricular septal defect, and the pericardial effusion that may be produced.

Medium-velocity injuries include bullet wound from handguns and air-powered pellet guns and are characterized by less primary tissue damage than PCT caused by high-velocity forces most often observed in military setting, involving high-velocity bullets from machine guns, rifles, grenades, and bombs. The high-velocity mechanism of military weapons causes more extensive damage to tissues in the path of the missile but also to remote organs by radiating shock waves.

Gunshot wounds to the heart are often immediately fatal, with high mortality rates of up to 96%.[1,35] This is due to bullets having deeper penetration, thus affecting more structures with direct perforating injuries and remote massive tissue destruction. It is essential that where a bullet entry site is located, exit site damage must be located and assessed. Bullet embolization should be suspected in patients with lack of exit wound. Artifacts from bullet fragments can obscure the pathway or exact positioning of the bullet on computed tomographic angiography, and echocardiography can play a key role in precisely locating retained bullet fragments within the heart, and for characterizing associated cardiac and vascular injury before and during surgical extraction.[36,37] Typically, most patients with venous bullet emboli are asymptomatic with the shrapnel migrating to the right heart, most commonly entrapped in tricuspid valve subvalvular apparatus and can be treated conservatively. Some venous bullet emboli will migrate to the pulmonary arterial tree and have the potential to cause pulmonary infarction or abscess. If the patient becomes symptomatic, or a missile is free or partially protruding into a left cardiac chamber it should managed with emergent removal, as the embolization of the object to the systemic arterial circulation may have a serious consequence of distal ischemia.

Clinical presentation of penetrating injuries

The two clinical manifestations of PCT are *hemorrhage* and *cardiac tamponade*. Hemorrhage can lead to shock with tachycardia and decreased systolic and mean arterial blood pressure (V16.7A, V16.7B).

The prognosis after a penetrating wound depends upon the nature and extent of the injuries, their rapid identification and assessment, and surgical correction as required. Cardiac decompensation may be difficult to appreciate clinically because of concomitant related injuries such as fractured ribs and pulmonary contusions. FoCUS and TTE may be easily available, but image quality may be challenging due to unfavorable acoustic windows from lung trauma, pneumothorax, and chest wall injuries. Therefore, TEE may be the imaging procedure of choice when former imaging options prove inadequate or inconclusive.[38]

Pericardial trauma and tamponade

The circumferential covering of the pericardium makes it almost impossible to avoid damage in the setting of a PCT. Pericardial injuries may result in the collection of pericardial fluid, slowly or rapidly, with subsequent tamponade, because the outer, parietal pericardial layer is fibrous and rigid and unable to accommodate sudden fluid accumulation.

Echocardiographic features of cardiac tamponade include right ventricular collapse during diastole and ventricular dyssynchrony related to pericardial constraint and ventricular interdependence. Fluctuating filling of the ventricles related to respiration suggest tamponade physiology with hemodynamic compromise (see Chapter 8).

There are *three important considerations* when examining for cardiac tamponade related to trauma. First, patients may initially be stable after trauma. Slow bleeding (often from pericardial laceration) or post-traumatic pericarditis may lead to tamponade developing late. It may therefore be necessary to repeat the echocardiogram over a number of hours, days, even weeks.[39] Second, pericardial hematomas after trauma may be loculated and localized (as is often the case after cardiac surgery), causing isolated compression of a single chamber, such as the right atrium (Figure 16.7) (V16.8A, V16.8B). Finally, pericardial wounds that open into the pleura may be associated with free bleeding into the pleural space. Such patients will experience signs and symptoms of hemothorax and loss of circulating blood volume with profound shock.

The management of PCT generally consists of immediate thoracotomy for resuscitation in the emergency room with subsequent definitive repair of cardiac injury in the operating room. While arrangements are being made for surgery, the blood volume should be expanded and pericardiocentesis may be performed, to provide time for resuscitation and surgical preparation. Echocardiographic-guided pericardiocentesis (see Chapter 8) minimizes the risks of pneumothorax and cardiac wall puncture by providing direct visualization of the fluid-filled space for assessment of size and distribution of the effusion, to select the proper entry site and needle trajectory for aspiration, and also to monitor the procedure.[40] Prompt confirmation that the needle tip is in fact positioned within the pericardial sac (not within the heart) is available by performing contrast echocardiography with injection of agitated saline contrast solution (V8.14 and V8.15).

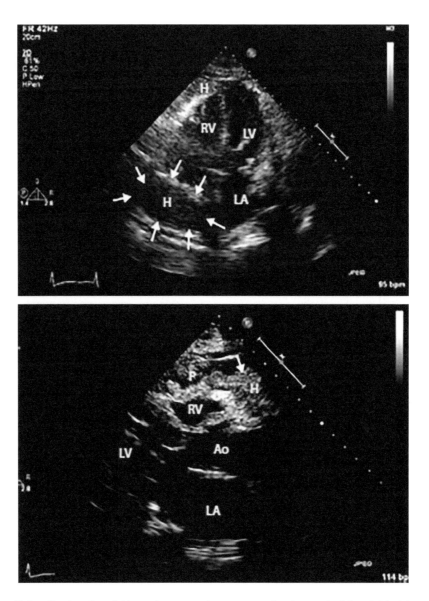

FIGURE 16.7   (A) Traumatic localized pericardial hematoma causing compression (arrows) of the right atrium (V16.8A). (B) Pericardial effusion and hematoma over the right ventricle are also present (V16.8B). Note small underfilled left ventricle. The patient presented in shock. Ao: aorta; LA: left atrium; LV: left ventricle; RV: right ventricle; P: pericardial effusion; H: hematoma.

Ventricular trauma

Most confrontations are fought head on, and as a result the free wall of the right ventricle is the most frequently wounded chamber. Myocardial laceration and perforations can occur, weakening the wall of the ventricle and contributing to the formation of ventricular aneurysms and ventricular arrhythmias. The presence of a left ventricular aneurysm following PCT is considered an indication for surgical intervention due to the risk of rupture.[41] Ventricular aneurysm formation also may cause blood flow stagnation with mural thrombus formation, which may be detectable by echocardiography. Imaging the apex of the left ventricle from the conventional echocardiographic windows does not always allow full appreciation of apical thrombus. By moving the ultrasound transducer one intercostal space higher than is used for the standard apical four-chamber window, and with steep inferior angulation, all four segments of the left ventricular apex can be well visualized in the so-called apical short-axis view.

Injury to the epicardium, myocardium, and endocardium may cause coronary artery injury and thrombosis with myocardial infarction.[42] Complications of penetrating injuries to the coronary arteries and myocardium are not always immediate. Premorbid ventricular function before trauma will influence the degree of hemodynamic compromise related to injury. Hemorrhage into a papillary muscle may cause late necrosis and delayed rupture, again highlighting the importance of careful patient monitoring after PCT.

Salvage rates are lower in patients with penetrating wounds involving thin-walled structures, such as the atria or the pulmonary artery (43% and 67%, respectively), as they rarely seal off spontaneously. Ventricular perforations are associated with higher survival rates, with the contractile properties of the ventricular wall acting to seal the perforation.[43]

Ventricular septal defect

Ventricular septal defects (VSD) occur in 1–5% of cases in PCT. Communication between the left and right ventricles is best detected using color Doppler imaging. Identifying the site and size of an acquired VSD will aid the surgical team in their approach. PCI causing a VSD usually will have an entry track through the right ventricular free wall which should be carefully examined during imaging to inspect for free-wall involvement. Due to the muscular properties of most of the ventricular septum, small acquired ventricular septal defects often seal off spontaneously,[44] however, close monitoring is essential. A traumatic VSD that disrupts the ventricular septum and atrioventricular junction can cause destabilization of the ventricular wall, and lead to full atrioventricular separation.[45] In contrast to congenital muscular VSDs, which are often obscured by ventricular trabeculae, acquired VSDs are usually readily visualized due to the fibrous rim and transected overlying trabeculae. Hemodynamically significant VSDs frequently present with coexistent injuries to the valvular and subvalvular apparatus and therefore should be carefully excluded[46] (Figures 16.8 and 16.9) (V16.13A, V16.13B).

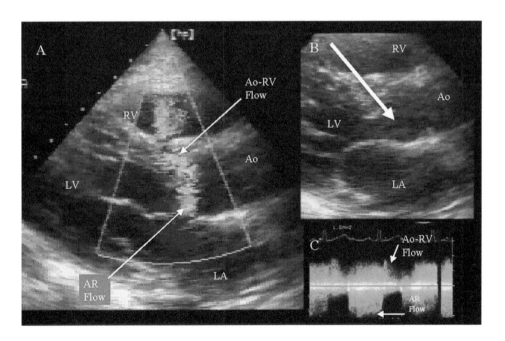

FIGURE 16.8   Knife stabbing injury. The entry wound through the right ventricle was closed urgently in the emergency room. A continuous machinery murmur was noted. Panel A shows jets of blood from aorta to right ventricle and aortic regurgitation. Panel B clearly demonstrates the knife track (white arrow) through the base of the ventricular septum, through the right coronary cusp of the aortic valve and into the aortic root. Panel C demonstrates continuous Ao-RV continuous-wave Doppler flow above the baseline and diastolic aortic regurgitation flow below the baseline. Ao: aorta, AR: aortic regurgitation; LA: left atrium; LV: left ventricle; RV: right ventricle.

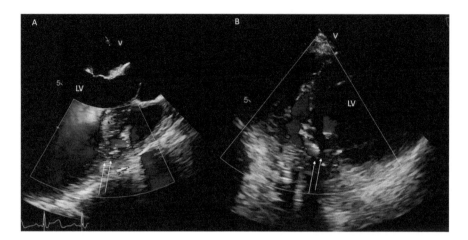

FIGURE 16.9 A 25-year-old male brought to the emergency room with a penetrating right parasternal chest wound. A midline sternotomy was performed, and the right ventricular free-wall perforation defect was repaired with a pledget, lacerated left anterior descending coronary artery was oversewn, and 2 liters of blood was evacuated from pericardium. Subsequent TEE demonstrated apico-septal VSD (white arrows indicates VSD flow) (V16.13A, V16.13B) and regional wall motion abnormalities, including dyskinetic mid to apical septum/anterior LV walls. It was deemed that the LAD infarct with anterior RWMA caused an ischemic ventricular septal defect not suitable for repair due to the friable myocardium. LV: left ventricle.

Valve trauma

Penetrating injuries to the heart are frequently complicated by valve leaflet perforation and laceration. Typically, valvular function (stenosis and regurgitation) is assessed using two-dimensional, color Doppler, and pulsed-wave and continuous-wave Doppler echocardiography. Mechanical complications such as papillary muscle laceration, transection of chordae and perforation of valvular leaflets can usually be imaged by two-dimensional echocardiography.

Valvular dysfunction can present with regurgitation, ranging from mild to severe.[47] Acute severe regurgitation of the atrioventricular valves will usually occur in the setting of a near normal-sized atrium (left atrial area ≤20cm², M-mode dimension ≤40 mm). The consequent rapid increase in volume loading of a small, non-compliant chamber can lead to abrupt, massive increases in filling pressure with secondary pulmonary edema and/or systemic congestion. This contrasts with the clinical setting of chronic valvular regurgitation, where the atria enlarge over time and filling pressures are only mildly elevated. Pre-existing valvular disease is not always known prior to injury, and it may therefore not always be possible to fully appreciate a cause-and-effect relationship between trauma and observed valve dysfunction. However, pre-existing valve disease will increase the risk of developing significant valvular pathology post-trauma (blunt and penetrating).[48]

PCT may cause minimal valvular regurgitation in the initial phase, which may over time develop into a significant regurgitant lesion requiring surgical intervention.[47] If clinically indicated, repeat transthoracic echocardiograms are useful in assessing the progression of valvular dysfunction following PCT. Echocardiographic calculations of regurgitant volumes and regurgitant fractions will aid in the quantitation of a progressive valvular lesion.

Great arteries

Penetrating injury to the great vessels should be suspected in any patient in whom a projectile traverses the mediastinum.[49] Presenting signs and symptoms of injury to the great vessels will depend on the size and site of the injury. The pericardium envelopes approximately 3–5 cm of the proximal ascending aorta and pulmonary artery as they spiral superiorly from the base of the heart. Damage to the great vessels in this area may cause communication between the artery and the pericardial space, frequently resulting in cardiac tamponade.

As mentioned, TEE is a valuable imaging option in the unstable polytrauma patient, however, should be performed by *highly experienced operator*. Penetrating wounds of the great vessels may result in the formation of a *pseudoaneurysm* with the possibility of subsequent rupture (Figure 16.10) (V16.9A, V16.9B). Echocardiographic features of pseudoaneurysm include the identification of a tear in the intima layer of the vessel and subsequent tearing along the length of the vessel until it comes to the origin of a communicating vessel. Rarely, aorto-cameral[50] or aorto-pulmonary communications[51] (fistulas) may complicate a penetrating injury to these vessels with possible resultant congestive cardiac failure.

IATROGENIC INJURIES

With the rapid development and evolution of both diagnostic and therapeutic intracardiac procedures and percutaneously implantable devices over the last few decades, there has been an inevitable increase in the occurrence of iatrogenic cardiac injuries (V16.10, V16.11). The majority of these injuries would be of

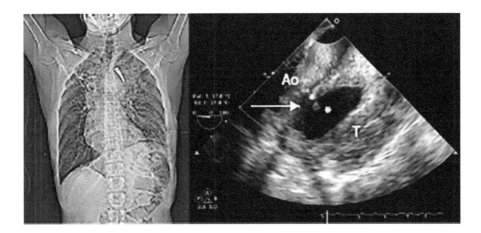

FIGURE 16.10 Aortic pseudoaneurysm caused by stabbing chest injury. A 43-year-old man presented in the emergency department with massive hemoptysis of more than 2 L during previous 24 hours. Hemoptysis had started 3 weeks earlier. He reported a knife-stabbing chest injury that had occurred 18 months earlier (left panel). This high transesophageal echocardiographic view of the aortic arch with color Doppler shows brisk flow in the true aortic lumen (Ao) and minimal flow in the partially thrombosed false lumen (*) (V16.9B). Note a narrow neck (tear of the aortic wall) of the pseudoaneurysm (arrow) (V16.9A). The patient underwent successful emergent surgical reconstruction of the aorta. T: thrombus.

(Images and videos provided by JS.)

a penetrating nature, such as with a guidewire, dilator, sheath, balloon or guiding catheter, pacemaker lead (V8.13), endomyo-cardial biopsy forceps, or excessive ablation energy.[52,53]

Echocardiography clearly will focus initially on the *detection of pericardial fluid*. Indeed, the request for echocardiography as an urgent procedure in the cardiac catheter lab when a patient experiences undue pain or hemodynamic instability is relatively common. The presentation may vary depending on the structure/s involved, the type and size of the device that caused the perforation, the baseline hemodynamic status of the patient, and the level of anticoagulation present. Early detection of pericardial fluid should prompt the operator to discontinue the intervention and, if appropriate, reverse the anticoagulation and/or proceed with pericardiocentesis. The patients are usually supine with their torso draped with sterile towels, and images are typically obtained from the subcostal imaging window.

The other iatrogenic cause of cardiac injury is *cardiopulmonary resuscitation* (CPR). The compressive nature of vigorous manual and mechanical CPR can cause a broad spectrum of cardiovascular injuries from low-velocity BCT to penetrating injuries from sternal or rib fractures caused by CPR.[54] As discussed in Chapter 5, there is a list of entities that needs to be excluded in such patients. It can be challenging to promptly differentiate and recognize cardiac abnormalities which are a consequential complication of CPR from those which were the initial cause of the cardiac arrest.

hospital or undergo imaging investigations. In those who do, echocardiography, particularly by the transesophageal route, offers an effective tool in rapidly and accurately evaluating the status of cardiac injury and providing anatomic and hemodynamic information at the patient's bedside. This early rapid detection and establishment of the patho-anatomy is crucial in allowing the treating team to assess stability and plan possible surgical management. The consequences of delays or errors in diagnosis can be immediate and drastic. *This is an area of echocardiography that should be undertaken by the most experienced operators where possible.* If doubt remains after echocardiography, particularly in situations with suspected trauma to the ascending aorta, there should be no hesitation for recommending supplementary investigations in these critically ill patients.

LIST OF VIDEOS

https://routledgetextbooks.com/textbooks/9781032157009/chapter-16.php

VIDEO 16.1A Traumatic right ventricular injury and pericardial effusion after blunt chest trauma (1/3): A 66-year-old woman was admitted to the hospital in shock after a high-speed motor vehicle

CONCLUSIONS

Thoracic trauma may be associated with potentially rapidly fatal injuries to the heart and great vessels that require prompt recognition and diagnoses. Many patients do not survive to reach accident. She sustained fractured pelvis and ribs. Transthoracic echocardiographic four-chamber view showing dilated poorly contracting right ventricle and hyperdynamic underfilled left ventricle. Note pericardial effusion over the right heart (see also Videos 16.1B and 16.1C). Six months before this presentation, she underwent cardiac investigation for chest pain syndrome, including transthoracic echocardiography, which showed structurally and functionally normal heart, and coronary angiography, which demonstrated normal coronary arteries.

VIDEO 16.1B   Traumatic right ventricular injury and pericardial effusion after blunt chest trauma (2/3): Transthoracic echocardiographic parasternal long-axis view showing a dilated, poorly contracting right ventricle and a hyperdynamic, underfilled left ventricle. Note pericardial effusion over posterior wall and the right ventricle (see also Videos 16.1A and 16.1C).

VIDEO 16.1C   Traumatic right ventricular injury and pericardial effusion after blunt chest trauma (3/3): Transthoracic echocardiographic parasternal short-axis view showing a dilated, poorly contracting right ventricle and a hyperdynamic, underfilled left ventricle in a patient with shock after blunt chest trauma. Note significant amount of pericardial effusion over the right ventricle and inferior wall (see also Videos 16.1A and 16.1B).

VIDEO 16.2A   Right ventricular contusion and pericardial effusion in a multitrauma patient (1/2): This midesophageal transesophageal echocardiographic four-chamber view shows dilated right ventricle with an akinetic distal half. Also, note significant pleural effusion (see also Video 16.2B). *(Video provided by JS.)*

VIDEO 16.2B   Right ventricular contusion and pericardial effusion in a multitrauma patient (2/2): Note venous extracorporeal membrane oxygenation (ECMO) cannula, which was inserted in the right atrium (see also Video 16.2A). *(Video provided by JS.)*

VIDEO 16.3A   Traumatic tricuspid valve injury after blunt chest trauma (1/2): A 25-year-old man presented to the hospital with a fractured sternum after a blow to the chest with a knee during an Australian Football League game. He had an unremarkable past medical history. At the time of his chest trauma, he experienced a syncopal episode. Investigations in the hospital revealed no evidence of myocardial contusion. His electrocardiogram showed sinus rhythm with heart rate of 82 bpm, with incomplete right bundle branch block. Transthoracic echocardiographic four-chamber view showed a rupture and flail of the anterior leaflet of the tricuspid valve (see also Video 16.3C). Color Doppler revealed severe tricuspid regurgitation (see Video 16.3B). Note the dilated, volume-overloaded right heart chambers. He sustained a fractured sternum and an avulsed papillary muscle of the tricuspid valve.

VIDEO 16.3B   Traumatic tricuspid valve injury after blunt chest trauma (2/3): A transthoracic echocardiographic four-chamber view showing severe tricuspid regurgitation by color Doppler caused by rupture and flail of the anterior leaflet of the tricuspid valve after blunt anterior chest trauma (see also Video 16.3A and 16.3C). Note the dilated, volume-overloaded right heart chambers.

VIDEO 16.3C   Traumatic tricuspid valve injury after blunt chest trauma (3/3): Transesophageal echocardiography showing ruptured chords with a muscle fragment (see also Videos 16.3A and 16.3B). Note the dilated, volume-overloaded right heart chambers.

VIDEO 16.4A   Tricuspid valve avulsion after car crash (1/2): Transthoracic echocardiographic four-chamber view showing avulsion and flail of the anterior leaflet of the tricuspid valve after blunt anterior chest trauma in car accident. Note akinesis of distal left ventricular septum and dyskinesis of the apex with thrombus (patient had a history of previous anteroseptal myocardial infarction). Note the bulging of the interatrial septum toward left atrium in systole, resulting from direct impact of regurgitant jet and higher right atrial pressure. Color Doppler reveals severe tricuspid regurgitation (see Video 16.4B).

VIDEO 16.4B   Tricuspid valve avulsion after car crash (2/2): Transthoracic echocardiographic four-chamber view showing severe tricuspid regurgitation by color Doppler caused by avulsion and flail of the anterior leaflet of the tricuspid valve (see also Video 16.4A) after blunt anterior chest trauma in car accident. Note the bulging of the interatrial septum toward left atrium in systole, resulting from direct impact of regurgitant jet and higher right atrial pressure. Note akinesis of distal left ventricular septum and dyskinesis of the apex with thrombus (patient had a history of previous anteroseptal myocardial infarction).

VIDEO 16.5A   Aortic transection (1/2): Transesophageal echocardiography. Pullback of transesophageal probe shows transection of the aorta in a 34-year-old woman after road traffic accident (see also Video 16.5B). *(Video provided by JS.)*

VIDEO 16.5B   Aortic transection (2/2): A large pleural effusion or hematoma can be seen by transesophageal echocardiography in front of the cross-section of the aorta (see also Video 16.5A). *(Video provided by JS.)*

VIDEO 16.6A   Traumatic aortic pseudoaneurysm (1/2): Three-dimensional transesophageal echocardiography (right panel) shows large pseudoaneurysm of the ascending aorta in a 75-year-old woman after a car accident (see also Video 16.6B). The patient received conservative treatment. *(Video provided by GA.)*

VIDEO 16.6B   Traumatic aortic pseudoaneurysm (2/2): Three-dimensional color Doppler transesophageal echocardiography (right panel) shows flow through the communication between the true and false lumina (see also Video 16.6A). *(Video provided by GA.)*

VIDEO 16.7A   Systolic anterior motion (SAM) of the mitral valve in the intensive care unit after trauma associated with hemorrhage (1/2): Left ventricular hypercontractility and SAM indicate the need for fluid administration (see also Video 16.7B). *(Video provided by JS.)*

VIDEO 16.7B   Systolic anterior motion (SAM) of the mitral valve in the intensive care unit after trauma associated with hemorrhage (2/2): Note the turbulence in the left ventricular outflow tract as a result of SAM. Left ventricular hypercontractility and SAM indicate the need for fluid administration (see also Video 16.7A). *(Video provided by JS.)*

VIDEO 16.8A   Traumatic localized pericardial hematoma (1/2): A 57-year-old man admitted to the hospital with progressive dyspnea and significant pitting pedal edema. Before the hospital presentation, the patient had sustained blunt chest trauma via a horse kick injury to the chest 3 weeks before the onset of symptoms. Transthoracic echocardiographic four-chamber view showing localized pericardial hematoma causing compression of the right atrium. Significant pericardial effusion and hematoma over the right ventricle are also present (see also Video 16.8B). Note the small underfilled left ventricle.

VIDEO 16.8B   Traumatic localized pericardial hematoma (2/2): Transthoracic echocardiographic parasternal long-axis view showing pericardial effusion and hematoma over the right ventricle (shown here). Compression of the right atrium with localized hematoma can be seen in four-chamber view (see Video 16.8A). Note the small underfilled left ventricle.

VIDEO 16.9A   Aortic pseudoaneurysm caused by a stabbing chest injury (1/2): A 43-year-old man presented in the emergency department with massive hemoptysis of more than 2 L during previous 24 hours. Hemoptysis had started 3 weeks earlier. He reported a knife stabbing chest injury that had occurred 18 months earlier (see Figure 16.8 in the book). This high transesophageal echocardiographic view of the aortic arch shows perivascular false lumen (pseudoaneurysm) with a narrow neck, partially filled with thrombus (see also Video 16.9B). The patient underwent successful emergent surgical reconstruction of the aorta. *(Video provided by JS.)*

VIDEO 16.9B   Aortic pseudoaneurysm caused by a stabbing chest injury (2/2): This high transesophageal echocardiographic view of the aortic arch with color Doppler view shows brisk flow in the true aortic lumen and minimal flow in the pseudoaneurysm. Note a narrow neck (tear of the aortic wall) of the pseudoaneurysm (see also Video 16.9A). The patient underwent successful emergent surgical reconstruction of the aorta. *(Video provided by JS.)*

VIDEO 16.10   Aortic dissection after coronary angiography: This transesophageal echocardiographic long-axis view of the aortic root shows localized iatrogenic aortic dissection in the right coronary sinus that occurred during diagnostic coronary angiography of the right coronary artery. *(Video provided by JS.)*

VIDEO 16.11   Free-floating Amplatzer atrial septal occluder device in the right ventricular outflow tract: After an unsuccessful attempt to deploy an atrial septal defect closure device, it was detached from the interatrial septum. This transesophageal echocardiographic long-axis view shows the device as an echogenic floating structure in the right ventricular outflow tract.

VIDEO 16.12   Cardiac tamponade after vigorous cardiopulmonary resuscitation and rib fracture. Subcostal view showing large pericardial effusion and a large pericardial hematoma. See also Figure 16.4 in the book.

VIDEO 16.13A   Ventricular septal rupture after penetrating cardiac injury (1/2): In a 25-year-old with a penetrating right parasternal chest wound TEE with color Doppler demonstrated turbulent flow through ventricular septal rupture (see also Video 16.13B). See also Figure 16.9 in the book.

VIDEO 16.13B   Ventricular septal rupture after penetrating cardiac injury (2/2): In a 25-year-old with a penetrating right parasternal chest wound TEE with color Doppler demonstrated turbulent flow through apico-septal ventricular septal rupture (see also Video 16.13A). See also Figure 16.9 in the book.

REFERENCES

1. Restrepo CS, Gutierrez FR, Marmol-Velez JA, Ocazionez D, Martinez-Jimenez S. Imaging patients with cardiac trauma. RadioGraphics. 2012;32(3):633–49.
2. Labovitz AJ, Noble VE, Bierig M, Goldstein SA, Jones R, Kort S, et al. Focused cardiac ultrasound in the emergent setting: a consensus statement of the American Society of Echocardiography and American College of Emergency Physicians. J Am Soc Echocardiogr. 2010;23(12):1225–30.
3. Plummer D, Brunette D, Asinger R, Ruiz E. Emergency department echocardiography improves outcome in penetrating cardiac injury. Ann Emerg Med. 1992;21(6):709–12.
4. Teixeira PG, Inaba K, Oncel D, Dubose J, Chan LS, Rhee P, et al. Blunt cardiac rupture: a 5-year NTDB analysis. J Trauma. 2009;67(4):788–91.
5. Zissimopoulos I, Tsoukas A, Koliandris I, Christakos S. Traumatic aortic transection. Echocardiography. 2005;22(1):35–8.
6. Kaye P, O'Sullivan I. Myocardial contusion: emergency investigation and diagnosis. Emerg Med J. 2002;2002(19):8–10.
7. Sybrandy KC, Cramer MJ, Burgersdijk C. Diagnosing cardiac contusion: old wisdom and new insights. Heart. 2003;89(5):485–9.
8. Bansal MK, Maraj S, Chewaproug D, Amanullah A. Myocardial contusion injury: redefining the diagnostic algorithm. Emerg Med J. 2005;22(7):465–9.
9. Moen J, Hansen W, Chandrasekaran K, Seward JB. Traumatic aneurysm and pseudoaneurysm of the right ventricle: a diagnosis by echocardiography. J Am Soc Echocardiogr. 2002;15(9):1025–6.
10. Maraqa T, Mohamed ATM, Wilson KL, Perinjelil V, Sachwani-Daswani GR, Mercer L. Isolated right atrial rupture from blunt trauma: a case report with systematic review of a lethal injury. J Cardiothor Surg. 2019;14(28).
11. Gelves J, Vasquez-Rodriguez JF, Medina HM, Marquez D, Jaimes C, Salazar G, et al. Severe aortic and tricuspid valve regurgitation after blunt chest trauma: an unusual presentation. CASE Cardiovasc Imaging Case Rep. 2020;4(4):230–5.
12. Goodman R, Mohananey D, Garster N, Gaglianello N. Incidental finding of traumatic papillary muscle rupture on intraoperative transesophageal echocardiogram following a motor vehicle accident. CASE (Phila). 2021;6(1):21–3.
13. Shaikh N, Ummunissa F, Abdel Sattar M. Traumatic mitral valve and pericardial injury. Case Rep Crit Care. 2013;2013:3.
14. Pandey Y, Owen B, Birnbaum G, Tabbaa R, Hamzeh I, Lakkis N, et al. Multivessel traumatic coronary artery dissection after a motor vehicle accident with successful percutaneous coronary intervention. JACC Case Rep. 2020;2(15):2295–8.
15. Lobay KW, MacGougan CK. Traumatic coronary artery dissection: a case report and literature review. J Emerg Med. 2012;43(4):e239–43.
16. Kurklu HA, Tan TS. Blast injury. JACC Case Rep. 2021;3(18):1898–902.

17. Sun L, Li Z-A, Zhao Y, Han J, Henein MY. Left anterior descending artery occlusion secondary to blunt chest trauma diagnosed by comprehensive echocardiography and coronary angiography. J Clin Ultrasound. 2012;40(6):370–4.

18. Okada M, Kamesaki M, Mikami M, Okura Y, Yamakawa J, Sugiyama K, et al. Evaluation of the outcome of traumatic thoracic aortic rupture in patients in a Trauma and Critical Care Center. Ann Vasc Dis. 2013;6(1):33–8.

19. Peterson BG, Matsumura JS, Morasch MD, West MA, Eskandari MK. Percutaneous endovascular repair of blunt thoracic aortic transection. J Trauma. 2005;59(5):1062–5.

20. Hunt JP, Baker CC, Lentz CW, Rutledge RR, Oller DW, Flowe KM, et al. Thoracic aortic injuries: management and outcome of 144 patients. J Trauma. 1996;40(4):547–55.

21. Benjamin MM, Roberts WC. Fatal aortic rupture from nonpenetrating chest trauma. Proc (Bayl Univ Med Cent). 2012;25(2):121–3.

22. Mouawad NJ, Paulisin J, Hofmeister S, Thomas MB. Blunt thoracic aortic injury—concepts and management. J Cardiothorac Surg. 2020;15.

23. Baqué P, Serre T, Cheynel N, Arnoux PJ, Thollon L, Behr M, et al. An experimental cadaveric study for a better understanding of blunt traumatic aortic rupture. J Trauma. 2006;61(3):586–91.

24. Karmy-Jones R, Jackson N, Long W, Simeone A. Current management of traumatic rupture of the descending thoracic aorta. Curr Cardiol Rev. 2009;5(3):187–95.

25. Vlahakes GJ, Warren RL. Traumatic rupture of the aorta. N Engl J Med. 1995;332(6):389–90.

26. McPherson SJ. Thoracic aortic and great vessel trauma and its management. Sem Interv Radiol. 2007;24(2):180–96.

27. Nzewi O, Slight RD, Zamvar V. Management of blunt thoracic aortic injury. Eur J Vasc Endovasc Surg. 2006;31(1):18–27.

28. Shiga T, Wajima Zi, Apfel CC, Inoue T, Ohe Y. Diagnostic accuracy of transesophageal echocardiography, helical computed tomography, and magnetic resonance imaging for suspected thoracic aortic dissection: systematic review and meta-analysis. Arch Intern Med. 2006;166(13):1350–6.

29. Smith MD, Cassidy JM, Souther S, Morris EJ, Sapin PM, Johnson SB, et al. Transesophageal echocardiography in the diagnosis of traumatic rupture of the aorta. N Engla J Med. 1995;332(6):356–62.

30. Shafaghi S, Behzadnia N, Sharif-Kashani B, Naghashzadeh F, Ahmadi ZH. Traumatic transection of descending thoracic aorta presenting as pseudo-coarctation. Tanaffos. 2018;17(4):295–8.

31. Vignon P, Gueret P, Vedrinne JM, Lagrange P, Cornu E, Abrieu O, et al. Role of transesophageal echocardiography in the diagnosis and management of traumatic aortic disruption. Circulation. 1995;92(10):2959–68.

32. Roisinblit JM, Allende NG, Neira JA, Torino AF, Karmazyn C, Pardo P, et al. Local thrombus as an isolated sign of traumatic aortic injury. Echocardiography. 2002;19(1):63–5.

33. Vignon P, Rambaud G, Francois B, Preux PM, Lang RM, Gastinne H. Quantification of traumatic hemomediastinum using transesophageal echocardiography: impact on patient management. Chest. 1998;113(6):1475–80.

34. Miglioranza MH, Proença Tavares Crespo AR. Focused ultrasound: a masterpiece in the puzzle of chest trauma evaluation. JACC Case Rep. 2020;2(4):565–7.

35. Okoye OT, Talving P, Teixeira PG, Chervonski M, Smith JA, Inaba K, et al. Transmediastinal gunshot wounds in a mature trauma centre: changing perspectives. Injury. 2013;44(9):1198–203.

36. Fry SJ, Picard MH, Tseng JF, Briggs SM, Isselbacher EM. The echocardiographic diagnosis, characterization, and extraction guidance of cardiac foreign bodies. J Am Soc Echocardiogr. 2000;13(3):232–9.

37. Yoon B, Grasso S, Hofmann LJ. Management of bullet emboli to the heart and great vessels. Mil Med. 2018;183(9–10):e307–e13.

38. Rywik T, Sitkowski W, Cichocki J, Rajecka A, Suwalski K. Acute mitral regurgitation caused by penetrating chest injury. J Heart Valve Dis. 1995;4(3):293–5.

39. Rendón F, Danés LHG, Castro M. Delayed cardiac tamponade after penetrating thoracic trauma. Asian Cardiovasc Thorac Ann. 2004;12(2):139–42.

40. Gumrukcuoglu HA, Odabasi D, Akdag S, Ekim H. Management of cardiac tamponade: a comperative study between echo-guided pericardiocentesis and surgery; a report of 100 patients. Cardiol Res Pract. 2011;2011.

41. Patanè F, Sansone F, Centofanti P, Rinaldi M. Left ventricular pseudoaneurysm after pericardiocentesis. Interact Cardiovasc Thorac Surg. 2008;7(6):1112–3.

42. Kumar S, Moorthy N, Kapoor A, Sinha N. Gunshot wounds causing myocardial infarction, delayed ventricular septal defect, and congestive heart failure. Texas Heart Inst J. 2012;39(1):129–32.

43. Wilson WR, Coyne JT, Greer GE. Mitral regurgitation as a late sequela of penetrating cardiac trauma. J Heart Valve Dis. 1997;6(2):171–3.

44. Dehghani P, Ibrahim R, Collins N, Latter D, Cheema AN, Chisholm RJ. Post-traumatic ventricular septal defects—review of the literature and a novel technique for percutaneous closure. J Invasive Cardiol. 2009;21(9):483–7.

45. Han FY, Reyes KG, Bleiweis MS. Managing extensive mitral valve and ventricular septal injuries secondary to penetrating trauma. Eur J Cardiothorac Surg. 2017;53(1):284–5.

46. Reddy D, Muckart DJJ. Holes in the heart: an atlas of intracardiac injuries following penetrating trauma. Interact Cardiovasc Thorac Surg. 2014;19(1):56–63.

47. Esfahanizadeh J, Abbasi Tashnizi M, Moeinipour AA, Sepehri Shamloo A. Undetected aorto-RV fistula with aortic valve injury and delayed cardiac tamponade following a chest stab wound: a case report. Trauma Mon. 2013;18(2):95–7.

48. Parmley LF, Manion WC, Mattingly TW. Nonpenetrating traumatic injury of the heart. Circulation. 1958;18(3):371–96.

49. O'Connor JV, Scalea TM. Penetrating thoracic great vessel injury: impact of admission hemodynamics and preoperative imaging. J Trauma. 2010;68(4):834–7.

50. Theron JP, Du Theron H, Long M, Marx JD. Late presentation of aorto-right ventricular fistula and associated aortic regurgitation following penetrating chest trauma. Cardiovasc J Africa. 2009;20(6):357–9.

51. Meel R, Govindasamy T, Gonçalves R. Traumatic aorto-pulmonary artery fistula: a case report. Eur Heart J Case Rep. 2019;3(3):ytz120.

52. Holmes Jr DR, Nishimura R, Fountain R, Turi ZG. Iatrogenic pericardial effusion and tamponade in the percutaneous intracardiac intervention era. JACC Cardiovasc Interv. 2009;2(8):705–17.

53. Alkhouli M, Rihal CS, Holmes DR. Transseptal techniques for emerging structural heart interventions. JACC Cardiovasc Interv. 2016;9(27):2465–80.

54. Miller AC, Rosati SF, Suffredini AF, Schrumpt DS. A systematic review and pooled analysis of CPR-associated cardiovascular and thoracic injuries. Resuscitation. 2014;85(6):724–31.

Stress echocardiography in the emergency department

17

Quirino Ciampi, George Athanassopoulos, and Eugenio Picano

Key Points

- In patients with chest pain, a resting, limited echocardiographic examination (even with a handheld imaging device) may provide invaluable information: a recent-onset regional wall motion abnormality of ischemic origin is frequently obvious when electrocardiographic changes are absent and cardiac enzymes (including high-sensitivity troponin) are not yet abnormal.
- The resting echocardiogram can document or raise suspicion of important nonischemic causes of chest pain, including pericardial effusion, pulmonary embolism, and acute aortic dissection.
- When resting echocardiography, electrocardiogram, and serial enzyme assay findings are negative and myocardial infarction has been ruled out, stress echo can be performed in patients with intermediate (30–60%) pretest probability, even at bedside, for risk stratification. If it is positive, hospital admission (in view of ischemia-driven angiography and revascularization in the presence of more extensive ischemia) is warranted. If it is negative with a comprehensive protocol (ideally including assessment of heart rate reserve and coronary flow velocity reserve), the patient can be safely discharged with very low probability of adverse outcome in the short- to medium-term follow-up.
- Acutely symptomatic patients should never be tested in the ED setting.

Approximately six million people annually undergo evaluation in the emergency department (ED) for acute chest pain, at a cost of several billion dollars in the United States.[1] Most of these patients are admitted to the hospital, and their average length of stay is 1.9 days. Nearly half of hospitalized patients with unstable angina eventually receive a noncardiac-related diagnosis[2]—most frequently panic attack,[3] gastroesophageal reflux, or musculoskeletal causes.[2]

The low-risk patients neither require nor benefit from management in a coronary care unit (CCU). In addition, unnecessary admission to a CCU is inordinately costly, over $2,000 per day, and it also reduces the availability of vital CCU beds. Finally, unnecessary CCU admission imposes both undue stress and potential morbidity. Although this low threshold for CCU admission results in a high ratio (4:1 to 5:1) of patients with nonischemic causes of chest pain to the number admitted with an ischemic event, 5% of patients with myocardial infarction are inappropriately discharged from the ED.[4]

In the United States, an estimated 25% of lawsuits concerning emergency care involve errors in the diagnosis of myocardial infarction.[5] In response to this need for improved emergency care, chest pain centers have been established, in which patients are monitored and observed for 24 hours. This observation protocol usually incorporates selective history, physical examination, and electrocardiographic variables, with the concomitant use of serum markers of myocardial cell death (usually

DOI: 10.1201/9781003245407-17

troponins). This primary risk stratification has limitations. Clinical variables have a low specificity, the electrocardiogram (ECG) has a high diagnostic accuracy in myocardial infarction but a low accuracy in unstable angina, and biochemical markers of cardiac damage are relatively late findings.[1,2] In this setting, the incremental value of imaging and stress-test techniques has been documented,[6–9] although the dramatic increase in resource use and intensity of cardiac imaging application does not seem to be matched by increased quality of care.[10]

RESTING ECHOCARDIOGRAPHY IN THE EMERGENCY DEPARTMENT

Transthoracic echocardiography (TTE) has universally recognized advantages over other imaging techniques: lower cost, use of nonionizing radiation, widespread availability, short imaging time, and online interpretation. These advantages are especially important in the ED setting, which is characterized by logistic restrictions and time constraints. TTE has several critical advantages in chest pain patients; identification of *resting wall motion abnormalities* is more sensitive in detecting acute myocardial infarction than the initial ECG. Echocardiography is readily accessible, portable, safe, radiation-free, and less expensive than myocardial perfusion imaging (MPI) and coronary multislice computed tomography (MSCT), and allows assessment of many non-ischemic causes of chest pain, including aortic dissection, hypertrophic cardiomyopathy, pulmonary embolism, and pericardial effusion.[6] Detection of reversible wall motion abnormality, occurring during chest pain attack and disappearing after cessation of chest pain spontaneously or after nitroglycerin administration, almost always suggests the presence of significant coronary artery disease (V17.1A, V17.1B). Moreover, the incremental diagnostic value of two-dimensional (2D) echo is additive to clinical parameters, ECG, and biochemical markers.[11–15] However, there are limitations to the 2D echo approach in the recognition of myocardial infarction. The sensitivity is higher in acute myocardial infarction but lower in unstable angina and non-Q-wave myocardial infarction. In addition, the technique is operator- and reader-dependent, and a poor acoustic window precludes diagnostic information in at least 10% of patients.[7] This percentage of uninterpretable studies can be further reduced with contrast echocardiography used for endocardial border recognition, recommended when two or more segments are unreadable.[7]

Early use of echocardiography is recommended by the current European Society of Cardiology (ESC) guidelines on acute coronary syndromes (ACSs).[9] Moreover, in patients who have still-undetermined chest pain, negative serial ECGs, negative serial enzymes, and even high sensitive (hs)-cTn and

negative baseline echocardiogram and who are free from chest pain for several hours, stress echocardiography may be an excellent option, especially in cases in which exercise ECG is unfeasible, uninterpretable, or submaximal.

STRESS ECHOCARDIOGRAPHY IN THE EMERGENCY DEPARTMENT

In the ED, baseline resting 2D echocardiography is indispensable, and both echocardiographic equipment and expertise must be available at the bedside. This means that when the resting echo is negative, the stress echo is already there at the bedside, with the 2D echo machine and the cardiologist who is able to interpret the regional wall motion in real time and ready to go with the stress echo. Certainly, at that point the stress chosen may be exercise (V17.2A, V17.2B, V17.2C), but the treadmill introduces additional noise and space requirements into the ED.[8] Pharmacologic stress echo with dobutamine or vasodilators is a more logistically convenient choice, because intravenous access has been previously established on arrival at the ED. The patient lies in a bed in the position most suitable for echo imaging, and the 2D echo instrument is already at the bedside (for the resting echocardiogram, the negativity of which is a logical prerequisite for further stress testing).

Stress echocardiography has been performed in the ED with several forms of testing,[16–29] including exercise,[17,20,24] dobutamine,[16,18,21,23,26–29] and dipyridamole.[19,22] Studies invariably show the very high feasibility of stress echo, higher with pharmacologic means than with exercise, with an excellent safety profile, better with dipyridamole than with dobutamine, and with very high negative predictive value of stress-echo results, further increased when wall motion negativity is coupled with perfusion negativity on myocardial contrast echocardiography (MCE)[26] (Table 17.1). One study reported the similar prognostic accuracy of stress echo and stress single-photon emission computed tomography (SPECT) scintigraphy simultaneously performed in the same patient.[23] It is important to note that the rate of positivity in the screened population varied considerably, from 3% to 45%. When the selection criterion is "any form of chest pain," typical or atypical, a very low positivity rate may be expected. If only patients with intermediate clinical risk are screened, the rate of positivity may be substantially higher.[20]

The high and low clinical scores may be identified based on chest pain characteristics: location, radiation, character, and associated symptoms.[23] The high-risk category corresponds to substernal chest pain with radiation (arm, shoulder, back, neck, or lower jaw), with a sensation of crushing, pressing, or heaviness, with associated dyspnea and nausea, or with a history of angina. At the opposite end of the clinical spectrum, a very low clinical score corresponds to a pain with apex location without radiation, with

TABLE 17.1   Prognostic Value of Stress Echo in Patients Presenting with Chest Pain to the Emergency Room

AUTHOR, YEAR	REFERENCE	STRESS OF CHOICE	NUMBER OF PATIENTS	MEAN FOLLOW-UP (MONTHS)	NEGATIVE PREDICTIVE VALUE (%)	RATE OF POSITIVITY
Trippi et al., 1997	16	Dobutamine	139	3	98.5	8/139 (6%)
Colon et al., 1998	17	Exercise	108	12.8	99	8/108 (7%)
Gelejinse et al., 2000	18	Dobutamine	80	6	95	36/80 (45%)
Orlandini et al., 2000	19	Dipyridamole	177	6	99	5/177 (3%)
Buchsbaum et al., 2001	20	Exercise	145	6	99.3	5/145 (3%)
Bholasingh et al., 2003	21	Dobutamine	377	6	96	26/377 (7%)
Bedetti et al., 2005	22	Dipyridamole	552	13±2	98.8	50/552 (9%)
Conti et al., 2005	23	Exercise	503	6	97	99/503 (20%)
Nucifora et al., 2007	24	Dobutamine	110	2	100	20/110 (18%)
Hong et al., 2011	25	Dobutamine	569	12–25	94.5[a]	64/569 (11%)
van der Zee et al., 2011	26	Dobutamine	524	9.4 years	NA[b]	23/350 (7%)
Hartlage et al., 2012	27	Dobutamine	255	299 days	99	2/166 (1%)
Shah et al., 2013	28	Exercise or dobutamine	811	1 year	99.5	98/802 (12%)

[a] Twenty-one cardiovascular deaths, with no difference between positive or negative dobutamine stress echo.

[b] 97.1% in negative stress echo also by perfusion (myocardial contrast echocardiography) criteria.

stabbing, pleuritic, pinprick character, without associated symptoms.[20] The rate of stress-echo positivity will be lower if all the patients with chest pain are evaluated and higher if only patients with medium to high probability on clinical grounds are selected.[23]

Positive stress echo indicates underlying coronary artery disease, and these patients should be admitted to the hospital (V17.3A, V17.3B, V17.3C, V17.3D, V17.3E). The efficiency of this algorithm has been shown not only in a single-center experiences but also in the large-scale, multicenter validation of the SPEED (Stress Pharmacological Echocardiography in the Emergency Department) trial, which analyzed more than 500 patients recruited from six centers in three different countries.[23] The negative predictive value of a negative algorithm is very high (99%) (V17.4A, V17.4B, V17.4C, V17.4D, V17.4E).

A randomized trial showed that stress echocardiography is more cost-effective than exercise-electrocardiography in predicting outcome and associated with less downstream resource utilization.[30]

However, there are occasional patients with negative stress test and early readmission for ACSs. This may be embarrassing for the physician but is unavoidable given the underlying pathophysiology of the disease. The specificity of stress echo based on RWMA is extremely high and superior to other techniques but the sensitivity for predicting events is suboptimal. This limitation is not surprising since events may occur independently of epicardial artery stenosis or missed myocardial infarction and can be due to other recognized vulnerabilities such as coronary microcirculatory dysfunction or altered cardiac autonomic balance.

The use of a comprehensive stress echocardiography with the ABCDE protocol allows to increase the sensitivity of the test and the positivity rate since it captures the sources of prognostic vulnerability of the patient beyond coronary artery stenosis: step A (for wall motion *a*bnormalities), step B (for *B*-lines on lung ultrasound, indicating pulmonary congestion), step C (for global left ventricular *c*ontractile reserve), step D (for *D*oppler-based assessment of coronary flow velocity reserve in left anterior descending coronary artery), and step E (*e*lectrocardiogram-based assessment of heart rate reserve and cardiac autonomic reserve). Each of them provides independent and incremental value in stratifying outcome.[31,32] This approach increases the capability of risk stratification of stress echocardiography without any significant increase in complexity and imaging time (Figure 17.1).

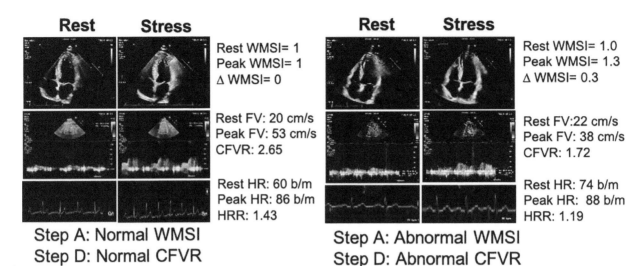

FIGURE 17.1 Comprehensive stress echocardiography ABCDE protocol. Steps A, D, and E of the ABCDE protocol are shown (see text). Left panel: normal 2D echo wall motion score index, coronary flow reserve and heart rate response during test. Right panel: increased 2D echo wall motion score index, reduced coronary flow reserve and blunted heart rate reserve during test, indicating presence of ischemia. CFVR: coronary flow velocity reserve; FV: flow velocity; HR: heart rate; HRR: heart rate reserve; WMSI: wall motion score index; Δ WMSI: delta wall motion score index.

IMAGING, APPROPRIATENESS, AND COST-EFFECTIVENESS IN THE EMERGENCY DEPARTMENT

A systematic search of the medical literature[32] and evidence-based guidelines[33] showed no significant differences among the three main modalities (MPI, stress echo, coronary MSCT) for the detection of coronary artery disease and events at follow-up. In a recent meta-analysis for patients in a low- to intermediate-risk category, the role of a negative stress echo was proven with only 1.68% major adverse events at 1 year.[34]

Stress echocardiography is equally effective and associated with less downstream resource utilization than noninvasive MSCT, with no difference in long-term cardiovascular outcomes.[33–41] Given the largely overlapping diagnostic and prognostic yield of the techniques (Table 17.2), practical aspects such as radiation exposure, cost and environmental impact become critical for decision-making. Direct cost is lowest for echo, intermediate for MSCT, and highest for MPI.[41] Radiation exposure is zero for echo, intermediate for MSCT (from 50 to 250 chest X-rays equivalent) and highest for MPI (from 250 to 500 chest X-rays).[42,43] Environmental impact is the lowest for echo (2 to 3 kg of CO_2 production per exam), intermediate for MSCT (20 to 30 kg of CO_2 per exam), and highest for cardiovascular magnetic resonance (200 to 300 kg of CO_2 per exam) or MPI (100 kg per exam excluding radioactive waste).[44,45]

The individual choice is also dictated by local practice, expertise available, medical facilities, and individual patient characteristics (Table 17.2). According to ESC guidelines on ACSs, TTE at rest is now mandatory.[9] When TTE is negative, the National Institute for Health and Care Excellence (NICE) guidelines recommend the use of stress imaging mainly in patients with a pretest probability between 30% and 60%, whereas patients in whom pretest probability is between 10% and 30% are recommended to have coronary MSCT.[46] However, also for stress echocardiography, the ED is a frequent source of inappropriate indications[7] (Table 17.3). The most appropriate indication remains the patient with intermediate pretest probability.[7] MSCT might be chosen as a second-line noninvasive test for intermediate-risk patients in whom stress echocardiography is unfeasible or gives ambiguous results. In high-risk patients, no further testing is recommended and direct referral to coronary angiography is warranted. The introduction of hsTn suggests the possibility of rapid direct discharge of hsTn-negative patients with acute chest pain, potentially without further stress ECG, functional, or anatomic testing in the ED.[37] The BEACON (Better Evaluation of Acute Chest Pain with Coronary Computed Tomography Angiography) trial concluded that when hsTn is available for ED evaluation of patients with acute chest pain, coronary CTA is associated with lower costs and less outpatient testing than standard of care that includes functional testing.[38] However, more data are also needed to support the extensive, aggressive use of imaging testing in patients presenting to the ED with chest pain.

Worth mentioning, acutely symptomatic patients should never be tested in the ED setting. The recommendation of

TABLE 17.2 Major Advantages and Disadvantages of Different Imaging Techniques for Detection of Presence of Acute Coronary Syndrome

IMAGING TECHNIQUE	MAJOR ADVANTAGES	MAJOR DISADVANTAGES
Echocardiography	Readily accessible Portable Safe Less expensive than MPI and MSCT Assessment of noncoronary conditions	Operator- and reader-dependent Poor acoustic window in 10% of patients (decreases with use of contrast) Suboptimal sensitivity (increase with HRR, MCE and/or CFR)
Radionuclide MPI	High sensitivity	Radiation exposure Expensive Low specificity Logistic barrier
Coronary MSCT	High sensitivity and high specificity Identification of noncoronary conditions Fast	Radiation exposure

Abbreviations: CFR, coronary flow reserve; HRR, heart rate reserve; MCE, myocardial contrast echocardiography; MPI, myocardial perfusion imaging; MSCT, multislice computed tomography.

(Modified from Dedic et al.[32])

TABLE 17.3 Role of Stress Echo in Acute Coronary Syndrome

	APPROPRIATE	UNCERTAIN	INAPPROPRIATE
Intermediate pretest probability (no dynamic ST changes, and serial cardiac enzymes negative)	✓		
Risk assessment without recurrent symptoms or signs of heart failure	✓		
Patient with prior positive MPI or positive MSCT		✓	
Low pretest probability of CAD, ECG interpretable, patient able to exercise			✓
High pretest probability of CAD			✓
ECG with ST elevation			✓

Abbreviations: CAD, coronary artery disease; ECG, electrocardiogram; MPI, myocardial perfusion imaging; MSCT, multislice computed tomography.

(Modified from Douglas et al.[7])

current guidelines is to use noninvasive cardiac testing for ED patients with negative serial electrocardiograms and cardiac troponins before or shortly after discharge from the emergency department.[47,48]

LIST OF VIDEOS

https://routledgetextbooks.com/textbooks/9781032157009/chapter-17.php

VIDEO 17.1A   Echocardiogram during anginal chest pain (1/2): Note an akinesis of the mid and apical part of the septum in the parasternal long-axis view of a patient with chest pain and nondiagnostic electrocardiogram. Initial and 6-hour follow-up troponin serum values were normal. After cessation of pain, contractility of the septum returned to normal (see also Video 17.1B). (*Video provided by VC.*)

VIDEO 17.1B   Echocardiogram during anginal chest pain (2/2): During an episode of anginal chest pain, akinesis of the septum was detected (see Video 17.1A). This follow-up echocardiogram recorded after cessation of the chest pain episode revealed normal contractility of the septum (shown here). These indicate the presence of significant stenosis and ischemia in the left anterior descending artery (LAD) territory. *Outcome:* Coronary angiography revealed 70% mid-LAD stenosis that was successfully stented. (*Video provided by VC.*)

VIDEO 17.2A   Positive exercise stress-echo test in the emergency department (ED) (1/3): A 45-year-old man was presented in the ED with atypical chest pain that had occurred during rest at home a few hours before and lasted about 5 minutes. He had no chest pain at the time of the presentation, the electrocardiogram was nondiagnostic, and the initial serum troponin level was normal. *Exercise stress-echo test* (using supine bicycle, workload 25–125 W, progression 25 W/2 min) was performed. Exercise-echo clips of the four-chamber view are presented: upper left, baseline; upper right, peak exercise; lower left, recovery. *Interpretation:* The test was stopped when a new akinesis of the distal half of the septum and the apex with left ventricular dilation was noted at peak exercise. The patient reported some chest discomfort. The contractility improved during recovery, but not completely. These findings indicate provocable ischemia in the left anterior descending artery (LAD) territory. *Outcome:* Immediate coronary angiography revealed 80% mid-LAD lesion, which was successfully stented (see also Videos 17.2B and 17.2C). *(Video provided by VC.)*

VIDEO 17.2B   Positive exercise stress-echo test in the emergency department (ED) (2/3): A 45-year-old man was presented in the ED with atypical chest pain that had occurred during rest at home a few hours before and lasted about 5 minutes. He had no chest pain at the time of the presentation, the electrocardiogram was nondiagnostic, and the initial serum troponin level was normal. *Exercise stress-echo test* (using supine bicycle, workload 25–125 W, progression 25 W/2 min) was performed. Exercise-echo clips of the two-chamber view are presented: upper left, baseline; upper right, peak exercise; lower left, recovery. *Interpretation:* The test was stopped when a new akinesis of the apex and distal two-thirds of the anterior wall with left ventricular dilation was noted at peak exercise. The patient reported some chest discomfort. The contractility improved during recovery, but not completely. These findings indicate provocable ischemia in the left anterior descending artery (LAD) territory. *Outcome:* Immediate coronary angiography revealed 80% mid-LAD lesion, which was successfully stented (see also Videos 17.2A and 17.2C). *(Video provided by VC.)*

VIDEO 17.2C   Positive exercise stress-echo test in the emergency department (ED) (3/3): A 45-year-old man was presented in the ED with atypical chest pain that had occurred during rest at home a few hours before and lasted about 5 minutes. He had no chest pain at the time of the presentation, the electrocardiogram was nondiagnostic, and the initial serum troponin level was normal. *Exercise stress-echo test* (using supine bicycle, workload 25–125 W, progression 25 W/2 min) was performed. Exercise-echo clips of the apical long-axis view are presented: upper left, baseline; upper right, peak exercise; lower left, recovery. *Interpretation:* The test was stopped when a new akinesis of the apex and distal two-thirds of the septum with left ventricular dilation were noted at peak exercise. The patient reported some chest discomfort. The contractility improved during recovery, but not completely. These indicate provocable ischemia in the left anterior descending artery (LAD) territory. *Outcome:* Immediate coronary angiography revealed 80% mid-LAD lesion, which was successfully stented (see also Videos 17.2A and 17.2B). *(Video provided by VC.)*

VIDEO 17.3A   Positive dobutamine stress-echo test in the emergency department (ED) (1/5): A 71-year-old man was presented in the ED with recurrent chest pain radiating to both shoulders, occurring at rest and lasting up to 10 minutes. There were no electrocardiographic changes, and his troponin levels at arrival and after 6 hours were both negative. Dobutamine stress-echo test was

performed using a standard protocol. *Interpretation:* Test was stopped before reaching 85% of predicted heart rate owing to development of regional wall motion abnormalities. Stress-echo test clips of the parasternal long-axis view are presented: upper left, baseline; upper right, low dose; lower left, peak dose; lower right, recovery. At this view, no new wall motion abnormalities were noted during the test (see also Videos 17.3B, 17.3C, 17.3D, and 17.3E). *(Video provided by PMM.)*

VIDEO 17.3B   Positive dobutamine stress-echo test in the emergency department (ED) (2/5): A 71-year-old man was presented in the ED with recurrent chest pain radiating to both shoulders, occurring at rest and lasting up to 10 minutes. There were no electrocardiographic changes, and his troponin levels at arrival and after 6 hours were both negative. Dobutamine stress-echo test was performed using a standard protocol. *Interpretation:* Test was stopped before reaching 85% of predicted heart rate owing to development of the regional wall motion abnormalities. Stress-echo test clips of the short-axis view are presented: upper left, baseline; upper right, low dose; lower left, peak dose; lower right, recovery. Note the hypokinesis of the septum (9–11 o'clock) during the peak dose compared with low dose (see also Videos 17.3A, 17.3C, 17.3D, and 17.3E). The patient was admitted to the hospital and coronary angiography revealed 85% mid-left anterior descending artery stenosis, which was successfully stented. *(Video provided by PMM.)*

VIDEO 17.3C   Positive dobutamine stress-echo test in the emergency department (ED) (3/5): A 71-year-old man was presented in the ED with recurrent chest pain radiating to both shoulders, occurring at rest and lasting up to 10 minutes. There were no electrocardiographic changes, and his troponin levels at arrival and after 6 hours were both negative. Dobutamine stress-echo test was performed using a standard protocol. *Interpretation:* Test was stopped before reaching 85% of predicted heart rate owing to development of regional wall motion abnormalities. Stress-echo test clips of the four-chamber view are presented: upper left, baseline; upper right, low dose; lower left, peak dose; lower right, recovery. Note a slight dilation of the left ventricle and hypokinesis of the septum and the apex during the peak dose compared with low dose. Note the aberrant chord in the left ventricular cavity (see also Videos 17.3A, 17.3B, 17.3D, and 17.3E). The patient was admitted to the hospital, and coronary angiography revealed 85% mid-left anterior descending artery stenosis, which was successfully stented. *(Video provided by PMM.)*

VIDEO 17.3D   Positive dobutamine stress-echo test in the emergency department (ED) (4/5): A 71-year-old man was presented in the ED with recurrent chest pain radiating to both shoulders, occurring at rest and lasting up to 10 minutes. There were no electrocardiographic changes, and his troponin levels at arrival and after 6 hours were both negative. Dobutamine stress-echo test was performed using a standard protocol. *Interpretation:* Test was stopped before reaching 85% of predicted heart rate owing to development of regional wall motion abnormalities. Stress-echo test clips of the two-chamber view are presented: upper left, baseline; upper right, low dose; lower left, peak dose; lower right, recovery. Note the hypokinesis of the distal half of the anterior wall during the peak dose compared with low dose. Note the aberrant chord in the left ventricular cavity (see also Videos 17.3A, 17.3B, 17.3C, and 17.3E). The patient was admitted to the hospital, and coronary angiography revealed 85% mid-left anterior descending artery stenosis, which was successfully stented. *(Video provided by PMM.)*

VIDEO 17.3E   Positive dobutamine stress-echo test in the emergency department (ED) (5/5): A 71-year-old man was presented in the ED with recurrent chest pain radiating to both shoulders, occurring at rest and lasting up to 10 minutes. There were no electrocardiographic changes, and his troponin levels at arrival and after 6 hours were both negative. Dobutamine stress-echo test was performed using a standard protocol. *Interpretation:* Test was stopped before reaching 85% of predicted heart rate owing to development of regional wall motion abnormalities. Stress-echo test clips of the apical long-axis view are presented: upper left, baseline; upper right, low dose; lower left, peak dose; lower right, recovery. Note the akinesis of the distal third of the septum and the apex during the peak dose compared with low dose. Note the aberrant chord in the left ventricular cavity (see also Videos 17.3A, 17.3B, 17.3C, and 17.3D). The patient was admitted to the hospital, and coronary angiography revealed 85% mid-left anterior descending artery stenosis, which was successfully stented. *(Video provided by PMM.)*

VIDEO 17.4A   Normal dobutamine stress-echo test in the emergency department (ED) (1/5): A 63-year-old woman was presented in the ED with atypical chest pain starting 4 hours before arrival. There was a stationary ST-segment depression up to 0.5 mV in electrocardiographic leads V_5 and V_6. Her troponin levels at arrival and after 2 hours were both negative. To further evaluate origin of chest pain, dobutamine stress-echo test was performed using a standard protocol. *Interpretation:* Test was stopped after reaching 85% of predicted heart rate. After images were obtained during peak dose, patient received slow intravenous injection of 5 mg of metoprolol. Patient did not experience worsening of chest pain during the test. Stress-echo test clips of the parasternal long-axis view are presented: upper left, baseline; upper right, low-dose dobutamine; lower left, peak dose; lower right, recovery. Note the absence of regional wall motion abnormalities during all stages of the test (see also Videos 17.4B, 17.4C, 17.4D, and 17.4E). The patient was sent home with the diagnosis of noncoronary chest pain. *(Video provided by PMM.)*

VIDEO 17.4B   Normal dobutamine stress-echo test in the emergency department (ED) (2/5): A 63-year-old woman was presented in the ED with atypical chest pain starting 4 hours before arrival. There was a stationary ST-segment depression up to 0.5 mV in electrocardiographic leads V_5 and V_6. Her troponin levels at arrival and after 2 hours were both negative. To further evaluate origin of chest pain, dobutamine stress-echo test was performed using a standard protocol. *Interpretation:* Test was stopped after reaching 85% of predicted heart rate. After images were obtained during peak dose, patient received slow intravenous injection of 5 mg of metoprolol. Patient did not experience worsening of chest pain during the test. Stressecho test clips of the short-axis view are presented: upper left, baseline; upper right, low-dose dobutamine; lower left, peak dose; lower right, recovery. Note the absence of regional wall motion abnormalities during all stages of the test (see also Videos 17.4A, 17.4C, 17.4D, and 17.4E). The patient was sent home with the diagnosis of noncoronary chest pain. *(Video provided by PMM.)*

VIDEO 17.4C   Normal dobutamine stress-echo test in the emergency department (ED) (3/5): A 63-year-old woman was presented in the ED with atypical chest pain starting 4 hours before arrival. There was a stationary ST-segment depression up to 0.5 mV in electrocardiographic leads V_5 and V_6. Her troponin levels at arrival and after 2 hours were both negative. To further evaluate origin of chest pain, dobutamine stress-echo test was performed

using a standard protocol. *Interpretation:* Test was stopped after reaching 85% of predicted heart rate. After images were obtained during peak dose, patient received slow intravenous injection of 5 mg of metoprolol. Patient did not experience worsening of chest pain during the test. Stress-echo test clips of the four-chamber view are presented: upper left, baseline; upper right, low-dose dobutamine; lower left, peak dose; lower right, recovery. Note the absence of regional wall motion abnormalities during all stages of the test (see also Videos 17.4A, 17.4B, 17.4D, and 17.4E). The patient was sent home with the diagnosis of noncoronary chest pain. *(Video provided by PMM.)*

VIDEO 17.4D   Normal dobutamine stress-echo test in the emergency department (ED) (4/5): A 63-year-old woman was presented in the ED with atypical chest pain starting 4 hours before arrival. There was a stationary ST-segment depression up to 0.5 mV in electrocardiographic leads V_5 and V_6. Her troponin levels at arrival and after 2 hours were both negative. To further evaluate origin of chest pain, dobutamine stress-echo test was performed using a standard protocol. *Interpretation:* Test was stopped after reaching 85% of predicted heart rate. After obtaining images during peak dose, patient received slow intravenous injection of 5 mg of metoprolol. Patient did not experienced worsening of chest pain during the test. Stress-echo test clips of the two-chamber view are presented: upper left, baseline; upper right, low-dose dobutamine; lower left, peak dose; lower right, recovery. Note the absence of regional wall motion abnormalities during all stages of the test (see also Videos 17.4A, 17.4B, 17.4C, and 17.4E). The patient was sent home with the diagnosis of noncoronary chest pain. *(Video provided by PMM.)*

VIDEO 17.4E   Normal dobutamine stress-echo test in the emergency department (ED) (5/5): A 63-year-old woman was presented in the ED with atypical chest pain starting 4 hours before arrival. There was a stationary ST-segment depression up to 0.5 mV in electrocardiographic leads V_5 and V_6. Her troponin levels at arrival and after 2 hours were both negative. To further evaluate origin of chest pain, dobutamine stress-echo test was performed using a standard protocol. *Interpretation:* Test was stopped after reaching 85% of predicted heart rate. After images were obtained during peak dose, patient received slow intravenous injection of 5 mg of metoprolol. Patient did not experience worsening of chest pain during the test. Stress-echo test clips of the apical long-axis view are presented: upper left, baseline; upper right, low-dose dobutamine; lower left, peak dose; lower right, recovery. Note the absence of regional wall motion abnormalities during all stages of the test (see also Videos 17.4A, 17.4B, 17.4C, and 17.4D). The patient was sent home with the diagnosis of noncoronary chest pain. *(Video provided by PMM.)*

REFERENCES

1. Farkouh ME, Smars PA, Reeder GS, et al. A clinical trial of a chest-pain observation unit for patients with unstable angina. N Engl J Med 1998; 339:1882–8.
2. Stein RA, Chaitman BR, Balady GJ, et al. Safety and utility of exercise testing in emergency room chest pain centers. An advisory from the committee on Exercise, Rehabilitation and Prevention, Council on Clinical Cardiology, American Heart Association. Circulation 2000; 102:1463–7.

3. Herlitz J, McGovern P, Dellborg M, et al. Comparison of treat-? ment and outcomes for patients with acute myocardial infarction in Minneapolis/St Paul, Minnesota, and Göteborg, Sweden. Am Heart J 2003; 146:1023–9.

4. Safavi KC, Li SX, Dharmarajan K, et al. Hospital variation in the use of noninvasive cardiac imaging and its association with downstream testing, interventions, and outcomes. JAMA Intern Med 2014; 174:546–53.

5. Flannery FT, Parikh PD, Oetgen WJ. Characteristics of medical professional liability claims in patients treated by family medicine physicians. J Am Board Fam Med 2010; 23:753–61.

6. Sechtem U, Achenbach S, Friedrich M, Wackers F, Zamorano JL. Non-invasive imaging in acute chest pain syndromes. Eur Heart J Cardiovasc Imaging 2012; 13:69–78.

7. Douglas PS, Garcia MJ, Haines DE, et al. ACCF/ASE/AHA/ ASNC/HFSA/HRS/SCAI/SCCM/SCCT/SCMR 2011 appropriate use criteria for echocardiography. A report of the American College of Cardiology Foundation Appropriate Use Criteria Task Force. J Am Coll Cardiol 2011; 57:1126–66.

8. Amsterdam EA, Aman E. The patient with chest pain: low risk, high stakes. JAMA Intern Med 2014; 174:553–4.

9. Byrne RA, Rossello X, Coughlan JJ, Barbato E, Berry C, Chieffo A, et al.; ESC Scientific Document Group. 2023 ESC Guidelines for the management of acute coronary syndromes. Eur Heart J 2023;44(38):3720–826.

10. Pines JM, Mullins PM, Cooper JK, Feng LB, Roth KE. National trends in emergency department use, care patterns, and quality of care of older adults in the United States. J Am Geriatr Soc 2013; 61:12–7.

11. Atar S, Feldman A, Darawshe A, Siegel RJ, Rosenfeld T. Utility and diagnostic accuracy of handcarried ultrasound for emergency room evaluation of chest pain. Am J Cardiol 2004; 94:408–9.

12. Hickman M, Swinburn JM, Senior R. Wall thickening assessment with tissue harmonic echocardiography results in improved risk stratification for patients with non-ST-segment elevation acute chest pain. Eur J Echocardiogr 2004; 5:142–8.

13. Loh IK, Charuzi Y, Beeder C, Marshall LA, Ginsburg JH. Early diagnosis of nontransmural myocardial infarction by two-dimensional echocardiography. Am Heart J 1982; 104:963–8.

14. Peels CH, Visser CA, Kupper AJ, Visser FC, Roos JP. Usefulness of two-dimensional echocardiography for immediate detection of myocardial ischemia in the emergency room. Am J Cardiol 1990; 65:687–91.

15. Sasaki H, Charuzi Y, Beeder C, Sugiki Y, Lew AS. Utility of echocardiography for the early assessment of patients with nondiagnostic chest pain. Am Heart J 1986; 112:494–97.

16. Trippi JA, Lee KS, Kopp G, Nelson DR, Yee KG, Cordell WH. Dobutamine stress tele-echocardiography for evaluation of emergency department patients with chest pain. J Am Coll Cardiol 1997; 30:627–32.

17. Colon PJ 3rd, Guarisco JS, Murgo J, Cheirif J. Utility of stress echocardiography in the triage of patients with atypical chest pain from the emergency department. Am J Cardiol 1998; 82:1282–4.

18. Gelejinse ML, Elhendy A, Kasprzak JD, et al. Safety and prognostic value of early dobutamine-atropine stress echocardiography in patients with spontaneous chest pain and a nondiagnostic electrocardiogram. Eur Heart J 2000; 21:397–405.

19. Orlandini A, Tuero E, Paolasso E, Vilamajo OG, Diaz R. Usefulness of pharmacologic stress echocardiography in a chest pain center. Am J Cardiol 2000; 86:1247–50.

20. Buchsbaum M, Marshall E, Levine B, et al. Emergency department evaluation of chest pain using exercise stress echocardiography. Acad Emerg Med 2001; 8:196–9.

21. Bholasingh R, Cornel JH, Kamp O, et al. Prognostic value of predischarge dobutamine stress echocardiography in chest pain patients with a negative cardiac troponin T. J Am Coll Cardiol 2003; 41:596–602.

22. Bedetti G, Pasanisi E, Picano F, et al. Stress echo in chest pain unit: the SPEED (Stress Pharmacological Echocardiography in Emergency Department) trial. Int J Cardiol 2005; 98:754–9.

23. Conti A, Sammicheli L, Gallini C, et al. Assessment of low risk pain patients in the emergency department: head to head comparison of exercise stress echocardiography and exercise myocardial SPECT. Am Heart J 2005; 150:123–7.

24. Nucifora G, Badano LP, Sarraf-Zadegan N, et al. Comparison of early dobutamine stress echocardiography and exercise electrocardiographic testing for management of patients presenting to the emergency department with chest pain. Am J Cardiol 2007; 100:1068–73.

25. Hong GR, Park JS, Lee SH, et al. Prognostic value of real time dobutamine stress myocardial contrast echocardiography in patients with chest pain syndrome. Int J Cardiovasc Imaging 2011; 27(Suppl 1):103–12.

26. van der Zee PM, Verberne HJ, Cornel JH, et al. GRACE and TIMI risk scores but not stress imaging predict long-term cardiovascular follow-up in patients with chest pain after a rule-out protocol. Neth Heart J 2011; 19:324–30.

27. Hartlage G, Janik M, Anadiotis A, et al. Prognostic value of adenosine stress cardiovascular magnetic resonance and dobutamine stress echocardiography in patients with low-risk chest pain. Int J Cardiovasc Imaging 2012; 28:803–12.

28. Shah BN, Balaji G, Alhajiri A, Ramzy IS, Ahmadvazir S, Senior R. Incremental diagnostic and prognostic value of contemporary stress echocardiography in a chest pain unit: mortality and morbidity outcomes from a real-world setting. Circ Cardiovasc Imaging 2013; 6:202–9.

29. Innocenti F, Lazzeretti D, Conti A, Zanobetti M, Vicidomini S, Pini R. Stress echocardiography in the ED: diagnostic performance in high-risk subgroups. Am J Emerg Med 2013; 3:1309–14.

30. Gurunathan S, Zacharias K, Akhtar M, et al. Cost-effectiveness of a management strategy based on exercise echocardiography versus exercise electrocardiography in patients presenting with suspected angina during long term follow up: a randomized study. Int J Cardiol 2018; 15;259:1–7.

31. Cortigiani L, Vecchi A, Bovenzi F, Picano E. Reduced coronary flow reserve and blunted heart rate reserve identify a higher risk group in patients with chest pain and negative emergency department evaluation. Intern Emerg Med 2022; 17(7):2103–11.

32. Ciampi Q, Zagatina A, Cortigiani L, et al. Prognostic value of ABCDE stress echocardiography. Eur Heart J 2021; 42:3869–78.

33. Sturts A, Ruzieh M, Dhruva SS, et al. Resource utilization following coronary computed tomographic angiography and stress echocardiography in patients presenting to the emergency department with chest pain. Am J Cardiol 2021. https:// doi.org/10.1016/j.amjcard.2021.09.043.

34. Mehta P, McDonald S, Hirani R, Good D, Diercks D. Major adverse cardiac events after emergency department evaluation of chest pain patients with advanced testing: systematic review and meta-analysis. Acad Emerg Med 2021. https://doi. org/10.1111/acem.14407.

35. Kargoli F, Levsky J, Bulcha N, et al. Comparison between anatomical and functional imaging modalities for evaluation of chest pain in the emergency department. Am J Cardiol 2020; 125(12):1809–14.

36. Levsky JM, Haramati LB, Spevack DM, et al. Coronary computed tomography angiography versus stress echocardiography in acute chest pain: a randomized controlled trial. JACC Cardiovasc Imaging 2018; 11(9):1288–97.
37. Haaf P, Reichlin T, Twerenbold R, et al. Risk stratification in patients with acute chest pain using three high-sensitivity cardiac troponin assays. Eur Heart J 2014; 35:365–75.
38. Dedic A, Lubbers MM, Schaap J, et al. Coronary CT angiography for suspected ACS in the era of high-sensitivity troponins: randomized multicenter study. J Am Coll Cardiol 2016; 67:16–26.
39. Foy AJ, Liu G, Davidson WR Jr, Sciamanna C, Leslie DL. Comparative effectiveness of diagnostic testing strategies in emergency department patients with chest pain: an analysis of downstream testing, interventions, and outcomes. JAMA Intern Med 2015; 175(3):428–36.
40. Romero J, Husain SA, Holmes AA, et al. Non-invasive assessment of low risk acute chest pain in the emergency department: A comparative meta-analysis of prospective studies. Int J Cardiol 2015; 187:565–80.
41. Iannaccone M, Gili S, De Filippo O, et al. Diagnostic accuracy of functional, imaging and biochemical tests for patients presenting with chest pain to the emergency department: a systematic review and meta-analysis. Eur Heart J Acute Cardiovasc Care 2019; 8(5):412–20.
42. Picano E, Vañó E, Rehani MM, et al. The appropriate and justified use of medical radiation in cardiovascular imaging: a position document of the ESC Associations of Cardiovascular Imaging, Percutaneous Cardiovascular Interventions and Electrophysiology. Eur Heart J 2014; 35:665–72.
43. Hirshfeld JW Jr, Ferrari VA, Bengel FM et al. 2018 ACC/HRS/NASCI/SCAI/SCCT Expert Consensus Document on Optimal Use of Ionizing Radiation in Cardiovascular Imaging-Best Practices for Safety and Effectiveness, Part 2: Radiological Equipment Operation, Dose-Sparing Methodologies, Patient and Medical Personnel Protection: A Report of the American College of Cardiology Task Force on Expert Consensus Decision Pathways. J Am Coll Cardiol 2018; 71(24):2829–55.
44. Marwick TH, Buonocore J. Environmental impact of cardiac imaging tests for the diagnosis of coronary artery disease. Heart 2011; 97(14):1128–31.
45. Picano E. Economic, ethical, and environmental sustainability of cardiac imaging. Eur Heart J 2022. https://doi.org/10.1093/eurheartj/ehac716. Online ahead of print.
46. Recent-onset chest pain of suspected cardiac origin: assessment and diagnosis. NICE Clinical guidelines, CG95—published: March 2010; last updated: November 2016. www.nice.org.uk/guidance/cg95 (last accessed November 19, 2022).
47. Amsterdam EA, Wenger NK, Brindis RG, et al. ACC/AHA Task Force Members. 2014 AHA/ACC guideline for the management of patients with non−ST-elevation acute coronary syndromes: executive summary: a report of the American College of Cardiology/American Heart Association Task Force on Practice Guidelines. Circulation 2014; 130:e344–e426.
48. Picano E, Pierard L, Peteiro J, Djordjevic-Dikic A, Sade LE, Cortigiani L, et al. The Clinical use of Stress Echocardiography in Chronic Coronary Syndromes and Beyond Coronary artery disease: A Clinical Consensus Statement from the European Association of Cardiovascular Imaging of the ESC. Eur Heart J Cardiovasc Imaging 2023 Oct 5:jead250. doi: 10.1093/ehjci/jead250. Online ahead of print.

Handheld ultrasound devices in the emergency setting

18

Ivan Stankovic and Nuno Cardim

The real value of any imaging technique is intimately dependent on our intellectual contributions:
how, when, and in what clinical situation will it have maximal clinical impact.
—JRTC Roelandt

Key Points

- Handheld ultrasound devices (HUDs) are powerful tools in the emergency setting for focused qualitative cardiac examinations of ventricular function, pericardial and pleural effusions, extravascular lung water, and intravascular volume assessment.
- The wide dissemination of HUDs and their use both by cardiologists and non-cardiologists has become a reality. This trend is expected to grow in the near future.
- Medical professionals using HUDs should receive appropriate education and training to avoid potentially catastrophic errors in the emergency setting. These include two components: competence in image acquisition and interpretation and specific education and training in HUD use.
- Examinations with current HUDs, owing to technical limitations, cannot replace a complete echocardiogram; they can only be reported as a complement to physical examination.

Ultrasound-based assessment of the heart with handheld ultrasound devices (HUDs) is an increasingly available imaging modality that may be used as an aid to rapid and accurate diagnosis of a variety of cardiac emergencies. In this chapter, we describe the technical aspects of these miniature ultrasound devices, review their usefulness in the emergency setting, and discuss limitations, potential pitfalls, and future perspectives.

Before the advent of portable and HUDs, emergency bedside echocardiography only was performed on bulky machines, wheeled to patient's bedside. Moving either a heavy machine to bedside or a critically ill patient to an echo lab is an unpractical, cumbersome, and time-consuming

task, so several attempts to make emergency echocardiography more portable have been made over the past few decades. The first HUD was introduced in 1978, and commercially available portable imaging devices became available in the late 1990s.[1,2] Currently, there are several truly portable echocardiographic systems that are substantially smaller (weighing 3.1 to 8.2 kg) and less expensive than full systems but still feature most of the advanced modalities to perform a comprehensive echo study. Some recent models of these devices also include a stress-echocardiography package, contrast imaging, and transesophageal echocardiography. Several reports have shown that important, although limited, information derived from hand-carried

DOI: 10.1201/9781003245407-18

devices permits faster clinical decisions than waiting for the formal, full echocardiographic examination and allow early detection of potentially serious cardiac conditions, leading to faster and more appropriate treatment.[3,4]

Recently, further advances in electronics and ultrasound technology have enabled the ultrasound industry to create true handheld imaging devices, small enough to fit in a physician's pocket. In comparison to portable and particularly to full echo systems, technical capabilities of these small echo scanners are currently still limited but sufficient to give the emergency physician accurate answers to simple but critical questions in acute settings.

TECHNICAL CHARACTERISTICS OF IMAGING WITH HANDHELD DEVICES

Currently, HUDs are available from several vendors and are capable of both cardiac and noncardiac (fetal, abdominal, pelvic, and peripheral vessel) imaging. Technical characteristics of some of currently marketed devices are summarized in Table 18.1.

All machines are battery operated and have a very short start-up time and user-friendly interfaces (V18.1A, V18.1B, V18.2A, V18.2B, V18.3A, V18.3B). All devices allow storage and retrieval of patient and study data and can connect to a personal computer or tablet (usually via a standard USB cable but some of them also wirelessly). Finally, all HUDs are far more affordable than full echo systems.

Available measurements are usually limited to simple distance and area assessments. While early devices allow data storage only in generic image or movie formats, some more recent machines support basic digital imaging and communications in medicine (DICOM) standards for downloading patient information upload images and perform offline measurements (such as LV ejection fraction). M-mode technology is not available in many, and simultaneous electrocardiogram (ECG) is lacking, so ECG triggering with precise end-diastole identification is not feasible. Nonetheless, one of the latest platforms offers full Doppler capabilities (color, pulsed-wave, and continuous-wave Doppler) and also artificial intelligence-driven automatic ejection fraction, stroke volume and cardiac output calculations. One of the probes from the same platform also offers integrated ECG and auscultation capabilities.

Recommendation documents from both the European Association of Cardiovascular Imaging (EACVI) and from the American Society of Echocardiography (ASE) underline that these devices do not provide a complete diagnostic capabilities of echocardiographic examination.[5,6] Instead, HUDs should be used only for a focused cardiac ultrasound (FoCUS) assessment, as a complement to physical examination, both in the out-of-hospital emergency context and in the hospital emergency setting (emergency rooms, intensive care units, etc.); this point should be always respected when discussing education, training and competence in HUDs.

The range of the EACVI-recommended indications for the use of HUDs is limited to the evaluation of (1) left ventricular (LV) and right ventricular (RV) global function and dimensions, (2) pericardial and pleural effusions, (3) pulmonary parenchyma and extravascular lung water, (4) respiratory variation of inferior vena cava size (intravascular volume

TABLE 18.1 Technical Characteristics of Handheld Ultrasound Devices*

DEVICE	IMAGING MODALITIES	DISPLAY (inches/cm)	TOTAL WEIGHT (G)	BATTERY CAPACITY	TRANSDUCER (MHz)
Vscan extend	2D, color Doppler	5.7/12.7	321	60 min	1.7–8 (dual) Phased array, Linear array
Lumify	2D, M-mode, color Doppler	Android-based smart device	96 (without cable)	Approx. the time of the tablet/ smartphone battery life	1–4 Phased array
Butterfly iQ	2D mode, biplane imaging, M-mode, color Doppler, PW Doppler	iOS- and Android-based mobile devices	309	≥120 min	1–10 MHz, depending on the selected exam preset
Kosmos	2D, M-mode, color Doppler, PW and CW Doppler, AutoEF	8/20.3 dedicated display unit (tablet)	227 (probe) 652 (display unit)	120 min	2–5 MHz
EagleView	2D, M-mode, color Doppler, PW Doppler	Smartphone-based (wireless connection)	260	2.5 h	3.5–10 (dual) Phased array Curvilinear

* For the latest technical characteristics, please visit the vendors' websites.

Abbreviations: 2D, two-dimensional; CW, continuous wave; EF, ejection fraction; CW, continuous wave; PW, pulsed wave.

assessment), (5) left and right atrial size, (6) gross valvular abnormalities, (7) large intracardiac masses, and (8) vascular assessment (thoracic and abdominal vessels).[5]

In emergency settings, HUDs can be used for point-of-care ultrasound (POCUS) in patients with acute dyspnea (lung and cardiac causes), with shock (cardiogenic, hypovolemic, distributive) and in cardiac arrest (Chapter 5), providing a fast diagnosis and clues to the adequate and early institution of therapy.[7] Lightweight HUD and POCUS protocols offer multiple capabilities to military clinicians of all types and levels in multiple environments. Its application in diagnostics, procedural guidance, and patient monitoring has recently started to be explored in the battlefield. Military clinicians demonstrated the ability to perform focused exams, including FAST exams (and fracture detection) with acceptable sensitivity and specificity. POCUS in the hands of trained military clinicians has the potential to improve diagnostic accuracy and ultimately care of the war fighter.[8]

The advantages of HUDs were also witnessed during the COVID-19 pandemic, both in emergency rooms and intensive care units. Used within different POCUS protocols, HUDs provide ultrasonic assessment from head to toe, sparing the use of stethoscope, chest X-ray, and computed tomography. Ideally, patients with COVID-19 should be examined using dedicated wireless machines (one multiple functionalities probe machine to each intensive care unit patient) and single-use ultrasound gel to avoid cross-contamination. A common scanning protocol should be defined for all patients in each environment.[9]

Although data demonstrating the usefulness of miniature echo machines in diagnosing cardiac emergencies are still scarce, there is a growing body of evidence that imaging capabilities of HUDs may be sufficient to provide emergency physicians with essential information by focused examinations performed at the point of care.[10–14] A great benefit of direct visualization of cardiac morphology and function by these devices should also be expected in remote areas or resource-constrained settings in which no other ultrasound machines are available.[15,16] However, because the space for echocardiographic examination in busy emergency departments is usually limited, HUDs may be useful for bedside examinations even in well-equipped hospitals.

The concordance between HUDs and high-end echo machines in terms of feasibility and accuracy was shown to be good[17–21]; intervendor comparison studies of currently available pocket-size devices have not been performed. Several recent publications[2–4,10–13,18,20,22,23] showing important diagnostic influence of focused cardiac examinations suggested that HUDs might be useful in emergency settings for (1) triaging patients, (2) making a crude but important diagnosis (ruling in and ruling out obvious but serious pathology), and (3) guiding procedures (e.g., pericardiocentesis, vascular access).

Although current ultrasound-based algorithms for assessment of cardiac emergencies are scarce,[24] several emergency conditions are much easier to recognize with ultrasound than with physical examination alone, which can be illustrated by the following cases from our cardiac emergency departments.

- A focused echocardiographic examination of an elderly patient admitted for presumed non-ST-segment elevation myocardial infarction is illustrated in Figure 18.1 (V18.4A, V18.4B). Although the chest pain and electrocardiographic changes were

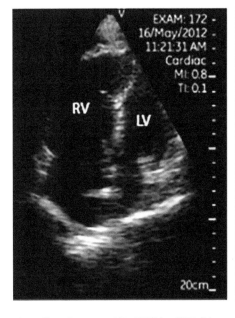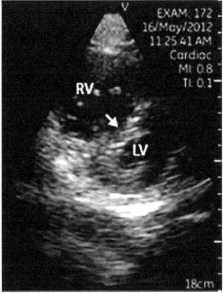

FIGURE 18.1   Focused cardiac ultrasound (FoCUS) by HUD (Vscan, GE Healthcare) in a patient admitted for presumed acute coronary syndrome. Dilation of the right ventricle (RV), hypokinesis of the right ventricular free wall (left panel, V18.4A), and flattening (arrow) of the interventricular septum causing D-shaped left ventricle (LV) (right panel, V18.4B) were all suggestive of pulmonary embolism, which was confirmed by pulmonary multislice computed tomography. A mobile, hyperechogenic right ventricular mass suggestive of a thrombus can also be seen (V18.4A).

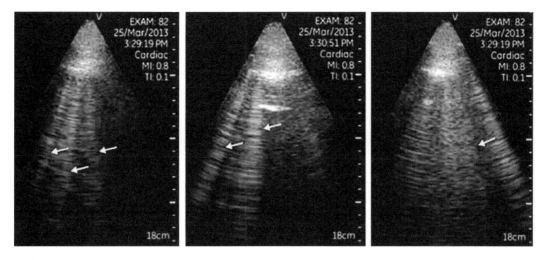

FIGURE 18.2 Lung ultrasound performed by an HUD showing multiple diffuse, hyperechogenic, vertical, bilateral B-lines (arrows, V18.5) in a patient with dyspnea caused by pulmonary congestion. B-lines ("comet tails," "lung comets") are consistent with the presence of extravascular lung water.

consistent with the admitting diagnosis, a 4-minute examination performed with an HUD allowed a rapid diagnosis of pulmonary embolism and initiation of appropriate treatment.

- Figure 18.2 illustrates the use of HUDs for the discrimination of cardiac and pulmonary dyspnea. The patient presented with shortness of breath and wheezing suggestive of an acute exacerbation of chronic obstructive pulmonary disease, but the point-of-care lung ultrasound revealed B-lines ("ultrasound comets"), which are a sensitive and specific sign of extravascular lung water (V18.5). Instead of being admitted to the pulmonary department and treated with bronchodilators, the patient was diagnosed with pulmonary congestion and admitted to the cardiology department.
- The unexpected finding of a cardiac myxoma in a patient with chest pain, dizziness, and palpitations is shown in Figure 18.3 (V18.6).
- Unexpected pericardial and pleural effusions in febrile patients with suspected endocarditis and sepsis are displayed in Figure 18.4 (V18.7A, V18.7B, V18.7C).

In addition to the emergency department, HUDs may find their place in many different environments in which ultrasound use was previously considered impractical. Figure 18.5 shows the images from an emergency examination performed in a cardiac catheterization room during coronary angiography in a patient with ST-segment elevation in the anterolateral leads who developed a sudden hemodynamic instability and a harsh systolic murmur. Examination performed with an HUD ruled out suspected mechanical complication of myocardial infarction and revealed that LV apical ballooning (V18.8A) and a dynamic left ventricular outflow tract obstruction (V18.8B, V18.8C) were true causes

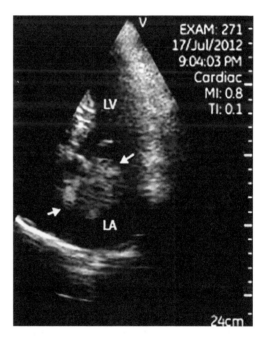

FIGURE 18.3 Apical four-chamber view showing left atrial echogenic mass (arrows) in a patient presenting to the emergency department with nonspecific complaints (V18.6). LA: left atrium; LV: left ventricle.

(Image and video provided by RV.)

of hemodynamic instability. Instead of inotropic agents, the patient was cautiously treated with intravenous betablockers, which reduced basal hypercontractility and normalized blood pressure.

Also, during electrophysiological procedures or complex percutaneous coronary interventions, these devices are often useful for early detection of iatrogenic pericardial effusion and cardiac tamponade.

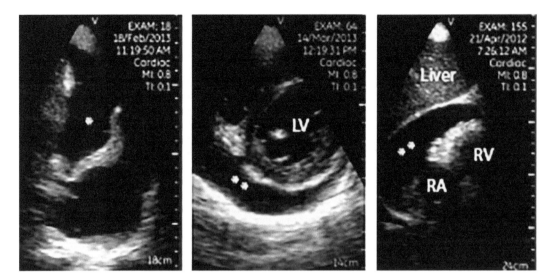

FIGURE 18.4   Unexpected pleural and pericardial effusions diagnosed with an HUD. Pleural effusion (*) in a patient with suspected endocarditis (left panel, V18.7A). Moderate pericardial effusion (**) in a patient with fever (middle panel, V18.7B). Large pericardial effusion (**) causing right ventricular collapse (cardiac tamponade) in a patient with sepsis (right panel, V18.7C). LV: left ventricle; RA: right atrium; RV: right ventricle.

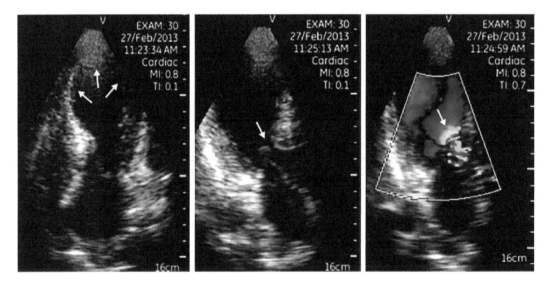

FIGURE 18.5   Examination performed with an HUD in a catheterization laboratory in a patient with a sudden unexplained hemodynamic instability and a new systolic murmur. Apical ballooning (arrows) and hypercontractility of the basal LV segments (left panel, V18.8A) caused dynamic left ventricular outflow tract (LVOT) obstruction (arrow, middle panel, V18.8B) as indicated by turbulent LVOT flow in the apical long-axis view (right panel, V18.8C).

TECHNICAL LIMITATIONS OF HANDHELD IMAGING DEVICES

Types of ultrasound examination of the heart (echocardiography, goal-oriented echocardiography, FoCUS) that can be performed by each type of ultrasound machines (stationary high-end, mobile systems, portable machines, or HUDs) are defined by their technological capabilities.[5] Thus, while FoCUS

examination can be performed with any type of ultrasound machine, a comprehensive or goal-oriented echocardiography can only be performed with fully equipped machines and not with HUDs.

A more convenient size and lower costs of HUDs have improved functionality at the patient's bedside, but these advances have come at a price of a lower image resolution and smaller screen and sector size. This is especially important in difficult cases and may result in technically suboptimal studies, leading to less reliable findings.[25] Furthermore, many other advanced features of full echo systems, including tissue Doppler, strain imaging, and three-dimensional echocardiography, are not available with miniature imaging devices. Currently, the most relevant technical limitation of HUDs in the emergency setting is lack of spectral Doppler, which is necessary for quantification of valvular lesion severity and the assessment of pulmonary hypertension, diastolic function, and pericardial constriction.[26] Nonetheless, full Doppler capabilities and artificial intelligence-driven calculations have already been included in the latest platforms, which may bring handheld devices closer to small high-end echocardiography machines available at a fraction of the cost of full platforms. Despite this, if HUDs are not used by fully trained operators, there is the potential for diagnostic errors which brings controversy in the echocardiographic community. Accordingly, the EACVI recommends that the use of these devices remain limited to the extension of the clinical assessment.[5]

COMPETENCE AND TRAINING OF THE USERS

Further technological progress in the ultrasound industry will result in a wide dissemination of miniature imaging devices, and like a stethoscope, in the future every physician may own a personal device. It is, therefore, of paramount importance that medical professionals using these devices receive appropriate training and understand the limitations of devices and focused cardiac examinations. Although emergency echocardiography is commonly performed by expert users (i.e., cardiologists with echocardiography expertise or experienced echosonographers), nowadays it is very likely that focused examinations with HUDs will be performed by the entire scale of non-experts (e.g., anesthesiologists, intensive care and emergency physicians, internal medicine specialists, cardiac surgeons, residents, fellows).

In the emergency settings, HUDs should be used only by appropriately trained operators irrespective of their professional background, who are familiar with the technical characteristics of the devices and aware of their diagnostic limitations.[5] To avoid potential harm to patients, both the ASE and EACVI have defined training requirements for the use of handheld imaging devices.[5,6] The process of education and training in HUDs recommended by the EACVI should include two steps (Figure 18.6): (1) competence in image acquisition and interpretation and (2) specific education and training in HUD use.[5]

In cardiology, competence in imaging acquisition and interpretation can be achieved by fulfilling current requirements for training and competence in echocardiography or FoCUS, described in detail in the respective EACVI and other documents.[25–27] This knowledge should always be complemented by additional specific education and training in HUDs (Figure 18.6). Except for expert echocardiographers, all other practitioners (i.e., cardiologists not fully trained in echocardiography and non-cardiologists) are required to reach and maintain a specific level of competence. According to the EACVI emergency echocardiography recommendations,[27] emergency echocardiography should be performed by anyone capable of acquiring and using valuable information from it for clinical decision-making (see Chapter 1), and requirements are the same for cardiologists and non-cardiologists. For FoCUS (see Chapter 19), the EACVI provided FoCUS core curriculum and core syllabus to define key principles and unifying framework for educational and training processes/programs that should result in competence in FoCUS for various medical professionals dealing with diagnostics and treatment of cardiovascular emergencies.[25] The document is prepared in close cooperation with the European Society of Anaesthesiology, the European Association of Cardiothoracic Anaesthesiology, the Acute Cardiovascular Care Association, and the World Interactive Network Focused On Critical Ultrasound (WINFOCUS).[25] Importantly, for focused cardiac ultrasound examinations,

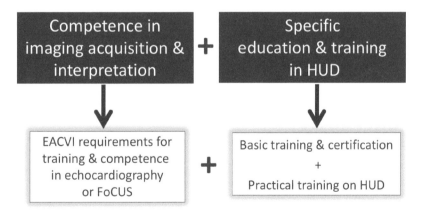

FIGURE 18.6 Education, training, and competence in HUDs.

(Modified with permission from Oxford University Press from Cardim N. et al.[5])

competence and training standards for non-cardiologists proposed by echocardiographic societies should ideally be elaborated by corresponding specialty societies and tailored to specific education programs of each specialty. One example are the recommendations for critical care basic ultrasound learning goals for American anesthesiology critical care trainees proposed by an expert group sponsored by the Society of Critical Care Anesthesiologists.[28] This document defined learning goals and recommended competencies concerning focused basic critical care ultrasound, including cardiac imaging, for critical care specialists in training. If similar teaching and training standards were released by other medical specialty societies, the achievement of necessary competencies for performing FoCUS by non-cardiologists would be greatly facilitated.

Of note, the competence in imaging acquisition and interpretation should always be complemented by additional specific education and training in HUDs (Figure 18.6). In this context, the feasibility and clinical accuracy of HUDs in the evaluation of cardiac morphology and function, their inherent technical limitations, and particular training on the specific ultrasound device in use are essential educational targets.[5]

POTENTIAL PITFALLS AND LIMITATIONS

Although primarily designed to reduce medical errors, under some circumstances, HUDs may become a source of errors themselves. Overreliance on ultrasound findings may sometimes either prematurely terminate needful diagnostic tests or lead to unnecessary testing, if information obtained with these devices is not interpreted together with other clinical and laboratory findings. To minimize the risk of potential pitfalls, HUDs should be used by experienced or properly trained users, and guideline-proposed algorithms for the diagnosis and treatment of cardiac emergencies must be strictly followed. Only in potentially life-saving circumstances, when expert users are not available in due course, might inexperienced users without supervision try to improve their diagnostic accuracy by using HUDs.[27] These situations should be exceptionally rare, and emergency ultrasound examination of the heart obtained by inexperienced users must be recorded and reviewed by experts as soon as possible.

FUTURE PERSPECTIVES

Many widely used diagnostic tools, including the stethoscope and electrocardiography, faced a deep skepticism at the time of their introduction; therefore, a fear that non-expert use of HUDs could endanger the reputation of echocardiography is somewhat expected.

However, these miniature imaging devices have a potential to make exciting changes in clinical medicine,[10,29] and their wide dissemination seems unstoppable. To ensure their proper use even in unexperienced hands, future medical students should learn not only gross anatomy during medical studies but also the ultrasound appearances of all organs the transducer can penetrate. It is encouraging that critical care basic ultrasound training was recently proposed as a formal part of an established anesthesiology—critical care medicine graduate medical education program.[28-31] This could speed up subsequent additional training tailored to specific needs of the users, and HUDs could indeed become "stethoscopes of the future" and an indispensable diagnostic tool in a wide range of clinical scenarios.[27,28]

It is, therefore, not difficult to envisage that many cardiac emergencies in the foreseeable future will accurately be recognized even by non-cardiologists using personal, smartphone-based, miniature ultrasound devices with or without the help of artificial intelligence (AI) algorithms.

As a matter of fact, many of the HUDs are now beginning to integrate AI for image analysis that may help clinicians in different parts of the examination:[32]

- *Image acquisition:* AI algorithms can assess image quality and provide feedback to the user through a real-time quality indicator.
- *Image quality:* AI algorithms reduce artifacts and improve image quality.
- *Image augmentation:* AI automatically increase the size of specific areas of interest allowing real-time highlighting of relevant anatomy or pathology.
- *Automatic calculation:* AI algorithms automatically assess LV ejection fraction, as well as regional function.

The following additional videos related to this chapter are available in the online resources: V18.9A, V18.9B, V18.9C, V18.9D, V18.9E; V18.10A, V18.10B, V18.10C; V18.11A, V18.11B, V18.11C, V18.11D; V18.12A, V18.12B, V18.12C; V18.13A, V18.13B, V18.13C, V18.13D, V18.13E; V18.14A, V18.14B; V18.15A, V18.15B, V18.15C, V18.15D, V18.15E; V18.16A, V18.16B, V18.16C, V18.16D, V18.17A, V18.17B, V18.17C, V18.18A, V18.18B, V18.18C, V18.18D, V18.19, V18.20A, V18.20B, V18.21, V18.22

LIST OF VIDEOS

VIDEO 18.1A   Comparison of image quality between high-end echo machine and handheld ultrasound devices in a patient with suboptimal echogenicity (1/2): A relatively poor left ventricular endocardial delineation with a handheld ultrasound device (shown here) can be overcome with a high-end scanner (see Video 18.1B).

VIDEO 18.1B   Comparison of image quality between high-end echo machine and handheld ultrasound devices in a patient with suboptimal echogenicity (2/2): A relatively poor left ventricular endocardial delineation with a handheld ultrasound device (see Video 18.1A) can be overcome with a high-end scanner (shown here).

VIDEO 18.2A   Comparison of color Doppler between high-end echo machine and handheld ultrasound devices (1/2): Regurgitant valve lesions (mitral regurgitation jet) may appear slightly more severe with handheld ultrasound devices (shown here) than with high-end echo machines (see Video 18.2B).

VIDEO 18.2B   Comparison of color Doppler between high-end echo machine and handheld ultrasound devices (2/2): Regurgitant valve lesions (mitral regurgitation jet) may appear slightly more severe with handheld ultrasound devices (see Video 18.2A) than with high-end echo machines (shown here).

VIDEO 18.3A   Comparison of image sector between high-end echo machine and handheld ultrasound devices (1/2): A wide image sector of high-end echo scanners allows the operator to encompass the entire heart in the apical four-chamber view (shown here) in contrast to a narrower image sector of handheld ultrasound devices (see Video 18.3B).

VIDEO 18.3B   Comparison of image sector between high-end echo machine and handheld ultrasound devices (2/2): A wide image sector of high-end echo scanners allows the operator to encompass the entire heart in the apical four-chamber view (see Video 18.3A) in contrast to a narrower image sector of handheld ultrasound devices (shown here).

VIDEO 18.4A   Focused cardiac ultrasound (FoCUS) by handheld ultrasound devices (Vscan, GE Healthcare) in a patient admitted for presumed acute coronary syndrome (1/2): Dilation of the right ventricle, hypokinesis of the right ventricular free wall and preserved contractility of the apical segment (McConnell's sign) (shown here), and flattening of the interventricular septum (D-shaped left ventricle) (see Video 18.4B) were all suggestive of pulmonary embolism, which was confirmed by pulmonary multislice computed tomography. Also note a mobile, hyperechogenic right ventricular mass suggestive of a thrombus (shown here).

VIDEO 18.4B   Focused cardiac ultrasound (FoCUS) by handheld ultrasound devices (Vscan, GE Healthcare) in a patient admitted for presumed acute coronary syndrome (2/2): Dilation of the right ventricle, hypokinesis of the right ventricular free wall and preserved contractility of the apical segment (McConnell's sign) (see Video 18.4A), and flattening of the interventricular septum (D-shaped left ventricle) (shown here) were all suggestive of pulmonary embolism, which was confirmed by pulmonary multislice computed tomography. Also note a mobile, hyperechogenic right ventricular mass suggestive of a thrombus (see Video 18.4A).

VIDEO 18.5   Lung comets: Ultrasound lung scan showing multiple diffuse bilateral B-lines in a patient with dyspnea caused by pulmonary congestion. Long hyperechogenic vertical lines (B-lines, comet tails, lung comets) are consistent with the presence of extravascular lung water.

VIDEO 18.6   Cardiac myxoma detected by focused cardiac ultrasound (FoCUS): FoCUS performed with a handheld ultrasound device in a patient presenting to the emergency department with nonspecific cardiorespiratory symptoms revealed in the apical four-chamber view left atrial echogenic mass attached to interatrial septum (cardiac myxoma), causing partial obstruction of the mitral valve in diastole. *(Video provided by RV.)*

VIDEO 18.7A   Unexpected finding of pleural effusion: Pleural effusion was diagnosed by a handheld ultrasound device in a patient with unexplained fever and suspected endocarditis.

VIDEO 18.7B   Unexpected finding of pericardial effusion: Pericardial effusion was diagnosed by a handheld ultrasound device from the parasternal short-axis view in a patient with fever.

VIDEO 18.7C   Unexpected finding of large pericardial effusion: Large pericardial effusion causing right ventricular collapse (cardiac tamponade) was diagnosed by a handheld ultrasound device in a patient with sepsis.

VIDEO 18.8A   Point-of-care ultrasound examination in a catheterization laboratory (1/3): Point-of-care ultrasound examination was performed with handheld ultrasound devices in a catheterization laboratory in a patient with a sudden unexplained hemodynamic instability and a new systolic murmur. Apical ballooning and basal hypercontractility of the left ventricle (shown here) caused dynamic left ventricular (LV) outflow obstruction (see Video 18.8B) as indicated by turbulent LV outflow tract flow in the apical long-axis view (see Video 18.8C).

VIDEO 18.8B   Point-of-care ultrasound examination in a catheterization laboratory (2/3): Point-of-care ultrasound examination was performed with a handheld ultrasound device in a catheterization laboratory in a patient with a sudden unexplained hemodynamic instability and a new systolic murmur. Apical ballooning and basal hypercontractility of the left ventricle (see Video 18.8A) caused dynamic left ventricular (LV) outflow obstruction (shown here) as indicated by turbulent LV outflow tract flow in the apical long-axis view (see Video 18.8C).

VIDEO 18.8C   Point-of-care ultrasound examination in a catheterization laboratory (3/3): Point-of-care ultrasound examination was performed with a handheld ultrasound device in a catheterization laboratory in a patient with a sudden unexplained hemodynamic instability and a new systolic murmur. Apical ballooning and basal hypercontractility of the left ventricle (see Video 18.8A) caused dynamic left ventricular (LV) outflow obstruction (see Video 18.8B) as indicated by turbulent LV outflow tract flow in the apical long-axis view (shown here).

VIDEO 18.9A   Focused cardiac ultrasound (FoCUS) after ventricular fibrillation (1/5): A 52-year-old woman with primary ventricular fibrillation during an acute inferior wall myocardial infarction. Bedside FoCUS with handheld ultrasound devices performed after defibrillation revealed inferoposterior wall asynergy (shown here; see also Video 18.9B), right ventricular dilation and free-wall akinesia (see Videos 18.9C and 18.9D), and an atrial septal defect (see Videos 18.9D and 18.9E), later confirmed later by transesophageal echocardiography.

VIDEO 18.9B   Focused cardiac ultrasound (FoCUS) after ventricular fibrillation (2/5): A 52-year-old woman with primary ventricular fibrillation during an acute inferior wall myocardial infarction. Bedside FoCUS with handheld ultrasound devices performed after defibrillation revealed inferoposterior wall asynergy (shown here; see also Video 18.9A), right ventricular dilation and free-wall akinesia (see Videos 18.9C and 18.9D), and an atrial septal defect (see Videos 18.9D and 18.9E), later confirmed by transesophageal echocardiography.

VIDEO 18.9C   Focused cardiac ultrasound (FoCUS) after ventricular fibrillation (3/5): A 52-year-old woman with primary ventricular fibrillation during an acute inferior wall myocardial infarction. Bedside FoCUS with handheld ultrasound devices performed after defibrillation revealed inferoposterior wall asynergy (see Videos 18.9A and 18.9B), right ventricular dilation and free-wall akinesia (shown here; see also Video 18.9D), and an atrial septal defect (see Videos 18.9D and 18.9E), confirmed later by transesophageal echocardiography.

VIDEO 18.9D   Focused cardiac ultrasound (FoCUS) after ventricular fibrillation (4/5): A 52-year-old woman with primary ventricular fibrillation during an acute inferior wall myocardial infarction. Bedside FoCUS with handheld ultrasound devices performed after defibrillation revealed inferoposterior wall asynergy (see Videos 18.9A and 18.9B), right ventricular dilation and free-wall akinesia (shown here; see also Video 18.9C), and an atrial septal defect (shown here; see also Video 18.9E), confirmed later by transesophageal echocardiography.

VIDEO 18.9E   Focused cardiac ultrasound (FoCUS) after ventricular fibrillation (5/5): A 52-year-old woman with primary ventricular fibrillation during an acute inferior wall myocardial infarction. Bedside FoCUS with handheld ultrasound devices performed after defibrillation revealed inferoposterior wall asynergy (see Videos 18.9A and 18.9B), right ventricular dilation and free-wall akinesia (see Videos 18.9C and 18.9D), and an atrial septal defect (shown here; see also Video 18.9D), confirmed later by transesophageal echocardiography.

VIDEO 18.10A   Inferior vena cava mass detected by Focused cardiac ultrasound (FoCUS) (1/3): FoCUS with a handheld ultrasound device showing a large, mobile, wormlike thrombus extending from the inferior vena cava into the right atrium (shown here) and further to the right ventricular outflow tract (see Videos 18.10B and 18.10C).

VIDEO 18.10B   Inferior vena cava mass detected by Focused cardiac ultrasound (FoCUS) (2/3): FoCUS using a handheld ultrasound device showing a large, mobile, wormlike thrombus extending from the inferior vena cava into the right atrium (see Video 18.10A) and further to the right ventricular outflow tract (shown here; see also Video 18.10C).

VIDEO 18.10C   Inferior vena cava mass detected by Focused cardiac ultrasound (FoCUS) (3/3): FoCUS with a handheld ultrasound device showing a large, mobile, wormlike thrombus extending from the inferior vena cava (see Video 18.10A) into the right atrium and further to the right ventricular outflow tract (shown here; see also Video 18.10B).

VIDEO 18.11A   Congenital apical ventricular septal defect in a patient with chest pain and murmur (1/4): Handheld ultrasound device examination in a patient with chest pain and a heart murmur demonstrating previously undiagnosed congenital apical ventricular septal defect (see also Videos 18.11B and 18.11C) with left-to-right shunt by color Doppler (see Video 18.11D). Note normal regional wall motion at the site of the defect.

VIDEO 18.11B   Congenital apical ventricular septal defect in a patient with chest pain and murmur (2/4): Handheld ultrasound device examination in a patient with chest pain and heart murmur demonstrating previously undiagnosed congenital apical ventricular septal defect (see also Videos 18.11A and 18.11C) with left-to-right shunt by color Doppler (see Video 18.11D). Note normal regional wall motion at the site of the defect.

VIDEO 18.11C   Congenital apical ventricular septal defect in a patient with chest pain and murmur (3/4): Handheld ultrasound device examination in a patient with chest pain and heart murmur demonstrating previously undiagnosed congenital apical ventricular septal defect (see also Videos 18.11A and 18.11B) with left-to-right shunt by color Doppler (see Video 18.11D). Note normal regional wall motion at the site of the defect.

VIDEO 18.11D   Congenital apical ventricular septal defect in a patient with chest pain and murmur (4/4): Handheld ultrasound device examination in a patient with chest pain and heart murmur demonstrating previously undiagnosed congenital apical ventricular septal defect (see Videos 18.11A, 18.11B, and 18.11.C) with left-to-right shunt by color Doppler (shown here). Note normal regional wall motion at the site of the defect.

VIDEO 18.12A   Lung comets in a patient with pulmonary edema (1/3): Lung ultrasound with a handheld ultrasound device showing vertical B-lines ("comet tails") in a patient with pulmonary edema and significant mitral regurgitation (see Videos 18.12B and 18.12C).

VIDEO 18.12B   Posterior wall hypokinesis in a patient with pulmonary edema (2/3): Posterior wall hypokinesis in a patient with pulmonary edema and significant mitral regurgitation (see Video 18.12C). Lung ultrasound with a handheld ultrasound device detected vertical B-lines ("comet tails"; see Video 18.12A).

VIDEO 18.12C   Significant mitral regurgitation in a patient with pulmonary edema (3/3): Significant mitral regurgitation in a patient with pulmonary edema and posterior wall hypokinesis (see also Video 18.12B). Lung ultrasound with a handheld ultrasound device revealed vertical B-lines ("comet tails"; see Video 18.12A).

VIDEO 18.13A   A patient with end-stage heart failure and hypotension (1/5): Biventricular systolic dysfunction (see also

Videos 18.13B and 18.13C) and pleural effusion (see Videos 18.13D and 18.13E) seen on handheld ultrasound device examination in a hypotensive patient with end-stage heart failure.

VIDEO 18.13B   A patient with end-stage heart failure and hypotension (2/5): Biventricular systolic dysfunction (see also Videos 18.13A and 18.13C) and pleural effusion (see Videos 18.13D and 18.13E) seen on handheld ultrasound device examination in a hypotensive patient with end-stage heart failure.

VIDEO 18.13C   A patient with end-stage heart failure and hypotension (3/5): Biventricular systolic dysfunction (see also Videos 18.13A and 18.13B) and pleural effusion (see Videos 18.13D and 18.13E) seen on handheld ultrasound device examination in a hypotensive patient with end-stage heart failure.

VIDEO 18.13D   A patient with end-stage heart failure and hypotension (4/5): Biventricular systolic dysfunction (see also Videos 18.13A, 18.13B, and 18.13C) and pleural effusion (shown here; see also Video 18.13E) seen on handheld ultrasound device examination in a hypotensive patient with end-stage heart failure.

VIDEO 18.13E   A patient with end-stage heart failure and hypotension (5/5): Biventricular systolic dysfunction (see also Videos 18.13A, 18.13B, and 18.13C) and pleural effusion (shown here; see also Video 18.13D) seen on handheld ultrasound device examination in a hypotensive patient with end-stage heart failure.

VIDEO 18.14A   A patient with hypotension and dyspnea (1/2): Focused cardiac ultrasound (FoCUS) by handheld ultrasound device examination showing previously undiagnosed severe left ventricular systolic dysfunction and moderate pericardial effusion in a patient evaluated for hypotension and dyspnea, as seen in the apical long-axis view (shown here) and the apical four-chamber view (see Video 18.14B).

VIDEO 18.14B   A patient with hypotension and dyspnea (2/2): Focused cardiac ultrasound (FoCUS) by handheld ultrasound device showing previously undiagnosed severe left ventricular systolic dysfunction and moderate pericardial effusion in a patient evaluated for hypotension and dyspnea, as seen in the apical long-axis view (see Video 18.14A) and the apical four-chamber view (shown here).

VIDEO 18.15A   A patient with worsening dyspnea after exertion (1/5): Focused cardiac ultrasound (FoCUS) with a handheld ultrasound device showing an eccentric mitral regurgitation jet (shown here; see also Video 18.15B) caused by a posterior leaflet flail (see Videos 18.15C, 18.15D, and 18.15E) in a patient presenting to the emergency department with worsening dyspnea after vigorous physical activity.

VIDEO 18.15B   A patient with worsening dyspnea after exertion (2/5): Focused cardiac ultrasound (FoCUS) with a handheld ultrasound device ce showing an eccentric mitral regurgitation jet (shown here; see Video 18.15A) caused by a posterior leaflet flail (see Videos 18.15C, 18.15D, and 18.15E) in a patient presenting to the emergency department with worsening dyspnea after vigorous physical activity.

VIDEO 18.15C   A patient with worsening dyspnea after exertion (3/5): Focused cardiac ultrasound (FoCUS) with a handheld ultrasound device showing an eccentric mitral regurgitation jet (see Videos 18.15A and 18.15B) caused by a posterior leaflet flail (shown here; see also Videos 18.15D and 18.15E) in a patient presenting to the emergency department with worsening dyspnea after vigorous physical activity.

VIDEO 18.15D   A patient with worsening dyspnea after exertion (4/5): Focused cardiac ultrasound (FoCUS) with a handheld ultrasound device showing an eccentric mitral regurgitation jet (see Videos 18.15A and 18.15B) caused by a posterior leaflet flail (shown here; see also Videos 18.15C and 18.15E) in a patient presenting to the emergency department with worsening dyspnea after vigorous physical activity.

VIDEO 18.15E   A patient with worsening dyspnea after exertion (5/5): Focused cardiac ultrasound (FoCUS) with a handheld ultrasound device showing an eccentric mitral regurgitation jet (see Videos 18.15A and 18.15B) caused by a posterior leaflet flail (shown here; see also Videos 18.15C and 18.15D) in a patient presenting to the emergency department with worsening dyspnea after vigorous physical activity.

VIDEO 18.16A   A patient with typical chest pain and T-wave inversions (1/4): Focused cardiac ultrasound (FoCUS) with a handheld ultrasound device showing extensive anteroapical left ventricular asynergy in a patient with typical chest pain and precordial T-wave inversions, as seen from the parasternal long-axis view (shown here), apical four-chamber view (see Video 18.16B), apical two-chamber view (see Video 18.16C), and apical long-axis view (see Video 18.16D).

VIDEO 18.16B   A patient with typical chest pain and T-wave inversions (2/4): Focused cardiac ultrasound (FoCUS) with a handheld ultrasound device showing extensive anteroapical left ventricular asynergy in a patient with typical chest pain and precordial T-wave inversions, as seen from the parasternal long-axis view (see Video 18.16A), apical four-chamber view (shown here), apical two-chamber view (see Video 18.16C), and apical long-axis view (see Video 18.16D).

VIDEO 18.16C   A patient with typical chest pain and T-wave inversions (3/4): Focused cardiac ultrasound (FoCUS) with a handheld ultrasound device showing extensive anteroapical left ventricular asynergy in a patient with typical chest pain and precordial T-wave inversions, as seen from the parasternal long-axis view (see Video 18.16A), apical four-chamber view (see Video 18.16B), apical two-chamber view (shown here), and apical long-axis view (see Video 18.16D).

VIDEO 18.16D   A patient with typical chest pain and T-wave inversions (4/4): Focused cardiac ultrasound (FoCUS) with a handheld ultrasound device showing extensive anteroapical left ventricular asynergy in a patient with typical chest pain and precordial T-wave inversions, as seen from the parasternal long-axis view (see Video 18.16A), apical four-chamber view (see Video 18.16B), apical two-chamber view (see Video 18.16C), and apical long-axis view (shown here).

VIDEO 18.17A   A young patient with stroke 10 days after mild COVID-19 (1/3): Focused cardiac ultrasound (FoCUS) with a handheld ultrasound device showing severe left ventricular systolic dysfunction in a patient with stroke shortly after mild COVID-19, as seen from the apical four-chamber view (shown here). An apical thrombus was observed in a modified apical view (see Video 18.17B) and short-axis view (see Video 18.17C).

VIDEO 18.17B   A young patient with stoke 10 days after mild COVID-19 (2/3): Focused cardiac ultrasound (FoCUS) with a handheld ultrasound device showing severe left ventricular systolic dysfunction in a patient with stroke shortly after mild COVID-19, as seen from the apical four-chamber view (see Video 18.17A). An apical thrombus was observed in a modified apical view (shown here) and short-axis view (see Video 18.17C).

VIDEO 18.17C   A young patient with stoke 10 days after mild COVID-19 (3/3): Focused cardiac ultrasound (FoCUS) with a handheld ultrasound device showing severe left ventricular systolic dysfunction in a patient with stroke shortly after mild COVID-19, as seen from the apical four-chamber view (see Video 18.17A). An apical thrombus was observed in a modified apical view (see Video 18.17B) and short-axis view (shown here).

VIDEO 18.18A   Acute pulmonary embolism in an elderly patient with COVID-19 (1/4): Seven days after the onset of the disease, the patient with COVID-19 was presented with acute dyspnea, hypoxemia, hypotension, and tachycardia. Chest X-ray was unremarkable. ECG was unremarkable (apart from tachycardia). In parasternal long-axis view, FoCUS performed with a handheld ultrasound device revealed right ventricular dilatation with underfilled, hypercontractile left ventricle (shown here; time: 9:37:01). In parasternal short-axis view, septal flattening ("D-shape sign") can be noted (see Video 18.18B; time: 9:37:12). A serpiginous, highly mobile thrombus was observed within dilated right heart chambers in a modified apical four-chamber view (see Video 18.18C; time: 9:38:06). It took 1 minute for the FOCUS exam and making the diagnosis! The effect of thrombolysis is shown on Video 18.18D.

VIDEO 18.18B   Acute pulmonary embolism in an elderly patient with COVID-19 (2/4): Seven days of the onset of the disease, the patient with COVID-19 was presented with acute dyspnea, hypoxemia, hypotension, and tachycardia. Chest X-ray was unremarkable. ECG was unremarkable (apart from tachycardia). In this parasternal short-axis view, FoCUS performed with a handheld ultrasound device revealed septal flattening ("D-shape sign"). A serpiginous, highly mobile thrombus was observed within dilated right heart chambers in a modified apical four-chamber view (see Video 18.18C). Dilatation of the right ventricle can be also appreciated from the parasternal long-axis view (see Video 18.18A). The effect of thrombolysis is shown on Video 18.18D.

VIDEO 18.18C   Acute pulmonary embolism in an elderly patient with COVID-19 (3/4): Seven days of the onset of the disease, the patient with COVID-19 was presented with acute dyspnea, hypoxemia, hypotension, and tachycardia. Chest X-ray was unremarkable. ECG was unremarkable (apart from tachycardia). In this modified apical four-chamber view, FoCUS performed with a handheld ultrasound device showed serpiginous, highly mobile thrombus within dilated

right heart chambers. In a parasternal short-axis view, septal flattening ("D-shape sign") can be noted (see Video 18.18B). Dilatation of the right ventricle can be also appreciated from the parasternal long-axis view (see Video 18.18A). It took one minute for the FOCUS exam and making the diagnosis (please note the time indicated on consecutive Videos 18.18A, 18.18B, and 18.18C)! Effect of thrombolysis is shown on Video 18.18D.

VIDEO 18.18D   Acute pulmonary embolism in an elderly patient with COVID-19 (4/4): Effect of thrombolysis in a patient with acute pulmonary embolism presented on Videos 18.18A, 18.18B, and 18.18C. Note that, 2 hours after alteplase administration (time: 11:27:47), thrombotic masses disappeared from the right heart chambers (which are still dilated), without clinical signs of recurrent pulmonary or systemic embolism.

VIDEO 18.19   Stress cardiomyopathy in a mechanically ventilated COVID-19 patient: Focused cardiac ultrasound (FoCUS), performed with a handheld ultrasound device, showing left ventricular apical ballooning and hypercontractility of basal segments (apical four-chamber view), consistent with stress cardiomyopathy, in a mechanically ventilated COVID-19 patient.

VIDEO 18.20A   Mitral valve endocarditis in an immunocompromised COVID-19 patient (1/2): Focused cardiac ultrasound (FoCUS) with a handheld ultrasound device showing large mitral valve vegetations in an immunocompromised COVID-19 patient, as seen in apical long-axis view (shown here). Color Doppler revealed significant mitral regurgitation (see Video 18.20B).

VIDEO 18.20B   Mitral valve endocarditis in an immunocompromised COVID-19 patient (2/2): Focused cardiac ultrasound (FoCUS) with a handheld ultrasound device showing large mitral valve vegetations in an immunocompromised COVID-19 patient, as seen in apical long-axis view (see Video 18.20A). Color Doppler revealed significant mitral regurgitation (shown here).

VIDEO 18.21   Large pericardial effusion in a patient with COVID-19: Focused cardiac ultrasound (FoCUS) with a handheld ultrasound device showing large pericardial effusion in a COVID-19 patient, as seen in parasternal short-axis view.

VIDEO 18.22   Hyperdynamic left ventricle in a hypotensive, mechanically ventilated COVID-19 patient: Focused cardiac ultrasound (FoCUS) with a handheld ultrasound device showing hyperdynamic left ventricle, as seen in subcostal short-axis view, in a mechanically ventilated, hypotensive COVID-19 patient. The subsequent work-up revealed that upper gastrointestinal bleeding was causing hemodynamic instability.

REFERENCES

1. Roelandt J., Wladimiroff J.W., Baars A.M. Ultrasonic real time imaging with a hand-held-scanner. Part II—initial clinical experience. Ultrasound Med Biol 1978; 4(2): 93–97.

2. Dalen H., Haugen B.O., Graven T. Feasibility and clinical implementation of hand-held echocardiography. Expert Rev Cardiovasc Ther 2013; 11(1): 49–54.

3. Rugolotto M., Chang C.P., Hu B., Schnittger I., Liang D.H. Clinical use of cardiac ultrasound performed with a hand-carried device in patients admitted for acute cardiac care. Am J Cardiol 2002; 90: 1040–1042.

4. Goodkin G.M., Spevack D.M., Tunick P.A., Kronzon I. How useful is hand-carried echocardiography in critically ill patients? J Am Coll Cardiol 2001; 37: 2019–2022.

5. Cardim N., Dalen H., Voigt J.U., et al. The use of handheld ultrasound devices: a position statement of the European Association of Cardiovascular Imaging (2018 update). Eur Heart J Cardiovasc Imaging. 2019; 20(3): 245–252.

6. Seward J.B., Douglas P.S., Erbel R., et al. Hand-carried cardiac ultrasound (HCU) device: recommendations regarding new technology. A report from the Echocardiography Task Force on New Technology of the Nomenclature and Standards Committee of the American Society of Echocardiography. J Am Soc Echocardiogr 2002; 15(4): 369–373.

7. Soliman-Aboumarie H., Breithardt O.A., Gargani L., Trambaiolo P., Neskovic A.N. How-to: focus cardiac ultrasound in acute settings. Eur Heart J Cardiovasc Imaging. 2022; 23(2): 150–153.

8. Savell S.C., Baldwin D.S., Blessing A., Medelllin K.L., Savell C.B., Maddry J.K. Military use of point of care ultrasound (POCUS). J Spec Oper Med. 2021; 21(2): 35–42.

9. Cheung J.C., Lam K.N. POCUS in COVID-19: pearls and pitfalls. Lancet Respir Med. 2020; 8(5): e34.

10. Testuz A., Müller H., Keller P.F., et al. Diagnostic accuracy of pocketsize handheld echocardiographs used by cardiologists in the acute care setting. Eur Heart J Cardiovasc Imaging 2013; 14(1): 38–42.

11. Biais M., Carrié C., Delaunay F., Morel N., Revel P., Janvier G. Evaluation of a new pocket echoscopic device for focused cardiac ultrasonography in an emergency setting. Crit Care 2012; 16(3): R82.

12. Lisi M., Cameli M., Mondillo S., et al. Incremental value of pocketsized imaging device for bedside diagnosis of unilateral pleural effusions and ultrasound-guided thoracentesis. Interact Cardiovasc Thorac Surg 2012; 15(4): 596–601.

13. Skjetne K., Graven T., Haugen B.O., Salvesen Ø., Kleinau J.O., Dalen H. Diagnostic influence of cardiovascular screening by pocketsize ultrasound in a cardiac unit. Eur J Echocardiogr 2011; 12(10): 737–743.

14. Culp B.C., Mock J.D., Ball T.R., Chiles C.D., Culp W.C., Jr. The pocket echocardiograph: a pilot study of its validation and feasibility in intubated patients. Echocardiography 2011; 28(4): 371–377.

15. Moore C.L., Copel J.A. Point-of-care ultrasonography. N Engl J Med 2011; 364(8): 749–757.

16. Choi B.G., Mukherjee M., Dala P., et al. Interpretation of remotely downloaded pocket-size cardiac ultrasound images on a webenabled smartphone: validation against workstation evaluation. J Am Soc Echocardiogr 2011; 24(12): 1325–1330.

17. Liebo M.J., Israel R.L., Lillie E.O., Smith M.R., Rubenson D.S., Topol E.J. Is pocket mobile echocardiography the next-generation stethoscope? A cross-sectional comparison of rapidly acquired images with standard transthoracic echocardiography. Ann Intern Med 2011; 155(1): 33–38.

18. Giusca S., Jurcut R., Ticulescu R., et al. Accuracy of hand-held echocardiography for bedside diagnostic evaluation in a tertiary cardiology center: comparison with standard echocardiography. Echocardiography 2011; 28(2): 136–141.

19. Mjølstad O.C., Andersen G.N., Dalen H., et al. Feasibility and reliability of point-of-care pocket-size echocardiography performed by medical residents. Eur Heart J Cardiovasc Imaging 2013; 14(12): 1195–1202.

20. Prinz C., Voigt J.U. Diagnostic accuracy of a hand-held ultrasound scanner in routine patients referred for echocardiography. J Am Soc Echocardiogr 2011; 24(2): 111–116.

21. Andersen G.N., Haugen B.O., Graven T., Salvesen O., Mjølstad O.C., Dalen H. Feasibility and reliability of point-of-care pocket-sized echocardiography. Eur J Echocardiogr 2011; 12(9): 665–670.

22. Lucas B.P., Candotti C., Margeta B., et al. Diagnostic accuracy of hospitalist-performed hand-carried ultrasound echocardiography after a brief training program. J Hosp Med 2009; 4(6): 340–349.

23. Galderisi M., Santoro A., Versiero M., et al. Improved cardiovascular diagnostic accuracy by pocket size imaging device in non-cardiologic outpatients: the NaUSiCa (Naples Ultrasound Stethoscope in Cardiology) study. Cardiovasc Ultrasound 2010; 8: 51.

24. Blanco P., Martínez Buendía C. Point-of-care ultrasound in cardiopulmonary resuscitation: a concise review. J Ultrasound. 2017; 20(3): 193–198.

25. Neskovic A.N., Skinner H., Price S., et al. Focus cardiac ultrasound core curriculum and core syllabus of the European Association of Cardiovascular Imaging European Heart Journal. Eur Heart J Cardiovasc Imaging 2018; 19: 475–481.

26. Spencer K.T., Kimura B.J., Korcarz C.E., Pellikka P.A., Rahko P.S., Siegel R.J. Focused cardiac ultrasound: recommendations from the American Society of Echocardiography. J Am Soc Echocardiogr 2013; 26(6): 567–581.

27. Neskovic A.N., Hagendorff A., Lancellotti P., et al. Emergency echocardiography: the European Association of Cardiovascular Imaging recommendations. Eur Heart J Cardiovasc Imaging 2013; 14(1): 1–11.

28. Fagley R.E., Haney M.F., Beraud A.S., et al. Critical care basic ultrasound learning goals for American anesthesiology critical care trainees: recommendations from an expert group. Anesth Analg 2015; 120(5): 1041–1053.

29. Roelandt J.R. Ultrasound stethoscopy. Eur J Intern Med 2004; 15: 337–347.

30. Panoulas V.F., Daigeler A.L., Malaweera A.S., et al. Pocket-size handheld cardiac ultrasound as an adjunct to clinical examination in the hands of medical students and junior doctors. Eur Heart J Cardiovasc Imaging 2013; 14(4): 323–330.

31. Solomon S.D., Saldana F. Point-of-care ultrasound in medical education—stop listening and look. N Engl J Med 2014; 370(12): 1083–1085.

32. Stewart J.E., Goudie A., Mukherjee A., Dwivedi G. Artificial intelligence-enhanced echocardiography in the emergency department. Emerg Med Australas 2021; 33(6): 1117–1120.

Focus cardiac ultrasound (FoCUS)

19

Guido Tavazzi, Costanza Natalia Julia Colombo, and Gabriele Via

Key Points

- Focus cardiac ultrasound (FoCUS) is a point-of-care, simplified, problem-oriented, goal-directed application of echocardiography aimed at detecting a limited number of critical cardiac conditions in critical scenarios for time-sensitive clinical decision-making.
- This limited approach is based on a "pattern recognition" interpretation, recognizing a few distinctive features of the cardiac ultrasonographic picture.
- FoCUS is typically performed by clinicians with cardiac ultrasound training that is limited in comparison to comprehensive echocardiography. It is done by using any ultrasound machine capable of basic cardiac ultrasound modalities, in any in-hospital or out-of-hospital critical scenario.
- The main goal of FoCUS is to uncover pathophysiology and mitigate diagnostic uncertainty and not necessarily reach a conclusive diagnosis.
- FoCUS should entail a low-threshold trigger for further testing, typically, but not exclusively, comprehensive echocardiography.

This chapter is aimed at providing the echocardiography beginner with theoretical and practical knowledge on focus cardiac ultrasound (FoCUS) and also at describing to clinicians competent in comprehensive echocardiography the specific features of this simplified cardiac ultrasound diagnostic test.

FOCUS: DEFINITION, AIMS, COMPETENCE, AND LIMITATIONS

FoCUS is a limited, point-of-care cardiac ultrasound examination, conforming to standardized, targeted scanning protocols, which represents an adjunct to the physical examination.[1–4]

FoCUS should be considered the cardiac application within the broader point-of-care ultrasound praxis[5,6]; in the last years, the European Association of Cardiovascular Imaging (EACVI) included lung ultrasound (LUS) in the FoCUS core curriculum[1] since it may help in narrowing down the differential diagnosis. Indeed, an International Evidence Based Consensus Conference promoted by the World Interactive Network Focused on Critical Ultrasound (WINFOCUS) and supported by multiple scientific bodies defined FoCUS nomenclature, scope of practice, indications, technique, targets of the exam, and the frameworks for education, quality assurance, credentialing and accreditation.[3] It is used in *critical scenarios*, where "critical" may either refer to the patient's compromised vital parameters but also to the discrepancy between the patient's needs and available resources (e.g., mass casualty scenarios, wherein patient screening

DOI: 10.1201/9781003245407-19

for triage purposes can be the critical issue, and/or austere, remote, or scarce-resource settings wherein patients deserve immediate critical decisions about their management and/or transport).

The essence of FoCUS lies in the following features: [1,2]

- *Performed at the point of care*—It is performed directly by the clinician attending the patient.
- *Adjunct to physical examination*—It does not replace physical examination, but it could be useful to guide clinical decision at the bedside.
- *Narrow in scope*—It aims to detect a limited number of critical cardiac conditions; it is not an exhaustive cardiac investigation and provides pathophysiologic insight on relevant clinical issues that require a rapid response. FoCUS hastens the diagnostic process by narrowing the differential diagnosis, mainly in a rule-in/rule-out (yes/no) fashion.
- *Problem-oriented*—It is dictated by the patient's symptoms.
- *Goal-directed*—Centered on clinically relevant question or problem (e.g., Why is the patient hypotensive? Might the patient benefit from fluid loading? Is major right ventricular [RV] systolic dysfunction responsible for the shock?).
- *Time-sensitive*—It is an abbreviated examination focused on a few targets and prioritized according to the critical patient's needs.
- *A simplified examination*—It is based on a limited number of transthoracic views, uses limited ultrasound modalities (two-dimensional [2D] and M-mode), and addresses an evidence-based restricted list of targets.
- *Provides qualitative or semiquantitative data*—Due to its limited scope, FoCUS examination collects mostly qualitative or semiquantitative findings of cardiac morphology and function.
- *Entails a low-threshold trigger for further testing*—FoCUS should always trigger additional testing (comprehensive echocardiography, angio-computed tomography, or cardiac catheterization) when it is inconclusive or nondiagnostic, when findings are discordant with the clinical picture or when cardiovascular abnormalities are detected and suspected cardiac disease goes beyond the diagnostic capabilities of this approach.

FoCUS is performed by appropriately trained clinicians to detect essential information in critical scenarios for time-sensitive clinical decision-making. Not only cardiologists but a wide range of medical professionals (anesthesiologists, intensive care specialists, emergency physicians, internists, pneumologists, cardiac surgeons, fellows, sonographers, and cardiac physiologists) are involved in the management of patients with emergencies. Although typically conducted in the emergency setting by non-cardiologists with limited echocardiography training, by means of portable or handheld ultrasound devices (HUDs), FoCUS is strictly related neither to the professional profile of the operator performing the examination nor to the type of ultrasound device used or the specific clinical scenario.[1–4] Thus, FoCUS can be performed *by any clinician appropriately trained* in FoCUS, *with any ultrasound machine capable of basic cardiac ultrasound modalities*, in any in-hospital or out-of-hospital *scenario where it is indicated.*

Compared with the demanding training required for competence in comprehensive echocardiography, competence in FoCUS can be achieved after a shorter, intensive, and narrow scope-oriented training.[7–10]

FoCUS should never be considered as an echocardiographic examination. The key distinction between FoCUS and comprehensive echocardiography lies in the *amount of information* obtained. Echocardiography refers to a comprehensive standard investigation of cardiac function and morphology. FoCUS examination provides information to identify basic cardiac conditions and gross pathologies, reported as absent or present (yes/no; i.e., qualitative assessment).[4] This makes awareness of the finite diagnostic capability of the application and of the operator's competence mandatory for the FoCUS practitioner. Neglecting the limitations of FoCUS carries the *risks of overlooking* important abnormalities beyond the scope of FoCUS and *misinterpretation* of an incomplete dataset. Clear definition of FoCUS purview and limitations should be incorporated into any FoCUS training curriculum.[4]

Performing FoCUS or using simplified ultrasound devices should never leave the patient without the opportunity of a better diagnostic test, where required. *Continuous supervision and quality control* are essential, and the established *emergency echocardiography service* in the hospital may provide professional, educational, and training support for non-cardiologists performing FoCUS, through 24-hour availability of second opinion and consultative or on-call services, teamwork (professional help, consultations, regular reviewing of cases), and continuous supervision.[1–4]

CLINICAL APPLICATIONS OF FOCUS

In several critical scenarios, FoCUS should become an essential part of the assessment of the patient with cardiopulmonary instability. It can help to narrow the differential diagnosis, uncover pathophysiology, identify reversible causes, guide therapeutic interventions, and monitor hemodynamic response to therapies. In addition, the assessment of gross signs of chronic heart disease with FoCUS is crucial to trigger further diagnostic tests like comprehensive echocardiography.[1,11]

Shock

FoCUS examination allows categorization into one of the main shock pathophysiologic subsets (hypovolemic, cardiogenic, obstructive, distributive) through detection of either the specific cardiac dysfunction involved (e.g., left ventricular [LV] or RV failure, cardiac tamponade, severe valvular dysfunction) or the consequences of disturbances in volume status or peripheral circulation at the level of the heart (e.g., hypovolemia, vasodilation).[11,12]

Identification of severe global right and left ventricular systolic dysfunction and pericardial effusion are all targets of FoCUS examination. In patients with circulatory shock, detection of severe global LV systolic dysfunction (V19.1) or biventricular failure (V19.3), due to myocardial ischemia, sepsis-related myocardial dysfunction, myocarditis, myocardial toxicity, or decompensation of chronic heart failure, suggests diagnosis of cardiogenic shock. The same categorization should be applied in case of severe acute valvular abnormalities and large intracardiac masses associated to severe cardiovascular compromise. Valvular assessment is potentially complex, entailing echocardiographic skills going beyond FoCUS competence; nevertheless, gross recognition of major valve disease on the basis of simple morphologic findings (leaflet or cusp flail, apparent severe valve thickening, evident disruption of the valvular apparatus, masses attached to valves) has been demonstrated as feasible[13] and should be part of a FoCUS examination (V19.8, V19.8.1).

FoCUS allows also the detection of free pericardial effusions (V19.5, V19.5.1) and their hemodynamic relevance; it hastens pericardiocentesis when tamponade is diagnosed (V19.6, V19.6.1), minimizing procedure-related complications and increasing success rate.[14,15]

Detection of RV dilation and hypokinesia (V19.2, V19.2.1) in a patient with shock may also suggest cardiogenic shock due to obstructive shock due to massive pulmonary embolism,[13] RV acute myocardial infarction [AMI], or decompensation of chronic RV failure (V19.9, V19.9.1),

Regarding the diagnosis of pulmonary embolism, FoCUS has high sensitivity for massive pulmonary embolism (acute cor pulmonale) in high-risk patients (see Chapter 7). In rare cases thrombus "in transit" can be detected in right-side cavities or in the inferior vena cava [IVC]. According to current guidelines, echocardiography is recommended as a first-step diagnostic test for investigation of suspected pulmonary embolism in patients with hemodynamic instability: the absence of signs of RV dysfunction allows the exclusion of pulmonary embolism as an actual cause of the circulatory shock. However, in hemodynamic stable patients, it does not allow ruling out thromboembolic disease.[16] In acute pulmonary embolism, venous ultrasound (see Chapter 7) may detect deep venous thrombosis, while LUS shows dry lungs pattern and/or consolidations due to pulmonary infarction.[11]

Current evidence suggests a role for FoCUS in identifying patients who may benefit from fluid loading, especially in pronounced states of hypovolemia (V19.4, V19.4.1). A typical "hyperdynamic pattern" characterized by small, hyperkinetic ventricles and small or collapsed IVC should prompt a diagnosis of severe hypovolemia (this evaluation should be assessed with normal RV function, as LV filling could be impaired by RV failure).[11,17]

Hypovolemia in hypotensive patients is also associated with reduced IVC diameter (dIVC), showing its maximum size at different phases of the respiratory cycle, according to intrathoracic pressure variation (maximum end-expiratory diameter in patients on spontaneous breathing, maximum end-inspiratory diameter in patients on mechanically ventilation).[18–20] Further investigations should include the assessment of caval indices, named "IVC collapsibility index" in spontaneous breathing (positive when at least 50% IVC size decrease at inspiration is demonstrated) or "IVC distensibility index" in mechanical ventilation (positive when at least 18% IVC size increase at inspiration is demonstrated). Both indices are calculated with the formula (dIVC maximum − dIVC minimum) / dIVC minimum × 100.[21,22] However, both these indices have shown conflicting results regarding their reliability as a diagnostic test for hypovolemia or fluid responsiveness.[23,24] Furthermore, ultrasound assessment of the IVC cannot estimate fluid responsiveness when mechanical ventilation is performed with assisted or non-invasive modalities and in other clinical conditions like lung hyperinflation (e.g., asthma or COPD exacerbation), significant inspiratory effort (producing markedly negative intrathoracic pressures), or in case of cardiac conditions, impeding venous return (e.g., cardiac tamponade, RV severe dysfunction).[25,26]

In distributive shock due to sepsis or anaphylaxis, characterized by low systemic vascular resistance (and reduced LV afterload), FoCUS may detect hyperdynamic LV with preserved biventricular systolic function and small LV end-systolic dimensions with normal end-diastolic size, according to pathophysiology. In some cases, FoCUS can detect cardiac cause of sepsis (e. g. valvular vegetation in case of infective endocarditis).[11,27]

The presence of complementary non-cardiac ultrasound findings, within a multi-organ point-of-care ultrasound examination (PoCUS) approach shock can add much to the FoCUS exam in terms of diagnostic yield.[28]

Cardiac arrest

International guidelines in advanced life support suggest that point-of-care ultrasound might be considered as adjunct to standard evaluation to identify treatable causes of cardiac arrest (see also Chapter 5). However, the priority during cardiac arrest is high-quality cardiopulmonary resuscitation with minimal interruptions to reduce the no-flow intervals: for this reason, guidelines strongly recommend that ultrasound examination should be performed by skilled operators, should neither cause prolonged interruption of chest compressions nor delay electrical treatment of ventricular arrhythmias.[29,30] One of the major components of practical training in FoCUS is specific training to use it as a part of ACLS algorithm, with an accent on the expected pathologies, communication of findings to the resuscitation team, and ACLS compliance.[1]

FoCUS is a valuable imaging technique to identify treatable causes of cardiac arrest during cardiopulmonary resuscitation, at the bedside.[11] As underlined before, the use of FoCUS in cardiac arrest should be preceded and followed by high-quality cardiopulmonary resuscitation (V5.11, audiovisual), timed to perfectly fit into the 10-second pulse check, within an effective, standardized, algorithmic execution scheme.[1–4,31]

Several observational trials have shown that the use of FoCUS in cardiac arrest identifies the presence or absence of organized myocardial mechanical activity, rapidly detects a potentially treatable cause, guides treatment and management, and predicts outcome.[31–35]

FoCUS goals in cardiac arrest resuscitation are multiple[11,33]:

- *Identifying the patterns of cardiac arrest in the setting of nonshockable rhythms*—The absence of organized cardiac contractility in the presence of undetectable electrocardiographic activity allows confirmation of asystole (V19.7)—In the presence of a potentially viable electrocardiographic rhythm, pulseless electrical activity (PEA), FoCUS identifies *true PEA* when demonstrating absent cardiac kinesis. The presence of ventricular contraction in PEA identifies an organized myocardial mechanical activity cardiac arrest pattern, also called *pseudo PEA* (a profound hypotension with an impalpable pulse). The detection of true PEA has been associated with an extremely poor outcome.[35]
- *Detection for the potentially reversible causes of cardiac arrest and guidance of consequent life-saving procedures*—Detection of organized myocardial contractility fosters identification of and therapy for some of the potentially treatable causes of cardiac arrest indicated by resuscitation guidelines (coronary thrombosis, pulmonary embolism, hypovolemia, tamponade). In case of cardiac kinetic activity in PEA, detection of severe LV systolic dysfunction with regional wall motion abnormalities and absence of signs of chronic LV disease suggests AMI. Detection of acute cor pulmonale presumptive diagnosis of massive pulmonary embolism. Pericardial effusion with signs of cardiac compression is diagnostic of tamponade. A hyperdynamic, small heart with a small, collapsible IVC should prompt aggressive volume resuscitation and a search for the cause of severe hypovolemia. Furthermore, LUS examination could identify pneumothorax as cause of cardiac arrest. Noticeably, of the main potentially treatable underlying causes of cardiac arrest, only three may otherwise be diagnosed at the bedside without FoCUS, using currently recommended monitoring and investigation (hypoxia, hypothermia, hypokalemia, or hyperkalemia).[29,30,33]

- *Role in the post-cardiac arrest setting*—FoCUS enables earlier detection of recovery of cardiac activity than simple pulse palpation. Furthermore, immediately after recovery of spontaneous circulation (ROSC), it can provide essential information in monitoring cardiac function and volume status, guide further therapeutic interventions and evaluate their efficacy.

An example of a FoCUS protocol for cardiac arrest, Focused Echocardiography Evaluation in Life Support (FEEL),[31] is described in Figure 19.1 and efficient ACLS-compliant teamwork during CPR is presented in V5.11 (audiovisual).

Trauma

Since early studies in 1992 showing decreased mortality with use of FoCUS in penetrating cardiac injury,[36] a large body of literature has been slowly added, making FoCUS an integral part of the evaluation of trauma patients. FoCUS for the *screening of hemopericardium* in penetrating and blunt chest injury (see Chapter 16) is incorporated into the Advanced Trauma Life Support (ATLS) training and practice, as a part of the Focused Assessment with Sonography for Trauma (FAST).[37]

FoCUS is also valuable in this context to diagnose blood loss associated hypovolemia, and even with negative results on a FAST examination is a strong predictor of hemorrhagic shock that will respond to volume.[20] Indeed, detection of a FoCUS pattern characterized by "empty or flat IVC" and small hyperdynamic ventricles (V19.4, V19.4.1) leads to better fluid management of shocked trauma patients.[38] Accuracy of IVC size may, however, be limited in milder degrees of hemorrhage.[39]

Finally, depressed myocardial contractility in the absence of signs of chronic cardiac disease may provide clues to *myocardial contusion* and trigger comprehensive echocardiography in due time. The recognition of signs of pre-existing cardiac disease may add information relevant for patient management.

Chest pain

FoCUS may be helpful also in the assessment of life-threatening chest pain syndromes.[1–4] As described earlier, FoCUS can rule out *massive embolism* when acute cor pulmonale is excluded, or it can raise suspicion for pulmonary embolism when acute cor pulmonale is detected, allowing immediate treatment if the patient is hemodynamic instable and computed tomography pulmonary angiography (CTPA) cannot be immediately performed.[12] In the suspicion of pulmonary embolism, FoCUS can be combined with compression venous ultrasound (VUS) to detect deep vein thrombosis: this finding in suspected pulmonary embolism is sufficient to start

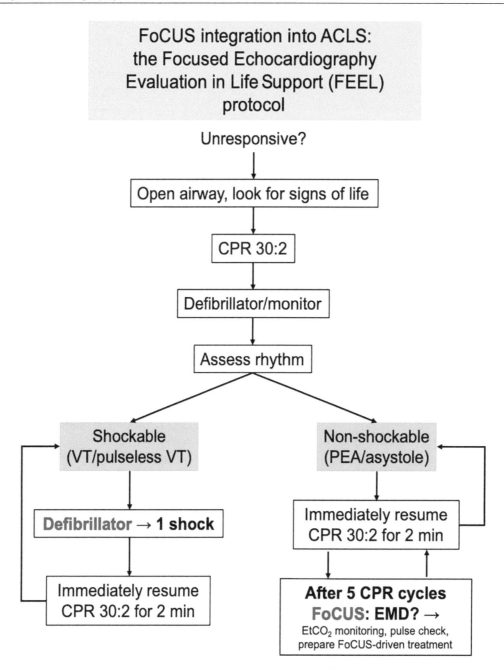

FIGURE 19.1 The Focused Echocardiography Evaluation in Life Support (FEEL) protocol. This is the paradigm of the protocol-based focused cardiac ultrasound (FoCUS) approach. It is conceived to be incorporated in an ACLS-conforming fashion into the extremely time-sensitive cardiac arrest scenarios. ACLS: Advanced Cardiac Life Support; CPR: cardiopulmonary resuscitation; EMD: electromechanical dissociation; ETCO2: end tidal carbon dioxide.[32]

anticoagulant treatment without further testing, after risk assessment evaluation.[16,40]

The role of FoCUS in the diagnosis of myocardial ischemia is more limited. Transthoracic echocardiography (see Chapter 2) is a class I indication in chest pain of suspected myocardial ischemic origin when the electrocardiogram (ECG) is nondiagnostic. The absence of regional wall motion abnormalities has a high negative predictive value for myocardial ischemia in chest pain patients, whereas its presence is not sufficiently specific.[41] However, accurate analysis of segmental wall motion and thickening is a highly technically demanding skill, falling well beyond the boundaries of FoCUS competence.[1–4]

In patients with suspected acute thoracic aorta dissection, FoCUS may raise clinical suspicion for the disease by detecting pericardial and/or pleural effusion, and/or a dilated aortic root (>4 cm) suggestive of aortic type A dissection. Of note, neither FoCUS nor comprehensive transthoracic echocardiography is sufficiently accurate to exclude aortic dissection, which remains within the diagnostic domain of transesophageal echocardiography and computed tomography (CT).

Dyspnea and respiratory failure

FoCUS provides useful information also in patients with acute respiratory symptoms. Furthermore, its *integration with LUS* allows a rapid evaluation of the cardiopulmonary conditions of the patient with acute dyspnea. According to the EACVI core curriculum, a FoCUS operator should be trained in basic LUS, becoming able to recognize pulmonary edema with interstitial syndrome (multiple diffuse bilateral B-lines—wet lung pattern) (V19.13) and pleural effusions[1] (V19.14).

In a patient with dyspnea, FoCUS may reveal *signs of pre-existing cardiac disease* LV (dilated heart chambers, hypertrophy—potentially suggesting decompensation of chronic heart failure), global LV systolic dysfunction, presence of acute cor pulmonale or pericardial effusion. These patients should always be referred for comprehensive echocardiography. In fact, full diagnostics of cardiac cause of dyspnea or respiratory failure, which usually includes the assessment of LV diastolic function, pulmonary pressure, and valvular function, goes far beyond the scope of the FoCUS.[1,11]

In patients with respiratory symptoms, *multi-organ point-of-care ultrasonography* (lung, cardiac, and deep venous ultrasound) has a high diagnostic potential and likely greater accuracy than sole FoCUS examination.[42] For example, in the presence of LV dysfunction, a diffuse lung ultrasound B-pattern may be detected with LUS (V19.13) and suggest diagnosis of congestive heart failure as cause of dyspnea.[11,43]

Syncope

FoCUS examination might be also useful in the evaluation of patients who present with *syncope*. It may detect any severe underlying cardiac lesions, such as gross valvular disease, a large cardiac mass, or severe LV dysfunction. As stressed earlier, cardiac causes of syncope are not always an appropriate target of a simplified cardiac ultrasound examination. In this case FoCUS may not be necessarily diagnostic, but it should help in identifying patients to be referred for comprehensive echocardiography.[1,44]

FOCUS TECHNIQUE

A FoCUS examination does not require the execution of all the views used in a comprehensive echocardiographic examination. Five views are suggested as a minimum dataset (Figure 19.2): parasternal long-axis, parasternal short-axis, apical four-chamber, subcostal long-axis, and subcostal IVC view.[1]

A systematic approach is recommended to increase the accuracy of FoCUS.[1] Going through most or all views in a standardized way increases FoCUS screening capabilities. In extreme situations with the greatest time sensitivity (e.g., the cardiac arrest scenario), the two combined subcostal views

may provide sufficient initial information, although the FoCUS examination should be completed as soon as the clinical situation permits. In fact, the subcostal window is the most easily accessible one (in the challenging mechanically ventilated patient it may be the only obtainable view), and with minimal probe manipulation, it quickly provides sonographic access also to the IVC.

The echocardiographic modalities applied in FoCUS are represented by 2D and M-mode, as current evidence does not support the use of Doppler-based techniques in this simplified application of echocardiography. For optimal FoCUS examination basic knowledge is required on ultrasound machine functioning and setting up (default settings, depth, gain, focus, zoom) and image storage.[1] Transthoracic cardiac phased-array transducer is the preferred probe for FoCUS examination.

When available and if compatible with the clinical scenario, ECG-gated acquisition during a FoCUS examination is advisable (although not indispensable), for a better timing of cardiac events. FoCUS examination may also be performed with respiratory cycle monitoring.

FOCUS FINDINGS AND PATTERNS

FoCUS includes the assessment of a narrow list (Table 19.1) of evidence-based detectable targets, including the following:[1–4]

- *Gross signs of chronic cardiac disease*—LV and left atrial (LA) major dilation (V19.10, V19.10.1) or pronounced LV hypertrophy (V19.11, V19.11.1) usually suggests pre-existing myocardial or valvular disease, right atrial (RA) major dilation suggests pre-existing right heart disease, and severe RV hypertrophy may suggest long-standing pulmonary hypertension. Screening for these findings represents the best start for the FoCUS examination because it allows correct interpretation of subsequent findings. The presence of chronic heart disease introduces a factor of complexity to the cardiac ultrasound evaluation, and the FoCUS practitioner should be aware of it. Overlooking this may compromise the correct interpretation of the examination.
- *LV systolic (dys)function and size*—Qualitative assessment of global and regional systolic function: visual ejection fraction, visual fractional area change (at mid-papillary short-axis view), and qualitative analysis of gross wall motion abnormalities (hyperkinesia, hypokinesia akinesia, dyskinesia) (V19.1). Of note, detection of subtle regional WMA is beyond the scope of FoCUS.[1,4]
- *RV systolic (dys)function and size*—Qualitative assessment with visual ejection fraction. RV dilatation, free-wall hypokinesia, and septal flattening are all hallmarks of RV dysfunction and overload (V19.2, V19.2.1). RV dilatation with marked RV

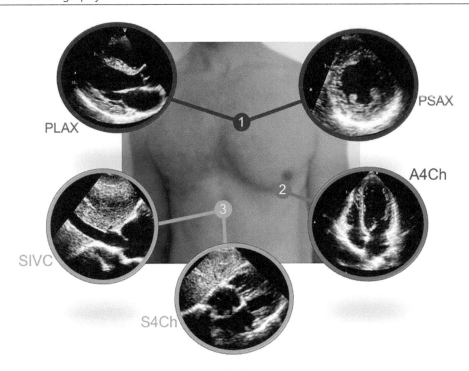

FIGURE 19.2   Suggested standard set of five views for FoCUS. Parasternal long-axis view (PLAX), parasternal short-axis view (PSAX), apical four-chamber view (A4Ch), subcostal four-chamber view (S4Ch), and subcostal inferior vena cava view (SIVC). Spots on the chest where transducer should be placed to obtain individual views are denoted by the corresponding numbers (1, 2, 3). If compatible with the clinical scenario, a systematic approach going through all these views is recommended.

(Modified from Stankovic I, Neskovic AN, Mladenovic Z (eds.), Clinical Cardiology, 2021, ECHOS, with permission.)

TABLE 19.1   Recommended Targets of the Focused Cardiac Ultrasound (FoCUS) Examination

- Gross signs of chronic heart disease
- Global left ventricular systolic function and size
- Global right ventricular systolic function and size
- Intravascular volume assessment
- Pericardial effusion, tamponade physiology
- Gross valvular abnormalities
- Large intracardiac masses

hypertrophy should steer to diagnosis of chronic pulmonary hypertension (V19.9, V19.9.1).

- *Pericardial effusion and its hemodynamic relevance*—Detection of echo-free or weakly echogenic pericardial space, semi-quantitative quantitation, and signs of compression of low-pressure chambers (RA systolic collapse, RV diastolic collapse, LA collapse, IVC plethora) (V19.5, V19.5.1, V19.6, V19.6.1).
- *Intravascular volume assessment*—Small, hyperkinetic RV and LV and small IVC are hallmarks of severe hypovolemia (V19.4, V19.4.1). *End-diastolic area* could help in distinguish hypovolemia and vasodilation (in both case end-systolic area is reduced): in case of *vasodilation*, end-diastolic area will be either normal or slightly reduced; in case

of *hypovolemia*, it will be much reduced. With the aforementioned limits, IVC indices of fluid responsiveness (collapsibility and distensibility index) can be assessed.

- *Gross valvular abnormalities*—The target findings are valve leaflet or cusp flail/prolapse (V19.8.1), valve thickening (V19.12.1), evident disruption of the valvular apparatus, and masses attached to valves (V19.8). The FoCUS aim is to trigger comprehensive echocardiographic evaluation when gross valve abnormalities are seen.
- *Large intracardiac masses*—Especially intracardiac thrombi or large valve vegetations (V19.8). FoCUS detection of large intracardiac masses should always trigger comprehensive echocardiography.

Recently, the EACVI provided FoCUS core curriculum and core syllabus to define key principles and unifying framework for educational and training processes/programs that should result in competence in FoCUS for various medical professionals dealing with diagnostics and treatment of cardiovascular emergencies.[1] The document is prepared in close cooperation with the European Society of Anaesthesiology, the European Association of Cardiothoracic Anaesthesiology, the Acute Cardiovascular Care Association, and the World Interactive Network Focused On Critical Ultrasound (WINFOCUS).[1] With appropriate, focused training (including exposure to video clips of normal and pathologic examples), detection of the aforementioned findings can be learned fast even by individuals with no or limited cardiac ultrasound competence.[3,7–9] This simplified approach is based on recognizing a few distinctive features and patterns of the cardiac ultrasonographic picture. A description of these *patterns* is shown in Table 19.2; each pattern is illustrated by corresponding video. For a better visual appreciation of structure size and systolic-diastolic size variation, please refer to the centimeter scale on one side of the sector; ECG tracing is not available in some clips because of either the time constraints of the emergency scenario or the use of an HUD.

Figure 19.3 provides clinical examples associated with common FoCUS patterns in shock; the same patterns, manifesting with greater severity, represent the four main patterns found in PEA cardiac arrest scenarios.

TABLE 19.2 Focus Cardiac Ultrasound (FoCUS) Patterns in Emergency Cardiac or Critical Care*

[1] Acute LV systolic dysfunction (V19.1)	*[2] Acute RV systolic dysfunction (V19.2, V19.2.1)*	*[3] Acute biventricular systolic dysfunction (V19.3)*
• LV global hypokinesia (visual estimation) • No signs of chronic LV disease • ± Regional wall motion abnormalities	• RV dilatation • RV hypokinesia (visual + reduced TAPSE) • No signs of chronic RV disease • ± Systolic septal flattening/dyskinesia (pressure overload) • ± Diastolic septal flattening/dyskinesia (volume overload)	• LV global hypokinesia • RV hypokinesia (visual + reduced TAPSE) • No signs of chronic RV or LV disease
[4] Severe hypovolemia (V19.4, V19.4.1)	*[5] Pericardial effusion (V19.5, V19.5.1)*	*[6] Cardiac tamponade (V19.6, V19.6.1)*
• Small LV end-diastolic & end-systolic size (hyperdynamic LV) • Small RV size, hyperdynamic RV • Small, collapsing IVC (spontaneous respiration) • Small IVC (mechanical ventilation)	• Anechoic/hypo-echoic pericardial free space	• Pericardial effusion • Signs of compression (collapse: RA systolic, RV diastolic, LA systolic, LV diastolic) • IVC plethora
[7] Cardiac standstill (V19.7)	*[8] Suspected severe acute valve dysfunction (V19.8, V19.8.1)*	*[9] Suspected chronic cor pulmonale (V19.9, V19.9.1)*
• Complete absence of cardiac wall motion (regardless of any valve motion)	• Abnormal valve motion (AV cusps flail; MV leaflet flail, prolapse, restriction) • And/or leaflets/cusps anatomical gaps • And/or mass(es) on leaflets/cusps	• RV dilatation • RV hypokinesia (visual + reduced TAPSE) • RV hypertrophy and RA dilatation • ± Septal flattening/dyskinesia
[10] Suspected chronic LV dysfunction (dilated cardiomyopathy) (V19.10, V19.10.1)	*[11] Suspected chronic LV dysfunction (hypertrophic/infiltrative cardiomyopathy) (V19.11, V19.11.1)*	*[12] Suspected chronic valve disease (V19.12, V19.12.1)*
• LV and LA dilatation • LV global hypokinesia • ± Regional wall motion abnormalities	• LV marked hypertrophy • LA dilatation • ± LV global hypokinesia • ± Regional WMA	• Abnormal valve thickening • Abnormal valve motion (AV cusps restricted motion; MV leaflets restricted motion; MV flail/prolapse) • LA dilatation ± LV dilatation or hypertrophy • ± LV global hypokinesia
[13] Wet lung pattern—Interstitial syndrome (pulmonary edema) (V19.13)	*[14] Pleural effusion (V19.14)*	
• Multiple diffuse bilateral B-lines	• Echo-free or weakly echogenic free fluid in pleural space	

* Common FoCUS patterns in adult shock states and cardiac arrest scenarios. Common cardiac arrest findings when electromechanical dissociation occurs are represented by dramatic acute LV systolic dysfunction, acute RV systolic dysfunction, severe hypovolemia, and cardiac tamponade (patterns 1, 2, *3, 4, and 6*). These are also common patterns in shock. Cardiac standstill (pattern 7) is another typical finding in cardiac arrest pulseless electrical activity or asystole rhythms. Importantly, patterns 8–12 should trigger comprehensive echocardiography referral within an appropriate time frame because their evaluation may go beyond FoCUS competency. Each pattern is illustrated by corresponding video.

Abbreviations: AV, aortic valve; IVC, inferior vena cava; LA, left atrial; LV, left ventricular; MV, mitral valve; RA, right atrial; RV, right ventricular; TAPSE, tricuspid annular plane systolic excursion; WMA, wall motion abnormalities.

(Modified from Reference 3)

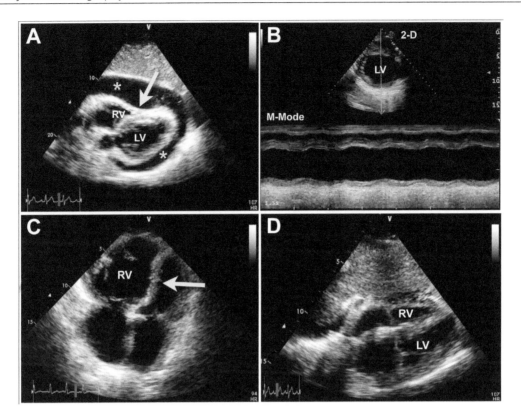

FIGURE 19.3 Common focused cardiac ultrasound (FoCUS) findings in shock. (A) *Cardiac tamponade.* Subcostal long-axis view in a patient with acute lymphatic leukemia in overt state of shock showing circumferential large pericardial effusion (*) exerting hemodynamic effects, as shown by compression of the right ventricle (RV) (yellow arrow) in mid-diastole. (B) *Severe global LV dysfunction.* Parasternal mid-papillary short-axis view (two-dimensional and M-mode evaluation) in a patient with autoimmune myocarditis showing severely reduced LV systolic function as evidenced by negligible inward systolic motion of left ventricular antero-septal and infero-lateral walls (M-mode tracing). (C) Apical four-chamber view in a patient with *suspected massive pulmonary embolism* 5 days after surgical colonic resection showing markedly *dilated RV compressing the left ventricle* (LV) and end-systolic septal dyskinesia (yellow arrow). (D) Subcostal long-axis view in a patient with sepsis due to community-acquired pneumonia showing *small RV and LV ventricular cavities at end-diastole.* The patient suddenly manifested extreme hypotension; severe hypovolemia was diagnosed and treated. LV: left ventricle; RV: right ventricle.

COMMON PITFALLS AND MISTAKES

If FoCUS is not practiced within the framework outlined earlier, its inherent limitations carry substantial risks of overlooking important abnormalities and/or misinterpreting the findings based on limited data set. The following are common pitfalls that the FoCUS practitioner should be aware of, and common mistakes that should be avoided:

- *Omitting the screening for signs of chronic cardiac disease*—Neglecting echocardiographic signs of chronic cardiac disease may lead to an erroneous diagnosis of acute LV or RV dysfunction in shock states in which cardiac disease is just an occasional comorbidity and may distract from the core pathophysiology (e.g., sepsis in a patient with chronic cor pulmonale mistaken for suspected massive pulmonary embolism).

- *Applying an out-of-clinical context interpretation of LV systolic function*—LV systolic function may be overestimated if LV contractility is interpreted without considering ongoing therapy (e.g., ongoing inotrope infusion or mechanical circulatory support). Caution in qualitative evaluation global LV systolic function is also required in case of bradycardia and tachycardia, severe hypotension and hypertension, mitral or aortic regurgitation, aortic stenosis or severe hypertrophy, mitral stenosis, ventricular septal defect, severe anemia, or other hyperdynamic states.

- *Having overconfidence in ruling out tamponade with FoCUS in the post-cardiac surgery patient*—FoCUS (and transthoracic echocardiography in general) is insufficiently accurate in diagnosing early postsurgical tamponade, which is frequently caused by loculated effusions or clots and not free effusions (i.e., FoCUS is useful only in diagnosing pericardial free fluid and providing clues to tamponade). In addition, tamponade remains a clinical diagnosis, although supported by echocardiographic findings.

- *Equating large effusion with tamponade*—A large pericardial effusion does not necessarily have hemodynamic effects if the fluid accumulates gradually. Tamponade is related to pericardial pressure (evidenced by ultrasound signs of cardiac compression) rather than to fluid amount.
- *Ruling out hypovolemia in the presence of non-small (normal or large) LV sizes*—Assessment of volume status with FoCUS (purely based on 2D modality) provides only a good rule-in criterion for hypovolemia: the hyperdynamic pattern with small ventricles is specific to severe hypovolemia but poorly sensitive (e.g., patients with a chronically dilated left ventricle and right ventricle will never have small ventricles despite relevant hypovolemia).
- *Diagnosing hypovolemia based exclusively on IVC respiratory variations*—IVC respiratory variability is determined not only by central volume status but also by the magnitude of the intrathoracic pressure variations (e.g., patients with respiratory distress and significative respiratory efforts). This may be misleading—that is, pronounced IVC inspiratory size reductions (IVC collapse) may coexist with systemic venous congestion and be related to vigorous inspiratory efforts rather than volume responsiveness; end-inspiratory IVC size (large in these cases) should never be disregarded.
- *Equating IVC plethora to absence of fluid responsiveness*—Separate interpretation of IVC size and respiratory behavior may be misleading: IVC plethora may coexist with volume responsiveness (e.g., in tamponade or RV AMI).
- *Equating a dilated, failing, right ventricle with signs of pressure overload to massive pulmonary embolism*—FoCUS allows diagnosis only of acute cor pulmonale and not of embolic disease, unless in-transit thrombi are detected in right heart cavities or pulmonary artery (very rarely). First, chronic cor pulmonale should always be ruled out. Second, computed tomography pulmonary angiography (CTPA) scan remains the diagnostic tool for suspected pulmonary thromboembolism, and specific treatment for it should be started based on FoCUS findings suggestive of acute cor pulmonale only in patients too unstable to be transferred for CTPA.
- *Considering McConnell's sign as specific for pulmonary embolism*—McConnell's sign (RV apex hyperkinesia in RV failure) is common to other etiologies of RV failure (e.g., RV AMI) and should not be considered as an exclusive hallmark of embolic disease.[16]
- *Ruling out the cardiogenic origin of pulmonary edema based on the finding of normal LV contractility*—In a relevant proportion of patients, cardiogenic pulmonary edema develops, in fact, in the absence of systolic LV dysfunction (e.g., diastolic dysfunction, acute valvular disease, hypertensive crisis, atrial fibrillation). Thus, FoCUS (and LUS) may only provide clues to the diagnosis of cardiogenic pulmonary edema and trigger comprehensive echocardiography.

FOCUS ARCHIVING AND REPORTING

Recording and storage of FoCUS studies should be accomplished for subsequent analysis, review, and comparison of findings.[1,3] Digital image and video archiving serves multiple objectives relevant to quality assurance of FoCUS, including case retrieval for confirmation of findings, information sharing, referral to experts, sequential patient assessment and medico-legal use.

Whenever FoCUS is performed, the findings of the examination should be appropriately documented, ideally in a report. The initial report may be extremely concise (written and/or verbal), concentrating on critical findings and integrated into the decision-making process, and must be followed by a final written report, interpreted, approved, and signed by the operators with adequate formal education.[1,3] For this reason, the use of simplified standardized report forms with minimal free text and box checking, in line with the speed of the FoCUS examination, is suggested. The report should ideally include sufficient clinical information for subsequent consistent interpretation of findings by the reader (vital signs, ongoing therapy, parameters of mechanical ventilation, indication for FoCUS). Potential indications for a second opinion, comprehensive echocardiography, and/or specification of the therapeutic interventions acted on should also be reported. An example of a FoCUS report form is presented in Figure 19.4.

FUTURE PERSPECTIVES AND CONCLUSION

A variety of medical professionals dealing with cardiovascular emergencies and critically ill patients will use FoCUS more and more to improve their diagnostic capabilities and to aid immediate decision-making and/or treatment. This growing use will be driven further by the wide availability of technically superior HUDs. However, proper training and education remain the keys for safe and efficient use of FoCUS in emergency settings.

For critically ill patients, it really does not matter whether the life-saving information is acquired by a non-cardiologist performing FoCUS or by an expert cardiologist performing echocardiography. When such information is available, for the benefit of the patient, it has to be used correctly, thoughtfully, and with care.[1–4]

Focused Cardiac UltraSound
(FoCUS)

PATIENT NAME: ....   DATE OF BIRTH: ....

OPERATOR: ....EXAM DATE: ....HOUR ....

INDICATION: ☐ PEA   ☐ Shock / Hypotension ☐ Resp. failure ☐ Oliguria ☐ Screening ☐ Other

HISTORY: ....

DRUGS/TREATMENT: ....

VENTILATION: ☐ Spontaneous ☐ MV passive   ☐ MV active   ☐ CPAP   PEEP/ Vt = .../..........

TYPE OF EXAM: ☐ FEEL (CPR/Peri-resuscitation)   ☐ Complete FoCUS   ☐ Repeated Assessment

WINDOWS, Used: ☐ SLAX ☐ SSAX ☐ SIVC ☐ PLAX ☐ PSAX   ☐ A4CH ☐ A2CH ☐ ALAX

Quality: S .... P .... A ....   (2 = optimal; 1= suboptimal; 0 = inadequate)

LEFT VENTRICLE

DIMENSION: ☐ Small ☐ Normal ☐ Dilated ☐ Markedly dilated   LA: ☐ Dilated   ☐ Non dilated

WALL THICKNESS: ☐ Normal   ☐ Markedly hypertrophied   RWMA: ☐ YES ☐ No

KINESIS: ☐ Hyper ☐ Normal ☐ Mild Hypo ☐ Moderate Hypo ☐ Severe Hypo ☐ Card. Standstill

---

RIGHT VENTRICLE

DIMENSION: ☐ Small   ☐ Normal   ☐ Dilated   ☐ Markedly dilated (bigger than LV)

KINESIS: ☐ Hyper ☐ Normal ☐ Hypo ☐ Cardiac Standstill   RA: ☐ Dilated   ☐ Non dilated

SEPTUM: ☐ Normal ☐ Flattened ☐ Paradoxical motion   WALL THIKNESS: ☐ Normal ☐ Hypertrophied

---

INFERIOR VENA CAVA

DIMENSION: ☐ ≤ 10mm   ☐ 10-15mm   ☐ 15-20mm   ☐ 20-25mm   ☐ >25mm

RESPIRATORY VARIATION: ☐ collapse ☐ >50% reduction   ☐ <50% reduction   ☐ absent

RESPIRATORY VARIATION (MV PASSIVE):   ☐ >20% distension   ☐ <20% distension   ☐ absent

---

VALVES & Intra-Cardiac MASSES

MITRAL LEAFLETS: ☐ Normal   ☐ Greatly thickened/calcified   ☐ Disrupted/Flail ☐ Hypomobile

AORTIC CUSPS: ☐ Normal ☐ Greatly thickened/calcified   ☐ Disrupted   ☐ Hypomobile

MASSES: ☐ None ☐ On Mitral valve ☐ On Aortic Valve ☐ In Right-side Cavities ☐ In the IVC

PERICARDIUM

☐ Normal ☐ Mild Effusion ☐ Larger Effusion   ☐ RA syst. collapse   ☐ RV diast. collapse

---

CHECK THAT ALL THE 6 TARGETS OF THE FOCUS EXAM HAVE BEEN ASSESSED:

1) Chronic Dysfunction? 2) Left Ventricle 3) Right Ventricle 4) Fluid Status 5) Pericardium 6) Valves/Masses

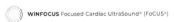

FIGURE 19.4 Simplified focused cardiac ultrasound (FoCUS) report. FoCUS reports should ideally be organized in different sections, including demographic data, minimal clinical data, findings, summary, date, and signature. Description of findings and summary should be consistent with goals and targets of FoCUS. The threshold for consultation by a more experienced operator or referrals for comprehensive echocardiography should be low and such requests should be clearly noted in the report.

(Modified with permission from the World Interactive Network Focused On Critical Ultrasound [WINFOCUS] from the document titled "Focused Cardiac Ultrasound Report Sheet.")

LIST OF VIDEOS

https://routledgetextbooks.com/textbooks/9781032157009/chapter-19.php

VIDEO 19.1 **Acute left ventricular systolic dysfunction:** Cardiogenic shock caused by extensive anterolateral myocardial infarction. In all three views, left ventricular global contractility appears very poor. The absence of left ventricular dilation, left ventricular severe hypertrophy, or major left atrial dilation suggests absence of chronic left-side disease. Regional wall motion abnormality is in this case visible, with a preserved contractility limited to the basal anterolateral (apical four-chamber view), posterior (parasternal long-axis view), and basal inferior (parasternal short-axis view) walls. Electrocardiogram tracing not available. LA: left atrium; LV: left ventricle; RA: right atrium; RV: right ventricle.

VIDEO 19.2 **Acute right ventricular systolic dysfunction:** Acute cor pulmonale caused by pulmonary embolism (subsequently diagnosed by pulmonary angio–computed tomography scan). The right ventricle (RV) is severely dilated (bigger than the left ventricle [LV]) and markedly hypokinetic (small reduction of its area from end-diastole to end-systole; shows negligible motion of the tricuspid annular plane in systole; markedly reduced tricuspid annular plane systolic excursion [TAPSE]) and compresses the LV. The interventricular septum (IVS) is flattened and shows a pathologic shift to the left at end-systole, which is a sign of pressure overload. No signs of chronic cor pulmonale are visible (no evident right ventricular hypertrophy is visible, despite these views not being the best ones for judging right ventricular thickness). Electrocardiogram tracing not available. LA: left atrium; RA: right atrium.

VIDEO 19.2.1 **Acute right ventricular systolic dysfunction.** Acute cor pulmonale caused by pulmonary embolism (subsequently diagnosed by pulmonary angio–computed tomography scan). The right ventricle (RV) is severely dilated (bigger than the left ventricle [LV]) and markedly hypokinetic (small reduction of its area from end-diastole to end-systole; shows negligible motion of the tricuspid annular plane in systole; markedly reduced tricuspid annular plane systolic excursion [TAPSE]) and compresses the LV. McConnell's sign, with RV apex hyperkinesia (red arrow) in RV failure, is visible in the second clip in apical four-chamber view. The interventricular septum (IVS) is flattened and shows a pathologic shift to the left at end-systole, which is a sign of pressure overload (systolic septal dyskinesia). No signs of chronic cor pulmonale are visible (no evident right ventricular hypertrophy is visible, despite these views not being the best ones for judging right ventricular thickness). LA: left atrium; RA: right atrium.

VIDEO 19.3 **Acute biventricular failure.** Cardiogenic shock caused by myocarditis. The left ventricle (LV) shows severely reduced contractility, visible both in the apical four-chamber view and in the

parasternal short-axis view. The right ventricle (RV) is dilated and severely hypokinetic (small reduction of its area from end-diastole to end-systole; negligible motion of tricuspid annular plane in systole; markedly reduced tricuspid annular plane systolic excursion [TAPSE]). The atria and the LV are not dilated (but rather at the upper limit of the range of normality), suggesting an exclusively acute condition. LA: left atrium; RA: right atrium.

VIDEO 19.4 **Severe hypovolemia:** Septic shock at onset in a neutropenic patient with bilateral pneumonia. Subcostal long-axis view shows small and hyperkinetic left ventricle (LV) and right ventricle (RV). Both left and right ventricular visual end-diastolic area and end-systolic area are small, indicating underfilled ventricles. The inferior vena cava (IVC) is extremely small and collapses with inspiration (the patient is in spontaneous respiration; this allows the derivation of reliable information on volume status also from the interpretation of IVC size and behavior). Apical four-chamber view confirms these findings, and parasternal short-axis view is quite eloquent regarding the hyperdynamic, underfilled state of the LV. Electrocardiogram tracing not available. LA: left atrium; LVEDA: left ventricular end-diastolic area; LVESA: left ventricular end-systolic area; RA: right atrium.

VIDEO 19.4.1 **Severe hypovolemia.** Septic shock at onset in a neutropenic patient with bilateral pneumonia. Subcostal long-axis view shows small and hyperkinetic left ventricle (LV) and right ventricle (RV). Both left and right ventricular visual end-diastolic area and end-systolic area are small, indicating underfilled ventricles. LA: left atrium; RA: right atrium.

VIDEO 19.5 **Pericardial effusion:** Patient in shock with severe trauma of the thorax and limbs after a car accident. An anechoic space is visible in the most dependent part of the pericardial sac sinus (red arrows), close to right ventricular free wall and right atrial wall; it identifies a pericardial effusion. The effusion is localized and does not circumferentially surround the heart. It separates the pericardial layers by no more than 1 cm; this indicates a small pericardial effusion. Regardless of the amount, the effusion does not cause any inward displacement of the right ventricular wall in diastole nor of the right atrial wall in systole; this indicates that there is no compressive effect of the effusion and that the cause of shock is not tamponade. Another sign confirming the absence of tamponade is visible in the subcostal inferior vena cava (IVC) view. The IVC diameter is roughly 1 cm, with pronounced respiratory collapse of the vessel (patient with spontaneous respirations). This suggests severe hypovolemia rather than tamponade as cause of the shock state. Electrocardiogram tracing not available. IVS: interventricular septum; LA: left atrium; LV: left ventricle; RA: right atrium.

VIDEO 19.5.1 **Pericardial effusion.** Patient with systemic lupus erythematosus. The anechoic space surrounding both left and right ventricle identifies the pericardial effusion. Regardless of the amount, the effusion does not cause any inward displacement of the right ventricular wall in diastole or of the right atrial wall in systole; this indicates that there is no compressive effect of the effusion and that the cause of shock is not tamponade. LA: left atrium; LV: left ventricle; RA: right atrium; RV: right ventricle

VIDEO 19.6 **Cardiac tamponade:** Shock in a patient with malignant pericardial disease. As in Video 19.5 and 19.5.1, a pericardial effusion is visible, but in this case, it shows a circumferential distribution (arrows) and a larger size. Regardless of the size of the effusion, the diagnosis of tamponade is made on clinical grounds (hypotension, jugular turgor, tachycardia) and the detection of cardiac ultrasound signs of compression of the "low pressure chambers": right atrial systolic collapse (inward displacement of right atrial wall) and right ventricular diastolic collapse (inward displacement of right ventricular free wall). The inferior vena cava is dilated and devoid of any respiratory variation, indicating systemic venous congestion. Electrocardiogram tracing not available. IVS: interventricular septum; LV: left ventricle; RA: right atrium; RV: right ventricle.

VIDEO 19.6.1   Cardiac tamponade. Shock in a patient with malignant pericardial disease. As in Videos 19.5 and 19.5.1, a pericardial effusion is visible, but in this case, the diagnosis of tamponade is made on clinical grounds (hypotension, jugular turgor, tachycardia) and the detection of cardiac ultrasound signs of compression of the "low pressure chambers": right atrial systolic collapse (inward displacement of right atrial wall) and right ventricular diastolic collapse (inward displacement of right ventricular free wall). LA: left atrium; LV: left ventricle; RA: right atrium; RV: right ventricle.

VIDEO 19.7   Cardiac standstill: Cardiac arrest: presentation rhythm was asystole. The electrocardiogram shows poorly organized broad-complex electrical activity. First part of the video clip is taken during chest compressions. Once the heart is better visualized (during the pulse check time), the subcostal view shows a complete absence of any cardiac mechanical activity. Regardless of the visible small valve motion (caused by blood displacement from the lung as an effect of the ventilation), left ventricular and right ventricular walls are immobile. LA: left atrium; LV: left ventricle; RA: right atrium; RV: right ventricle.

VIDEO 19.8   Suspected acute valve dysfunction: Acute endocarditis causing cardiogenic shock. The apical four-chamber view shows a thickened anterior mitral leaflet (red arrow), with a distorted morphology, small globular masses attached, and also a visible interruption in leaflet integrity. In the parasternal long-axis view, similar findings pertaining to the anterior mitral leaflet are shown (inferior red arrow); in addition, the aortic cusps appear completely disrupted (superior red arrow) and "bounce" to and fro between the left ventricular outflow tract and the ascending aorta (Asc Ao). This is altogether likely to cause massive mitral and aortic valve regurgitations (the existence of "anatomical gaps" detectable with simple two-dimensional modality is the hallmark of a severe regurgitation). Comprehensive echocardiography confirmed the diagnosis. Electrocardiogram tracing not available. LA: left atrium; LV: left ventricle; RA: right atrium; RV: right ventricle.

VIDEO 19.8.1   Suspected acute valve dysfunction. Complete posterior mitral leaflet prolapse complicating acute myocardial infarction. The apical four-chamber view shows a thickened posterior mitral leaflet (red arrow), with a distorted morphology and prolapse. In the parasternal long-axis view, similar findings pertaining to the posterior mitral leaflet are shown (inferior red arrow). This is altogether likely to cause massive mitral and aortic valve regurgitations (the existence of "anatomical gaps" detectable with simple two-dimensional modality is the hallmark of a severe regurgitation). Comprehensive echocardiography confirmed the diagnosis. LA: left atrium; LV: left ventricle; RA: right atrium; RV: right ventricle.

VIDEO 19.9   Suspected chronic cor pulmonale: Shock in a patient with pulmonary fibrosis. The right ventricle (RV) is dilated and hypokinetic and compresses the left ventricle (LV), as visible in this apical four-chamber view. The interventricular septum (IVS) is flattened. As opposed to Video 19.2 and 19.2.1, the presence of right ventricular free-wall hypertrophy (subcostal long-axis view, arrow) suggests the existence of a chronic cor pulmonale. The cause of shock in this case was not right ventricular failure per se but septic shock and decompensating chronic cor pulmonale. Comprehensive echocardiography confirmed the diagnosis. Electrocardiogram tracing not available. LA: left atrium; RA: right atrium.

VIDEO 19.9.1   Suspected chronic cor pulmonale. Shock in a patient with decompensated chronic cor pulmonale. The right ventricle (RV) is dilated and hypokinetic and compresses the left ventricle (LV), as visible in this apical four-chamber view. The interventricular septum (IVS) is flattened. As opposed to Video 19.2 and 19.2.1, the presence of right ventricular free-wall hypertrophy (arrow) suggests the existence of a chronic cor pulmonale. The cause of shock in this case was not right ventricular failure per se but septic shock and decompensating chronic cor pulmonale. Comprehensive echocardiography confirmed the diagnosis. LA: left atrium; RA: right atrium.

VIDEO 19.10   Suspected chronic left ventricular failure (dilated cardiomyopathy): Shock in a patient with dilated cardiomyopathy. Similar to the case presented in Video 19.1, the left ventricle (LV) appears severely hypokinetic in the apical four-chamber view and the parasternal short- and long-axis views. However, in this case signs of preexisting cardiac disease are visible: the LV is dilated, with the end-diastolic diameter reaching 6 cm, and the left atrium (LA) is dilated, too. Left ventricular and left atrial dilation indicate a long-standing pressure overload of these heart chambers. Asc Ao: ascending aorta; LA: left atrium; RA: right atrium; RV: right ventricle.

VIDEO 19.10.1   Suspected chronic left ventricular failure (dilated cardiomyopathy). Shock in a patient with dilated cardiomyopathy. As in Video 19.1, the left ventricle (LV) appears severely hypokinetic in the parasternal long-axis view and apical four-chamber view. However, in this case, signs of pre-existing cardiac disease are visible: the LV is dilated, with the end-diastolic diameter reaching 6 cm, and the left atrium (LA) is dilated, too. Left ventricular and left atrial dilation suggest a long-standing pressure overload of these heart chambers. LA: left atrium; RA: right atrium; RV: right ventricle.

VIDEO 19.11   Suspected chronic left ventricular failure (hypertrophic or infiltrative cardiomyopathy): Hypotension and pulmonary edema in a patient with no previous history of cardiac disease and known chronic kidney failure. In all views the left ventricle shows a strikingly small cavity and marked concentric hypertrophy. Its wall thickness, in each segment, is much more than 1 cm (rough reference value for normality). The left ventricle (LV), as can be judged in these views, is hyperdynamic. The right ventricle (RV) shows increased thickness of its free wall. The myocardium, to a more expert eye, shows a peculiar texture. In this case the pathologic pattern corresponded to decompensation in a patient with cardiac amyloidosis, subsequently confirmed by a comprehensive echocardiogram and endomyocardial biopsy. Asc Ao: ascending aorta; LA, left atrium; RA, right atrium.

VIDEOS 19.11.1   Suspected chronic left ventricular failure (hypertrophic or infiltrative cardiomyopathy). Patient admitted for out-of-hospital cardiac arrest with ventricular fibrillation and restoration of spontaneous circulation after Advanced Cardiac Life Support (ACLS). FoCUS confirmed severe concentric ventricular hypertrophy with increased septum and posterior wall thickness. In fact, the apical four-chamber view and the parasternal views the left ventricle shows a strikingly small cavity and marked concentric hypertrophy; its wall thickness, in each segment, is much more than 1 cm (rough reference value for normality). Subsequent comprehensive echocardiogram confirmed diagnosis of hypertrophic obstructive cardiomyopathy. Asc Ao: ascending aorta; LA, left atrium; RA, right atrium.

VIDEO 19.12   Suspected chronic valvular disease: The patient was presented with severe dyspnea. Mitral valve leaflets (arrow) are thickened, hyperechoic (likely calcified), and scarcely mobile, with no visible opening (apical four-chamber view). Signs of chronic disease are present: the left atrium (LA) is dilated. These mitral valve findings (inferior red arrow) are confirmed in the parasternal long-axis view, and the evidence of diseased aortic withs thickened cusps showing limited mobility in systole (superior red arrow). Left atrial dilation suggests a long-standing atrial pressure overload. The diagnosis of decompensation of chronic severe mitral and aortic stenoses was subsequently confirmed clinically and by comprehensive echocardiography. Asc Ao: ascending aorta; LV: left ventricle; RA: right atrium; RV: right ventricle.

VIDEO 19.12.1   Suspected chronic valvular disease. Respiratory failure in a patient with mitral stenosis and aortic stenosis. Posterior mitral valve leaflet (inferior red arrow) is thickened, hyperechoic (likely calcified), and scarcely mobile, causing reduced opening of the valve (parasternal long-axis view). Signs of chronic disease are present: the left atrium (LA) is dilated. In parasternal long-axis view, thickened cusps of the aortic valve can be noted showing limited opening in systole (superior red arrow). Left atrial dilation suggests a long-standing atrial pressure overload. The diagnosis of decompensation of chronic valvular disease was subsequently confirmed clinically and by comprehensive echocardiography. Asc Ao: ascending aorta; LV: left ventricle; RA: right atrium; RV: right ventricle.

VIDEO 19.13   Wet lungs. Respiratory failure in a patient with acute decompensated heart failure. Ultrasonographic evaluation of the chest showed multiple diffuse bilateral B-lines. B-lines are the vertical, hyperechoic image that arises from the pleural line; they are synchronous with respiration and extend to the bottom of the screen. Diffuse B-line pattern (also called "wet lungs" pattern, "lung comets") indicates increased extracellular lung water is typical for acute decompensated heart failure (pulmonary oedema).

VIDEO 19.14   Pleural effusion. Pleural effusion causing dyspnea. Lung ultrasound at bilateral inferior fields showed anechoic space surrounding the lung, identifying the pleural effusion.

REFERENCES

1. Neskovic AN, Skinner H, Price S, et al. Focus cardiac ultrasound core curriculum and core syllabus of the European Association of Cardiovascular Imaging European Heart Journal. Eur Heart J Cardiovasc Imaging 2018; 19:475–81.

2. Spencer KT, Flachskampf FA. Focused cardiac ultrasonography. JACC Cardiovasc Imaging 2019; 12(7):1243–53.

3. Via G, Hussain A, Wells M, et al. International evidence-based recommendations for focused cardiac ultrasound. J Am Soc Echocardiogr 2014; 27(7):683.e1–.e33.

4. Neskovic AN, Edvardsen T, Galderisi M, et al. Focus cardiac ultrasound: the European Association of Cardiovascular Imaging viewpoint. Eur Heart J Cardiovasc Imaging 2014; 15(9):956–60.

5. Neri L, Storti E, Lichtenstein D. Toward an ultrasound curriculum for critical care medicine. Crit Care Med 2007; 35(5 Suppl):S290–304.

6. Martin LD, Mathews S, Ziegelstein RC, et al. Prevalence of asymptomatic left ventricular systolic dysfunction in at-risk medical inpatients. Am J Med 2013; 126(1):68–73.

7. Vignon P, Dugard A, Abraham J, et al. Focused training for goaloriented hand-held echocardiography performed by non-cardiologist residents in the intensive care unit. Intensive Care Med 2007; 33(10):1795–9.

8. Ferrada P, Anand RJ, Whelan J, et al. Limited transthoracic echocardiogram: so easy any trauma attending can do it. J Trauma 2011; 71(5):1327–31; discussion 31.

9. Jones AE, Tayal VS, Kline JA. Focused training of emergency medicine residents in goal-directed echocardiography: a prospective study. Acad Emerg Med 2003; 10(10):1054–8.

10. Neskovic AN, Hagendorff A, Lancellotti P, et al. Emergency echocardiography: the European Association of Cardiovascular Imaging recommendations. Eur Heart J Cardiovasc Imaging 2013; 14(1):1–11.

11. Soliman-Aboumarie H, Breithardt OA, Gargani L, et al. How-to: focus cardiac ultrasound in acute settings. Eur Heart J Cardiovasc Imaging 2022; 23(2):150–3.

12. Via G, Braschi A. Echocardiographic assessment of cardiovascular failure. Minerva Anestesiol 2006; 72(6):495–501.

13. Shmueli H, Burstein Y, Sagy I, et al. Briefly trained medical students can effectively identify rheumatic mitral valve injury using a hand-carried ultrasound. Echocardiography 2013; 30(6):621–6.

14. Tayal VS, Kline JA. Emergency echocardiography to detect pericardial effusion in patients in PEA and near-PEA states. Resuscitation 2003; 59(3):315–8.

15. Mazurek B, Jehle D, Martin M. Emergency department echocardiography in the diagnosis and therapy of cardiac tamponade. J Emerg Med 1991; 9(1–2):27–31.

16. Konstantinides SV, Meyer G, Becattini C, et al. 2019 ESC guidelines for the diagnosis and management of acute pulmonary embolism developed in collaboration with the European Respiratory Society (ERS). Eur Heart J 2020; 41(4):543–603.

17. Leung JM, Levine EH. Left ventricular end-systolic cavity obliteration as an estimate of intraoperative hypovolemia. Anesthesiology 1994; 81(5):1102–9.

18. Zengin S, Al B, Genc S, et al. Role of inferior vena cava and right ventricular diameter in assessment of volume status: a comparative study: ultrasound and hypovolemia. Am J Emerg Med 2013; 31(5):763–7.

19. Dipti A, Soucy Z, Surana A, Chandra S. Role of inferior vena cava diameter in assessment of volume status: a meta-analysis. Am J Emerg Med 2012; 30(8):1414–9.e1.

20. Yanagawa Y, Sakamoto T, Okada Y. Hypovolemic shock evaluated by sonographic measurement of the inferior vena cava during resuscitation in trauma patients. J Trauma 2007; 63(6):1245–8.

21. Weekes AJ, Tassone HM, Babcock A, et al. Comparison of serial qualitative and quantitative assessments of caval index and left ventricular systolic function during early fluid

resuscitation of hypotensive emergency department patients. Acad Emerg Med 2011; 18(9):912–21.

22. Barbier C, Loubières Y, Schmit C, et al. Respiratory changes in inferior vena cava diameter are helpful in predicting fluid responsiveness in ventilated septic patients. Intensive Care Med 2004; 30(9):1740–6.

23. Muller L, Bobbia X, Toumi M, et al. Respiratory variations of inferior vena cava diameter to predict fluid responsiveness in spontaneously breathing patients with acute circulatory failure: need for a cautious use. Crit Care 2012; 16(5):R188.

24. Corl K, Napoli AM, Gardiner F. Bedside sonographic measurement of the inferior vena cava caval index is a poor predictor of fluid responsiveness in emergency department patients. Emerg Med Australas 2012; 24(5):534–9.

25. Juhl-Olsen P, Frederiksen CA, Sloth E. Ultrasound assessment of inferior vena cava collapsibility is not a valid measure of preload changes during triggered positive pressure ventilation: a controlled cross-over study. Ultraschall Med 2012; 33(2):152–9.

26. Via G, Tavazzi G, Price S. Ten situations where inferior vena cava ultrasound may fail to accurately predict fluid responsiveness: a physiologically based point of view. Intens Care Med. 2016; 42(7):1164–7.

27. Via G, Price S, Storti E. Echocardiography in the sepsis syndromes. Crit Ultrasound J 2011; 3(2):71–85.

28. Volpicelli G, Lamorte A, Tullio M, et al. Point-of-care multiorgan ultrasonography for the evaluation of undifferentiated hypotension in the emergency department. Intensive Care Med 2013; 39(7):1290–8.

29. Soar J, Böttiger BW, Carli P, et al. European Resuscitation Council Guidelines 2021: adult advanced life support. Resuscitation 2021; 161:115–51.

30. Panchal AR, Bartos JA, Cabañas JG, et al. Part 3: adult basic and advanced life support: 2020 American Heart Association guidelines for cardiopulmonary resuscitation and emergency cardiovascular care. Circulation 2020; 142(16 Suppl 2):S366–468.

31. Breitkreutz R, Price S, Steiger HV, et al. Focused echocardiographic evaluation in life support and peri-resuscitation of emergency patients: a prospective trial. Resuscitation 2010; 81(11):1527–33.

32. Breitkreutz R, Walcher F, Seeger FH. Focused echocardiographic evaluation in resuscitation management: concept of an advanced life support-conformed algorithm. Crit Care Med 2007; 35(5 Suppl):S150–61.

33. Price S, Uddin S, Quinn T. Echocardiography in cardiac arrest. Curr Opin Crit Care 2010; 16(3):211–5.

34. Balderston JR, You AX, Evans DP, Taylor LA, Gertz ZM. Feasibility of focused cardiac ultrasound during cardiac arrest in the emergency department. Cardiovasc Ultrasound. 2021; 19(1):19.

35. Flato UA, Paiva EF, Carballo MT, et al. Echocardiography for prognostication during the resuscitation of intensive care unit patients with non-shockable rhythm cardiac arrest. Resuscitation. 2015; 92:1–6.

36. Plummer D, Brunette D, Asinger R, Ruiz E. Emergency department echocardiography improves outcome in penetrating cardiac injury. Ann Emerg Med 1992; 21(6):709–12.

37. American College of Surgeons. Committee on Trauma. *Advanced Trauma Life Support: Student Course Manual.* Tenth edition. Chicago, IL: American College of Surgeons, 2018.

38. Ferrada P, Evans D, Wolfe L, et al. Findings of a randomized controlled trial using limited transthoracic echocardiogram (LTTE) as a hemodynamic monitoring tool in the trauma bay. J Trauma Acute Care Surg 2014; 76(1):31–8.

39. Juhl-Olsen P, Vistisen ST, Christiansen LK, Rasmussen LA, Frederiksen CA, Sloth E. Ultrasound of the inferior vena cava does not predict hemodynamic response to early hemorrhage. J Emerg Med 2013; 45(4):592–7.

40. Nazerian P, Vanni S, Volpicelli G, et al. Accuracy of point-of-care multiorgan ultrasonography for the diagnosis of pulmonary embolism. Chest 2014; 145(5):950–7.

41. Byrne RA, Rossello X, Coughlan JJ, Barbato E, Berry C, Chieffo A, et al.; ESC Scientific Document Group. 2023 ESC Guidelines for the management of acute coronary syndromes. Eur Heart J 2023;44(38):3720–826.

42. Laursen CB, Sloth E, Lassen AT, et al. Point-of-care ultrasonography in patients admitted with respiratory symptoms: a single-blind, randomised controlled trial. Lancet Respir Med 2014; 2(8):638–46.

43. Picano E, Pellikka PA. Ultrasound of extravascular lung water: a new standard for pulmonary congestion. Eur Heart J 2016; 37(27):2097–104.

44. Ghani AR, Ullah W, Abdullah HMA., et al. The role of echocardiography in diagnostic evaluation of patients with syncope—a retrospective analysis. Am J Cardiovasc Dis 2019; 9(5):78–83.

Lung ultrasound in emergency cardiac care

20

Luna Gargani

Key Points

- Lung ultrasound (LUS) can provide useful information in emergency cardiac care, especially for the differential diagnosis of life-threatening conditions, such as acute respiratory and circulatory failure.
- Acute cardiogenic pulmonary edema can be easily recognized by LUS through the detection of multiple diffuse bilateral B-lines.
- An integrated cardiopulmonary ultrasound assessment, combining LUS with focus cardiac ultrasound (FoCUS) examination, can empower the diagnostics, management, and risk stratification in cardiac emergencies.

In the recent years, lung ultrasound (LUS) has been increasingly used to support the management of patients in different emergency scenarios because its high versatility. LUS can be easily applied at the bedside in a point-of-care approach and can provide useful information about lung aeration in a timely manner, allowing a rapid rule-in and rule-out of many critical conditions.

LUS is especially powerful when coupled with echocardiography or focus cardiac ultrasound (FoCUS) in an *integrated cardiopulmonary evaluation*. The availability of portable, handheld, low-cost ultrasound machines and the diffusion of the use of point-of-care ultrasound outside the cardiology community have further spread this tool, which is now regularly employed in emergency departments, intensive care units, and internal medicine wards.

In this chapter, the role of LUS in diagnostics and management of the common cardiac or cardiac-like emergencies is discussed.

ACUTE CARDIOGENIC PULMONARY EDEMA

Diagnosis

In an acute cardiogenic pulmonary edema, LUS reveals *multiple diffuse bilateral B-lines* over the anterolateral chest (Figure 20.1) (V20.1).[1] *Multiple* refers to the presence of at least 3 B-lines in a single scanning site, *diffuse* refers to the presence of at least 3 B-lines in at least two adjacent scanning sites, and this pattern must be *bilateral*. These three characteristics are needed to be present at the same time because a few B-lines, especially at the lung bases, can be seen even in normal subjects, likely representing trivial gravity-related de-aerated areas. Patients with exacerbation of chronic obstructive pulmonary disease (COPD),

DOI: 10.1201/9781003245407-20

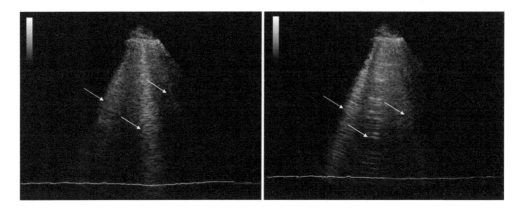

FIGURE 20.1   Multiple diffuse bilateral B-lines (arrows) in a patient with cardiogenic pulmonary edema (V20.1).

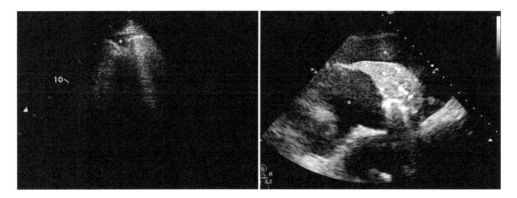

FIGURE 20.2   Left panel: trivial pleural effusion (*) at the costophrenic angle. Right panel: large pleural effusion (*) with compression atelectasis (V20.2).

which represents the main differential diagnosis with cardiogenic pulmonary edema in patients with acute dyspnea, do not show multiple diffuse bilateral B-lines,[2] making LUS a very suitable tool to support the clinical evaluation in this frequent scenario.

Combining cardiac and lung assessment is especially useful in patients with suspected acute cardiogenic pulmonary edema because the *integrated cardiopulmonary ultrasound approach* provides information on the likely cause of the ongoing heart failure (HF) and, on the other side, on the presence and degree of decompensation, manifests as pulmonary interstitial edema.[3] Even in the presence of a severe cardiac dysfunction, the absence of multiple diffuse bilateral B-lines make the diagnosis of cardiogenic pulmonary edema very unlikely.

In the evaluation of patients with suspected cardiogenic pulmonary edema, adding LUS to the clinical evaluation has resulted in a higher accuracy compared to clinical evaluation combined with chest X-ray and natriuretic peptides (LUS AUC of 0.95 vs. chest X-ray/NTproBNP 0.87, p<0.01); moreover, this approach is quicker to reach the correct diagnosis, with 5 minutes median time with LUS (25th–75th percentiles: 4–9 minutes) and 104 minutes median time with chest X-ray/NTproBNP (25th–75th percentiles: 80–131.5 minutes).[4]

LUS is also useful for the assessment of *pleural effusion* in patients with cardiogenic pulmonary edema.[5] Pleural effusion is often present in these patients, especially in patients with long-lasting HF, and may range from a trivial effusion limited to the costophrenic angle, to large effusions with compression atelectasis of the lung parenchyma (Figure 20.2) (V20.2).[6] Some formulas have been proposed to quantify the amount of fluid, although none of these is universally accepted, and most of them have been derived from studies in patients on mechanical ventilation.[6] A simple way to semi-quantify pleural effusion is to count the number of intercostal spaces in which the effusion is visible (Table 20.1).[7]

Monitoring

Once the diagnosis of cardiogenic pulmonary edema is established, LUS can be useful to monitor decongestion during hospitalization.[8,9] Assessing *dynamic changes of B-lines* is an additional parameter to evaluate diuretic response, which may be useful to better determine an effective diuretic dose and may be integrated with the clinical assessment, diuresis, and natriuresis estimation. Some preliminary data show that patients in which the diuretic therapy has been guided also

TABLE 20.1 Semi-Quantification of Pleural Effusion by Ultrasound

GRADING	INTERCOSTAL SPACES
Grade 1: Trivial	Limited to costophrenic angle
Grade 2: Small	1 Intercostal space
Grade 3: Small to medium	2–3 Intercostal spaces
Grade 4: Medium	3–4 Intercostal spaces
Grade 5: Large	4 Intercostal spaces or more

(Adapted from Reference 7.)

TABLE 20.2 Lung Ultrasound Features to Differentiate Acute Heart Failure from Acute Lung Injury/Acute Respiratory Distress Syndrome

LUS FEATURES	ACUTE HEART FAILURE	ALI/ARDS
B-lines	Multiple, diffuse, bilateral	Multiple, patchy, usually bilateral
Distribution of B-lines in a single scanning area	Quite homogenous	Spared areas
Distribution of B-lines over the whole chest	Gravity-related	Patchy
Pleural line	Regular, thin appearance	Irregular
Small peripheral consolidations	Usually absent	Present
Larger consolidations	Usually absent (possible compression atelectasis with large pleural effusion)	Usually present

Abbreviations: ALI, acute lung injury; ARDS, acute respiratory distress syndrome; LUS, lung ultrasound.

by LUS have a shorter length of hospital stay, compared to patients in which diuretic therapy is guided by chest X-ray.[10] Thus, the concept of LUS as a time-saving exam may hold for both diagnostic and monitoring purposes. However, more definite studies are needed to better understand the additional value of an LUS-guided versus a standard approach.

Risk stratification

Many different studies demonstrated that patients still showing B-lines on the day of discharge after a hospitalization for acute HF have a significantly higher risk of being readmitted for a new episode of decompensated HF in the following 3 months.[11–14] This aspect has been underlined in the latest ESC (European Society of Cardiology) Guidelines, which recommended (class I recommendation) that patients hospitalized for HF should be carefully evaluated to exclude persistent signs of congestion before discharge and to optimize oral treatment.[15]

The *number of B-lines* can stratify the risk even when assessed at admission, and more B-lines at admission predict further acute heart HF rehospitalization independently of the initial ejection fraction (EF) and independently of actual symptoms and signs.[16]

Randomized studies have shown that guiding diuretic therapy by LUS in outpatients with HF improve outcomes, in terms of death, rehospitalization for acute HF, and urgent visit for acute HF.[17–19]

NON-CARDIOGENIC PULMONARY EDEMA

Acute respiratory distress syndrome (ARDS) and acute lung injury (ALI) are frequent in patients with respiratory failure. LUS features of ALI/ARDS include those of a pulmonary edema, thus multiple diffuse bilateral B-lines, but with some substantial differences compared to cardiogenic pulmonary edema (Table 20.2).[20]

Cardiogenic pulmonary edema has a more homogenous distribution, both in the single scanning area and on the whole chest, where B-lines are more numerous at the lung bases and less numerous at the apexes; also, in a patient who's lying down they are more numerous in the lower/posterior part of the chest, compared to the upper/anterior part of the chest.

The distribution of B-lines in ALI/ARDS is instead inhomogeneous and patchy, both in the single scanning area where we can appreciate "spared areas" (an abrupt alternation of a normal LUS pattern with a completely abnormal pattern, with several B-lines with or without pleural line alterations and/or small peripheral consolidations) (Figure 20.3) (V20.3A, V20.3B), as well as on the whole chest—similar to irregular and patchy distribution that can be noted on the chest computed tomography (CT) scan.[3,21]

Both in ARDS and cardiogenic pulmonary edema, LUS can be used not only for supporting the diagnosis but also for monitoring – LUS can help in assessing recruitment and to

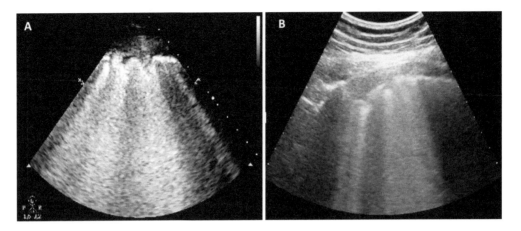

FIGURE 20.3　(A) Typical LUS pattern of non-cardiogenic pulmonary edema due to ALI/ARDS with a cardiac probe (V20.3A). (B) Typical LUS pattern of non-cardiogenic pulmonary edema due to ALI/ARDS with a convex probe (V20.3B).

TABLE 20.3　Semi-Quantification of Recruited Lung Areas

POINTS	LUS PATTERN	LUNG AERATION
0	No significant B-lines	Normal aeration (cannot distinguish normal aeration from over-aeration)
1	Multiple B-lines covering ≤50% of the screen	Mild to moderate loss of aeration
2	Multiple, coalescent B-lines covering >50% of the screen	Moderate to severe loss of aeration
3	Consolidation	Complete loss of aeration

(Modified from Bouhemad B, et al. Bedside ultrasound assessment of positive end-expiratory pressure-induced lung recruitment. *Am J Respir Crit Care Med* 2011;183:341–7.)

predict post-extubation distress during a weaning trial. If we grade deaeration from 0 to 3 in 6 thoracic area per hemithorax (Table 20.3),[22] we can assign an *LUS score*, which can predict the likelihood of a successful extubation with good accuracy, as well as provide a semi-quantification of the recruited lung areas.[23] Patients with higher LUS scores have an increased deaeration status, whereas a lower LUS score indicates a more aerated lung parenchyma. Switching from a higher to a lower score indicates an active recruitment of the pulmonary parenchyma and can help to better select therapeutic options and follow-up. Moreover, a lower LUS score should also warn about the risk of overdistention; therefore, more caution should be taken in increasing positive end-expiratory pressure (PEEP) values.[22,24]

The ultrasonographic *evaluation of the weaning process from mechanical ventilatory support* may be further enriched by the additional information on systolic and diastolic left ventricular (LV) function and from the *excursion of diaphragm*. Hence, LVEF <40%, E/A >2, E/e' >12, and diaphragmatic excursion <11 mm during a spontaneous breathing trial all indicate probable failing of the weaning process. The changes in cardiac output after a *passive leg raise* is an additional parameter that can enrich this evaluation: no increase in cardiac output after a passive leg raise is indicative of an increased likelihood of failure of the spontaneous breathing trial.[25]

CARDIOGENIC SHOCK

Patients in shock (see also Chapters 4 and 21) can be assessed by LUS to better understand the etiology of the shock.[20,26] Again, *integrated cardiopulmonary ultrasound* (Figure 20.4) is powerful tool to rule-in or rule-out some of the main causes of shock.[27]

Some algorithms have been proposed for a step-by-step POCUS evaluation of these patients. The SESAME (Sequential Emergency Scanning Assessing Mechanism Or Origin of Shock Indistinct Cause) and the FALLS protocols are useful schematic decision trees to progressively exclude or rule-in the main etiologies of shock.[28,29] An integration of a FoCUS scanning with a simple LUS scanning of the upper anterior quadrants would provide many information to support the differential diagnosis of undifferentiated shock/circulatory failure (Table 20.4). The FoCUS scanning includes a quick visual assessment of the parasternal long and short axes views, then moving to the apical four-chamber view and lastly to the subcostal view.[30] From these acquisitions the presence of a severe LV systolic dysfunction and/or the suspicion of a severe valvular heart disease can be raised. From the subcostal view, we can exclude the presence of pericardial effusion with echo signs of tamponade

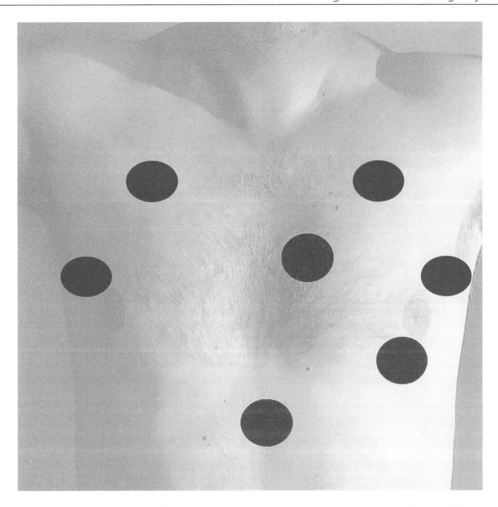

FIGURE 20.4 Proposed positions on the chest for the placement of an ultrasound transducer to obtain individual FoCUS (red circles) and LUS views (blue circles—apical and lateral scanning bilaterally) in the evaluation of patients with suspected cardiac emergencies (see also Figure 19.2).

TABLE 20.4 FoCUS and LUS Findings Useful for Rule-In/Rule-Out of Some of the Main Causes of Shock

FoCUS/LUS	FINDINGS	CONDITION
FoCUS	Severe LV systolic dysfunction)	Cardiogenic shock
FoCUS	Pericardial effusion with tamponade physiology	Cardiac tamponade
FoCUS	Dilated right heart chambers	Pulmonary embolism
FoCUS	"Kissing" LV walls	Hypovolemic shock
LUS	Multiple bilateral diffuse B-lines with homogenous distribution	Cardiogenic pulmonary edema
LUS	Multiple bilateral diffuse B-lines with patchy distribution, irregular pleural line, small consolidations	Non-cardiogenic pulmonary edema
LUS	Absence of lung sliding and absence of B-lines +/− lung point	Pneumothorax

Abbreviations: FoCUS, focus cardiac ultrasound; LV, left ventricular; LUS, lung ultrasound.

physiology, which would support the diagnosis of cardiac tamponade, and exclude the presence of a dilated right heart, which would support the diagnosis of pulmonary embolism. Then, the lungs should be scanned at the upper anterior chest to search the LUS pattern of acute pulmonary edema, which would support the diagnosis of cardiogenic shock (integrated with the previous cardiac scanning). This LUS scanning would also yield the diagnosis of pneumothorax in case of an absent lung sliding or the presence of a lung point. If a normal LUS pattern is identified at the upper anterior chest quadrants, other potential causes of shock include either septic shock or hypovolemic shock (if not excluded by

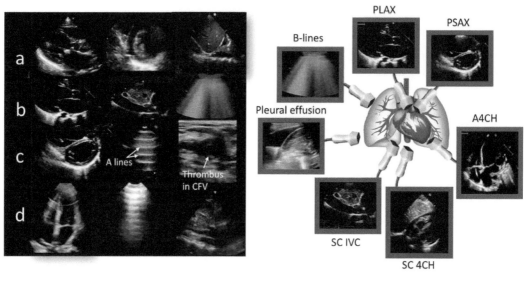

Panel A   Panel B

FIGURE 20.5   Panel A: Various scenarios for the use of FoCUS in shock states: (a) Leftward image: PLAX view showing a large hyperechoic mass at the anterior mitral leaflet (vegetation). Middle image: PLAX view showing hyperdynamic LV activity with pre-served LV end-diastolic volume (vasoplegia). Rightward image: LUS assessment of the right costo-phrenic angle at the mid-axillar line shows evidence of a basal lung consolidation. Findings are supportive of a diagnosis of septic shock due to infective endocarditis and bacterial pneumonia. (b) Leftward image: PLAX view showing dilated LV cavity. Middle image: Subcostal IVC view showing dilated IVC. Rightward image: LUS shows multiple B-lines. Findings are supportive of a diagnosis of cardiogenic shock due to acute decompensated heart failure in a patient with dilated cardiomyopathy. (c) Leftward image: Left parasternal short-axis view show-ing dilated RV with flattening of the IVS leading to D-shaped LV. Middle image: LUS shows predominant A-lines. Rightward image: ultrasound of deep lower limb veins shows a thrombus in the CFV. Findings are supportive of a diagnosis of obstructive shock due to pulmonary thromboembolism. (d) Leftward image: A4CH view showing hyperdynamic LV with small RV and LV cavity size. Middle image: LUS shows predominant A-lines. Rightward image: Subcostal IVC view showing collapsed IVC in a spontaneously ventilated patient. Findings are supportive of a diagnosis of hypovolemic shock. Panel B: Suggested scanning protocol for FoCUS and LUS in the acute settings.

(Modified with permission from Oxford University Press from Soliman-Aboumarie H et al.[20])

other assessments). The clinical response to fluid administra-tion could also help in differentiating these two conditions, with likely no clinical benefit and appearance of pulmonary B-lines in case of septic shock and with clinical benefit in case of hypovolemic shock.

Various scenarios for the use of FoCUS and LUS in shock states are illustrated in Figure 20.5.

ACUTE PULMONARY EMBOLISM

Acute pulmonary embolism can be totally missed by ultra-sound examination of the heart when there is no hemodynamic compromise, but in the presence of hypotension or shock car-diac, alterations are usually present and visible (see Chapter 7). The FoCUS can reveal a dilated and/or dysfunctional right ventricle (RV), with a ratio between the basal RV to LV diam-eter in apical four-chamber view >1, a flattened interventricu-lar septum in parasternal short axes view (D-shape of the LV), and a dilated inferior vena cava in subcostal view. The worse

is the hemodynamic profile, the more likely cardiac ultrasound will show some abnormalities.

LUS in acute pulmonary embolism can show the *pulmo-nary infarction* as an oval or polygonal pulmonary consolida-tion; often multiple small consolidations can be detected by LUS.[31] However, the sensitivity of LUS in pulmonary embo-lism to detect the pulmonary infarction is rather low, and the added value of LUS in patients with suspected pulmonary embolism is more related to the possibility of excluding other life-threatening conditions than to the ruling-in of pulmo-nary embolism itself. Compression venous ultrasound (VUS) Doppler examination of the leg veins is also useful in this sce-nario, although still with a high specificity, but low sensitiv-ity. Nazerian et al. reported rather low sensitivity of the single typical ultrasound findings of pulmonary embolism, whereas specificity was very high. However, when combining FoCUS, LUS, and VUS in a *multiorgan examination*, the sensitivity significantly increases with a small reduction of specificity (reported sensitivity and specificity for diagnosis of acute pul-monary embolism are 33% and 91% for FoCUS, 61% and 96% for LUS, 53% and 93% for VUS, and 90% and 86% for multi-organ ultrasound, respectively).[32]

ACUTE CORONARY SYNDROMES

Ultrasound is extremely useful in acute coronary syndromes (see also Chapters 2 and 3) and for the differential diagnosis of acute chest pain.[27] Echocardiography can reveal regional wall motion abnormalities, raising the suspicion of an ischemic etiology. However, although trained FoCUS operators may identify striking asynergy, subtle regional wall motion abnormalities are not evidence-based targets for FoCUS. Therefore, patients with chest pain and suspected acute coronary syndrome and acute aortic syndrome should be referred to comprehensive echocardiography as soon as possible.[30] It should be also underlined that many patients with non-ST elevation acute myocardial infarction (NSTEMI) have no visible regional wall motion abnormalities at initial presentation and that in patients with chronic coronary artery disease and a previous myocardial infarction, it might be difficult to differentiate new asynergy from existing one.

In these patients, LUS can easily detect pulmonary congestion, especially in those with large anterior myocardial infarctions.[33] By using ultrasound, it is possible to perform *a kind of Forrester's classification assessment*, where the presence of multiple diffuse bilateral B-lines identifies "wet" patients. It has been shown that the presence of B-lines in patients with acute coronary syndromes is associated with worse prognosis (Table 20.5).[34]

Since the velocity-time integral (VTI) of the left ventricular outflow tract (LVOT) is a non-invasive estimation of the cardiac output, it could be a used as a surrogate of perfusion, although this kind of evaluation is beyond the scope of FoCUS and requires comprehensive echocardiography evaluation.

PNEUMONIA

Although not strictly the part of emergency cardiac care, pneumonia is a very frequent condition in hospitalized cardiac patients. It is often associated with HF, being a typical precipitant of acute HF episode. Also, acute HF may facilitate immunodepression and consequent pneumonia.[35] A diagnosis of pneumonia during HF hospitalization is independently associated with in-hospital mortality. As rales and dyspnea are cardinal signs and symptoms of both diseases, the clinical diagnosis of the association of acute HF and pneumonia is usually challenging, especially in the elderly population, who less often present respiratory and non-respiratory symptoms of pneumonia.[36-38] According to the current guidelines, the presence of infiltrates demonstrated by imaging is mandatory for diagnosis of pneumonia.[39,40] LUS can be used for detection of parenchymal consolidations, which are not typical in acute HF unless the compression atelectasis concomitant with a large pleural effusion occurs.[1,24]

The sonographic appearance of pneumonia is either an *echo-poor region* (usually for non-translobar consolidations) (Figure 20.6) (V20.4) or *tissue-like echo texture* (usually in translobar consolidations). A sonographic *focal interstitial syndrome* can indicate pneumonia: a focal interstitial syndrome refers to multiple B-lines localized in only one thoracic scanning area. These multiple localized B-lines pattern can represent the early phase of the partial pulmonary deaeration preceding the complete deaeration that is going to follow soon or the perilesional edema of a consolidation that is too deep in the pulmonary parenchyma to be detected by ultrasound.[1,3] *Pleural effusion* can be also present, visible at the costophrenic angles.

TABLE 20.5 Studies Addressing the Prognostic Value of Lung Ultrasound in Acute Coronary Syndromes

PAPER	YEAR	TYPE OF ACUTE CORONARY SYNDROME	NUMBER OF PATIENTS	OUTCOME
Bedetti et al.	2010	STEMI, NSTEMI, UA	470	All-cause death or non-fatal MI
Ye et al.	2019	STEMI	96	*In-hospital:* Symptomatic HF *Out-hospital:* All-cause death or HF-rehospitalization
Araujo et al.	2020	STEMI	215	In-hospital mortality
Parras et al.	2021	STEMI, NSTEMI	200	In-hospital new HF
Araujo et al.	2021	STEMI	218	*In-hospital:* MACE *Out-hospital:* MACE at 30 days

Abbreviations: HF, heart failure; MACE, major adverse cardiac event; NSTEMI, non-ST elevation acute myocardial infarction; STEMI, ST-elevation acute myocardial infarction; UA, unstable angina.

(Adapted from Reference 34)

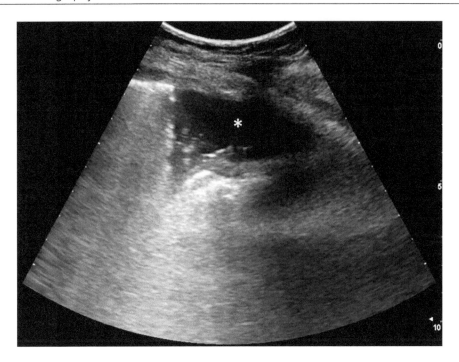

FIGURE 20.6 LUS pattern of a non-translobar pneumonic consolidation displayed as an echo-poor region (*) (V20.4).

LIST OF VIDEOS

https://routledgetextbooks.com/textbooks/9781032157009/chapter-20.php

VIDEO 20.1 LUS showing multiple diffuse bilateral B-lines in a patient with cardiogenic pulmonary edema.

VIDEO 20.2 LUS showing large pleural effusion with compression atelectasis.

VIDEO 20.3A Typical LUS pattern of non-cardiogenic pulmonary edema due to acute lung injury or ARDS performed with a cardiac probe. Note the irregular pleural line and multiple diffuse bilateral B-lines.

VIDEO 20.3B Typical LUS pattern of non-cardiogenic pulmonary edema due to acute lung injury or ARDS performed with a convex probe. Note the irregular pleural line and multiple diffuse bilateral B-lines.

VIDEO 20.4 Lung ultrasound showing echo-poor region indicating non-translobar pneumonic consolidation.

REFERENCES

1. Volpicelli G, Elbarbary M, Blaivas M, et al. International evidence-based recommendations for point-of-care lung ultrasound. *Intensive Care Medicine* 2012;38(4):577–91.
2. Lichtenstein D, Mezière G. A lung ultrasound sign allowing bedside distinction between pulmonary edema and COPD: the comet-tail artifact. *Intensive Care Medicine* 1998;24(12):1331–4.
3. Gargani L. Ultrasound of the lungs: more than a room with a view. *Heart Failure Clinics* 2019;15(2):297–303.
4. Pivetta E, Goffi A, Nazerian P, et al. Lung ultrasound integrated with clinical assessment for the diagnosis of acute decompensated heart failure in the emergency department: a randomized controlled trial. *European Journal of Heart Failure* 2019;21(6):754–66.
5. Lindner M, Thomas R, Claggett B, et al. Quantification of pleural effusions on thoracic ultrasound in acute heart failure. *European Heart Journal: Acute Cardiovascular Care* 2020;9(5):513–21.
6. Brogi E, Gargani L, Bignami E, et al. Thoracic ultrasound for pleural effusion in the intensive care unit: a narrative review from diagnosis to treatment. *Critical Care* 2017;21(1):325.
7. Smargiassi A, Inchingolo R, Zanforlin A, Valente S, Soldati G, Corbo GM. Description of free-flowing pleural effusions in medical reports after echographic assessment. *Respiration* 2013;85(5):439–41.
8. Volpicelli G, Caramello V, Cardinale L, Mussa A, Bar F, Frascisco MF. Bedside ultrasound of the lung for the monitoring of acute decompensated heart failure. *The American Journal of Emergency Medicine* 2008;26(5):585–91.
9. Gargani L. Lung ultrasound: a new tool for the cardiologist. *Cardiovascular Ultrasound* 2011;9:6.
10. Mozzini C, Di M, Perna D, et al. Lung ultrasound in internal medicine efficiently drives the management of patients with

heart failure and speeds up the discharge time Inferior Cave Vein Collassability index. *Internal and Emergency Medicine* 2018;13(1):27–33.

11. Gargani L, Pang PS, Frassi F, et al. Persistent pulmonary congestion before discharge predicts rehospitalization in heart failure: a lung ultrasound study. *Cardiovascular Ultrasound* 2015;13:40.

12. Coiro S, Rossignol P, Ambrosio G, et al. Prognostic value of residual pulmonary congestion at discharge assessed by lung ultrasound imaging in heart failure. *European Journal of Heart Failure* 2015;17(11):1172–81.

13. Cogliati C, Casazza G, Ceriani E, et al. Lung ultrasound and short-term prognosis in heart failure patients. *International Journal of Cardiology* 2016;218:104–8.

14. Gargani L, Ferre RM, Pang PS. B-lines in heart failure: will comets guide us? *European Journal of Heart Failure* 2019;21(12):1616–8.

15. McDonagh TA, Metra M, Adamo M, et al. 2021 ESC guidelines for the diagnosis and treatment of acute and chronic heart failure: Developed by the Task Force for the diagnosis and treatment of acute and chronic heart failure of the European Society of Cardiology (ESC) with the special contribution of the Heart Failure Association (HFA) of the ESC. *European Heart Journal* 2021;42(36):3599–726.

16. Gargani L, Pugliese NR, Frassi F, et al. Prognostic value of lung ultrasound in patients hospitalized for heart disease irrespective of symptoms and ejection fraction. *ESC Heart Failure* 2021;8(4):2660–9.

17. Marini C, Fragasso G, Italia L, et al. Lung ultrasound-guided therapy reduces acute decompensation events in chronic heart failure. *Heart* 2020;106(24):1934–9.

18. Araiza-Garaygordobil D, Gopar-Nieto R, Martinez-Amezcua P, et al. A randomized controlled trial of lung ultrasound-guided therapy in heart failure (CLUSTER-HF study). *American Heart Journal* 2020;227:31–9.

19. Rivas-Lasarte M, Álvarez-García J, Fernández-Martínez J, et al. Lung ultrasound-guided treatment in ambulatory patients with heart failure: a randomized controlled clinical trial (LUS-HF study). *European Journal of Heart Failure* 2019;21(12):1605–13.

20. Soliman-Aboumarie H, Breithardt OA, Gargani L, Trambaiolo P, Neskovic AN. How-to: focus cardiac ultrasound in acute settings. *European Heart Journal: Cardiovascular Imaging* 2022;23(2):150–3.

21. Gargani L, Soliman-Aboumarie H, Volpicelli G, Corradi F, Pastore MC, Cameli M. Why, when, and how to use lung ultrasound during the COVID-19 pandemic: enthusiasm and caution. *European Heart Journal: Cardiovascular Imaging* 2020;21(9):941–8.

22. Bouhemad B, Mongodi S, Via G, Rouquette I. Ultrasound for "lung monitoring" of ventilated patients. *Anesthesiology* 2015;122(2):437–47.

23. Soummer A, Arbelot C, Lu Q, et al. Ultrasound assessment of lung aeration loss during a successful weaning trial predicts postextubation distress. *Critical Care Medicine* 2012;40(7):2064–72.

24. Bouhemad B, Liu ZH, Arbelot C, et al. Ultrasound assessment of antibiotic-induced pulmonary reaeration in ventilator-associated pneumonia. *Critical Care Medicine* 2010;38(1):84–92.

25. Mayo P, Volpicelli G, Lerolle N, Schreiber A, Doelken P, Vieillard-Baron A. Ultrasonography evaluation during the weaning process: the heart, the diaphragm, the pleura and the lung. *Intensive Care Medicine* 2016;42(7):1107–17.

26. Volpicelli G, Lamorte A, Tullio M, et al. Point-of-care multiorgan ultrasonography for the evaluation of undifferentiated hypotension in the emergency department. *Intensive Care Medicine* 2013;39(7):1290–8.

27. Lancellotti P, Price S, Edvardsen T, et al. The use of echocardiography in acute cardiovascular care: recommendations of the European Association of Cardiovascular Imaging and the Acute Cardiovascular Care Association. *European Heart Journal: Acute Cardiovascular Care* 2015;16(2):119–46.

28. Lichtenstein D, Malbrain MLNG. Critical care ultrasound in cardiac arrest. Technological requirements for performing the SESAME-protocol—a holistic approach. *Anaesthesiology Intensive Therapy* 2015;47(5):471–81.

29. Lichtenstein D. Fluid administration limited by lung sonography: the place of lung ultrasound in assessment of acute circulatory failure (the FALLS-protocol). *Expert Review of Respiratory Medicine* 2012;6(2):155–62.

30. Neskovic AN, Skinner H, Price S, et al. Focus cardiac ultrasound core curriculum and core syllabus of the European Association of Cardiovascular Imaging. *European Heart Journal: Cardiovascular Imaging* 2018;19(5):475–81.

31. Reissig A, Kroegel C. Transthoracic ultrasound of lung and pleura in the diagnosis of pulmonary embolism: a novel non-invasive bedside approach. *Respiration* 2003;70(5):441–52.

32. Nazerian P, Vanni S, Volpicelli G, et al. Accuracy of point-of-care multiorgan ultrasonography for the diagnosis of pulmonary embolism. *Chest* 2014;145(5):950–7.

33. Bedetti G, Gargani L, Sicari R, Gianfaldoni ML, Molinaro S, Picano E. Comparison of prognostic value of echographic [corrected] risk score with the Thrombolysis in Myocardial Infarction (TIMI) and Global Registry in Acute Coronary Events (GRACE) risk scores in acute coronary syndrome. *American Journal of Cardiology* 2010;106(12):1709–16.

34. Lindner M, Lindsey A, Bain PA, Platz E. Prevalence and prognostic importance of lung ultrasound findings in acute coronary syndrome: a systematic review. *Echocardiography* 2021;38(12):2069–76.

35. Mazzola M, Pugliese NR, Zavagli M, et al. Diagnostic and prognostic value of lung ultrasound B-lines in acute heart failure with concomitant pneumonia. *Frontiers in Cardiovascular Medicine* 2021;8:693912.

36. Metlay JP, Schulz R, Li YH, et al. Influence of age on symptoms at presentation in patients with community-acquired pneumonia. *Archives of Internal Medicine* 1997;157(13):1453–9.

37. Ware LB, Matthay MA. Acute pulmonary edema. *New England Journal of Medicine* 2005;353(26):2788–96.

38. Jobs A, Simon R, de Waha S, et al. Pneumonia and inflammation in acute decompensated heart failure: a registry-based analysis of 1939 patients. *European Heart Journal Acute Cardiovascular Care* 2018;7(4):362–70.

39. Metlay JP, Waterer GW, Long AC, et al. Diagnosis and treatment of adults with community-acquired pneumonia. *American Journal of Respiratory and Critical Care Medicine* 2019;200(7):E45–E67.

40. Woodhead M, Blasi F, Ewig S, et al. Guidelines for the management of adult lower respiratory tract infections—full version. *Clinical Microbiology and Infection* 2011;17:E1–E59.

Echocardiography-guided patient management in the intensive care unit

21

Valentino Dammassa, Guido Tavazzi, and Susanna Price

Key Points

- As a first-line tool for the diagnosis and management of acute cardiovascular and respiratory failure, echo-cardiography is essential in evaluating critically ill patients in the intensive care unit (ICU).
- Assessment of ICU patients is *complex*: the ventricular systolic and diastolic function parameters must be contextualized with volume and inotropic conditions and the presence of respiratory and/or mechanical circulatory support.
- The *integrative multi-parametric approach*, including assessment of commonly used indices (left ventricular ejection fraction and congestion indices) along with electro-mechanical and systo-diastolic synchrony (total isovolumic time and mitral annular plane systolic excursion), is important to define not only the global ventricular function but also the underlying mechanism limiting cardiac output.

Echocardiography is the first-line tool for the diagnosis and management of acute cardiovascular and respiratory failure. Standardized restrictive imaging protocols, such as focus cardiac ultrasound (FoCUS), are currently widely used in both pre-hospital and emergency department settings to assist decision-making in hemodynamically instable acutely ill patients.[1] Advanced critical care echocardiography (transthoracic [TTE] and transesophageal [TEE]), is an essential tool for diagnosis, decision-making, and monitoring critically ill patients in both cardiac and general intensive care units (ICUs).[2]

As there are no indices specifically validated in this population, the contextualization with loading and inotropic conditions and with an actual type of organ support (respiratory and/or mechanical circulatory) is of utmost importance.[3,4]

In this chapter, we aim to discuss usefulness and limitations of long-established parameters of ventricular function

along with some less commonly used indices that may help in defining the hemodynamic profile and underlying patho-physiological mechanism leading to cardiovascular failure, highlighting their strengths, limitations, and some of the potential pitfalls in their use.

HYPOVOLEMIA AND FLUID RESPONSIVENESS

Hypovolemia, defined as the depletion of effective intravascular volume, is a common cause of shock with numerous potential underlying causes, frequently requiring rapid fluid administration to achieve hemodynamic stability. After this

DOI: 10.1201/9781003245407-21

TABLE 21.1   Static Echocardiographic Indices for Assessment of Volume Status with Respective Reference Values and Limitations

STATIC PARAMETER	MEASUREMENT	REFERENCE VALUES	PITFALLS AND LIMITATIONS
Inferior vena cava (IVC) diameter	TTE—subcostal view	Suggestive of severe hypovolemia: • <10 mm in spontaneous breathing • <15 mm on positive-pressure ventilation	• Poor correlation with fluid responsiveness • Confounding factors: mechanical ventilation (especially if high PEEP), respiratory pathologies (COPD and asthma), RV dysfunction, TR, tamponade mechanisms (cardiac tamponade and tension pneumothorax), mechanical obstruction (cannulation for ECMO), and increase in intra-abdominal pressure.
Left ventricular end-diastolic volume (LVEDV)	TTE— apical four- and two-chamber view (method of disc summation)	34–74 mL/m² for males 29–61 mL/m² for females	• Requires adequate definition of endocardial borders • Pre-existing cardiomyopathies and previous myocardial infarction may present with altered dimensions and geometry secondary to ventricular remodeling
Left ventricular end-diastolic area (LVEDA)	TTE—parasternal short-axis view (level of papillary muscles) TEE—trans-gastric mid-papillary short-axis view (include papillary muscles and trabeculations)	*Normal values:* 13 ± 2 cm/m² *Severe hypovolemia:* <6 cm/m² and end-systolic obliteration of LV cavity	• Requires adequate definition of endocardial borders • Pre-existing cardiomyopathies and previous myocardial infarction may present with altered dimensions and geometry secondary to ventricular remodeling

Abbreviations: ECMO, extracorporeal membrane oxygenation; COPD, chronic obstructive pulmonary diseases; LV, left ventricle; PEEP, positive end-expiratory pressure; RV, right ventricle; TEE, transesophageal echocardiography; TR, tricuspid regurgitation; TTE, transthoracic echocardiography.

initial resuscitative phase, more cautious fluid management is advocated, as excessive volume resuscitation is associated with worse outcomes.[5]

Echocardiography can be used as a first-line imaging tool for the recognition of hypovolemia and to evaluate whether the patient with shock might benefit from fluid administration. Here, the ability to increase stroke volume by 15% or more in response to volume loading is defined as *volume responsiveness*. Several static and dynamic echocardiographic indices provide useful insight into the volume status and may predict fluid responsiveness.[6] However, a number of clinical and management conditions may represent pitfalls and limitations in fluid responsiveness evaluation (Tables 21.1 and 21.2). Therefore, a thoughtful evaluation of cardiac morphology and function (i.e., chronic pathophysiology) and contextualization of existing cardiovascular and respiratory conditions, along with ongoing supports (vasopressors/inotropes, mechanical ventilation, mechanical circulatory devices), must be taken in consideration.

Static parameters of fluid responsiveness

Evaluated at end-expiration, these measurements generally provide an unreliable estimation of preload and fluid responsiveness but nonetheless are widely used. Static parameters, with their relative pitfalls and limitations, are summarized in Table 21.1. For all the reasons described in the Table 21.1, they cannot be considered as reliable indices for the assessment of volume status and fluid responsiveness,[7] with an exception

of patients with extremely low preload (severe hypovolemia) (Figure 5.5) (V5.9A, V5.9B, V5.9C, V5.9D).

Dynamic parameters of fluid responsiveness

Assessed under different cardiac-loading conditions generated by a fluid challenge, postural changes, or heart-lung interactions (variation in intrathoracic pressure during the respiratory cycle), these indices can be evaluated *both* in mechanically ventilated and spontaneously breathing patients.

Fluid responsiveness during mechanical ventilation

In mechanically ventilated patients, cyclical changes in intrathoracic pressures, determined by positive-pressure inspiration and passive expiration, affect preload and afterload of both right and left ventricles (for further details see the following paragraphs) (Figure 21.1). The variation of left ventricular (LV) stroke volume in response to these changes can be used to predict response to fluid administration. Left ventricular outflow (LVOT) velocity-time integral (VTI) can be measured with both TTE and TEE and used to estimate LV stroke volume. Cyclical variation of LVOT VTI (ΔVTI) under positive-pressure ventilation has proven to be related to response to volume loading, with a ΔVTI >10% being predictive of fluid responsiveness. In a similar way, variation of LVOT peak velocity (ΔV_{peak}) can predict fluid responsiveness if ΔV_{peak} is >12% (Figure 21.2).

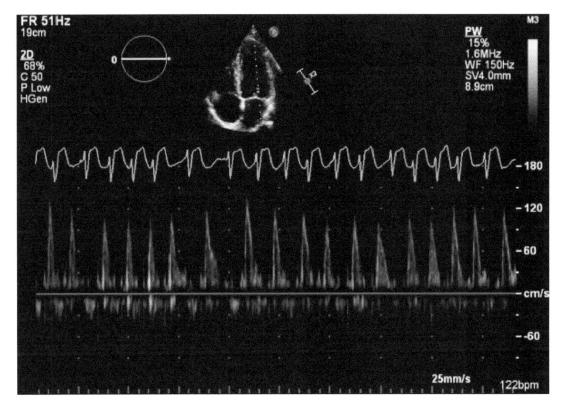

FIGURE 21.1   Pulsed-wave Doppler of mitral inflow showing respiratory variations of the E-wave velocity throughout the respiratory cycle.

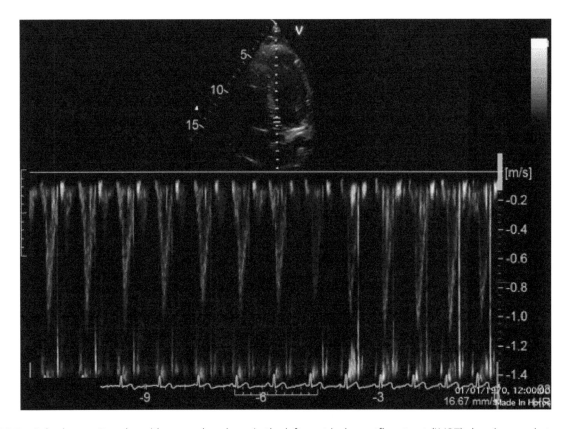

FIGURE 21.2   Pulsed-wave Doppler with a sample volume in the left ventricular outflow tract (LVOT) showing respiratory variations of the LVOT VTI and LVOT peak velocity.

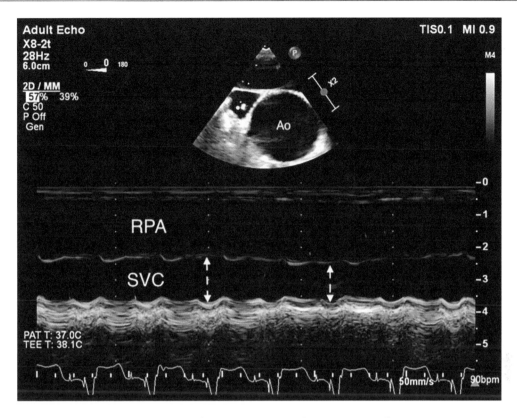

FIGURE 21.3 Assessment of respiratory variations of superior vena cava by TEE. Arrows denote SVC diameter on M-mode display during respiratory cycle. Ao: aorta; RPA: right pulmonary artery; SVC: superior vena cava.

TEE allows the measurement of superior vena cava (SVC) diameter (Figure 21.3). Being intrathoracic, the SVC is not influenced by intra-abdominal pressure, and its dimension is directly affected by cycling of intrathoracic pressure throughout the respiratory cycle. A respiratory variation of SVC >36% has been proposed as a predictor of fluid responsiveness.[8]

Inferior vena cava (IVC) diameter can be easily measured with TTE (1–2 cm upstream to atrio-caval junction in subcostal view). IVC is an intra-abdominal vessel and for this reason, an increase in intrathoracic pressure determined by positive-pressure inspiration causes an increase in IVC diameter (in contrast to what happens with an inspiration during spontaneous breathing); for the similar reason, a high intra-abdominal pressure represents a pitfall (Table 21.2). Similar to SVC, IVC variation during respiratory cycle (*IVC distensibility index*) has been validated for the evaluation of fluid responsiveness with two different proposed thresholds (12% and 18%).[9] In order to predict fluid responsiveness according to respiratory variations of LVOT VTI, SVC, and IVC, the patient must be completely passive on mechanical ventilation and should be in sinus rhythm (to avoid beat-to-beat variations of the LVOT VTI and ΔV_{peak} generated by irregular cardiac rhythms).

It has to be kept in mind that none of the fluid challenge parameters, including IVC variations, have been validated in patients with cardiomyopathies, cardiogenic shock, right ventricular dysfunction, pulmonary hypertension, and acute/

advanced heart failure.[7] Therefore, their use in acute cardiac care may be limited and must be contextualized.

Fluid responsiveness in spontaneously breathing patients

Passive leg raising (PLR) is an alternative for the assessment of fluid responsiveness in spontaneously breathing patients and in those with irregular heart rhythm. PLR results in the reversible transfer of blood from the venous system in lower limbs to central circulation—equivalent to a fluid bolus of ~300 mL. The advantage is the possibility of rapid reversal, avoiding the risk of inadvertent overload when the patient is not volume responsive. The starting patient position should be semi-recumbent (45°) and the bed moved to a supine position with legs at 45°, thus creating a 90° postural change. A positive response is a >10–15% variation of the LVOT VTI after one minute.[10]

Table 21.2 summarizes the pitfalls and limitations of dynamic indices of fluid responsiveness.

CARDIOGENIC SHOCK

Cardiogenic shock (CS) is defined as a critical state of end-organ hypoperfusion and hypoxia caused by a primary cardiac

TABLE 21.2 Limitations and Pitfalls of Dynamic Parameters for the Assessment of Fluid Responsiveness

DYNAMIC PARAMETER	LIMITATIONS AND PITFALLS
Respiratory variations of LVOT VTI	• Spontaneous respiratory efforts (dyspnea, tachypnea, respiratory distress) and arrhythmias • Respiratory-induced changes in LVOT VTI are dependent on tidal volume; hence, tidal volumes <7 mL/kg may yield false-negative results • RV failure (e.g., acute cor pulmonale related to acute pulmonary embolism or ARDS) can cause false-positive dynamic changes in LVOT VTI, not related to volume depletion but to cyclic changes in RV stroke volume (reduction during inspiratory peak pressure)
Respiratory variations of IVC and SVC diameters	• Spontaneous respiratory efforts and arrhythmias • High intra-abdominal pressure • High PEEP/intrathoracic pressure and low tidal volume • Moderate to severe tricuspid regurgitation • RV failure and/or tamponade physiology • Not investigated in pulmonary hypertension patients • Not investigated in cardiogenic shock and cardiomyopathies • Assessment of respiratory variations of SVC requires TEE
Passive leg raising	• Contraindicated in patients with intracranial hypertension • The response to centralization of blood volume may be reduced in the presence of intra-abdominal hypertension (false-negative response) • Unfeasible in patients with mechanical circulatory support

Abbreviations: ARDS, acute respiratory distress syndrome; IVC, inferior vena cava; LVOT, left ventricular outflow tract; PEEP, positive end-expiratory pressure; RV, right ventricle; SVC, superior vena cava; TEE, transesophageal echocardiography; VTI, velocity-time integral.

disorder potentially leading to multiorgan failure, which is associated with high mortality (in-hospital mortality of 40–50%) and morbidity. In CS, comprehensive TTE is recommended as the first-line non-invasive imaging technique,[11,12] providing useful information regarding the diagnosis of the underlying cause, as well as hemodynamic status and guidance of interventions (see Chapter 4). TEE should be performed if the image quality of TTE is poor and/or if the diagnosis remains uncertain.

Ventricular performance

As the epidemiology of cardiogenic shock is changing over time, roughly 30% of cases are related to acute myocardial infarction (AMI) (V4.7), whereas 35–40% are seen in patients with acute decompensated heart failure (ADHF) (V4.6).[13] Importantly, AMI-CS and ADHF-CS have different pathophysiology, the former mostly related to abrupt hypoperfusion and the latter to the long-standing congestion. Therefore, the echocardiographic parameters to assess them should *encompass indices reflecting both perfusion and congestion.*

Left ventricular ejection fraction (LVEF) is a widely used parameter to assess global LV function with well-known advantages. However, LVEF is highly dependent on (1) loading conditions, (2) heart rate, (3) extent of dyssynchrony, and (4) end-diastolic volumes. Additionally, it has lower accuracy for subtle and early alteration of systolic function, and it falsely overestimates global LV systolic function in case of severe mitral regurgitation.[14] Although LVEF is a key parameter to define global LV function, it may be less accurate in defining which are the underlying

causes leading to ventricular dysfunction and limiting cardiac output.

Longitudinal function may be assessed by measuring mitral annular plane systolic excursion (MAPSE) using M-mode and by measuring S′ wave using tissue Doppler imaging or strain. Longitudinal myocardial fibers are located more subendocardial and in papillary muscles, and, therefore, they are exquisitely sensitive to perfusion mismatch. Indeed MAPSE alteration occurs earlier as compared to LVEF in case of perfusion mismatch (e.g., ischemia). Additionally, during ischemia, besides the reduction of longitudinal fibers shortening, prolongation of shortening time may also be observed—named "*post-ejection shortening*," which is defined as the systolic shortening peak occurring beyond the T-wave of the superimposed ECG (Figure 21.4); this results in a consequent reduction of the ventricular filling period and stroke volume.[15,16]

Systo-diastolic interaction may be reliably evaluated with the calculation of *total isovolumic time* (t-IVT). t-IVT is calculated as the sum of total filling time (t-FT) and total ejection time (t-ET), which are normalized by the heart rate, subtracted by 60, and expressed as second/minutes (Figure 21.5). This index has demonstrated high sensitivity in differentiating between left bundle branch block due to ischemia or pure conduction abnormalities.[17] Moreover, it has been shown to be the best echocardiographic index identifying the optimal heart rate and hemodynamic profile in patients with medical and post-cardiotomy CS or hemodynamic instability.[18,19]

LV stroke work index has been tested in a retrospective population of CS patients demonstrating good predictability of mortality and the *cardiac power output* in patients with heart failure with reduced LVEF.[20,21]

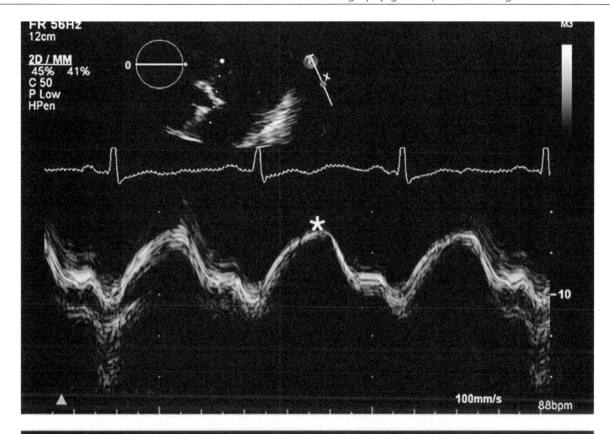

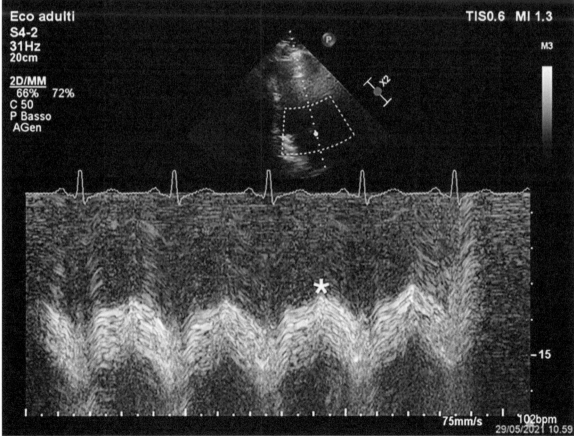

FIGURE 21.4 Post-ejection shortening. Upper panel: M-mode of the septal wall showing normal longitudinal function with the peak of systolic shortening (*) occurring within the end of the T-wave on the ECG. Lower panel: M-mode of anterior wall showing occurrence of longitudinal shortening beyond the end of the T-wave (*)—post-ejection shortening.

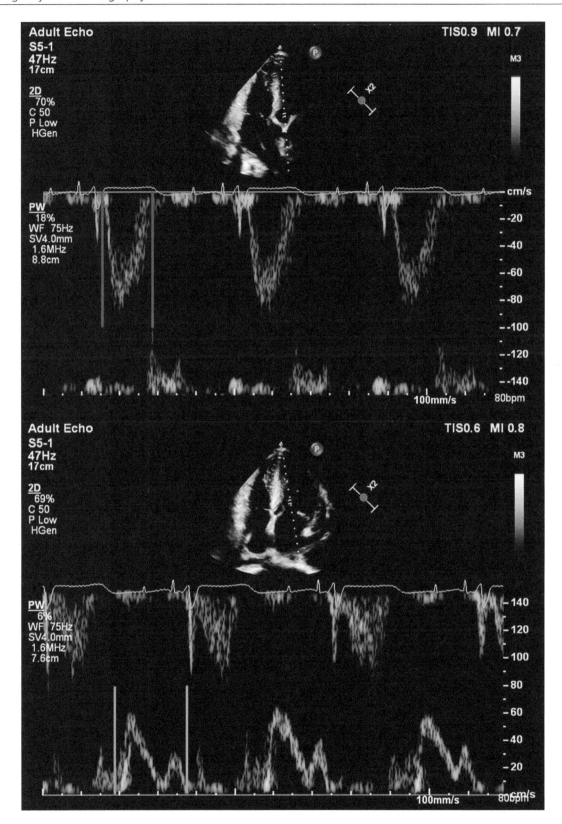

FIGURE 21.5   Total isovolumic time (t-IVT). Upper panel: Aortic ejection flow sampled with pulsed-wave (PW) Doppler in transthoracic apical five-chamber view. The ejection time (ET) is measured from the onset of the aortic flow to the aortic artifact closure (between red lines). RR interval is measured on the ECG trace, and the total ET (t-ET) is obtained applying the following formula: t-ET = [(60,000 / RR) × ET] / 1,000. Lower panel: Mitral inflow sampled with PW Doppler in transthoracic apical four-chamber view. The filling time (FT) (between green lines) is measured from the onset of the E-wave to the end of A-wave. Similar to t-ET, RR interval is measured on the superimposed ECG and the total FT (t-FT) is obtained applying the following formula: t-FT = [(60,000 / RR) × FT] / 1,000. The t-IVT is calculated as: t-IVT (s/min) = 60 − (t-FT + t-ET).

For the *assessment of right ventricular (RV) function in the acute setting*, typical echocardiographic parameters with good reproducibility at bedside are RV size, tricuspid annular plane systolic excursion (TAPSE), and tricuspid annular S' velocity.[22]

Valves and congestion

Acute mitral regurgitation in the context of AMI (see Chapters 3 and 10) may be either caused by functional ischemic mechanism (V4.8A, V4.8B) and/or by papillary muscle rupture (V21.1). Reliance on color Doppler alone for evaluation of MR severity is not recommended because in case of complete flail or severe coaptation defect regurgitant flow can be almost laminar between the LV and left atrium (LA), and consequently, the severity of MR might be underestimated. In addition, MR jets are often eccentric (with Coanda effect), which makes the assessment of the severity of actual MR even more difficult (V21.2). Once recognized, comprehensive assessment of the mitral valve, including making decisions regarding potential surgical or percutaneous interventions, is needed.

The pathophysiology of secondary MR entails a complex interplay between reduced closing forces (generated by impairment of LV systolic function) and increased tethering forces (related to LV dimensions, LV systolic dysfunction and displacement of papillary muscles). These result in a "dynamic" condition with a severity of MR dependent on loading conditions. For example, due to suddenly increased afterload after successful mitral valve repair, severe postoperative low-cardiac output state may occur in the cardiothoracic ICU (V4.4A, V4.4B). Similarly, secondary MR may not be clinically significant in sedated and mechanically ventilated patients but becoming evident during weaning from mechanical ventilation or immediately after extubation (phase characterized by increased oxygen consumption and loss of unloading effect of positive-pressure ventilation on LV).

The *assessment of congestion* mostly relies on the evaluation of left and right atrial pressures. *Left atrial pressure (LAP)* and assessment of LV diastolic function are discussed in Chapter 4. *Estimation of right atrial pressure (RAP)* is mostly based on the evaluation of IVC diameter and its respiratory collapsibility, although with the limitations mentioned earlier. It is important to note that the correlation between noninvasive indices and invasively measured end-diastolic pressure/LAP was at best low to moderate in most of the existing studies.[23] However, using the available indices to assess the diastolic function and estimating the LAP should be routinely used not to derive a single value but rather to estimate weather they are normal or elevated and their *trend* in response to therapy.

An intriguing index is the ratio between the *time of onset* of early diastolic mitral annular velocity (e') by tissue Doppler imaging (TDI) and E-wave of transmitral flow by pulsed-wave Doppler. According to physiology, e' at TDI occurs earlier that E-wave, whereas when LAP is severely elevated, the e' and E-wave occur at the same time (a sign of diastolic dysfunction),

reflecting very low compliance of the LA unable to tolerate further filling.[24]

Along with rupture of papillary muscle leading to severe MR, other mechanical complications of AMI are rare, and often associated with high mortality (see Chapter 3). Ventricular septal rupture (VSR) has a bimodal peak being more common within the first 24 hours or after 3–5 days, but it can occur within 2 weeks from the onset of AMI (V21.3A, V21.3B). The rupture more commonly involves the apical septum and is associated with anterior myocardial infarction. Less frequently it involves the basal segment of inferior septum (in inferior myocardial infarction), but it is linked to grim prognosis (V21.4A, V21.4B, V21.4C. V21.4D) Echocardiography plays a key role in the diagnosis of VSR by revealing defect across the interventricular septum with the presence of left-to-right shunt (identified by color Doppler), signs of RV overload, and the estimation the Qp/Qs by assessing LV VTI and RV VTI.

Absence of improvement in cardiac output with increasing dosage of inotrope(s) should raise the suspicion of *dynamic LVOT obstruction*. The presence of septal hypertrophy in context of hypovolemia and high adrenergic stimulation (both endogenous and exogenous) may cause systolic anterior motion (SAM) of the mitral valve and LVOT obstruction, with characteristic echocardiographic findings. Echocardiography can provide prompt diagnosis revealing typical dagger-shaped continuous-wave Doppler signal in LVOT, SAM of anterior leaflet of the mitral valve, and associated eccentric mitral regurgitation jet (Figure 4.3) (V4.10). Fluid administration, reduction in inotrope dose, and increase in vasopressor support (in case of coexistence of reduced afterload) represent the mainstem therapeutic interventions. A similar kind of dynamic obstruction can be generated at *mid-ventricular level* in patients with hyperkinetic function during septic shock.

Echocardiography and mechanical circulatory support

In recent years, the implantation of short-term percutaneous mechanical circulatory support (MCS) devices has been increasingly used in patients with CS refractory to conventional critical care interventions (fluid optimization and vasopressor/inotropic support) (see Chapter 15). The aim of MCS devices is to restore adequate tissue perfusion and to buy time to allow intervention to reverse the underlying cause, to allow the heart to recover (bridge to recovery), or to serve as a bridge to definitive longer-term support/transplantation (bridge to bridge or bridge to transplant).[25] MCS can be classified according to the mechanism of action (counterpulsation, axial flow pump, and centrifugal flow pump) and the ability to provide mono- or biventricular support and eventually oxygenation in case of respiratory failure (Figures 15.1 and 15.6). Some forms of MCS, such as venoarterial extracorporeal membrane oxygenation (VA ECMO), provide not only support to cardiovascular system but also oxygenation and decarboxylation of the blood, entirely supplying the gas exchanges when respiratory function is impaired. Each category of MSC has different impact on native cardiac function and circulation.[26]

Echocardiography has a pivotal role throughout the process of MCS placement,[27] including the following:

- Validation of contraindications (moderate/severe aortic regurgitation, aortic dissection, right/left side thrombosis, severe preload deficit)
- Assessment during process of implantation by identification of guidewire and/or correct position of the cannula (VA ECMO) or device (IABP/Impella®)
- Evaluation of cardiac adaptation to device flows (ventricular size, aortic opening, mitral regurgitation, LAP assessment)
- Assessment of potential discontinuation from MCS (weaning trials) or need to upscale to another off-loading/long-term device(s)

After MCS device implantation, echocardiography should be used as a monitoring tool at least daily and whenever significant hemodynamic variation occurs.[28,29]

OBSTRUCTIVE SHOCK

Obstructive shock is caused by critical *impairment of cardiac filling* (cardiac tamponade, tension pneumothorax, acute severe asthma, and mediastinal and cardiac masses) *or emptying* (acute pulmonary embolism and aortic stenosis). In most of these clinical scenarios, echocardiography plays a crucial role, enabling diagnosis and guiding prompt therapeutic interventions.

Cardiac tamponade

Cardiac tamponade is a life-threatening condition caused by slow or rapid accumulation of fluid, blood, pus, or gas in the pericardial space, leading to increased intrapericardial pressure with consequent impairment of diastolic filling and reduction in cardiac output. Echocardiography allows the evaluation of the size and location of pericardial effusion/collection and degree of hemodynamic compromise (Figure 8.5 and 8.6) (V8.5, V8.6).[30] Of note, the rate of accumulation will determine the rise of intrapericardial pressure. Thus, a relatively small collection of fluid (Figure 8.12) (V8.12A) developing over a short period of time can cause tamponade.[31]

Echocardiographic features of tamponade are well-documented (see Chapter 8). However, *in critical care, two situations necessitate consideration*. First, during positive pressure ventilation, the alteration in transvalvular flows is reversed (compared with spontaneous ventilation—see Figure 8.1) Second, in post-cardiotomy patients, pericardial collections can be small, localized, and exerting compression on a single chamber or vessel, often without typical Doppler findings suggestive of tamponade physiology (V14.13B, V14.13C). In this

clinical context, TEE performs better than TTE to identify the presence of localized collection. Importantly, the absence of characteristic echocardiographic signs does not exclude cardiac tamponade, which is fundamentally a clinical diagnosis.[32]

Echocardiography-guided pericardiocentesis could be performed in the ICU, especially in extreme emergency situations such as cardiac arrest (V21.5A, V21.5B, V21.5C).

Acute pulmonary embolism

Acute pulmonary embolism is one of the most common causes of RV failure and acute cor pulmonale. Sudden increase in RV afterload triggers a cascade of events, leading to RV dilatation, tricuspid regurgitation, RV ischemia, and RV systolic dysfunction, which ultimately result in obstructive shock. Echocardiographic findings in acute pulmonary embolism[33,34] are discussed in detail in Chapter 7. Echocardiography plays a crucial role during the initial assessment of suspected acute pulmonary embolism, especially in those patients who are too unstable to safely undergo immediate CT scan, justifying emergency reperfusion treatment in case of high clinical probability and unequivocal signs of RV pressure overload (with no other obvious causes). Decision-making in acute pulmonary embolism in the ICU might be challenging and the management of an individual patient might be critically influenced by actual echocardiographic findings (V21.6A, V21.6B, V21.6C, V21.6D, V21.6E, V7.22A, V7.22B). It is also worth mentioning compression venous ultrasound (VUS) in the differential diagnosis of suspected pulmonary embolism. Diagnosis of venous thromboembolism (and pulmonary embolism) could be made if VUS reveals proximal deep venous thrombosis in a patient with high clinical suspicion for pulmonary embolism.[35]

SEPSIS AND SEPTIC SHOCK

In septic shock, echocardiography is not only useful for the hemodynamic optimization but may also reveal a cardiac source of infection (V21.7A, V21.7B). The diagnosis of infective endocarditis in the critical care setting is complex, but standard guidelines apply.[36]

Sepsis-related cardiac dysfunction

Sepsis-related cardiac dysfunction is described in up to 60% of patients admitted with septic shock within 3 days from the onset and may affect one or both ventricles. The cause is not completely elucidated but is mainly reversible in those who survive.[37]

Reversal of vasodilation (with vasopressor medications) and optimization of circulating volume may unmask *LV dysfunction*. Interest has been focused on global longitudinal strain (GLS) as an imaging technique to assess LV function in sepsis. However, it requires high-quality images, which are not always obtainable in ICU patients, especially if they are on positive-pressure mechanical ventilation.

LV diastolic dysfunction is described in 40–50% of patients with septic shock, where the degree of diastolic dysfunction may directly influence fluid tolerance, and it is related to mortality.[38] The incidence of *RV dysfunction* in sepsis varies from 30% to 80% and is more commonly associated with acute respiratory distress syndrome (ARDS).[39]

ACUTE RESPIRATORY FAILURE AND MECHANICAL VENTILATION

Acute respiratory failure is a frequent cause of ICU admission. The initial assessment of dyspneic patient should be focused on differentiation between cardiac and non-cardiac (pulmonary) etiology of respiratory failure, to direct the patient to proper diagnostic and therapeutic pathway. Thoracic ultrasonography, the combination of cardiac and lung ultrasound (LUS), represents a valuable and reliable tool for the clinician facing acute respiratory failure. Of note, LUS can detect lung congestion (V20.1), pleural effusion (V20.2), and pneumothorax (V2.16) with high accuracy (see Chapter 20).

Acute respiratory distress syndrome and acute cor pulmonale

Acute cor pulmonale (ACP) is defined as an acute right heart failure related to sudden increase of afterload leading to RV dilatation. Most common causes of ACP are acute pulmonary embolism and ARDS. The incidence of ACP in ARDS patients is reduced to 25% with the application of lung protective ventilation. ARDS-related ACP encompasses a combination of RV pressure overload, leading to systolic dysfunction, and RV volume overload, causing diastolic dysfunction.[40]

The echocardiographic pattern is characterized by RV dilatation, septal flattening, and paradoxical septal motion with or without longitudinal systolic dysfunction (TAPSE ≤16 mm).[41,42] LUS reveals multiple diffuse bilateral B-lines similar to cardiogenic pulmonary edema pattern but typically with irregular pleural line (see Table 20.3, V20.3A, and V20.3B in Chapter 20). The changes of RV size and function have a negative impact on LV because of ventricular interdependence. The combination of reduced pulmonary venous return (due to RV systolic dysfunction) and LV diastolic compression (determined by interventricular septal shift) causes decrease in LV stroke volume. The reduction in cardiac output determines further impairment of right coronary artery perfusion, which is already blunted in systole, which, along with hypoxemia due to ARDS, may eventually lead to RV ischemia.[43]

The presence of *pre-systolic A-wave* (an anterograde flow through the pulmonary valve during atrial contraction) is a sensitive marker of low RV diastolic compliance (restrictive physiology) occurring when diastolic pressure exceeds 20 mmHg, and it was shown to be related with increased ventilatory pressure and hypercapnia (Figure 21.6).[44]

In order to prevent the onset or exacerbation of RV dysfunction, it has been suggested that in ARDS, intensivists should not aim at lung protective ventilation only but also at RV-protective ventilatory strategy. The key components of the RV-protective ventilatory strategy are (1) limiting plateau and driving pressures to minimize lung stress, (2) preventing or reversing pulmonary vasoconstriction by improving oxygenation and controlling capnia, and (3) using the prone position in moderate to severe hypoxemia to unload RV.[45]

Mechanical ventilation and weaning from mechanical ventilation

The application of *positive-pressure ventilation* has different effects on the cardiovascular system.[46,47] The main effects on ventricular function are summarized as follows:

Effects on RV

1. Decrease of preload due to increase of intrathoracic pressure and consequent impediment of venous return (by reducing intrathoracic and intra-abdominal pressure gradient) and, therefore, RV stroke volume
2. Increase in afterload, determined by direct compression of pulmonary vasculature, which leads to a rise of pulmonary vascular resistance
3. The last effect is counterbalanced by an improvement in gas exchanges, with attenuation/resolution of hypoxia-mediated vasoconstriction and better control of CO_2 level, resulting in decrease in pulmonary vascular resistances

Effects on LV

1. Decrease in LV preload (mediated by reduction of RV output and ventricular interdependence)
2. Improvement of LV afterload by reduction of transmural pressure
3. Improvement of oxygenation and ratio between oxygen delivery and consumption (DO_2/VO_2) by alveolar recruitment

The *process of weaning* from positive-pressure mechanical ventilation to negative-pressure spontaneous breathing has profound physiological effects on both respiratory and cardiovascular system. The primary result of reduction/interruption of positive intrathoracic pressure is an increment in venous return, which increases cardiac preload and filling pressures. In addition, the loss of positive intrathoracic pressure leads to an increase in transmural pressure, hence a rise in LV afterload. The combination of these two mechanisms may have detrimental effect on

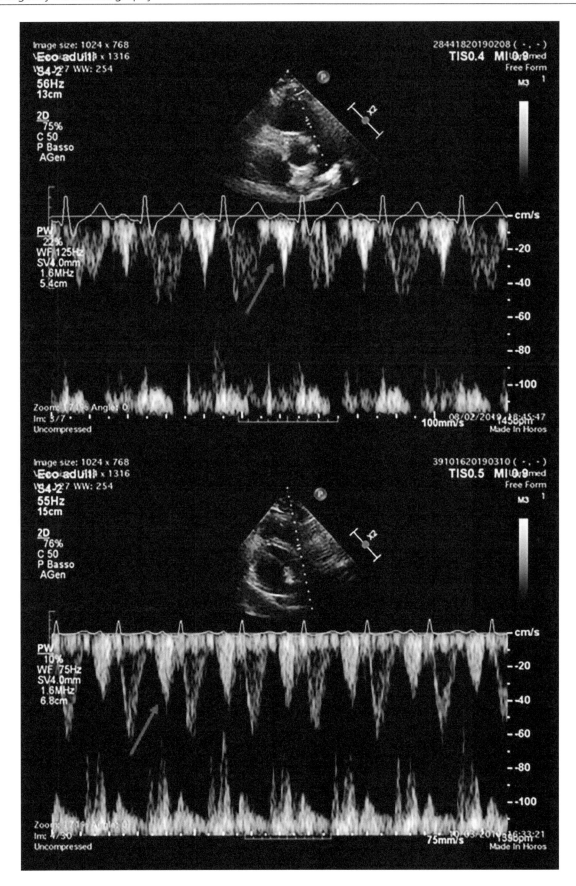

FIGURE 21.6 Pre-systolic A-wave. Pulsed-wave Doppler with a sample volume in the pulmonary artery (upper panel) and right ventricular outflow tract (lower panel). Note the presence of anterograde flow through the pulmonary valve during atrial contraction (red arrows).

LV performance, which is particularly evident when systolic and/or diastolic function are impaired. The increase in LV afterload negatively impacts the *severity of MR* (especially in context of secondary and dynamic MR), which may cause the development of pulmonary edema. During the weaning process and after discontinuation of mechanical ventilation, the respiratory muscles are no more unloaded, which results in increase of body oxygen consumption and adds further workload to the heart with possible development of weaning-induced myocardial ischemia.[48]

An *integrated ultrasound approach* based on both echocardiography and LUS is advised to monitor the weaning from mechanical ventilation (see also Chapter 20), assessing both systolic and diastolic ventricular function, as well as diaphragmatic and lung function, during a spontaneous breathing trial.[49,50] The presence of diastolic dysfunction has been proven to be associated with weaning failure. In patients without significant mitral valve abnormalities, and mitral valve repair or replacement, the integration of mitral inflow (measured by pulsed-wave Doppler) and relaxation velocities (measured by TDI) enables assessing diastolic function and estimation of LV filling pressures/LAP. A worsening of mitral inflow pattern (from impaired relaxation [E/A ≤0.8] to pseudo-normalization [E/A 0.8–2.0] or from pseudo-normalization to restrictive [E/A >2]) and an increase in estimated LV filling pressures (E/e′ >13) are warning signs of possible weaning failure during a spontaneous breathing trial.[51,52] Of note, E/e′ ratio is the strongest predictor of weaning failure among echocardiographic parameters.[53] Alongside with ECG monitoring, echocardiography allows identification of early signs of *weaning-induced myocardial ischemia* by detecting the presence of post-ejection shortening and/or regional wall motion abnormalities. Finally, diaphragmatic excursion of <11 mm as assessed by LUS during weaning attempt indicates probable weaning failure.

LIST OF VIDEOS

https://routledgetextbooks.com/textbooks/9781032157009/chapter-21.php

VIDEO 21.1 Partial papillary muscle rupture. TEE mid-esophageal mitral commissural (on the left) and long-axis (on the right) views showing partial rupture of the papillary muscle.

VIDEO 21.2 Posterior mitral leaflet prolapse. TEE mid-esophageal four-chamber view showing prolapse of the posterior mitral leaflet with severe mitral regurgitation. Note the anteriorly directed eccentric jet with Coanda effect in the left atrium.

VIDEO 21.3A Postinfarction ventricular septal rupture (1/2). Deep transgastric TEE four-chamber view showing infarcted inferior septum with large apical rupture (see also Video 21.3B).

VIDEO 21.3B Postinfarction ventricular septal rupture (2/2). Transgastric TEE mid-papillary short-axis view showing rupture of inferior septum with left-to-right shunt on color Doppler (see also Video 21.3A).

VIDEO 21.4A Postinfarction ventricular septal rupture (1/4). In a postinfarction patient with a new holosystolic murmur, parasternal short-axis view at mid-papillary level showing discontinuation of the myocardium of the inferior septum (at 11 o'clock) indicating ventricular septal rupture (see also Videos 21.4B, 21.4C, and 21.4D). *(Video provided by AZ.)*

VIDEO 21.4B Postinfarction ventricular septal rupture (2/4). In a postinfarction patient with a new holosystolic murmur, color Doppler in parasternal short-axis view at mid-papillary level showing turbulent flow across the ruptured inferior interventricular septum (see also Videos 21.4A, 21.4C, and 21.4D). *(Video provided by AZ.)*

VIDEO 21.4C Postinfarction ventricular septal rupture (3/4). In a postinfarction patient with a new holosystolic murmur, subcostal four-chamber view showing discontinuation of the myocardium of the inferior septum, indicating ventricular septal rupture (see also Videos 21.4A, 21.4B and 21.4D). *(Video provided by AZ.)*

VIDEO 21.4D Postinfarction ventricular septal rupture (4/4). In a postinfarction patient with a new holosystolic murmur, color Doppler in subcostal four-chamber view showing turbulent flow across the ruptured inferior interventricular septum (see also Videos 21.4A, 21.4B and 21.4C). *(Video provided by AZ.)*

VIDEO 21.5A Cardiopulmonary resuscitation (CPR) and pericardiocentesis in a patient with cardiac tamponade (1/3). Note huge pericardial effusion with "swinging heart" detected by FoCUS in a subcostal view during CPR pulse check, indicating tamponade as a possible cause of cardiac arrest (see also Videos 21.5B and 21.5C). *(Video provided by MS.)*

VIDEO 21.5B Cardiopulmonary resuscitation (CPR) and pericardiocentesis in a patient with cardiac tamponade (2/3). In attempt to perform urgent pericardiocentesis during CPR (note chest compressions), a small amount of agitated saline was administered (note bubbles) to check the proper needle position within the pericardial space (see also Videos 21.5A and 21.5C). *(Video provided by MS.)*

VIDEO 21.5C Cardiopulmonary resuscitation (CPR) and pericardiocentesis in a patient with cardiac tamponade (3/3). After needle aspiration of around 800 mL of bloody fluid from pericardial space, CPR was successfully completed, with return of spontaneous circulation (ROSC). Note fair global LV function and still large pericardial effusion but without echocardiographic signs of tamponade physiology (there is no diastolic collapse of the right ventricle) (see also Videos 21.5A and 21.5B). *(Video provided by MS.)*

VIDEO 21.6A   Acute massive pulmonary embolism treated by percutaneous catheter aspiration and intrapulmonary fibrinolysis (1/5). A 76-year-old lady was admitted in the ICU due to dyspnea, chest pain, and fall on the head due to syncope. Heart rate was 100 beats/min, blood pressure was 90/60 mmHg, and oxygen saturation was 72%. There was a visible bump on the forehead due to head injury. Emergency FoCUS with a handheld imaging device (shown here), TTE (see Video 21.6B), and TEE (see Video 21.6C) revealed dilated right heart with a large worm-like, highly mobile mass in the right atrium and moderate tricuspid regurgitation, with estimated right ventricular systolic pressure of around 45 mmHg and TAPSE 15 mm. Patient was considered as having high-risk acute pulmonary embolism. In view of recent head injury and possibility of thrombus dislodgement by fibrinolysis administration that might lead to potentially fatal recurrent episode of pulmonary embolism, patient was urgently transferred to cardiac surgery center for emergent pulmonary embolectomy. Instead of open-heart surgery, successful percutaneous catheter aspiration of right atrial thrombus and intrapulmonary administration of alteplase was done (see Videos 21.6D and 21.6E). *(Video provided by AZ.)*

VIDEO 21.6B   Acute massive pulmonary embolism treated by percutaneous catheter aspiration and intrapulmonary fibrinolysis (2/5). Following FoCUS (see Video 21.6), emergency TTE (shown here) and TEE (see Video 21.6C) revealed dilated right heart with a large worm-like, highly mobile mass in the right atrium, and moderate tricuspid regurgitation, with estimated right ventricular systolic pressure of around 45 mmHg (see Videos 21.6D and 21.6E). *(Video provided by AZ.)*

VIDEO 21.6C   Acute massive pulmonary embolism treated by percutaneous catheter aspiration and intrapulmonary fibrinolysis (3/5). Following FoCUS and TTE (see Videos 21.6A and 21.6B), emergency TEE was performed, which confirmed the presence of large, mobile mass in the right atrium (shown here) and intact interatrial septum (see also Videos 21.6D and 21.6E). *(Video provided by AZ.)*

VIDEO 21.6D   Acute massive pulmonary embolism treated by percutaneous catheter aspiration and intrapulmonary fibrinolysis (4/5). A 65 cm long 8F sheath was introduced into the right atrium (shown here by fluoroscopy) via femoral vein and several attempts of manual thrombus aspiration was done under echocardiographic guidance (see Videos 21.6A, 21.6B, 21.6C, and 21.6E). *(Video provided by SO.)*

VIDEO 21.6E   Acute massive pulmonary embolism treated by percutaneous catheter aspiration and intrapulmonary fibrinolysis (5/5). Thrombotic material removed from the right atrium by aspiration is shown here. Following thrombus aspiration, head CT was performed. Since no signs of intracerebral bleeding was reported, a pigtail catheter was introduced into pulmonary artery and 25 mg of alteplase was administered locally during next 10 hours (2.5 mg/h). The patient gradually hemodynamically improved and survived (see Videos 21.6A, 21.6B, 21.6C, and 21.6D). *(Video provided by SO.)*

VIDEO 21.7A   Infective endocarditis of the implantable cardioverter defibrillator (ICD) lead with purulent pericarditis (1/2). In a septic patient, TEE bicaval view showing the part of the ICD lead in the right atrium coated with adherent, warm-like echogenic structures, indicating vegetations due to infective endocarditis. Blood cultures revealed *Staphylococcus haemolyticus* as a cause of sepsis. The infection spread toward pericardium causing purulent pericarditis,

which was confirmed later by pericardiocentesis and blood cultures (see Video 21.7B). *(Video provided by MS.)*

VIDEO 21.7B   Infective endocarditis of the implantable cardioverter defibrillator (ICD) lead with purulent pericarditis (2/2). Transthoracic modified four-chamber view showing ICD lead in the right heart chambers coated with echogenic material. In addition, a large, echodense pericardial effusion and thickened right atrial wall can be noted. The infection was presumable spread through right atrial wall toward pericardium, causing purulent pericarditis—confirmed later by pericardiocentesis and blood cultures (see also Video 21.7A). *(Video provided by MS.)*

REFERENCES

1. Neskovic AN, Skinner H, Price S, et al. Focus cardiac ultrasound core curriculum and core syllabus of the European Association of Cardiovascular Imaging. Eur Heart J Cardiovasc Imaging. 2018;19:475–81.
2. Vieillard-Baron A, Millington SJ, Sanfilippo F, et al. A decade of progress in critical care echocardiography: a narrative review. Intensive Care Med. 2019;45:770–88.
3. Frankel HL, Kirkpatrick AW, Elbarbary M, et al. Guidelines for the appropriate use of bedside general and cardiac ultrasonography in the evaluation of critically ill patients-part I: general ultrasonography. Crit Care Med. 2015;43:2479–502.
4. Levitov A, Frankel HL, Blaivas M, et al. Guidelines for the appropriate use of bedside general and cardiac ultrasonography in the evaluation of critically ill patients-part II: cardiac ultrasonography. Crit Care Med. 2016;44:1206–27.
5. Vincent JL. Fluid management in the critically ill. Kidney Int. 2019;96:52–57.
6. Monnet X, Marik PE, Teboul JL. Prediction of fluid responsiveness: an update. Ann Intensive Care. 2016;6:111.
7. Via G, Tavazzi G, Price S. Ten situations where inferior vena cava ultrasound may fail to accurately predict fluid responsiveness: a physiologically based point of view. Intensive Care Med. 2016;42:1164–7.
8. Vieillard-Baron A, Chergui K, Rabiller A, et al. Superior vena caval collapsibility as a gauge of volume status in ventilated septic patients. Intensive Care Med. 2004;30:1734–9.
9. Feissel M, Michard F, Faller JP, Teboul JL. The respiratory variation in inferior vena cava diameter as a guide to fluid therapy. Intensive Care Med. 2004;30:1834–7.
10. Monnet X, Marik P, Teboul JL. Passive leg raising for predicting fluid responsiveness: a systematic review and meta-analysis. Intensive Care Med. 2016;42:1935–47.
11. van Diepen S, Katz JN, Albert NM, et al. Contemporary management of cardiogenic shock: a scientific statement from the American Heart Association. Circulation. 2017;136:e232–68.
12. Tehrani BN, Truesdell AG, Psotka MA, et al. A Standardized and comprehensive approach to the management of cardiogenic shock. JACC Heart Fail. 2020;8:879–91.
13. Sinha SS, Rosner CM, Tehrani BN, et al. Cardiogenic shock from heart failure versus acute myocardial infarction: clinical characteristics, hospital course, and 1-year outcomes. Circ Heart Fail. 2022;15:e009279.
14. Marwick TH. Ejection fraction pros and cons: JACC state-of-the-art review. J Am Coll Cardiol. 2018;72:2360–79.
15. Henein MY, Gibson DG. Long axis function in disease. Heart. 1999;81:229–31.

16. Tavazzi G, Via G, Braschi A, Price S. An 82-year-old woman with ongoing dyspnea. Chest. 2016;150:e9–11.
17. Duncan AM, Francis DP, Henein MY, Gibson DG. Limitation of cardiac output by total isovolumic time during pharmacologic stress in patients with dilated cardiomyopathy: activation-mediated effects of left bundle branch block and coronary artery disease. J Am Coll Cardiol. 2003;41:121–8.
18. Tavazzi G, Kontogeorgis A, Bergsland NP, Price S. Resolution of cardiogenic shock using echocardiography-guided pacing optimization in intensive care: a case series. Crit Care Med. 2016;44:e755–61.
19. Tavazzi G, Kontogeorgis A, Guarracino F, et al. Heart rate modification of cardiac output following cardiac surgery: the importance of cardiac time intervals. Crit Care Med. 2017;45:e782–8.
20. Jentzer JC, Anavekar NS, Burstein BJ, et al. Noninvasive echocardiographic left ventricular stroke work index predicts mortality in cardiac intensive care unit patients. Circ Cardiovasc Imaging. 2020;13:e011642.
21. Pugliese NR, Fabiani I, Mandoli GE, et al. Echo-derived peak cardiac power output-to-left ventricular mass with cardiopulmonary exercise testing predicts outcome in patients with heart failure and depressed systolic function. Eur Heart J Cardiovasc Imaging. 2019;20:700–8.
22. Soliman-Aboumarie H, Joshi SS, Cameli M, et al. EACVI survey on the multi-modality imaging assessment of the right heart. Eur Heart J Cardiovasc Imaging. 2022;23:1417–22.
23. Gillebert TC. Estimating LV filling pressures noninvasively: a word of caution. JACC Cardiovasc Imaging. 2022;15:1692–95.
24. Diwan A, McCulloch M, Lawrie GM, et al. Doppler estimation of left ventricular filling pressures in patients with mitral valve disease. Circulation. 2005;111:3281–9.
25. Chieffo A, Dudek D, Hassager C, et al. Joint EAPCI/ACVC expert consensus document on percutaneous ventricular assist devices. EuroIntervention. 2021;17:e274–86.
26. Bouchez S, Van Belleghem Y, De Somer F, et al. Haemodynamic management of patients with left ventricular assist devices using echocardiography: the essentials. Eur Heart J Cardiovasc Imaging. 2019;20:373–82.
27. Donker DW, Meuwese CL, Braithwaite SA, et al. Echocardiography in extracorporeal life support: a key player in procedural guidance, tailoring and monitoring. Perfusion. 2018;33:31–41.
28. Douflé G, Roscoe A, Billia F, Fan E. Echocardiography for adult patients supported with extracorporeal membrane oxygenation. Crit Care. 2015;19:326.
29. Aissaoui N, Luyt CE, Leprince P, et al. Predictors of successful extracorporeal membrane oxygenation (ECMO) weaning after assistance for refractory cardiogenic shock. Intensive Care Med. 2011;37:1738–45.
30. Adler Y, Charron P, Imazio M, et al. 2015 ESC guidelines for the diagnosis and management of pericardial diseases: the Task Force for the Diagnosis and Management of Pericardial Diseases of the European Society of Cardiology (ESC) Endorsed by: the European Association for Cardio-Thoracic Surgery (EACTS). Eur Heart J. 2015;36:2921–64.
31. Spodick DH. Acute cardiac tamponade. N Engl J Med. 2003;349:684–90.
32. Price S, Prout J, Jaggar SI, et al. 'Tamponade' following cardiac surgery: terminology and echocardiography may both mislead. Eur J Cardiothorac Surg. 2004;26:1156–60.
33. Harjola VP, Mebazaa A, Čelutkienė J, et al. Contemporary management of acute right ventricular failure: a statement from the Heart Failure Association and the working group on pulmonary circulation and right ventricular function of the European Society of Cardiology. Eur J Heart Fail. 2016;18:226–41.
34. Vieillard-Baron A, Naeije R, Haddad F, et al. Diagnostic workup, etiologies and management of acute right ventricle failure: a state-of-the-art paper. Intensive Care Med. 2018;44:774–90.
35. Konstantinides SV, Meyer G, Becattini C, et al. 2019 ESC guidelines for the diagnosis and management of acute pulmonary embolism developed in collaboration with the European Respiratory Society (ERS). Eur Heart J. 2020;41:543–603.
36. Habib G, Badano L, Tribouilloy C, et al. Recommendations for the practice of echocardiography in infective endocarditis. Eur J Echocardiogr. 2010;11:202–19.
37. Vieillard-Baron A, Cecconi M. Understanding cardiac failure in sepsis. Intensive Care Med. 2014;40:1560–3.
38. Landesberg G, Gilon D, Meroz Y, et al. Diastolic dysfunction and mortality in severe sepsis and septic shock. Eur Heart J. 2012;33:895–903.
39. Ehrman RR, Sullivan AN, Favot MJ, et al. Pathophysiology, echocardiographic evaluation, biomarker findings, and prognostic implications of septic cardiomyopathy: a review of the literature. Crit Care. 2018;22:112.
40. Vieillard-Baron A, Schmitt JM, Augarde R, et al. Acute cor pulmonale in acute respiratory distress syndrome submitted to protective ventilation: incidence, clinical implications, and prognosis. Crit Care Med. 2001;29:1551–5.
41. Jardin F, Dubourg O, Bourdarias JP. Echocardiographic pattern of acute cor pulmonale. Chest. 1997;111:209–17.
42. Jardin F, Vieillard-Baron A. Acute cor pulmonale. Curr Opin Crit Care. 2009;15:67–70.
43. Zochios V, Parhar K, Tunnicliffe W, et al. The right ventricle in ARDS. Chest. 2017;152:181–93.
44. Tavazzi G, Bergsland N, Alcada J, Price S. Early signs of right ventricular systolic and diastolic dysfunction in acute severe respiratory failure: the importance of diastolic restrictive pattern. Eur Heart J Acute Cardiovasc Care. 2020;9:649–56.
45. Repessé X, Charron C, Vieillard-Baron A. Acute respiratory distress syndrome: the heart side of the moon. Curr Opin Crit Care. 2016;22:38–44.
46. Alviar CL, Miller PE, McAreavey D, et al. Positive pressure ventilation in the cardiac intensive care unit. J Am Coll Cardiol. 2018;72:1532–53.
47. Pinsky MR. The right ventricle: interaction with the pulmonary circulation. Crit Care. 2016;20:266.
48. Tavazzi G. Mechanical ventilation in cardiogenic shock. Curr Opin Crit Care. 2021;27:447–53.
49. Mayo P, Volpicelli G, Lerolle N. Ultrasonography evaluation during the weaning process: the heart, the diaphragm, the pleura and the lung. Intensive Care Med. 2016;42:1107–17.
50. Haaksma ME, Tuinman PR, Heunks L. Weaning the patient: between protocols and physiology. Curr Opin Crit Care. 2021;27:29–36.
51. Santangelo E, Mongodi S, Bouhemad B, Mojoli F. The weaning from mechanical ventilation: a comprehensive ultrasound approach. Curr Opin Crit Care. 2022;28:322–30.
52. Moschietto S, Doyen D, Grech L, et al. Transthoracic echocardiography with Doppler tissue imaging predicts weaning failure from mechanical ventilation: evolution of the left ventricle relaxation rate during a spontaneous breathing trial is the key factor in weaning outcome. Crit Care. 2012;16:R81.
53. Sanfilippo F, Di Falco D, Noto A, et al. Association of weaning failure from mechanical ventilation with transthoracic echocardiography parameters: a systematic review and meta-analysis. Br J Anaesth 2021;26:319–30.

Echocardiography in complications of percutaneous interventions

22

Fabian Knebel, Nicolas Merke, Elena Romero Dorta, and Sebastian Spethmann

> **Key Points**
> - Most percutaneous procedures in contemporary cardiology practice rely on echocardiographic assessment before and during interventions.
> - The role of echocardiography is not only to guide interventions but also to identify acute, early, and late procedure-related complications.

Since Andreas Grüntzig founded interventional cardiology with the first percutaneous transluminal coronary angioplasty (PTCA) of a left anterior descending artery (LAD) stenosis over 40 years ago, complications have continued to occur despite continuous development of techniques and material. In an aging society with many comorbidities that often prohibit cardiac surgical therapy, there is a growing need for more complex percutaneous treatment of heart diseases, increasing the risk of procedure-related complications.

It is imperative for interventional cardiologists to be familiar with the entire spectrum of potential periprocedural complications and be equipped with the tools to manage both common and rare events. Of note, targeted treatment of complications of percutaneous interventions depends critically on prompt and correct diagnosis. Echocardiography is routinely used as a guiding tool during many percutaneous interventional procedures and has a central role for diagnosis of complications.

This chapter summarizes the typical complications sorted by intervention that can be detected and assessed by echocardiography.

The role of echocardiography in mechanical circulatory support is discussed in detail in Chapter 15.

COMPLICATIONS FOLLOWING PERCUTANEOUS CORONARY INTERVENTIONS

The history of percutaneous coronary interventions (PCI) is a success story. Due to the continuous development of new interventional techniques accompanied by advances in stent design and adjunctive technology, the success rate has been substantially improved over time. Additionally, the incidence of periprocedural complications associated with PCI has decreased, even for highly complex procedures, such as retrograde recanalization of chronic total occlusions (CTO) or rotablation and atherectomy in severely calcified vessels. The overall complication risk is ~3% but varies widely between studies and increases with higher

DOI: 10.1201/9781003245407-22

lesion complexity.[1] Although angiography is the imaging of choice for the diagnosis of the vast majority of PCI complications, echocardiography can provide additional information in the cath lab and is crucial for detection of complications that develop later.

ACUTE CORONARY SYNDROMES

Emergency echocardiography should be performed in patients with an inconclusive diagnosis of acute coronary syndrome (ACS) and in patients with cardiac arrest, hemodynamic instability, or suspected mechanical complications. However, it should not be performed before emergency revascularization if it delays reperfusion. It seems reasonable to perform transthoracic echocardiography shortly after PCI to determine, at a minimum, LV and RV systolic function and detect possible valve dysfunction and pericardial effusion. However, it should be always done immediately upon hemodynamic deterioration to diagnose new regional wall motion abnormality, mechanical complications (e.g., ventricular septal defect, papillary muscle rupture), or tamponade. In rural or underserved areas where primary PCI is not widely available, delayed reperfusion may be more common, resulting in a higher rate of infarct-related complications and mortality.[2] The role of echocardiography in detection of complications of acute myocardial infarction is discussed in detail in Chapter 3.

CHRONIC CORONARY SYNDROMES

Besides in ACS, PCI is also indicated in individuals with chronic stable angina and ischemia that is refractory to optimal medical therapy. In the case of elective PCI, complications are mainly related to the procedure itself.

Coronary perforation is an important complication with an estimated incidence of 0.5%.[3,4] It is associated with a fivefold increase of 30-day mortality.[3] Risk factors are balloon or stent mismatch, severe arterial calcification, use of atherectomy devices or cutting balloons.[5] Severe perforations can lead to cardiac tamponade. Importantly, due to the acute nature of the pericardial effusion, even relatively small amounts of blood (<200 mL) can result in severe hemodynamic deterioration (Figure 8.12) (V8.12A, V8.12B). Delayed development of pericardial effusion or even tamponade can also be caused by inadvertent migration of the tip of the coronary wire.

A very rare, but often fatal complication after PCI is *stent infection leading to stent abscess*, presented as echolucent or echodense myocardial mass (Figure 22.1) (V22.1) Since the introduction of coronary stents in 1987, only a few cases of infection have been published.[6] In most cases, anti-infective therapy was not sufficient and cardiac surgery was required to remove the abscess and perform coronary artery bypass grafting.

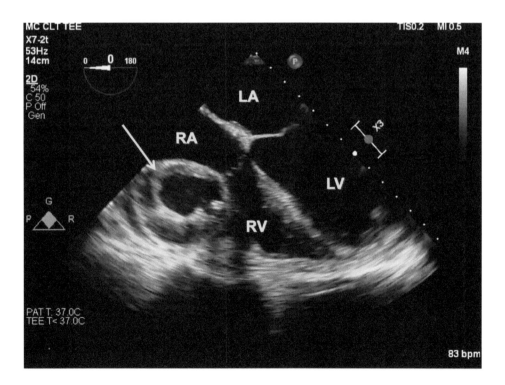

FIGURE 22.1 Stent abscess. Transesophageal echocardiography showing round echolucent mass (arrow) in the RV myocardium consistent with abscess formation (V22.1). LA: left atrium; LV: left ventricle; RA: right atrium; RV: right ventricle.

(Image and video provided by GNR.)

COMPLICATIONS FOLLOWING TRANSCATHETER AORTIC VALVE IMPLANTATION (TAVI)

Transcatheter aortic valve implantation (TAVI) has become the standard treatment of patients with severe aortic stenosis at increased surgical risk and in older patients (≥75 years).[7] Since recent studies have reported noninferiority of TAVI in low- and intermediate-risk patients,[8,9] it is increasingly adopted in this patient population in clinical routine.[10] This expansion of TAVI was only possible because the incidence of severe complications has decreased in recent years.[11] However, as always, a new therapy also results in new complications that require rapid diagnosis and appropriate treatment. In addition to vascular complications due to access route, complications from balloon aortic valvuloplasty or valve deployment, as well as long-term aspects of transcatheter heart valves (THV) function, must be considered. Table 22.1 summarizes acute and long-term complications of TAVI.

Complications during TAVI

Incomplete valve expansion, migration, and embolization

Immediately after deployment of the valve *incomplete expansion* of the device could be detected by TEE (see Figure 12.8). *Valve migration and embolization* are rare but relevant complications of TAVI, associated with a significant increase in mortality. Notably, the incidence of valve embolization has decreased over the years to less than 0.5%, reflecting the growing experience of institutions and operators, as well as the availability of preplanning imaging and newer generation valves.[12] THV can migrate either into the aorta or into the left ventricle (V14.10A, V14.10B). Aortic embolization is usually the result of deployment in a high position and/or poor coaxial alignment of the device to the annulus plane during implantation of self-expanding valves ("pop-up") or due to loss of capture during deployment of balloon-expandable valves.[13] Caudal migration toward the left ventricle (Figure 22.2) (V22.2) usually occurs

TABLE 22.1 Acute and Long-Term Complications Related to TAVI

Prosthesis dislocation

Endocarditis

LV perforation

Annulus rupture

HALT

Paravalvular leakage

Abbreviations: HALT, hypoattenuated leaflet thickening; LV, left ventricular.

because of shallow implantation depth, eccentric and asymmetric calcification, and device undersizing.[14]

Ventricular perforation

During TAVI, a stiff guidewire is commonly placed in the left ventricle (LV) to support the valve system. The use of a stiff guidewire poses numerous risks, including perforation of the LV—the leading cause for emergent cardiac surgery. Risk factors for LV perforation during TAVI are a small LV cavity, a hypercontractile state, a thin muscular wall, and a narrow aorto-mitral angle.[15] In case of hemodynamic instability, pericardial drainage is mandatory (see Figure 12.9). If bleeding persists, surgery must follow.

Aortic annulus rupture

Rupture of the device landing zone is a rare but feared complication of TAVI, with a mortality of up to 75% in cases of uncontrolled rupture.[16] The most common anatomic site of rupture is the aortic annulus, although the sinus of Valsalva and left ventricular outflow tract (LVOT) have also been described.[16] Rupture is usually related to the use of a balloon-expandable valve but can also occur with self-expanding systems during postdilation, particularly with >20% area oversizing.[17] Therefore, a self-expanding valve is preferable in high-risk LVOT calcification cases and shallow sinuses of Valsalva. *Limited rupture* causing periaortic hematoma has a less dramatic appearance. In cases with limited injury and a non-catastrophic clinical presentation, pericardial drainage and/or observation might be considered initially. Depending on the calcium distribution, perforation into the right ventricle may also occur (V22.3). In the event of an *uncontrolled rupture*, conversion to emergency surgery is often the only possible solution. Nevertheless, there are case reports of successful sealing of an annulus rupture by implantation of a second THV as a valve-in-valve (ViV) procedure.[18]

Long-term complications of TAVI

Paravalvular leaks

In the beginning of TAVI, acute peri-prosthetic aortic regurgitation (AR) was detected in a significant proportion of patients (V14.9A, V14.9B).[19] However, with next-generation valves, advances have been made in reducing residual AR after TAVI.[20] There are three important factors associated with paravalvular AR: undersizing of the prosthesis, severity of aortic calcification, and prosthesis position in relation to the annulus.[21] Grading of the severity of paravalvular AR by echocardiography (Figure 22.3) (V22.4) is often difficult because of the different anatomy and course of regurgitant jets compared to those seen after conventional surgical aortic valve replacement (SAVR) with a sewing ring.[22] Severe AR after implantation of a self-expanding valve can be solved by implantation of an additional balloon-expanding THV if postdilation is not sufficient (V14.9B).

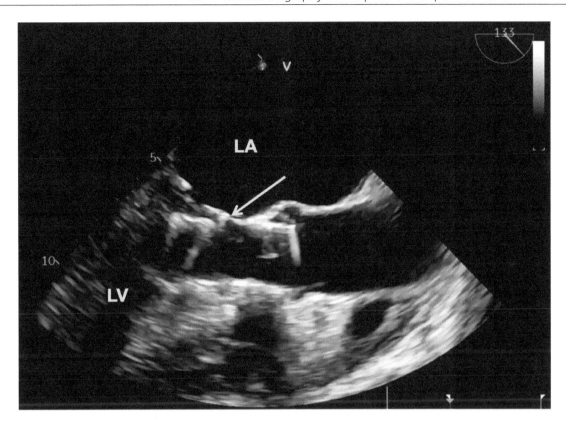

FIGURE 22.2 Migration of the implanted aortic valve after TAVI. Mid-esophageal long-axis view showing a caudal dislocation of balloon-expanding valve in the direction of LVOT/LV, causing impaired opening of the anterior mitral leaflet (arrow) (V22.2). LA: left atrium; LV: left ventricle.

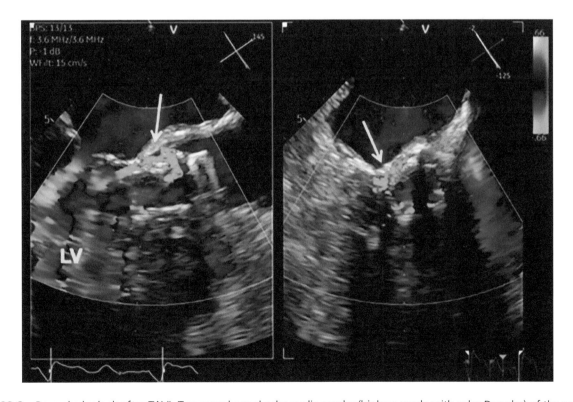

FIGURE 22.3 Paravalvular leak after TAVI. Transesophageal echocardiography (biplane mode with color Doppler) of the aortic valve showing paravalvular leakage (arrows) into the left ventricular outflow tract during diastole (V22.4). LV: left ventricle.

Infective endocarditis

Infective endocarditis is a serious complication after both TAVI and SAVR resulting in high mortality. However, it is a relatively rare condition with an incidence of 0.2–3.1% within 1 year after TAVI,[23] and there is no evidence of a significant difference in incidence compared to patients undergoing SAVR.[24] Diagnostics do not differ between THV and surgical prosthetic valves endocarditis (see Chapter 12) and comprise an integrative approach, including imaging (V22.5A, V22.5B), mainly transesophageal echocardiography (TEE), as well as clinical and microbiological findings.[25]

Valve durability and function

Similar to biologic surgical prosthetic valves, THV can degenerate over time due to calcifications or pannus. While longitudinal echocardiographic data show stable hemodynamic outcomes after TAVI,[26] similarly robust data on the durability of THV over more than a decade (as with surgical bioprostheses) are needed. A transcatheter ViV procedure may be the solution for the treatment of both degenerated THV and surgically implanted bioprostheses.[27]

Recently, *hypoattenuated leaflet thickening (HALT)* of bioprosthetic aortic valves have been reported to be associated with a risk for increased transvalvular gradients, which was observed in 40% of patients in a clinical trial cohort and 13% of patients in two registries.[28] Until further data are available, a selective strategy of anticoagulation may be appropriate in patients with marked increase of transvalvular gradient.

COMPLICATIONS FOLLOWING PERCUTANEOUS MITRAL VALVE REPAIR

Valvular heart disease (VHD) represents a major burden in terms of mortality and morbidity worldwide, with a preponderance of degenerative and functional disease in higher income countries over the greater prevalence of a rheumatic etiology in developing countries.[29] Mitral valve disease is the second most prevalent valvulopathy in Europe. The paradigm of treatment is still surgical mitral valve repair or replacement. Nevertheless, the growing number of patients with a high surgical risk and symptomatic severe mitral regurgitation (MR) in last decade forced major developments in transcatheter therapies,[30] becoming effective and safe for suitable patients. Nowadays, two-dimensional (2D) and three-dimensional (3D) TEE are the most important tools for patient selection and guiding the interventionist during percutaneous mitral valve repair. Echocardiography is also the technique of choice for anticipating and detecting potential complications of the procedure.

In this chapter, we summarized the role of echocardiography in detecting the most frequent complications of the currently most established percutaneous mitral valve procedures, such as transcatheter edge-to-edge repair (TEER), percutaneous mitral valve annuloplasty (PMVA), and transcatheter mitral valve-in-ring and valve-in-valve procedure (TMVIR, MVIV).

Mitral valve transcatheter edge-to-edge repair (TEER)

Percutaneous mitral valve TEER with MitraClip (Abbott Vascular, Menlo Park, CA) or PASCAL (Edwards Lifesciences, Irvine, CA, USA) device has been established as a valid and secure treatment for symptomatic MR in eligible patients.[31] Nearly 50% of patients with severe symptomatic MR are refused for surgery because of advanced age or comorbidities. TEER has been associated with a relevant reduction of the rate of hospitalization and all-cause mortality compared with medical therapy alone.[32]

Although safety of the procedure has been well established, up to 4.35% of the patients experience major complications,[30,33] which can be divided into device- or procedure-related (Table 22.2).

Single leaflet detachment, also known as *partial clip detachment*, is the most frequent structural device complication, occurring in approximately 1.9% of the cases.[33] It describes the complete separation of the clip to one leaflet (V22.6A, V22.6B, V22.6C), and it happens more often in complex lesions. On most occasions, the detachment occurs acutely (during the implantation) or subacutely (in the first few days after).[33,34] To try to minimize this complication, the echocardiographer who is guiding the procedure needs to provide a good visualization of both leaflets for an adequate grasping. The standard views are the TEE mid-esophageal biplane intercommissural (60°) and long-axis views (120°), focused on the mitral valve. After grasping and before releasing, it must be checked that both leaflets show a deep insertion, being embraced by the clip from the tip to the body (Figure 22.4), forming a "V." When proper vision is hindered by artifacts in the classical grasping views, transgastric short-axis view could be used. The single leaflet detachment that does not follow insufficient grasping is due to *leaflet tear or perforation*. Over the years, there has been a continual lowering the incidence of a single leaflet detachment due to developments in the device systems, optimal TEE imaging guiding and improvement in the interventionists' learning curve. If technically feasible, re-treatment of the regurgitation with another device should be attempted.

The *complete detachment of both leaflets*, which leads to *clip embolization*, is extremely rare (up to 0.7%).[34] In the few published case reports, the device embolized into the left ventricle and was retrogradely removed,[35] or it ended up in the right axillary artery without symptoms and no requirement for further therapy.[36]

Valve damage is commonly discovered in patients with persistent mitral regurgitation after TEER. Grasping the leaflets may injure the tissue, causing a *leaflet perforation* by the

TABLE 22.2 Complications Detected by Echocardiography during Percutaneous Mitral Valve Procedures and Tips and Tricks to Minimize or Detect Them Rapidly

PROCEDURE	COMPLICATION DETECTED BY ECHOCARDIOGRAPHY	TIPS AND TRICKS (HOW TO MINIMIZE OR DETECT RAPIDLY COMPLICATIONS)
Mitral valve (MV) edge-to-edge	**Procedure-related** • Atrial or ventricular perforation	• If possible, always keep the tip of the device/sleeve on sight and communicate with the interventionist if it seems close to the atrial, ventricular, or aortic wall (caution: transseptal puncture).
	• Pericardial effusion, cardiac tamponade	• Rule out preexisting effusion at the beginning of the procedure; re-evaluate and compare if hemodynamic instability occurs.
	• Iatrogenic ASD	• Document the iatrogenic ASD at the end of the procedure.
	• Acute RV failure	• Fast detection when hemodynamic instability can determine the need for inotropic agents and foresee require of resuscitation.
	• Infective endocarditis	• Challenging diagnosis; multimodality image may be needed.
	• Thrombosis	• Despite the intraprocedural administration of heparin, acute thrombi formation can be detected at the transseptal puncture site or at the device itself—rapid detection to cancellation of procedure, thrombolysis, or thrombectomy.
	Device-related • Single leaflet detachment	• Good visualization of both leaflets during grasping; use different views to evaluate the attachment before and after releasing the device (biplane, transgastric short axis); look for the V-morphology of the leaflets; always apply color Doppler.
	• Clip embolization	• Advance the device slightly in ventricular direction during clip closure and invert the arms each time to remove the clip back to the left atrium.
	• Leaflet injury, chordal rupture	• Preprocedural evaluation of mitral valve area, mean gradient, and annular diameter using 2D and 3D TEE.
	• Mitral stenosis	• The implanter's and echocardiographer's expertise play a crucial role to identify an optimal approach for each patient and select the most beneficial clip size to minimize residual MR; detailed evaluation of the residual regurgitation after device(s) release; pulmonary vein flow profile assessment.
	• Residual mitral regurgitation	
Indirect MV Annuloplasty (Carillon)	• Coronary sinus dissection or perforation	• Rule out pericardial effusion; definitive diagnosis can be made through fluoroscopy (CS venogram).
	• Extrinsic coronary artery compression (Caution: LCA due to its close relation to the CS)	• Detect wall motion abnormalities if there is persistent compression (the implantation should be terminated); simultaneous coronary angiogram and CS venogram is mandatory.
	• Partial device dislodgment or fracture	• Comprehensive assessment using 2D and 3D TEE before release of the system to identify possible dislodgment or fracture.
Direct MV annuloplasty (Cardioband)	• LCA obstruction or perforation (direct damage by the anchors, coronary kinking cinching-related)	• Rule out pericardial effusion; detect wall motion abnormalities.
	• Anchor disengagement, partial device detachment	• Assure the correct position and angle of the sheath at the hinge point (enough tissue); push-pull testing before releasing every anchor (special attention in the P2 area); use biplane 2D or 3D reconstruction if needed to localize the tip of the implant catheter.

(Continued)

TABLE 22.2 Complications Detected by Echocardiography during Percutaneous Mitral Valve Procedures and Tips and Tricks to Minimize or Detect Them Rapidly (continued)

PROCEDURE	COMPLICATION DETECTED BY ECHOCARDIOGRAPHY	TIPS AND TRICKS (HOW TO MINIMIZE OR DETECT RAPIDLY COMPLICATIONS)
MV-in-ring and valve-in-valve	• Transseptal puncture, septostomy and iatrogenic ASD	• Keep the tip of the sheath, dilators, etc., on sight (at best in a biplane view) to ensure there is no unintended injury of aorta or cardiac perforation. Unlike other percutaneous MV procedures using transseptal approach, the septostomy with 12 or 14 Fr balloon causes a large iatrogenic ASD, which needs percutaneous closure by the end of the procedure.
	• Leaflet rupture, ventricular rhythm disorders	• Keep the tip of the stiff wire on sight to guide the interventionist during manipulation; use a 3D full-volume approach to assist in orientation of the catheter trajectory; check for leaflet rupture and significant regurgitation while handling through the valve, especially if signs of acute pulmonary congestion.
	• LVOT obstruction	• Infer the maximal LVOT gradient after valve deployment from a deep transgastric view using CW-Doppler; notice the difference between transaortic (early systolic peak) and LVOT flow pattern (end-systolic peak).
	• Paravalvular leak	• Intraprocedural quantification to evaluate the result and decide if the implantation of a second valve is needed after postdilation; use 3D color—you may need to planimetry the vena contracta in a triplane reconstruction and evaluate hemodynamic parameters (pulmonary vein flow).
	• Dislodgement, acute or delayed embolization of the valve	• During deployment, consider valve depth and axiality according to mitral annulus (generally guided by fluoroscopy); evaluate the correct position and function of the valve after release using 2D and 3D TEE.

Abbreviations: 2D, two-dimensional; 3D, three-dimensional; ASD, atrial septal defect; CS, coronary sinus; LCA, left coronary artery; LVOT, left ventricular outflow tract; MV, mitral valve; MR, mitral regurgitation; RV, right ventricle; P2, P2 scallop of the posterior mitral leaflet; TEE, transesophageal echocardiography.

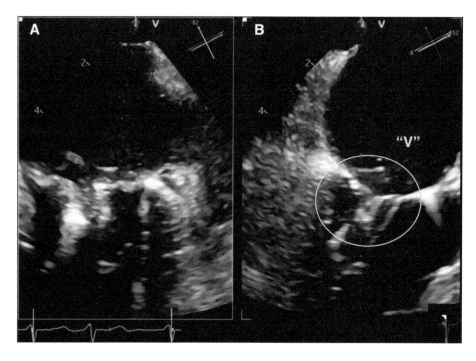

FIGURE 22.4 Echo-checking after grasping and before releasing the device. Both leaflets show a deep insertion being embraced by the clip from the tip to the body forming a "V".

end of the clip arm or a *leaflet tear* parallel to the clip arm. An incidence of 0–2% of leaflet injury has been described in the literature.[34] Manipulating the device on the ventricular side of the valve may also lead to *chordal rupture*. An important safety measure is to advance the device slightly in ventricular direction during clip closure and invert the arms each time the manipulator removes the clip back to the left atrium.

In addition to structural device problems, we can encounter functional system failures, such as *device-related stenosis* or *persistent regurgitation*. Relevant stenosis after TEER is defined by a mean transvalvular diastolic pressure gradient (MPG) >5 mmHg, and it is associated with higher mortality and worse long-term outcomes.[33] Several anatomic and technical features have been related to higher risk of stenosis.[36] The meticulous preprocedural evaluation of mitral valve area (MVA), mean gradient, and annular diameter using 2D and 3D TEE is essential to decide the approach in order to keep this risk low. Even with a two-clip approach, grasping at the "hot zone," and generating a triple orifice, the postprocedural MPG can remain <5 mmHg if the anatomic characteristics are suitable. The *remaining regurgitation* after TEER of the mitral valve has also prognostic value.[33,34] Due to the technical improvements of the devices and gaining experience of the operators a considerable increase of cases with mild or trace residual MR has been described.[37] Quantification might be challenging, and hemodynamic parameters, such as the pulmonary vein flow before and after implantation, can be used in addition to visually graduated residual regurgitation by color Doppler.

Percutaneous mitral valve annuloplasty (PMVA)

Nowadays, the *indirect percutaneous mitral valve annuloplasty through the coronary sinus (CS)* using the Carillon Mitral Contour System (Cardiac Dimension Inc., Kirkland, WA, USA) is indicated for symptomatic patients with dilated cardiomyopathy and severe functional MR, which are still on NYHA III–IV despite optimal medical therapy.[38] It is a right-heart transcatheter device conceived to adjust the anatomy of the mitral valve apparatus from the coronary sinus, reducing the regurgitation without involving the valve and therefore without compromising future therapeutic options. The device comprises two anchors, proximal and distal, connected by a shaping ribbon with semi-helical shape. In contrast to direct annuloplasty using Cardioband (Edwards Lifesciences, Irvine, CA), the Carillon system can be retrieved and removed before being released. Both safety and efficacy of the system have been assessed at the TITAN and TITAN II trials (Transcatheter Implantation of Carillon Mitral Annuloplasty Device) and, lately, at the REDUCE FMR (Carillon system for reducing functional mitral regurgitation),[39] first sham-controlled randomized double-blinded study in valve therapy. The trial showed that the Carillon system remarkably diminished MR and LV volumes. The procedure is done under general anesthesia and guided through TEE and fluoroscopy.

Several complications which can be detected by echocardiography have been described.[30] While cannulating and during guidewire/delivery system forwarding, *dissection or perforation of the coronary sinus* may occur. In most cases, it does not lead to a major bleeding with cardiac tamponade but rather shows a self-limiting course. When there is the suspicion of dissected or perforated CS, the echocardiographer must rule out pericardial effusion. The definitive diagnosis can be done through CS venogram on the fluoroscopy. If the patient is hemodynamic stable and in good general clinical conditions, the interventionist may decide not to break off the procedure. Since the Carillon system does not entail a transseptal access, the risk of puncture-related pericardial effusion or cardiac tamponade is not present.

Due to the adjacency of the CS with the left circumflex artery (LCx), *extrinsic coronary artery compression* after device deployment and tensioning may occur.[39] It is obligatory to perform a concurrent coronary angiogram and CS venogram at the start and just before releasing the system to exclude eventual coronary artery compression. If there are persistent ECG changes and regional wall motion abnormalities after tension reduction or repositioning of the device, the implantation should be terminated (17% in the TITAN II trial).[30]

After the modifications of the first-generation device, the cases of *device dislodgment or fracture* have been significantly reduced (one case reported in the TITAN II trial without clinical consequences). Although the need for conversion to open surgery has not been described so far,[38,39] an emergency surgical back-up is needed in case of complications.

The indirect percutaneous mitral valve annuloplasty with the Carillon system could be considered as the initial interventional approach in the effective management path of the patient with symptomatic functional MR because of the less invasiveness, positive impact on left ventricular volumes, and the opportunity to correct the remaining insufficiency with other interventions, like the TEER.[40]

Direct percutaneous valve annuloplasty can be performed using the Cardioband (Edwards Lifesciences, Irvine, CA) catheter-delivered system to improve leaflet coaptation, which resembles the surgical approach.[41] It consists of the supra-annular fixation of sequential stainless-steel anchors from trigone to trigone under fluoroscopic and TEE guidance, which are later cinched through the wire to reduce MV annulus dimensions. It is implanted through venous femoral access and a 25F transseptal steerable sheath, so the same *interatrial septum puncture-related complications* can occur as described for the TEER. Invigorating results with safe deployment in patients with clinically significant functional MR, lasting MR reduction, better quality of life, and improved exercise capacity at 1-year follow-up was lately published,[42] even though several complications have been described.[30]

The ongoing Edwards Cardioband System ACTIVE Pivotal Clinical Trial is designed to confirm the safety and effectiveness of the system, enrolling over 350 patients with functional MR and heart failure, with an estimated release date in September 2024. Edwards Lifesciences has recently reported a higher-than-expected rate of *coronary artery injuries* (5.7%) during placement of the system, mainly due to direct interaction between the anchors and the LCx.[41] Coronary kinking while cinching of the band with transitory LCx occlusion has also been described. Stent implantation at the proximal LCx and cinching reduction from 4.5 to 3.5 cm are possible solutions to prevent ischemic myocardial damage. A good screening process based on computed tomography (CT) is mandatory to assess the distance between the LCx and theoretical hinge point (anchor releasing zone). Messika-Zeitoun et al. reported one case of myocardial infarction and one with cardiac arrest because of ventricular fibrillation,[42] both events associated to LCx injuries and successfully fixed.

Insufficient anchor insertion can cause *anchor disengagement* and consequent *partial device detachment*, which may result in significant MR recurrence. The disengaged anchors remain within the band, so there is no risk of embolization or migration. Improvements in the device design (anchor length increased from 4 to 6 mm) and in the imaging techniques, using multiple 2D and 3D TEE views, made the intervention safer and increased the device success rate. Close echocardiographic controls are of cardinal importance at follow-up because of the *risk of delayed dehiscence.*

Transcatheter mitral valve-in-ring (TMVIR) and mitral valve-in-valve (MVIV) procedures

The treatment of aortic valve dysfunction via TAVI is nowadays a cornerstone in patients with intermediate, high, and prohibitive surgical risk. This has result in its implementation to treat other conditions, such as degenerated biological aortic prothesis (valve-in-valve).[29] On this basis, transcatheter treatment has become a prospective alternative to surgery for patients with unsuccessful mitral valve annuloplasty rings and degenerated mitral biological valve replacements.[43]

Although there is a less experience than in the field of the aortic valve, mitral valve-in-valve (MVIV) and mitral valve-in-ring (MVIR) procedures gain ground lately. Due to more heterogeneity in properties and dimensions of rings, MVIR shows poorer outcomes than MVIV. Being aware of the features of rings and bioprostheses and knowing the procedure steps and the complications that can potentially occur are crucial to perform the procedure with minimal risk and the best results.

SAPIEN balloon expandable platform (SAPIEN, SAPIEN XT, and SAPIEN 3, Edwards Lifesciences, Irvine USA) with transseptal approach is used in majority of cases.[43] An ideal location for septal puncture for TMVIR and MVIV is postero-inferior, at least 3.5 cm from the annulus. Once the septum is crossed and over the guidewire placed into the left atrium, a steerable guide catheter is inserted and hooked toward the mitral valve, which allows the interventionist to get through the valve. After the catheter has been advanced, a stiff wire is placed into the left ventricle (LV) to give support for delivering the valve. For facilitating the visualization of the distal tip

of the wire by either 2D or 3D TEE, a pigtail configuration of the guidewire is preferable since it is difficult to identify the tip of any straight guidewire.[44] Despite careful management of the various catheters and guidewires to prevent LV damage, complications associated with the manipulation during procedure can occur. When crossing the valve, the valve can be injured, resulting in massive regurgitation due to *leaflet rupture* (Figure 22.5) (V22.7), pulmonary congestion, and hemodynamic compromise. Maneuvering the stiff wire inside the LV can trigger ventricular arrhythmias, such as sustained ventricular tachycardia degenerating into ventricular fibrillation, with the need of intraprocedural defibrillation (V22.8). Septostomy is needed to allow the passage of the valve delivery system, commonly using a 12 or 14 Fr balloon.[43] The valve is then advanced and positioned through the ring or bioprosthesis. During deployment, the main imaging considerations are valve depth and axiality relating to mitral annulus, as well as the full expansion of the device within the native or prosthetic tissue. Rapid pacing is suggested, generally around 140 beats per minute. Device depth may be checked by TEE but is generally guided by fluoroscopy since prosthetic material

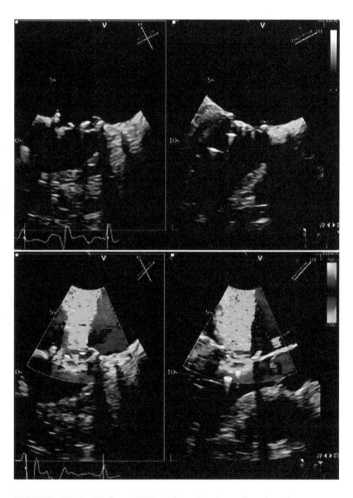

FIGURE 22.5 Biplane TEE with color Doppler showing severe mitral regurgitation. Leaflets can be injured after crossing the valve (V22.7), causing a massive regurgitation due to leaflet rupture.

is well visualized. The aim is to implant nearly 20% of the valve in the left atrium and 80% in the ventricle;[44] this height provides better transvalvular gradients, although the risk of *left ventricular outflow tract (LVOT) obstruction* is greater in a more ventricular position, especially when the anterior leaflet was not resected at the time of previous surgery. After MVIR, the anterior mitral leaflet shelters the transcatheter valve, and it is consequently pushed toward LVOT. In addition to the depth of the implanted device, other factors associated with an increased risk of LVOT obstruction after MVIV and MVIR include a large septal bulge and a less obtuse aortomitral annular angle.[43]

Following MVIR deployment, the occurrence of a *significant paravalvular leak* is not surprising due to the lack of ability of rings to become circular. The paravalvular leak can be effectively treated by postdilation and, in some cases, with a second valve implantation as a valve-in-valve procedure (Figure 22.6) (V22.9A, V22.9B). Of note, paravalvular leaks detected after cardiac surgery could also be closed by percutaneous intervention (Figure 14.8) (V14.11A, V14.11B, V14.11C, V14.11D).

The risk of *valve dislodgement* (Figure 22.7) or even *acute/delayed embolization* of an improperly sized transcatheter valve is higher after MVIR or MVIV procedure as compared with aortic VIV procedure due to higher pressure on the closed mitral valve leaflets.[44]

Different from other percutaneous MV procedures using transseptal approach, the large iatrogenic atrial septal defect (ASD) caused by the septostomy needs percutaneous closure by the end of the procedure, using the ASD closure device.

COMPLICATIONS FOLLOWING PERCUTANEOUS TRICUSPID VALVE REPAIR

For a long time, tricuspid valve (TV) has been defined as the "forgotten valve." However, in the last few years, tricuspid regurgitation (TR) has gained attention due to its high prevalence, its progressive association with mortality as severity increases, and a limited implementation of surgical treatment in the setting of the late presentation of the disease and consequently elevated in-hospital mortality.[45] Transcatheter solutions for management of TR have emerged as a safe and effective alternative to surgery, for which survival benefits have been reported in this high-risk population in comparison to medical treatment alone.[46] Up to 90% of these patients have secondary/functional TR as a result of annular dilation and leaflet tethering.[47] In comparison to MV disease, the TV and right ventricular (RV) anatomy show greater variability, which makes understanding of disease pathophysiology, evaluation, and patient selection challenging for a cardiac imager. Thinner leaflets, hard visualization of the TV apparatus, and a usually large coaptation gap are contributing factors to the demanding skills of the examiner. Though a

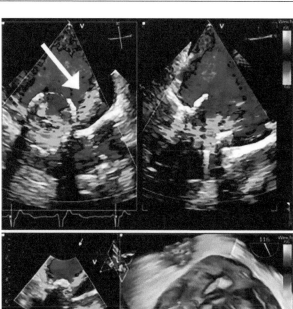
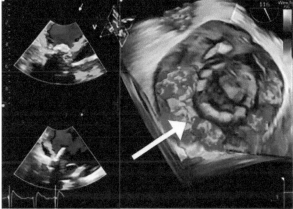
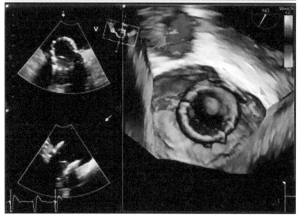

FIGURE 22.6 Significant paravalvular leak after MVIR implantation successfully treated with MVIV procedure. 2D (upper panels) and 3D TEE (middle panels) with color Doppler showing significant paravalvular regurgitation after MVIR implantation (V22.9A). Postdilation and insertion of the second valve (MVIV procedure) was performed, resulting in insignificant residual mitral regurgitation (lower panel) (V22.9B).

multimodality imaging approach is often needed, 2D and 3D TTE and TEE remain the most important instruments for screening and selecting patients for transcatheter tricuspid valve repair (TTVr).[48] Echocardiography is also crucial for guiding the interventionist through the procedure and diagnosing acute and delayed complications related to intervention (Table 22.3).

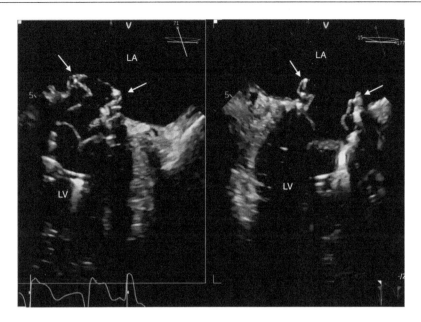

FIGURE 22.7   Mitral valve dislodgement. Biplane TEE showing a dislodgement (arrows) of the prosthetic valve toward the left atrium. LA: left atrium; LV: left ventricle.

TABLE 22.3   Complications Detected by Echocardiography during Tricuspid Valve Percutaneous Procedures and Tips and Tricks to Minimize or Detect Them Rapidly

PROCEDURE	COMPLICATION DETECTED BY ECHOCARDIOGRAPHY	TIPS AND TRICKS (HOW TO MINIMIZE OR DETECT RAPIDLY COMPLICATIONS)
TV edge-to-edge	• Single leaflet detachment; clip embolization	• Keep both leaflets on sight while grasping; standard "grasping view" (mid-esophageal biplane RV inflow-outflow, 60°/150°); confirm correct attachment in different views before releasing the device (biplane, transgastric short-axis); apply color Doppler; independent leaflet grasping if needed.
	• Leaflet injury, chordal rupture	• Provide views with enough depth to see the TV apparatus, invert device arms to remove the clip back to the right atrium.
	• Tricuspid stenosis	• Assess mean gradient before and after the procedure; rare complication due to tricuspid annular dilation in the vast majority of patients.
	• Tricuspid regurgitation	• Compare multiple views before and after leaflet approximation; be aware of eccentric jets; use hemodynamic parameters as hepatic vein flow.
Direct TV annuloplasty (Cardioband)	• RCA complications (extrinsic compression, perforation)	• Simultaneous coronary angiogram is mandatory; CT evaluation distance of RCA to hinge point in screening; detect wall motion abnormalities; detect acute decrease in RV systolic function; the view of the vessel by TEE during last anchors may be possible from transgastric view.
	• Partial device dislodgment or fracture	• Provide a sharp echocardiographic view during anchoring to make sure the tip of the sheath is at the hinge point and there is enough tissue under each screw; you may need multiplanar 3D reconstruction for the posterior anchors; proof stability of the anchors during push-pull test
	• Tricuspid regurgitation	• Comprehensive assessment including accurate quantification of the remaining regurgitation during and after completing the cinching; in patients with a reduced, though still large, residual gap, edge-to-edge as a second procedure is possible.

Abbreviations: 3D, three-dimensional; CT, computed tomography; RCA, right coronary artery; TV, tricuspid valve; TEE, transesophageal echocardiography.

Tricuspid valve transcatheter edge-to-edge repair (TEER)

Tricuspid valve transcatheter edge-to-edge repair (T-TEER) is the most frequently used TTVr-technique worldwide because it is widely available, easy to perform, safe, and efficient.[49] The TriClip (Abbott Vascular, Santa Clara, CA, USA) and the PASCAL systems (Edwards Lifesciences, Irvine, CA, USA) are approved in the Europe for T-TEER.

After initial experience with the available systems a greater risk of *single leaflet detachment* compared to MV procedures was recognized (nearly 7% in the TRILUMINATE study). With the development of the devices with different implant sizes and possibility of independent grasping, the frequency of detachment has been reduced. A non-anteroseptal position (Figure 22.8) and a coaptation gap >8 mm have been associated with device failure.[46] During the procedure, the visualization of both leaflets during the grasping is the key. Standard TEE grasping view is mid-esophageal biplane RV inflow-outflow, usually at 60°/150°. Before release of the device, correct attachment in different views and the result in terms of TR reduction should be confirmed.

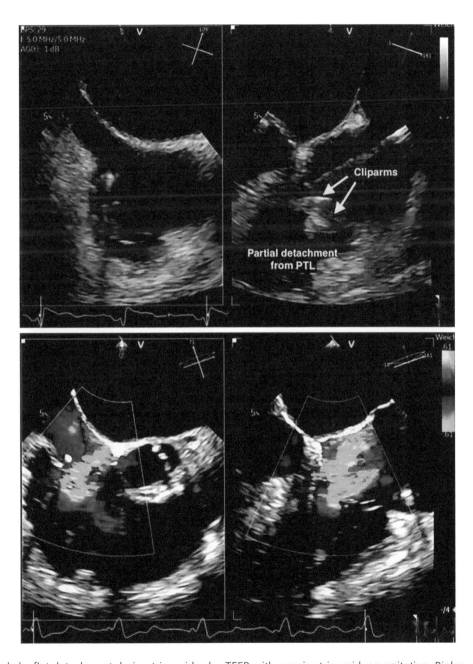

FIGURE 22.8 Single leaflet detachment during tricuspid valve TEER with massive tricuspid regurgitation. Biplane TEE without (upper panels) and with color Doppler (lower panels) illustrating massive tricuspid regurgitation after TEER of the tricuspid valve due to partial detachment from PTL (arrows). To avoid this, it is mandatory to visualize by TEE that both leaflets are safely grasped by the device used. PTL: posterior tricuspid leaflet.

Detachment as a consequence of *leaflet perforation* and complete loss of insertion with *clip embolization* are far less common complications.[48]

Compared to the MV, *device-related stenosis* is not an issue in most of the cases due to frequent annular dilation. Relevant tricuspid stenosis, defined as a transtricuspid mean diastolic pressure gradient (MPG) >5 mmHg, is rare.[49]

Quantification of *residual regurgitation* after T-TEER could be challenging. It is suggested to use multiple views to detect eccentric jets and to compare findings with images taken before leaflet approximation (Figure 22.8). Additional parameters can be used, such as the hepatic vein flow profile.

Percutaneous tricuspid valve direct annuloplasty

The Cardioband direct annuloplasty system (Edwards Lifesciences) is indicated for the treatment of patients with chronic functional TR, which is symptomatic despite diuretic therapy. The device consists of a screw-anchored adjustable band, which is implanted in counterclockwise direction along TV annulus.[47] The position of the catheter is checked under TEE and fluoroscopy. The real challenge for the echocardiographer is to provide good quality images at every anchoring position, using often modified approaches to visualize the hinge point at difficult positions for the direction of the beam, such as the posterior part of the annulus.

Right coronary artery (RCA) complications (perforation, extrinsic compression) have been described in up to 15% of the patients in real-world experience multicenter studies, which sometimes require coronary stent implantation.[50] The distance from the hinge point to the vessel is carefully measured in the screening CT along the whole annulus to evaluate the feasibility of the procedure and, therefore, the interventionist can know in advance which region can be particularly problematic for potential RCA complications. In a TEE transgastric view during the last anchors, when getting closer to the coronary sinus, the RCA may be very well visualized (V22.10).

To avoid *anchor disengagement* with possible *device dislodgment or fracture*, the accurate sight of the hinge point is critical. It must be confirmed that the anchor is being screwed into the tissue and proved its stability by push-pull test.

A substantial and sustained reduction of functional TR in around 70% of the patients has been reported in both the European approval study (TRI-REPAIR) and the post-market TriBAND study.[51] *Residual significant regurgitation* is more frequent in candidates with more advanced disease, whose RV shows already a marked remodeling with pronounced dilation. In cases in which the gap has been reduced with annuloplasty but remaining TR is still clinically relevant, patients become candidates for T-TEER in a second procedure (Figure 22.9).

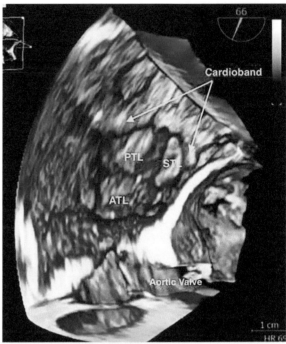
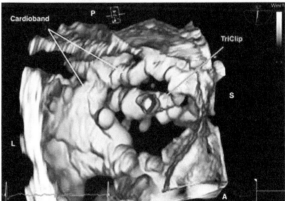

FIGURE 22.9 T-TEER in a second procedure for residual tricuspid regurgitation after direct tricuspid annuloplasty with Cardioband. 3D TEE imaging of the tricuspid valve. In patients with dilated RV, there is the option to first perform a TV annuloplasty (in this case Cardioband, yellow arrows, upper panel) and, in case of residual TR, to perform a TEER procedure (in this case TriClip, green arrow, lower panel). ATL: anterior tricuspid leaflet; STL: septal tricuspid leaflet; PTL: posterior tricuspid leaflet.

COMPLICATIONS FOLLOWING ELECTROPHYSIOLOGY PROCEDURES

Pacemaker and ICD implantation

Pacemaker and implantable cardioverter defibrillator (ICD) implantations are usually low-risk procedures. However, complications can occur in the different stages of the procedure.

Echo guidance for the implantation of a pacemaker is not routinely performed. However, it is advised to have an echo machine available in the electrophysiology laboratory to diagnose acute complications quickly. Long-term complications include infection of the pacemaker and endocarditis of the pacemaker leads.

TEE is mandatory in suspected *pacemaker lead endocarditis* (V21.7A, V21.7B). The examiner must follow and document the entire lead, starting from the vena cava superior to the tip of the lead. Biplane imaging is very helpful in this setting. In case of multiple leads, the probe should be adjusted so that each lead can be visualized. Frequently, it is difficult to differentiate thrombus from vegetations by echocardiography alone. The integration of clinical information (inflammatory parameters, blood cultures, fever) is mandatory to make the diagnosis of pacemaker lead infection (Figure 22.10) (V13.25).

A special constellation is cardiac resynchronization therapy (CRT) lead endocarditis in which the visualization of the coronary sinus must be performed.

Perforation of the myocardium by the pacemaker lead can be observed acutely after implantation (V8.13) or during follow-up. A transthoracic echo focused on the RV should be performed. The beam width should be narrowed in order to increase spatial and temporal resolution. Echocardiographic findings suggestive to lead perforation are pericardial effusion and visualization of the tip of the lead outside of the RV myocardium.

Pacemaker lead detachment can be seen as well. It is a rare complication and can be visualized by TTE.

Electrophysiology procedures

Electrophysiological (EP) procedures are generally performed with a very low risk of complications. In most cases, a TEE is performed prior to every procedure, especially for atrial fibrillation. Therefore, the electrophysiologist is aware of the anatomy of the interatrial septum (IAS) and the left atrial appendage (LAA). It should be part of every EP procedure to look at the TEE images before intervention.

The interatrial septum must be crossed for pulmonary vein ablations. Usually, the transseptal puncture is performed with fluoroscopy and not by echo-guidance. In hypermobile IAS, echocardiography might help to ensure the correct position of transseptal puncture. The electrophysiologist should inform the echocardiographer when transseptal puncture gets difficult. Usually, there is no residual left-to-right shunt after EP procedures compared to iatrogenic ASD after procedures with a large guide (e.g., MitraClip).

The most common complications of EP procedures are *acute and subacute pericardial effusions.* An acute pericardial effusion during an EP procedure may be associated with acute hemodynamic compromise of the patient. An ultrasound machine should always be in the EP room, and the diagnosis can usually be made quickly. The best approach is to look at the heart from the subcostal view immediately. In most cases, the right atrium (RA) is the first structure to be affected. Urgent pericardiocentesis may be needed and in some cases autotransfusion should be performed.

COMPLICATIONS FOLLOWING STRUCTURAL INTERVENTIONS

Patent foramen ovale and atrial septal defect occluders implantation

The implantation of patent foramen ovale (PFO) and ASD occluders are usually low-risk procedures. It is mandatory to perform a TEE prior to the procedure in order to describe the shape, size, and hemodynamic relevance of the defect.

In case of an ASD, it has to be made clear if the ASD is a single or multifenestrated lesion. Three-dimensional TEE can help to analyze the anatomy. It should be avoided to perform ASD closure intervention without detailed prior planning of the procedure. Furthermore, the size of the aortic rim should be measured. If the rim is not sufficiently large or too floppy, the dislocation of the occluder is more likely.

In case of a PFO, the relevance of the PFO and the atrial septal aneurysm should be diagnosed prior to PFO closure. Usually, both PFO with a relevant shunt (>30 bubbles during Valsalva maneuver) and an atrial septal aneurysm >10 mm should be present to justify the procedure.[52]

The worst complication besides *incomplete closure* of the defect is the *dislocation of the implanted device.* In most

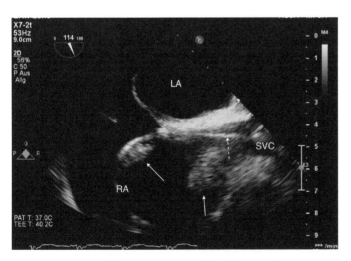

FIGURE 22.10 Pacemaker lead infective endocarditis. TEE bicaval view showing a mobile mass (white arrows) attached to the pacemaker lead (dotted arrow). Although this is not diagnostic for endocarditis, it is highly suggestive finding in case the patient has fever, positive blood cultures, or elevated inflammatory markers. A differential diagnosis is thrombus. LA: left atrium; RA: right atrium; SVC: superior vena cava.

cases this is due to incorrect sizing or malpositioning of the device. This is usually seen immediately by the echocardiographer (Figure 22.11) (V22.11A, V22.11B, V16.11). The consequence is usually urgent cardiac surgery referral of the patient.

Late complications are *erosions*, *thrombi*, or *endocarditis*, all of which can be identified by TEE.

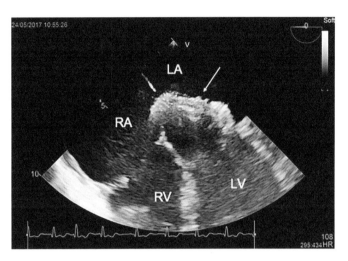

FIGURE 22.11 Dislocation of the ASD occluder detected by TEE during procedure. TEE image showing ASD occluder (arrow) migrated into the left atrium shortly after percutaneous implantation (V22.11A, V22.11B). LA: left atrium; LV: left ventricle; RA: right atrium; RV: right ventricle.

(Image and videos provided by MK.)

Left atrial appendage occluder implantation

The implantation of a left atrial appendage (LAA) occluder is an echo-guided procedure. Prior to the implantation, it is mandatory to perform a TEE with two goals: exclusion of LAA thrombus and the analysis of the shape and size of the LAA.

The occluder systems have fundamental differences. While both widely used devices seal the LAA, the mechanism is different. The Amulet LAA occluder closes the LAA by lobe and disc; the LAA ostium is closed with the disc. In contrast, the Watchman device fills only the body of the LAA.

Complications include *pericardial effusion* during the implantation, which can be easily detected by echocardiography

In rare cases the device is completely or partially *detached*. Therefore, it is mandatory to perform the "tug test" in order to make sure that the occluder is well attached to the LAA tissue before deployment. The dislocation of the occluder can be observed by TEE immediately. The occluder will dislocate into the left atrium (V22.12). Then, a transmitral dislocation can occur and the occluder could pass into the left ventricle. Depending on the size and the aortic valve, the occluder could also pass aortic valve and even be dislocated into the aorta (V22.13, V22.14). In the case of dislocation of the LAA occluder, a surgical removal is usually the only solution.

A complication of LAA occluder implantation is the formation of *thrombi* on the occluder. Especially in patients with thrombogenic diseases (e.g., malignancies), the diagnosis of a thrombus on an LAA occluder might lead to the continuation of oral anticoagulation (Figure 22.12).[53]

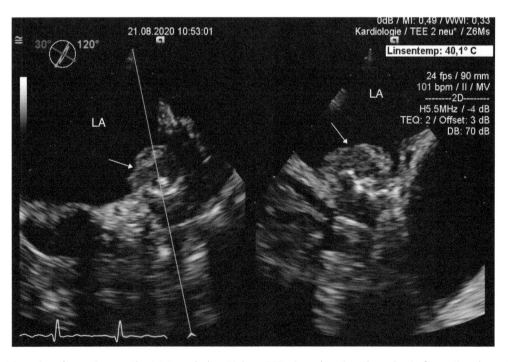

FIGURE 22.12 Thrombus formation on the LAA occluder. Biplane TEE view showing thrombotic formation (arrow) over the LAA occluder (Watchman device). This was seen during the follow-up TEE examination. LA: left atrium.

Endocarditis of the LAA occluder is another complication after LAA occlusion. Of note, the implantation should be performed only in patients that are free of infection.

LIST OF VIDEOS

https://routledgetextbooks.com/textbooks/9781032157009/chapter-22.php

VIDEO 22.1   Stent abscess. Transesophageal echocardiography in a mid-esophageal four-chamber view showing an echolucent mass in the coronary sulcus between the right atrium and right ventricle. *(Video provided by GNR.)*

VIDEO 22.2   Migration of transcatheter aortic heart valve during TAVI. Transesophageal echocardiography in a mid-esophageal long-axis view showing a caudal dislocation of balloon-expanding valve toward the LVOT, causing impaired opening of the anterior mitral leaflet.

VIDEO 22.3   Annulus perforation into the right ventricle during TAVI. Transesophageal echocardiography in a mid-esophageal long-axis view with color Doppler showing a turbulent jet indicating perforation into the right ventricle.

VIDEO 22.4   Paravalvular leak after TAVI. Transesophageal echocardiography in a mid-esophageal long-axis view showing a severe paravalvular aortic regurgitation.

VIDEO 22.5A   Endocarditis after TAVI with balloon-expanding valve (1/2). Transthoracic parasternal long-axis view showing a vegetation in the left ventricular outflow tract after implantation of a balloon-expanding valve (see also Video 22.5B).

VIDEO 22.5B   Endocarditis after TAVI with balloon-expanding valve (2/2). Transthoracic parasternal short-axis view showing a vegetation inside the balloon-expanding valve (see also Video 22.5A).

VIDEO 22.6A   Single leaflet detachment (1/3). TEE showing acute single leaflet detachment after MitraClip implantation. Loss of leaflet insertion on the anterior mitral leaflet can be seen in mid-esophageal four-chamber view (see also Videos 22.6B and 22.6C).

VIDEO 22.6B   Single leaflet detachment (2/3): TEE in the "grasping view" (biplane intercommissural and mid-esophageal long-axis views) showing acute single leaflet detachment after MitraClip implantation (see also Videos 22.6A and 22.6C).

VIDEO 22.6C   Single leaflet detachment (3/3): TEE 3D volume acquisition obtained using 3D zoom mode. Mitral valve is displayed centrally with the aortic valve inferiorly (6 o'clock). The MitraClip shows a single leaflet attachment on the posterior leaflet at the central segment (P2) (see also Videos 22.6A and 22.6B).

VIDEO 22.7   Mitral injury during transcatheter mitral valve procedure shown by 3D TEE. Three-dimensional full-volume TEE oriented en face as the "surgical view" during a mitral valve-in-ring procedure with the aortic valve at 12 o'clock, the interatrial septum on the right side, and the mitral valve after repair with annuloplasty at 6 o'clock (not fully represented in the 3D data set). Across the interatrial septum, a steerable guide catheter hooked toward the mitral valve and the stiff guidewire crossed the mitral valve.

VIDEO 22.8   Ventricular fibrillation during transcatheter deployment of the mitral valve. Manipulation of the wire and catheters through the valve and inside the left ventricle during MVIR may cause ventricular tachycardia with degeneration into ventricular fibrillation and need for intraprocedural defibrillation.

VIDEO 22.9A   3D TEE showing paravalvular leak after mitral valve-in-ring implantation (MVIR) (1/2). Severe paravalvular mitral regurgitation after the implantation of the first 26 mm SAPIEN 3 in a 30 mm semi-rigid complete Medtronic CG Future ring presented in 3D zoom with color (see also Video 22.9B)

VIDEO 22.9B   3D TEE showing result of second valve-in-valve implantation (MVIV) (2/2). Result after postdilation and insertion of a second 26 mm SAPIEN 3, valve-in-valve, showing a mild paravalvular regurgitation with two small jets, at 10 and 2 o'clock of the circumference of the prosthesis (see also Video 22.9A).

VIDEO 22.10   Transgastric TEE view of the right coronary artery during tricuspid valve direct annuloplasty. Transgastric modified reverse RV inflow-outflow view with right and anteflexion of the probe at 180° during tricuspid valve direct annuloplasty (Cardioband). The 12th anchor is already firmly placed inside the tissue, not released yet (at the tip of the sheath). Notice the cross-section of the right coronary artery right to the anchor, with the guidewire (safety marker) inside the vessel.

VIDEO 22.11A   Dislocation of the ASD occluder detected by TEE during procedure (1/2). During the attempt of percutaneous closure of the ASD (measured 28 mm prior to intervention), shortly after implantation of the ASD occluder Figulla Flex N°33 (shown here, in place), migration of the occluder into the left atrium was detected by TEE (see Video 22.11B). The patient was referred to emergent cardiac surgery, the occluder was removed and ASD was closed by the patch. *(Video provided by MK.)*

VIDEO 22.11B   Dislocation of the ASD occluder detected by TEE during procedure (2/2). During the attempt of percutaneous closure of the ASD (measured 28 mm prior to intervention), shortly after implantation of the ASD occluder Figulla Flex N°33 (see Video 22.11A), migration of the occluder into the left atrium was detected by TEE (shown here). The patient was referred to emergent cardiac surgery, the occluder was removed and ASD was closed by the patch. *(Video provided by MK.)*

VIDEO 22.12 Dislocated LAA occluder freely moving in the left atrium. TEE showing a dislocation of LAA occluder (Watchman). The swirling device is seen in the LA.

VIDEO 22.13 Dislocated LAA occluder moving through the aortic valve into the aorta. TEE showing the LAA occluder in the left ventricular outflow tract and subsequent passage through the aortic valve into the aorta.

VIDEO 22.14 Dislocated LAA occluder detected in the aortic arch. Biplane TEE showing the LAA occluder dislocated in the aortic arch.

REFERENCES

1. Brilakis ES, Mashayekhi K, Tsuchikane E, Rafeh NA, Alaswad K, Araya M, et al. Guiding Principles for Chronic Total Occlusion Percutaneous Coronary Intervention. Circulation. 2019;140(5):420–33.
2. Vallabhajosyula S, Dunlay SM, Barsness GW, Rihal CS, Holmes DR, Jr., Prasad A. Hospital-Level Disparities in the Outcomes of Acute Myocardial Infarction with Cardiogenic Shock. Am J Cardiol. 2019;124(4):491–8.
3. Kinnaird T, Kwok CS, Kontopantelis E, Ossei-Gerning N, Ludman P, deBelder M, et al. Incidence, Determinants, and Outcomes of Coronary Perforation during Percutaneous Coronary Intervention in the United Kingdom Between 2006 and 2013: An Analysis of 527 121 Cases drom the British Cardiovascular Intervention Society Database. Circ Cardiovasc Interv. 2016;9(8).
4. Shimony A, Joseph L, Mottillo S, Eisenberg MJ. Coronary Artery Perforation during Percutaneous Coronary Intervention: A Systematic Review and Meta-Analysis. Can J Cardiol. 2011;27(6):843–50.
5. Giannini F, Candilio L, Mitomo S, Ruparelia N, Chieffo A, Baldetti L, et al. A Practical Approach to the Management of Complications during Percutaneous Coronary Intervention. JACC Cardiovasc Interv. 2018;11(18):1797–810.
6. Elieson M, Mixon T, Carpenter J. Coronary Stent Infections: A Case Report and Literature Review. Tex Heart Inst J. 2012;39(6):884–9.
7. Vahanian A, Beyersdorf F, Praz F, Milojevic M, Baldus S, Bauersachs J, et al. 2021 ESC/EACTS Guidelines for the Management of Valvular Heart Disease. Eur J Cardiothorac Surg. 2021;60(4):727–800.
8. Mack MJ, Leon MB. Transcatheter Aortic-Valve Replacement in Low-Risk Patients. Reply. N Engl J Med. 2019;381(7):684–5.
9. Popma JJ, Deeb GM, Yakubov SJ, Mumtaz M, Gada H, O'Hair D, et al. Transcatheter Aortic-Valve Replacement with a Self-Expanding Valve in Low-Risk Patients. N Engl J Med. 2019;380(18):1706–15.
10. Voigtlander L, Seiffert M. Expanding TAVI to Low and Intermediate Risk Patients. Front Cardiovasc Med. 2018;5:92.
11. Walther T, Hamm CW, Schuler G, Berkowitsch A, Kotting J, Mangner N, et al. Perioperative Results and Complications in 15,964 Transcatheter Aortic Valve Replacements: Prospective Data from the GARY Registry. J Am Coll Cardiol. 2015;65(20):2173–80.
12. Scarsini R, De Maria GL, Joseph J, Fan L, Cahill TJ, Kotronias RA, et al. Impact of Complications during Transfemoral Transcatheter Aortic Valve Replacement: How Can They be Avoided and Managed? J Am Heart Assoc. 2019;8(18):e013801.
13. Fournier S, Monney P, Roguelov C, Ferrari E, Eeckhout E, Muller O, et al. How Should I Treat an Edwards SAPIEN 3 Aortic Valve Embolisation during a Transaortic Transcatheter Aortic Valve Implantation? EuroIntervention. 2017;13(4):495–8.
14. Barbash IM, Bogdan A, Fefer P, Spiegelstein D, Raanani E, Beinart R, et al. How Should I Treat a Left Ventricular Outflow Tract-Migrated Balloon-Expandable Transcatheter Heart Valve? EuroIntervention. 2016;11(12):1442–5.
15. Owais T, El Garhy M, Fuchs J, Disha K, Elkaffas S, Breuer M, et al. Pathophysiological Factors Associated with Left Ventricular Perforation in Transcatheter Aortic Valve Implantation by Transfemoral Approach. J Heart Valve Dis. 2017;26(4):430–6.
16. Barbanti M, Yang TH, Rodes Cabau J, Tamburino C, Wood DA, Jilaihawi H, et al. Anatomical and Procedural Features Associated with Aortic Root Rupture during Balloon-Expandable Transcatheter Aortic Valve Replacement. Circulation. 2013;128(3):244–53.
17. Aksoy O, Paixao AR, Marmagkiolis K, Mego D, Rollefson WA, Cilingiroglu M. Aortic Annular Rupture during TAVR: Mini Review. Cardiovasc Revasc Med. 2016;17(3):199–201.
18. Kellogg MS, Tuttle MK, Sharma RK, et al. Percutaneous Management of a Contained Annular Rupture Occurring With Self-Expanding Transcatheter Aortic Valve Replacement. JACC Case Rep 2020;2:1852–1858.
19. Sinning JM, Hammerstingl C, Vasa-Nicotera M, Adenauer V, Lema Cachiguango SJ, Scheer AC, et al. Aortic Regurgitation Index Defines Severity of Peri-Prosthetic Regurgitation and Predicts Outcome in Patients after Transcatheter Aortic Valve Implantation. J Am Coll Cardiol. 2012;59(13):1134–41.
20. Thourani VH, Kodali S, Makkar RR, Herrmann HC, Williams M, Babaliaros V, et al. Transcatheter Aortic Valve Replacement Versus Surgical Valve Replacement in Intermediate-Risk Patients: A Propensity Score Analysis. Lancet. 2016;387(10034):2218–25.
21. Athappan G, Patvardhan E, Tuzcu EM, Svensson LG, Lemos PA, Fraccaro C, et al. Incidence, Predictors, and Outcomes of Aortic Regurgitation After Transcatheter Aortic Valve Replacement: Meta-Analysis and Systematic Review of Literature. J Am Coll Cardiol. 2013;61(15):1585–95.
22. Onishi T, Sengoku K, Ichibori Y, Mizote I, Maeda K, Kuratani T, et al. The Role of Echocardiography in Transcatheter Aortic Valve Implantation. Cardiovasc Diagn Ther. 2018;8(1):3–17.
23. Harding D, Cahill TJ, Redwood SR, Prendergast BD. Infective Endocarditis Complicating Transcatheter Aortic Valve Implantation. Heart. 2020;106(7):493–8.
24. Allen CJ, Patterson T, Chehab O, Cahill T, Prendergast B, Redwood SR. Incidence and Outcomes of Infective Endocarditis Following Transcatheter Aortic Valve Implantation. Expert Rev Cardiovasc Ther. 2020;18(10):653–62.
25. Delgado V, Ajmone Marsan N, de Waha S, Bonaros N, Brida M, Burri H, et al.; ESC Scientific Document Group. 2023 ESC Guidelines for the management of endocarditis. Eur Heart J 2023;44(39):3948–42.

26. Spethmann S, Dreger H, Baldenhofer G, Pflug E, Sanad W, Stangl V, et al. Long-Term Doppler Hemodynamics and Effective Orifice Areas of Edwards SAPIEN and Medtronic CoreValve Prostheses after TAVI. Echocardiography. 2014;31(3):302–10.

27. Vrachatis DA, Vavuranakis M, Tsoukala S, Giotaki S, Papaioannou TG, Siasos G, et al. TAVI: Valve in Valve. A New Field for Structuralists? Literature Review. Hellenic J Cardiol. 2020;61(3):148–53.

28. Goel K, Lindman BR. Hypoattenuated Leaflet Thickening after Transcatheter Aortic Valve Replacement: Expanding the Evidence Base but Questions Remain. Circ Cardiovasc Imaging. 2019;12(12):e010151.

29. Coffey S, Roberts-Thomson R, Brown A, Carapetis J, Chen M, Enriquez-Sarano M, et al. Global Epidemiology of Valvular Heart Disease. Nat Rev Cardiol. 2021;18(12):853–64.

30. Gheorghe L, Ielasi A, Rensing B, Eefting FD, Timmers L, Latib A, et al. Complications Following Percutaneous Mitral Valve Repair. Front Cardiovasc Med. 2019;6:146.

31. Schneider LMS, Markovic S, Mueller K, Felbel DF, Gercek GM, Friedrichs K, et al. Mitral Valve Transcatheter Edge-to-Edge Repair Using MitraClip or PASCAL: A Multicenter Propensity Score-Matched Comparison. JACC Cardiovasc Interv. 2022;15(24):2554–67.

32. Shah MA, Dalak FA, Alsamadi F, Shah SH, Qattea MB. Complications Following Percutaneous Mitral Valve Edge-to-Edge Repair Using MitraClip. JACC Case Rep. 2021;3(3):370–6.

33. Eggebrecht H, Schelle S, Puls M, Plicht B, von Bardeleben RS, Butter C, et al. Risk and outcomes of complications during and after MitraClip implantation: Experience in 828 patients from the German TRAnscatheter mitral valve interventions (TRAMI) registry. Catheter Cardiovasc Interv. 2015;86(4):728–35.

34. Schnitzler K, Hell M, Geyer M, Kreidel F, Münzel T, von Bardeleben RS. Complications Following MitraClip Implantation. Curr Cardiol Rep. 2021;23(9):131.

35. Sticchi A, Bartkowiak J, Brugger N, Weiss S, Windecker S, Praz F. Retrograde Retrieval of a Novel Large Mitral Clip After Embolization Into the Left Ventricle. JACC Case Rep. 2021;3(14):1561–8.

36. Bilge M, Alsancak Y, Ali S, Duran M, Biçer H. An extremely rare but possible complication of MitraClip: embolization of clip during follow-up. Anatol J Cardiol. 2016;16(8):636–8.

36. Kassar M, Praz F, Hunziker L, Pilgrim T, Windecker S, Seiler C, et al. Anatomical and Technical Predictors of Three-Dimensional Mitral Valve Area Reduction After Transcatheter Edge-To-Edge Repair. J Am Soc Echocardiogr. 2022;35(1):96–104.

37. Praz F, Winkel MG, Fam NP. A New Age for Transcatheter Mitral Valve Repair: The Complexity of Choice. JACC Cardiovasc Interv. 2020;13(20):2415–7.

38. Anker SD, Starling RC, Khan MS, Friede T, Filippatos G, Lindenfeld J, et al. Percutaneous Mitral Valve Annuloplasty in Patients With Secondary Mitral Regurgitation and Severe Left Ventricular Enlargement. JACC Heart Fail. 2021;9(6):453–62.

39. Witte KK, Lipiecki J, Siminiak T, Meredith IT, Malkin CJ, Goldberg SL, et al. The REDUCE FMR Trial: A Randomized Sham-Controlled Study of Percutaneous Mitral Annuloplasty in Functional Mitral Regurgitation. JACC Heart Fail. 2019;7(11):945–55.

40. Lainscak M, Böhm M. Embracing Secondary Mitral Regurgitation with Carillon: Past, Present, and Future. ESC Heart Fail. 2020;7(6):3268–70.

41. Miller M, Thourani VH, Whisenant B. The Cardioband Transcatheter Annular Reduction System. Ann Cardiothorac Surg. 2018;7(6):741–7.

42. Messika-Zeitoun D, Nickenig G, Latib A, Kuck KH, Baldus S, Schueler R, et al. Transcatheter Mitral Valve Repair for Functional Mitral Regurgitation using the Cardioband System: 1 Year Outcomes. Eur Heart J. 2019;40(5):466–72.

43. Pirelli L, Hong E, Steffen R, Vahl TP, Kodali SK, Bapat V. Mitral Valve-in-Valve and Valve-in-Ring: Tips, Tricks, and Outcomes. Ann Cardiothorac Surg. 2021;10(1):96–112.

44. Little SH, Bapat V, Blanke P, Guerrero M, Rajagopal V, Siegel R. Imaging Guidance for Transcatheter Mitral Valve Intervention on Prosthetic Valves, Rings, and Annular Calcification. JACC Cardiovasc Imaging. 2021;14(1):22–40.

45. Hahn RT, Badano LP, Bartko PE, Muraru D, Maisano F, Zamorano JL, et al. Tricuspid Regurgitation: Recent Advances in Understanding Pathophysiology, Severity Grading and Outcome. Eur Heart J Cardiovasc Imaging. 2022;23(7):913–29.

46. Taramasso M, Benfari G, van der Bijl P, Alessandrini H, Attinger-Toller A, Biasco L, et al. Transcatheter versus Medical Treatment of Patients with Symptomatic Severe Tricuspid Regurgitation. J Am Coll Cardiol. 2019;74(24):2998–3008.

47. Praz F, Muraru D, Kreidel F, Lurz P, Hahn RT, Delgado V, et al. Transcatheter Treatment for Tricuspid Valve Disease. EuroIntervention. 2021;17(10):791–808.

48. Hahn RT, Saric M, Faletra FF, Garg R, Gillam LD, Horton K, et al. Recommended Standards for the Performance of Transesophageal Echocardiographic Screening for Structural Heart Intervention: From the American Society of Echocardiography. J Am Soc Echocardiogr. 2022;35(1):1–76.

48. Lurz P, Stephan von Bardeleben R, Weber M, Sitges M, Sorajja P, Hausleiter J, et al. Transcatheter Edge-to-Edge Repair for Treatment of Tricuspid Regurgitation. J Am Coll Cardiol. 2021;77(3):229–39.

49. Lee H, Kim J, Oh SS, Yoo JS. Long-term Clinical and Hemodynamic Outcomes of Edge-to-Edge Repair for Tricuspid Regurgitation. Ann Thorac Surg. 2021;112(3):803–8.

50. Korber MI, Landendinger M, Gercek M, Beuthner BE, Friedrichs KP, Puls M, et al. Transcatheter Treatment of Secondary Tricuspid Regurgitation with Direct Annuloplasty: Results from a Multicenter Real-World Experience. Circ Cardiovasc Interv. 2021;14(8):e010019.

51. Nickenig G, Friedrichs KP, Baldus S, Arnold M, Seidler T, Hakmi S, et al. Thirty-Day Outcomes of the Cardioband Tricuspid System for Patients with Symptomatic Functional Tricuspid Regurgitation: The TriBAND Study. EuroIntervention. 2021;17(10):809–17.

52. Silvestry FE, Cohen MS, Armsby LB, Burkule NJ, Fleishman CE, Hijazi ZM, et alE. Guidelines for the Echocardiographic Assessment of Atrial Septal Defect and Patent Foramen Ovale: From the American Society of Echocardiography and Society for Cardiac Angiography and Interventions. J Am Soc Echocardiogr. 2015;28(9):910–58.

53. Palios J, Paraskevaidis I. Thromboembolism Prevention via Transcatheter Left Atrial Appendage Closure with Transeosophageal Echocardiography Guidance. Thrombosis. 2014; 2014:832752.

Index

Note: Page numbers in *italic* indicate a figure and page numbers in **bold** indicate a table on the corresponding page.

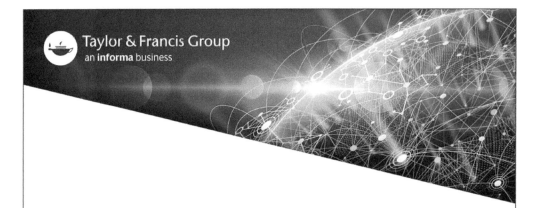
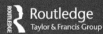
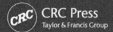